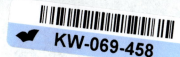

Drugs in Cardiology

A Comprehensive Guide to Cardiovascular Pharmacotherapy

Edited by

Juan Carlos Kaski

Professor of Cardiovascular Science
Head, Cardiovascular Sciences Research Centre
St George's, University of London
London, UK

Associate editors

Stuart Baker

General Practitioner
Musgrove Park Hospital,
Taunton, UK

Carl Hayward

Cardiology Registrar
North East Thames
Training Rotation
London, UK

Teck K. Khong

Senior Lecturer in Clinical
Pharmacology
Basic Medical Sciences
St George's University of
London
London, UK

Saagar Mahida

Cardiology Registrar
Leeds General Infirmary
Leeds, UK

Juan Tamargo

Professor of Pharmacology
Head, Department of
Pharmacology
School of Medicine
Universidad Complutense
Madrid, Spain

OXFORD
UNIVERSITY PRESS

OXFORD
UNIVERSITY PRESS

Great Clarendon Street, Oxford OX2 6DP

Oxford University Press is a department of the University of Oxford.
It furthers the University's objective of excellence in research, scholarship,
and education by publishing worldwide in

Oxford New York

Auckland Cape Town Dar es Salaam Hong Kong Karachi
Kuala Lumpur Madrid Melbourne Mexico City Nairobi
New Delhi Shanghai Taipei Toronto

With offices in

Argentina Austria Brazil Chile Czech Republic France Greece
Guatemala Hungary Italy Japan Poland Portugal Singapore
South Korea Switzerland Thailand Turkey Ukraine Vietnam

Oxford is a registered trade mark of Oxford University Press
in the UK and in certain other countries

Published in the United States
by Oxford University Press Inc., New York

© Oxford University Press, 2010

British Library Cataloguing in Publication Data
Data available

Library of Congress Cataloging-in-Publication-Data
Data available

Typeset by Glyph International, Bangalore, India
Printed in Great Britain
on acid-free paper by
Ashford Colour Press Ltd., Gosport, Hampshire

ISBN 978-0-19-955746-2

10 9 8 7 6 5 4 3 2 1

RM
345
<2

OXFORD MEDICAL PUBLICATIONS

Drugs in Cardiology

Foreword by John Camm

Drug therapy for cardiovascular disease has taken many giant steps forward in the last decade and the process is still ongoing. Although statins, ACE inhibitors and angiotensin receptor blockers, aldosterone inhibitors and numerous therapies for heart failure and hypertension have now largely matured, a number of new therapeutic targets are still being explored. Anticoagulants, antiarrhythmics, HDL therapies and a variety of anti-diabetic agents amongst others have taken on a new lease of life and have been recently or will soon be released into the therapeutic arena. In any event, the range and diversity of drugs used for the treatment of patients with cardiovascular disease is now enormous. Cardiologists and physicians involved with the broader aspects of cardiovascular medicine (including diabetes, hypertension, metabolic syndrome, heart failure, chronic arrhythmias, etc.) have many therapies from which to choose. It is therefore important that there is now a modern and comprehensive textbook on this subject to assist them to rapidly discover the relevant facts and important details of these many potential drug treatments.

JC Kaski has put together a compendium of information about drugs for cardiovascular therapy. The book is divided into two large sections: a catalogue of drugs, and a series of conditions for which these drugs are prescribed. The process for assembling these data was to ask busy cardiology/cardiovascular medicine practitioners what was important for the everyday medical management of their patients, and to derive theoretical background information from expert clinical scientists. The book is therefore both academic dealing with the evidence base, and practical concentrating on guideline mandated therapy. The section on drugs allows the various applications of each drug to be appreciated simultaneously, and the discussion on disease processes and pathophysiologies exposes the variety of therapies which is available for any one condition or group of pathologies.

This is a fast moving field. Information derived from the Internet is often fresh but raw. Textbook information can be old and stale. The content of this new book is ideal, at once both up-to-date and fully contextualized. The combination of practising cardiologists and seasoned academics is a perfect mix of authors that can distil this ideal blend of practical and educational information.

John Camm
Professor Of Clinical Cardiology,
St. George's University of London,
United Kingdom

Foreword by Jay N. Cohn

We are in the era of drug therapy to treat and prevent cardiovascular disease. Although invasive management with surgery and devices has garnered much attention in recent years, the major clinical benefit of treatment has resulted from drugs. Clinical trials have provided a vast body of knowledge about the proper use of these powerful agents. Nonetheless, a comprehensive unbiased source of this information has been lacking.

Drugs in Cardiology by Kaski and his colleagues is aimed at closing the gap between what is known and what is properly employed in management. Selection of the right drug or combination of drugs in the right dosages requires insight and experience. The authors of *Drugs in Cardiology* set out to provide the background and overview that should allow health care providers to optimize care of patients with a wide range of clinical conditions.

One of the strengths of this book is its blending of pharmacology and clinical medicine. Knowledgeable application of pharmacotherapy requires knowledge about both disciplines. The authors have attempted to provide the framework for optimal and evidence-based therapy. If the readers integrate this information into their management strategies, the cause of national therapeutics should be advanced.

Jay N. Cohn, M.D.
Professor of Medicine
University of Minnesota Medical School
Minneapolis, Minnesota

Foreword by Bill Louis

One of the difficulties associated with the rapid emergence of new drugs and the rapid changes in treatment in modern medicine, is to find text-books which keep pace with this change and provide clear and authoritative treatment plans which can be easily modified as new information becomes available. Nowhere is this more obvious than in the field of cardiology where there are now available a wide range of effective drugs, guidelines and treatment plans.

In my nearly 60 years as a student and then in academic clinical practice there has been a therapeutic explosion. From a situation where we essentially had digitalis, diet, ganglion blocking drugs and mercurial diuretics we now have drugs which act on most elements of the renin–angiotensin system, sophisticated diuretics, beta-blockers, calcium antagonists, numerous antiarrhythmics, statins, platelet aggregation inhibitors, nitrates etc as well interventions such as PCI, stents, bypass surgery and cardiac transplantation. All of these are associated with trial data given exotic names such as COMMIT, COMET, BEAUTIFUL, ISIS, ONTARGET, TRANSCEND, PRoFESS, ALL HAT, CAMELOT, EUROPA and so the list goes on. As well we have numerous guidelines: Heart Foundation guidelines, WHO guidelines, AHA guidelines, ACC guidelines, joint AHA/ACC guidelines and ESC guidelines.

Led by Prof Kaski, the authors of *Drugs in Cardiology* provide us with a comprehensive yet clear way through this mass of information. It is strongly evidence based using current classifications with short medical summaries of the individual diseases and associated risk factors. It summarizes key trials and relevant guidelines; all well referenced. Its focus is on proven benefits rather than potential theoretical advantages thus eliminating much of the confusion generated by the marketing arms of drug companies. The authors provide simple flow diagrams for individual patient management which incorporate the current treatment options and drug doses together with key adverse reactions, all of which can be easily updated as new information becomes available.

They also provide sensible non-pharmacological advice and basic clinical pharmacology important for the proper use of the various drugs in different population groups: the young, the elderly, males, females, patients with renal failure etc. In addition there is in Section 2 a comprehensive A–Z of cardiac drugs and in the Appendix a list of non-cardiac drugs with significant cardiac actions or interactions.

The book provides all this information in a form which is easily accessible by the reader and in a style which is easy to read and even easier to understand. This is not to say that I agree with all its recommendations. Experts in individual areas often argue about the relative merits of different pieces of information. The beauty of this volume is that it allows one to participate in this argument and hopefully further improve management.

Drugs in Cardiology is a book which will become essential reading for students and resident staff and for the specialist in the areas outside their immediate areas of specialization.

Bill Louis
Prof. Emeritus Univ. of Melbourne
Formerly Foundation Professor of Clinical Pharmacology and
Therapeutics Univ. of Melbourne and Director of Cardiac Services
and Head of the Joint Hospital/University Department of Clinical
Pharmacology and Hypertension Services, Austin Health, Melbourne

Preface

Despite the tremendous advances in interventional cardiology in recent years, cardiovascular pharmacotherapy can genuinely claim a major role among both life-saving and quality of life enhancer therapies. Over the past decade physicians have witnessed the arrival of a large number of pharmacological agents tested in well designed clinical studies and are likely to see many others entering the clinical arena in the near future in fields as diverse as hypertension, dyslipidaemia, coronary artery disease, heart failure, and arrhythmias.

A major challenge facing the busy practising physician exposed to the relentless emergence of new pharmacological agents and treatment guidelines is to keep up to date with this progress. Not only have they to be conversant with the indications and dosages of the new drugs but also with their adverse effects, interactions with other drugs and actions on other organs and systems. Evidence-based therapeutic decisions are critical nowadays and physicians are expected to be aware also of at least the basic pharmacological characteristics of the drugs they prescribe. Guidelines from cardiac societies are becoming extremely complex in their attempt to cover all possible situations but they usually do not deal with issues such as individual patient responsiveness, polypharmacy, drug classes, and dosing.

Pharmacological knowledge and drug management of these specific diseases is commonly relegated to 'disease specific' experts. Facilitating access to clinically useful information on pharmacotherapy can help physicians in their difficult task of prescribing wisely.

Together with my co-editors we have produced a volume aimed at providing comprehensive, evidence based, easily accessible information on cardiovascular pharmacotherapy. On preparing this book we had in mind several groups of physicians who might find it useful to have access to up to date guidance on cardiovascular pharmacotherapy. Cardiologists, cardiology trainees, internal medicine specialists, anaesthetists, clinical pharmacologists, obstetricians, and general physicians—we believe—may find this monographic work of interest.

We have subdivided the book into two sections: Section 1, where we provide a brief description of cardiovascular diseases requiring drug treatment and current management guidelines, and Section 2, edited by Dr T Khong and Prof J Tamargo, that contains an 'A–Z' of cardiac drugs where pharmacological information together with advice on dosage is provided. There is also an Appendix where we have included a large list of non-cardiac drugs with cardiac actions or interactions. Tackling the complex issue of cardiovascular pharmacotherapy has not been an easy task, particularly when dealing with a field that moves so rapidly. There is always room for improvement in first editions and we hope in future editions to polish our work if required. Reader feedback in this regard will be very welcome indeed.

Perhaps unusual, a characteristic of this book is that editors, chapter authors and chapter advisors, represent a large clinical–academic spectrum encompassing from physicians in training up to senior academics and experienced clinical consultants. This, we hope, has allowed us to identify both what is useful information for day-to-day practice as well as important scientific data.

The editors will be delighted and truly feel that their task has been accomplished if the content of this book helps physicians in their endeavours to serve their patients better.

JC Kaski, on behalf of the editors

Contents

Detailed contents

Section 2 **A–Z of cardiac drugs**   327

Editors: Teck K. Khong and Juan Tamargo

Contributors

Mohammed Majid Akhtar

Foundation Year 2 Doctor
Southend University Hospital,
Department of Neurology and
Stroke, Southend-on-Sea,
Essex, UK

Luciano Candilio

Cardiology Specialist
Registrar, Blood Pressure Unit,
St George's Hospital, London, UK

Nihil Chitalia

Clinical Teaching Research Fellow,
Department of Renal Medicine,
St George's Hospital and Division
of Cardiac and Vascular Sciences,
St George's, University of London,
UK

Graciana Ciambrone

Cardiovascular Biology Research
Centre, Division of Cardiac and
Vascular Sciences, St George's,
University of London, UK

Inaki Marina Clopes

Academic Visitor, Cardiovascular
Biology Research Centre, Division
of Cardiac and Vascular Sciences,
St George's, University of
London, UK

Lourdes Garcia Bueno

Cardiovascular Biology Research
Centre, Division of Cardiac and
Vascular Sciences, St George's,
University of London, UK

Yassir Iqbal

Foundation Year 2 Doctor
Department of Cardiothoracid
Surgery, St George's Hospital,
London

Mohammed Khanji

Specialist Registrar in Cardiology,
St George's Hospital, University of
London, UK

Ammar Killu

Foundation Year 1 Doctor
St George's Hospital,
University of London, UK

Fu Liang Ng

Academic Clinical Fellow
St George's Hospital,
University of London, UK

Ketna Patel

Specialist Registrar
Chest Medicine
Papworth Hospital, UK

Mike Purkiss

Registrar in Cardiology
Queen Alexandra Hospital,
Portsmouth, UK

Jonathan Sandoe

Consultant Microbiologist
Leeds General Infirmary, UK

Juan-Antonio Sieira

Academic Visitor, Division of
Cardiac and Vascular Sciences,
St George's, University of
London, UK

George Siotis

Academic Visitor, Division of
Cardiac and Vascular Sciences,
St George's, University of
London, UK

Jason Tarkin

Foundation Year 2 Doctor
Central Middlesex Hospital,
North West London NHS Trust, UK

Advisors

Dawn Adamson
Consultant Interventional
Cardiologist, University Hospital of
Coventry and Warwickshire, UK

Lisa Anderson
Consultant in Cardiology
St George's Hospital, London, UK

Tarek Francis Antonios
Senior Lecturer and Consultant
Physician in Cardiovascular and
General Medicine
St George's, University of
London, UK

Elijah R. Behr
Senior Lecturer and Honorary
Consultant Electrophysiologist
St George's, University of
London, UK

Richard Bogle
Consultant in Cardiology
St George's Hospital, London, UK

Stephen J.D. Brecker
Consultant Cardiologist and
Cardiology Care Group Lead
St George's Hospital, London, UK

Nicholas Bunce
Consultant Cardiologist,
St George's Hospital,
London, UK

Anne H. Child
Reader in Cardiovascular Genetics
and Honorary Consultant
Cardiology and Genetics
St George's Hospital, University of
London, UK

Paul Collinson
Consultant Chemical Pathologist
St George's Hospital, London, UK

Perry Elliott
Reader and Consultant
Cardiologist
The Heart Hospital, London, UK

Colin Forfar
Consultant Physician/Cardiologist,
John Radcliffe Hospital, Oxford;
Senior Lecturer in Medicine,
University of Oxford, UK

Marjan Jahangiri
Professor of Cardiac Surgery
St George's Hospital, London, UK

Charles Knight
Consultant Cardiologist
London Chest Hospital, UK

Pitt Lim
Consultant Cardiologist
St George's Hospital, University of
London, UK

Brendan Madden
Professor of Cardiothoracic
Medicine
St George's Hospital, London, UK

M.M. Thompson
Professor of Vascular Surgery
St George's Hospital Medical
School, London, UK

David E. Ward
Consultant in Cardiology and
Electrophysiology,
St George's Hospital, London, UK

Symbols and abbreviations

♂	doses
☻	side effects
📖	cross reference
1°	primary
2°	secondary
α	alpha
β	beta
~	approximately
≈	approximately equal to
3-KAT	3-ketoacyl coenzyme A thiolase
6MWT	6-minute walk time
AA	2° amyloidosis
AAA	abdominal aortic aneurysm
ABG	arterial blood gas
ABPI	ankle–brachial pressure index
ACC	American College of Cardiology
ACCP	American College of Chest Physicians
ACE	angiotensin-converting enzyme
ACEI	angiotensin-converting enzyme inhibitor
ACHD	adult congenital heart disease
AChE	acetylcholinesterase
ACLS	advanced cardiac life support
ACS	acute coronary syndrome
ACT	activated clotting time
ACTH	adrenocorticotrophic hormone
ADH	antidiuretic hormone
ADHD	attention deficit hyperactivity disorder
ADP	adenosine diphosphate
AF	atrial fibrillation
AHA	American Heart Association
AL	1° amyloidosis
ALT	alanine aminotransferase
AMI	acute myocardial infarction
APAH	pulmonary arterial hypertension associated with another disorder
APD	action potential duration
ApoB	apolipoprotein B

APTT	activated partial thromboplastin time
AR	aortic regurgitation
ARB	angiotensin receptor blocker
ARVC	arrhythmogenic right ventricular cardiomyopathy
AS	aortic stenosis
ASD	atrial septal defect
AST	aspartate aminotransferase
AT	antithrombin
ATC	Antithrombotic Trialists' Collaboration
ATP	adenosine triphosphate
AV	atrioventricular
AVNRT	atrioventricular nodal reciprocating tachycardia
AVP	arginine vasopressin, antidiuretic hormone
AVRT	atrioventricular reciprocating tachycardia
BAV	bicuspid aortic valve
bd	twice a day
BHS	British Hypertension Society
BMI	body mass index
BMS	bare-metal stent
BNP	B-type natriuretic peptide
BP	blood pressure
bpm	beats per minute
BRCP	breast cancer resistance protein
BSAC	British Society of Antimicrobial Chemotherapy
Ca^{2+}	calcium
CABG	coronary artery bypass graft
CAD	coronary artery disease
cAMP	cyclic adenosine monophosphate
CCB	calcium-channel blocker
CCF	congestive cardiac failure
CCTGA	congenitally corrected transposition of the great arteries
cGMP	cyclic guanosine monophosphate
CHD	coronary heart disease
CI	confidence interval
C_{max}	maximum plasma concentration
CML	chronic myeloid leukaemia
CMR	cardiac magnetic resonance
CMV	cytomegalovirus
CNE	culture-negative endocarditis
CNS	central nervous system

CO	cardiac output
COMT	catechol-O-methyltransferase
CONS	coagulase-negative staphylococci
COPD	chronic obstructive pulmonary disease
COX	cyclo-oxygenase
CPK	creatine phosphokinase
CPR	cardiopulmonary resuscitation
CPVT	catecholaminergic polymorphic ventricular tachycardia
CrCl	creatinine clearance
CRF	chronic renal failure
CRP	C-reactive protein
CRT-D	cardiac resynchronization therapy with ICD
CRT-P	cardiac resynchronization therapy–pacing
CSM	Committee on Safety of Medicines
CT	computed tomography
CTD	connective tissue disease
CV	cardiovascular
CVA	cerebrovascular accident
CVAD	central venous access device
CVD	cardiovascular disease
CXR	chest X-ray
DA	dopamine
DALY	disability adjusted life-year
DBP	diastolic blood pressure
DCCV	direct current cardioversion
DCM	dilated cardiomyopathy
DCP	dual chamber pacemaker
DES	drug-eluting stent
DHA	docosahexaenoic acid
dL	decilitre/s
DOPA	3,4-dihydroxyphenylalanine
DOPAC	3,4-dihydroxyphenylacetic acid
DTGA	dextro-transposition of the great arteries
DVT	deep vein thrombosis
EBV	Epstein–Barr virus
ECG	electrocardiogram
ECT	ecarin clotting time
EECP	enhanced external counterpulsation
EF	ejection fraction
eGFR	estimated glomerular filtration rate
ENaC	epithelial sodium channel

EP	electrophysiological
EPA	eicosapentanoic acid
ER	extended-release
ERP	effective refractory period
ESC	European Society of Cardiology
ESH	European School of Haematology
ESR	erythrocyte sedimentation rate
ESRD	end-stage renal disease
ETT	exercise tolerance testing
FA	fatty acid
FBC	full blood count
FDA	Food and Drug Administration
FFA	free fatty acid
FiO_2	fraction of inspired oxygen
FPAH	familial pulmonary arterial hypertension
G6PD	glucose-6-phosphate dehydrogenase
GCA	giant cell arteritis
GCS	Glasgow Coma Scale
GFR	glomerular filtration rate
GI	gastrointestinal
GITS	gastrointestinal therapeutic system
GL-3	globotriaosylceramide
GP	glycoprotein
GTN	glyceryl trinitrate
GU	genitourinary
h	hour/s
Hb	haemoglobin
HACA	human anti-chimeric antibody
HACEK	*Haemophilus*, *Actinobacillus*, *Cardiobacterium*, *Eikerella*, and *Kingella*
HbA_{1c}	glycosylated haemoglobin
HCM	hypertrophic cardiomyopathy
HCTZ	hydrochlorthiazide
HDL	high-density lipoprotein
HDL-C	high-density lipoprotein-cholesterol
HEFH	heterozygous familial hypercholesterolaemia
HF	heart failure
H-ISDN	hydralazine and ISDN
HIT	heparin-induced thrombocytopaenia
HITT	heparin-induced arterial thrombosis

HMG-CoA	3-hydroxy-3-methyl-glutaryl-coenzyme A
HOCM	hypertrophic obstructive cardiomyopathy
HR	hazard ratio
HRT	hormone replacement therapy
HVA	homovanillic acid
IABP	intra-aortic balloon pump
IART	intra-atrial re-entry tachycardia
ICD	implantable cardiac defibrillator
IE	infective endocarditis
IFG	impaired fasting glucose
IGT	impaired glucose tolerance
IHD	ischaemic heart disease
IM	intramuscular
INR	international normalized ratio
IP3	inositol triphosphate
IPAH	idiopathic pulmonary arterial hypertension
IR	immediate release
ISA	intrinsic sympathomimetic activity
ISDN	isosorbide dinitrate
ISH	isolated systolic hypertension
ISMN	isosorbide mononitrate
ITU	intensive therapy unit
IUGR	intrauterine growth restriction
IV	intravenous
IVC	inferior vena cava
IVUS	intravascular ultrasound
JVP	jugular venous pressure
K^+	potassium
L	litre/s
LA	left atrial/atrium
LBBB	left bundle branch block
LDL	low-density lipoprotein
LDL-C	low-density lipoprotein-cholesterol
LFT	liver function test
LLD	lipid-lowering drug
LMWH	low-molecular-weight heparin
LPL	lipoprotein lipase
LQTS	long QT syndrome
LTOT	long-term oxygen therapy
LV	left ventricle/ventricular

LVAD	left ventricular assist device
LVEF	left ventricular ejection fraction
LVF	left ventricular failure
LVH	left ventricular hypertrophy
LVOT	left ventricular outflow tract
MAC	minimum active concentration
MACE	major adverse cardiac events
MAO	monoamine oxidase
MAOI	monoamine oxidase inhibitor
MBC	minimum bactericidal concentration
mcg	microgram/s
MHPG	methoxyhydroxyphenyl glycol
MI	myocardial infarction
MIC	minimum inhibitory concentration
min	minute/s
mL	millilitre/s
MMP	matrix metalloproteinase
MMSE	Mini Mental State Examination
MPS	mucopolysaccaridosis
MR	mitral regurgitation
MRI	magnetic resonance imaging
ms	millisecond/s
MS	mitral stenosis
MVO_2	myocardial oxygen demand
MVP	mitral valve prolapse
MW	molecular weight
Na^+	sodium
NADP	nicotinamide adenine dinucleotide phosphate
NAION	non-arteritic anterior ischaemic optic neuropathy
NAPA	N-acetylprocainamide
NCT	narrow complex tachycardia
NDCCB	non-dihydropyridine calcium-channel blockers
NICE	National Institute for Health and Clinical Excellence
NIV	non-invasive ventilation
NNH	number needed to harm
NNT	number needed to treat
NO	nitric oxide
NSAID	non-steroidal anti-inflammatory drug
NSTEACS	non-ST-segment elevation acute coronary syndrome
NSTEMI	non-ST-segment elevation myocardial infarction

NSVT	non-sustained ventricular tachycardia
NT-proBNP	N-terminal prohormone brain natriuretic peptide
NVE	native valve endocarditis
NYHA	New York Heart Association
OA	osteoarthritis
OAC	oral anticoagulation
OCP	oral contraceptive pill
od	once a day
OGTT	oral glucose tolerance test
PAD	peripheral arterial disease
PAF	paroxysmal atrial fibrillation
PAH	pulmonary arterial hypertension
PaO_2	partial pressure of oxygen in arteries
PAP	pulmonary artery pressure
PASP	pulmonary artery systolic pressure
PAV	per cent atheroma volume
PCI	percutaneous coronary intervention
PCR	polymerase chain reaction
PCWP	pulmonary capillary wedge pressure
PDA	patient ductus arteriosus
PDE-5	phosphodiesterase-5
PDEI	phosphodiesterase inhibitor
PE	pulmonary embolism
PEA	pulseless electrical activity
PEEP	positive end-expiratory pressure
PF	platelet factor
PH	pulmonary hypertension
PM	poor metabolizer
PLE	protein-losing enteropathy
PO	by mouth
PO_2	partial pressure of oxygen
POTS	paroxysmal orthostatic tachycardia syndrome
PPAR	peroxisome proliferator-activated receptor
PPI	proton pump inhibitor
PR	pulmonary regurgitation
PRA	plasma renin activity
PS	pulmonary stenosis
PT	prothrombin time
PVC	premature ventricular complex
PVD	peripheral vascular disease

PVE	prosthetic valve endocarditis
PVR	pulmonary vascular resistance
qds	four times a day
QoL	quality of life
RA	right atrial/atrium *or* rheumatoid arthritis
RAAS	renin–angiotensin–aldosterone system
RAP	right arterial pressure
RAS	renin–angiotensin system
RBBB	right bundle branch block
RCOG	Royal College of Obstetricians and Gynaecologists
RCT	randomized controlled trial
RDA	recommended daily amount
RHC	right heart catheter
RR	relative risk
RRR	relative risk reduction
rTPA	recombinant tissue plasminogen activator
RV	right ventricle/ventricular
RVOT	right ventricular outflow tract
s	second/s
SA	sinoatrial
SaO_2	arterial oxygen saturation
SBP	systolic blood pressure
SC	subcutaneous
SGOT	serum glutamic oxaloacetic transaminase
SGPT	serum glutamic pyruvic transaminase
SIADH	syndrome of inappropriate antidiuretic hormone
SIGN	Scottish Intercollegiate Guidelines Network
SK	streptokinase
SLE	systemic lupus erythematosus
SND	sinus node dysfunction
SpO_2	oxygen saturation measured by pulse oximetry
SSRI	selective serotonin reuptake inhibitor
stat	immediately
STEMI	ST-segment elevation myocardial infarction
SVC	superior vena cava
SVR	systemic vascular resistance
SVT	supraventricular tachycardia
$t_{1/2}$	half-life
T3	triiodothyronine
T4	thyroxine

TC	total cholesterol
tds	three times a day
TFT	thyroid function test
TG	triglyceride
TGA	transposition of the great arteries
TIA	transient ischaemic attack
TNF	tumour necrosis factor
TOE	transoesophageal echocardiogram
TOF	tetralogy of Fallot
tPA	tissue plasminogen activator
TR	tricuspid regurgitation
TS	tricuspid stenosis
TSH	thyroid-stimulating hormone
TT	thrombin time
TTE	transthoracic echocardiogram
TXA_2	thromboxane
U&Es	urea and electrolytes
UA	unstable angina
UCAR	urinary creatinine:albumin ratio
UFH	unfractionated heparin
UGT	uridine 5'-diphosphate glucuronosyl transferases
ULN	upper limit of normal
VASP	vasodilator-stimulated phosphoprotein
V_d	volume of distribution
VF	ventricular fibrillation
VLDL	very low-density lipoprotein
VMA	vanillyl mandelic acid
$\dot{V}O_{2max}$	maximal oxygen consumption
VSD	ventricular septal defect
VT	ventricular tachycardia
VTE	venous thromboembolic event
VZV	varicella zoster virus
WHO	World Health Organization
WPW	Wolff–Parkinson–White

Characterization of the evidence available regarding the usefulness of pharmacological agents mentioned in the book

Throughout the book we have used the ACC/AHA classification system to characterize the efficacy/usefulness of pharmacological agents mentioned in the text. The ACC/AHA classifications I, II, and III summarize both the evidence and expert opinion. Briefly:

Class I: It is considered that there is evidence and/or general agreement that the pharmacological agent is useful and effective.

Class II: There is conflicting evidence and/or a divergence of opinion about the usefulness/efficacy of the treatment.

Class IIa: Weight of evidence/opinion is in favour of usefulness/efficacy.
Class IIb: Usefulness/efficacy is less well established by evidence/opinion.

Class III: There is evidence and/or general agreement that the treatment is not useful/effective and in some cases may be harmful.

As per ACC/AHA recommendations, the weight of the evidence was ranked highest (A) if the data were derived from multiple randomized clinical trials that involved large numbers of patients and intermediate (B) if the data were derived from a limited number of randomized trials that involved small numbers of patients or from careful analyses of nonrandomized studies or observational registries. A low rank (C) was given when expert consensus was the primary basis for the recommendation.

(Data from ACC/AHA Guidelines for the Management of Patients With Unstable Angina and Non-ST-Segment Elevation Myocardial Infarction: Executive Summary and Recommendations. A Report of the American College of Cardiology/American Heart Association Task Force on Practice Guidelines (Committee on the Management of Patients With Unstable Angina) *Circulation* 2000; **102**:1193–209.)

Clinical conditions

Heart failure

Introduction

Heart failure (HF) is a complex condition that results from cardiac functional and/or structural abnormalities that affect the ability of the heart to pump blood, and is often defined as the inability of the heart to adequately perfuse the organs of the body. Symptoms of HF vary depending on several factors but the most common manifestations of HF are dyspnoea and fatigue. Of importance, HF is not necessarily associated with a reduced ejection fraction (EF) (systolic HF), as up to 50% of cases occur in the presence of a preserved systolic function (diastolic dysfunction).

HF can be classified as acute or chronic, depending on how quickly symptoms and signs develop; systolic or diastolic, depending on whether patients have a reduced left ventricular ejection fraction (LVEF) as opposed to a preserved LVEF and high- vs. low-output HF. Right and left HF are terms that indicate whether symptoms predominantly suggest right ventricular failure with peripheral oedema, raised JVP and hepatomegaly, or predominantly left ventricular failure with pulmonary oedema and hypotension.

The severity of HF can be assessed objectively with an echocardiogram, cardiac magnetic resonance (CMR), or nuclear imaging. It is not clear what the best objective measure of LV function is, but as EF has been used systematically as a major inclusion criterion in most HF trials, it has become one of the most commonly used measurements for assessment of the severity of HF.

Although the severity of LV dysfunction does not necessarily correlate with symptoms, useful grading systems exist in the clinical setting that are based on symptoms, i.e. the New York Heart Association (NHYA) classification (see Table 1.1).

The present chapter discusses, separately, three subgroups of HF patients:
• chronic HF with impaired LVEF (systolic HF).
• chronic HF with normal LVEF (diastolic HF).
• acute HF.

NYHA class and symptoms (Table 1.1)

Table 1.1 NYHA classification I–IV

Class	Symptoms
I	No limitation to physical activity. Ordinary physical activity does not cause fatigue, breathlessness, or palpitations (asymptomatic HF)
II	Slight limitation to physical activity. Such patients are comfortable at rest. Ordinary physical activity results in fatigue, palpitations, breathlessness, or angina pectoris (mildly symptomatic HF)
III	Marked limitation of physical activity. Although patients are comfortable at rest, less than ordinary physical activity will lead to symptoms (symptomatically 'moderate' HF)
IV	Inability to carry on any physical activity without discomfort. Symptoms are even present at rest (symptomatically 'severe' HF)

Data from ACC/AHA Guidelines for the Management of Patients With Unstable Angina and Non–ST-Segment Elevation Myocardial Infarction: Executive Summary and Recommendations A Report of the American College of Cardiology/American Heart Association Task Force on Practice Guidelines (Committee on the Management of Patients With Unstable Angina) *Circulation*. 2000;**102**:1193–1209.

Chronic heart failure with reduced LVEF (systolic heart failure)

Incidence and prognosis

HF is a common condition whose incidence increases with age and, due to demographic trends of an ageing population, is increasing in prevalence.

There are an estimated 934,000 people over the age of 45 who have diagnosed or suspected HF in the UK.

Mortality has been quoted as high as 30% at 1 year after diagnosis but survival has improved with newer HF treatments.

Aetiology

The most common causes are:
- ischaemic heart disease; the most common cause in developed countries (50–70% of cases)
- systemic hypertension, which often causes HF with preserved LVEF
- the cardiomyopathies, including dilated cardiomyopathy, hypertrophic cardiomyopathy, restrictive cardiomyopathy, peripartum cardiomyopathy, and arrhythmogenic cardiomyopathy.

- Other common causes include: alcohol consumption, the use of certain drugs (i.e. chemotherapy), valvular heart disease, infiltrative disorders (amyloid and sarcoid), diabetes, and rhythm disturbances such as chronic uncontrolled tachycardia.
- High-output cardiac failure is a less common form of presentation and can be caused by thyrotoxicosis, beri-beri, Paget's disease, sepsis, anaemia, and some arrhythmias.
- The most common causes for an acute decompensation in a patient with chronic HF include myocardial ischaemia or infarction, arrhythmias, inappropriate or insufficient drug therapy, infection, anaemia, etc.

Symptoms and signs of HF

The cardinal symptoms of HF are dyspnoea at rest or on exertion, orthopnoea, paroxysmal nocturnal dyspnoea, and fatigue. Signs of HF include those attributable to left ventricular failure such as pulmonary oedema, cold extremities, hypotension, a third heart sound, and those of right HF such as a raised JVP, peripheral oedema, hepatomegaly, and ascites, among others.

Useful investigations

- *Blood tests.* In addition to routine blood tests including FBC, U&Es, urinalysis, fasting glucose, lipids, LFTs and TFTs, the measurement of B-type natriuretic peptide (BNP) is very important. BNP can help not only in the diagnosis and prognosis of patients with HF but also in the assessment of the response to treatment.
- *A normal BNP concentration* in an untreated patient makes the diagnosis of HF unlikely whereas a high BNP level despite maximal medical treatment often indicates a poor prognosis. Conditions other than

HF that can lead to a raised BNP include: sepsis, renal dysfunction, LV hypertrophy (LVH), myocardial ischaemia, and advanced age.

- *The resting 12-lead ECG* (electrocardiogram) may show signs of ischaemic heart disease, such as an old infarction or left bundle branch block (LBBB), LVH, conduction disturbances (important to note that a QRS >120ms is one of the criteria for cardiac resynchronization therapy), or cardiac arrhythmias. Holter monitoring might be considered, to look for ventricular tachycardia (VT) in high-risk patients.
- *The chest X-ray* provides evidence for cardiomegaly, pulmonary venous congestion, pulmonary oedema, pleural effusion, and lung disease.
- *Transthoracic echocardiography* is essential in the assessment of patients with symptoms/signs of HF.
- LVEF is used to classify HF as diastolic or systolic and the echocardiogram may establish the aetiology of HF in the individual patient, e.g. valvular heart disease, myocardial infarction (MI), LVH, or global LV dysfunction associated with dilated cardiomyopathy.
- *Stress echocardiography* can be used to detect reversible myocardial ischaemia, to assess myocardial hibernation, valvular abnormalities, and the response to cardiac resynchronization therapy.
- *Coronary angiography* should be performed in patients presenting with HF who have angina or significant myocardial ischemia on non-invasive testing. Unfortunately, controlled trials have not addressed the issue of whether coronary revascularization can improve clinical outcomes in patients with HF who do not have angina pectoris.
- *Magnetic resonance imaging* (MRI) is the gold standard for evaluating ventricular dimensions as it has a high degree of reproducibility. It is also extremely useful for the assessment of ventricular function and wall motion abnormalities, myocardial viability, and scar tissue. It can also be useful for detecting right ventricular (RV) dysplasia, and identifying the presence of pericardial disease.
- $\dot{V}_{O_2max}$ *(maximal oxygen consumption) exercise testing* can give useful information in patients presenting with HF who may be candidates for cardiac transplantation or device implantation.

Pharmacological management of chronic heart failure

The recommendations that follow are based on National Institute for Health and Clinical Excellence (NICE), European Society of Cardiology (ESC), and American Heart Association (AHA) guidelines. Of importance, the NICE guidelines apply only to patients who already have HF. AHA guidelines take into account patients without HF but who have risk factors for HF, including known coronary artery disease, hypertension, diabetes mellitus, and a family history of cardiomyopathy. These high-risk patients require treatment with disease-modifying agents. There is substantial trial evidence for the treatment of HF but it must be remembered that women and the elderly are not well represented in these trials.

Pharmacological treatment

This can be divided into:

- treatments that prolong life in patients with HF and should be prescribed to all patients with HF—predominantly angiotensin-converting enzyme inhibitors (ACEIs), angiotensin receptor blockers (ARBs), aldosterone antagonists (i.e. spironolactone and eplerenone), and β-blockers
- treatments that improve symptoms only (i.e. diuretics and digoxin).

See the flow chart in Fig. 1.1 for a summary of the pharmacological management of chronic systolic HF.

All patients with LV dysfunction should receive treatment with:

An **ACEI** (do not wait for the patient to develop symptoms before commencing ACEI therapy. An ARB can be used if ACEI treatment is not well tolerated) and
A **β-blocker** (do not wait for maximum titration dose of ACEI before commencing β-blocker therapy)

Diuretics: for symptomatic relief only
Used at lowest possible dose to treat fluid overload, either pulmonary oedema or peripheral oedema. Loop diuretics: *furosemide* (dose can vary from 40mg in mild oedema up to 120mg bd in severe cases), or *bumetanide* (1mg equivalent to 40mg furosemide). Thiazide diuretics are particularly potent when used with a loop diuretic. *Bendroflumethiazide* use 2.5mg daily. In severe cases use one-off 2.5mg dose of *metolazone*

In patients with moderate to severe symptoms despite treatment with ACEI and β-blockers add:

Spironolactone (or eplerenone)—spironolactone is first choice among aldosterone antagonists but eplerenone is used following a MI and in patients who develop gynaecomastia on spironolactone

Mortality benefit

No mortality benefit

Digoxin should be considered in all patients in atrial fibrillation. If the patient is in sinus rhythm, digoxin can be added as a final step if the patient is still symptomatic despite maximal treatment.
AHA guidelines are similar to those above, except for their recommendation of the addition of **hydralazine** and **isosorbide dinitrate (ISDN)** in severe HF.

Fig. 1.1 Pharmacological treatment of chronic systolic heart failure.

ACEI or ARB (class I evidence A) (Table 1.2)

ACEIs are recommended as first-line therapy in all patients with EF <40% irrespective of symptoms. In patients with risk factors for HF who have a normal LVEF, AHA guidelines recommend starting an ACEI or ARB as a preventative action (class IIa evidence). Multiple trials have shown that ACEIs improve survival and functional capacity, delay the onset of symptoms, and reduce adverse LV remodelling in patients with HF. However, many patients are excluded from these trials, such as those with hypotension, renal failure, or normal EF, and the very elderly.

Some patients improve within 48h of starting ACEI therapy but most patients only get benefit after several weeks or months of treatment. A meta-analysis of short-term, placebo-controlled trials reported a clear reduction in mortality within 3 months.

SAVE was the first large trial of ACEI in LV dysfunction following MI. Over 2000 patients with an EF <40% 3–16 days following MI were randomized to either placebo or captopril. All-cause mortality was 19% lower in the ACEI group. There was also a 37% reduction in the development of severe HF.

CONSENSUS and SOLVD randomized patients with mild to severe HF to treatment with placebo or enalapril. There was a reduction in mortality of 27% in CONSENSUS and 16% in SOLVD.

The SOLVD-Prevention trial showed that patients with low EF but no symptoms benefited from ACEI with a 20% relative risk reduction (RRR) in death or hospitalization with HF. This emphasises the importance of starting ACEI therapy in patients with HF, even before they become symptomatic.

A meta-analysis of three large trials (SAVE, AIRE, and TRACE) showed an absolute risk reduction of 2.3%. The number needed to treat (NNT) to achieve this goal was 43.

ARBs

ACEIs are always used as first line in preference to ARBs. This is because there is more clinical experience and weight of trials behind their use compared to ARBs. It is reasonable to use an ARB when a patient develops a significant ACEI-induced cough.

CHARM-Alternative was a placebo-controlled trial with candesartan in patients with a LVEF <40%, who were intolerant to ACEI. Candesartan resulted in a RRR of death from a cardiovascular cause or hospital admission for worsening HF, of 23%.

An important question has been raised as to whether the addition of an ARB to a patient already on an ACEI and β-blocker would be beneficial. There is some evidence (CHARM–Added and Val-HeFT) that patients who are NYHA III or IV despite ACEI and β-blocker therapy do benefit from the addition of candesartan or valsartan, mainly in terms of a lower risk of death or hospitalization. Both trials showed a reduction in hospital admissions for worsening HF: RRR 24% in Val-HeFT and 17% in CHARM-Added. There was a 16% RRR in the risk of death from cardiovascular causes with candesartan in CHARM-Added.

AHA guidelines therefore suggest that it is reasonable to add an ARB in patients who are persistently symptomatic despite ACEI and β-blockers (class IIb evidence B). This recommendation is also given in the ESC guidelines but not in the NICE guidelines. This guidance is complicated by the fact that in the VALIANT study (captopril vs. valsartan vs. a combination of both) there was no significant difference in all-cause mortality between valsartan and captopril. The combination of both drugs did not reduce mortality and was associated with an increase in adverse events.

Many patients with NYHA III or IV have difficulty in achieving target doses of ACEI and β-blockers due to the occurrence of hypotension.

Initiation of treatment and uptitration
Prior to initiation of ACEI/ARB treatment, renal function and electrolytes should be assessed and then rechecked 1–2 weeks after starting treatment. ACEI/ARBs should be commenced at a low dose and titrated up at 2-weekly intervals with the aim of reaching target doses. Uptitration is dependent on blood pressure (BP) response. Hypotension is acceptable if systolic BP (SBP) is >90mmHg and asymptomatic. Symptomatic hypotension can be minimized by nocturnal dosing. In hospitalized patients ACEIs should be started prior to discharge.

ACEIs and β-blockers should always be titrated up to the maximum tolerated dose.

Contraindications
History of angio-oedema, bilateral renal artery stenosis, serum potassium >5mmol/L, serum creatinine >220μmol/L, severe aortic stenosis.

Side effects
- *Cough*: a dry cough related to the use of ACEIs is the most common reason for the withdrawal of long-term treatment. It occurs in 5–10% of white patients and up to 50% of Chinese patients. It usually appears within the first month of treatment and disappears within 1–2 weeks of discontinuing treatment. Given the known benefits of ACEIs, it is important to try and persist with treatment unless the cough is severe, particularly since the cough may be coincidental as found in many studies. If a significant cough does develop on an ACEI, then an ARB should be used instead.
- *Hypotension*: if a patient develops symptomatic hypotension, reduce the dose of any other antihypertensives before reducing the dose of the ACEI.
- *Hyperkalaemia*: may be managed by stopping potassium supplements or potassium-sparing diuretics. If the potassium still rises above 5.5mmol/L, halve the dose of the ACEI. If the potassium rises above 6.0mmol/L then stop the ACEI.
- *Deterioration in renal function*: some increase in urea and creatinine can be expected after starting an ACEI. An increase of 50% in creatinine from baseline or to an absolute concentration of 265μmol/L may be acceptable but must be carefully monitored.
  - If the creatinine rises above 310μmol/L then the ACEI should be stopped and renal function carefully monitored. It may be necessary to reduce the dose of ACEI or discontinue it altogether.
- *Angio-oedema* is a very serious side effect and if this occurs then the ACEI must be stopped immediately.

Table 1.2 ACEIs and ARBs with the largest evidence in HF trials

	Starting dose (mg)	Target dose (mg)
ACEI		
Captopril	6.25 tds	50–100 tds
Enalapril	2.5 od	10–20 bd
Lisinopril	2.5 od	20–35 od
Ramipril	1.25–2.5 od	10 od
ARB		
Candesartan	4 or 8 od	32 od
Valsartan	40 bd	160 bd

β-blockers (class I evidence A)

β-blockers should be used in all patients with impaired LV function unless there are compelling contraindications. They have been shown to improve mortality, reduce hospitalization, and improve functional class.

Evidence to support the use of β-blockers derives from the following trials: CIBIS II (bisoprolol), COPERNICUS (carvedilol), and MERIT-HF (sustained-release metoprolol). These trials randomized nearly 9000 patients with HF to either placebo or β-blocker therapy; 90% of these patients were on an ACEI or ARB. Each of these trials showed that β-blockers reduced mortality (RRR about 34% in each trial) and hospital admissions for worsening HF (RRR 28–36%).

There are very few trials in HF that included elderly patients. SENIORS was a randomized controlled trial (RCT) in elderly (>70 years old) patients with HF. Treatment with nebivolol resulted in an RRR of 14% in the primary composite endpoint of death or hospital admissions for a cardiovascular reason.

Not all β-blockers have the same effect. Metoprolol tartrate, as opposed to the sustained-release metoprolol succinate, does not confer as much benefit as carvedilol (COMET trial). There is no evidence of benefit for bucindolol (increases death in African Americans), and xamoterol has been found to be harmful in this context. As such, the only recommended β-blockers for management of HF patients are bisoprolol, carvedilol, nebivolol, and sustained-release metoprolol (not available in the UK).

Commencing therapy and uptitration (Table 1.3)

β-blockers should be commenced at a low dose and titrated up to target doses at 2-week intervals. They should usually be initiated in stable patients and only with caution in recently decompensated patients. Titrate up every 2–4 weeks. Do not increase dose if signs of worsening HF and symptomatic hypotension appear, or the heart rate is <50bpm.

In patients admitted with a decompensation of HF and hypotension, β-blockers may need to be discontinued temporarily. However, a recent study has shown increased mortality in HF patients who have their β-blockers stopped.

Contraindications

- Obstructive airways disease (not chronic obstructive pulmonary disease (COPD) per se).
- 2nd- or 3rd-degree heart block.
- Sinus bradycardia (<50bpm), symptomatic hypotension.
- Peripheral vascular disease (this is a relative contraindication as benefits may outweigh a potential deterioration in symptoms of peripheral vascular disease).

☺ Side effects

Symptomatic hypotension is relatively common and often improves over time. If hypotension appears, reduce doses of other BP-lowering medications (except ACEI/ARB) before reducing the dose of β-blocker. Asymptomatic hypotension does not require intervention.

If HF does deteriorate on β-blockers, it is possible to try and remain on the β-blocker but temporarily increase the dose of diuretics.

Table 1.3 β-blockers used in the management of HF

β-blocker	Starting dose (mg)	Target dose (mg)
Bisoprolol	1.25 od	10 od
Carvedilol	3.125 bd	25–50 bd
Metoprolol succinate	12.5 od	200 od
Nebivolol	1.25 od	10 od

Aldosterone antagonists (class I evidence B) (Table 1.4)

Aldosterone antagonists are used in patients with moderate to severe symptomatic HF (NYHA class III and IV) with a LVEF <35%, in combination with ACEIs, β-blockers, and diuretics. Spironolactone has been demonstrated to improve survival and morbidity in these patients.

RALES trial: treatment with spironolactone led to a 30% RRR of death and a 35% RRR in hospital admissions for worsening HF compared to placebo.

Eplerenone is a selective aldosterone antagonist shown to be of benefit in patients with symptomatic LV impairment following a recent MI (EPHESUS), and should be used in this group of patients. The EPHESUS trial enrolled patients 3–14 days after an acute MI with an EF <40% and HF or diabetes. Patients were randomized to placebo or eplerenone. Eplerenone lead to a RRR in death of 15%

There are no randomized clinical trials comparing eplerenone with spironolactone and there is no evidence for spironolactone in the post-MI group of patients studied on EPHESUS. However, there is not enough evidence to say if aldosterone antagonists are also beneficial in HF patients with only mild symptoms.

Cautions/contraindications

Cautions for starting treatment include hyperkalaemia and renal impairment. Check renal function prior to starting therapy and again at 1 and 4 weeks after starting treatment. Increase dose after 4–8 weeks. Recheck renal function and potassium at 1 and 4 weeks after each dose increase and 3-monthly thereafter.

Should not be prescribed if a patient is receiving combined treatment with an ACEI and an ARB.

Side effects

- *Hyperkalaemia*: if the potassium rises to >5.5mmol/L the dose of spironolactone (or eplerenone) should be halved and potassium levels monitored. If potassium rises to 6.0mmol/L, stop spironolactone (or eplerenone) and monitor carefully.
- *Worsening renal function*: if creatinine rises to >220µmol/L, halve the dose of spironolactone (or eplerenone). If creatinine rises to >310µmol/L then stop the spironolactone/eplerenone.
- *Gynaecomastia*: this occurs in about 10% of patients given spironolactone. These patients should be switched to eplerenone.

Table 1.4 Aldosterone antagonists

	Starting dose (mg)	Target dose (mg)
Spironolactone	12.5 od	50 od
Eplerenone	12.5 od	50 od

Digoxin (class IIa evidence B for reducing hospital admissions)

Digoxin is of particular benefit in patients with atrial fibrillation (AF) and HF. It slows down ventricular rate, leading to increased filling time and has a positive inotropic effect. If a patient is in sinus rhythm, digoxin can still be beneficial if symptoms persist despite maximum treatment, by reducing hospital admissions, although there is no effect on mortality. Loading doses are not generally required in stable patients. A daily dose of 125–250mcg is appropriate in the context of normal renal function. In the elderly and those with renal impairment, a smaller dose may be required.

Contraindications

2nd- or 3rd-degree heart block and pre-excitation syndromes. Caution is required in patients with renal dysfunction.

Diuretics (symptomatic improvement only) (Table 1.5)

Diuretics are used in HF to alleviate symptoms by reducing fluid overload but have not been shown to improve mortality. Diuretics reduce hospital admissions for worsening HF and improve exercise capacity. Commonly used diuretics include loop diuretics and thiazides. Thiazide diuretics may be preferred in hypertensive patients with HF.

Patients who are in decompensated HF can develop resistance to oral diuretics due to reduced drug absorption. These patients often require admission to hospital for IV diuretics.

Table 1.5 Diuretics used in the management of HF

	Initial dose (mg)	Usual dose (mg)
Loop diuretics		
Furosemide	20–40	40–240
Bumetanide	0.5–1	1–5
Thiazide diuretics		
Bendroflumethiazide	2.5	2.5–10
Metolazone	2.5	2.5–10

Side effects associated with use of diuretics
- Hypokalaemia, hyponatraemia, hypocalcaemia, hypomagnesaemia
- Hypotension
- Ototoxicity
- Hyperuricaemia

Combination of hydralazine and ISDN (H-ISDN) (class IIa evidence A)

Recommendations for the use of a combination of nitrates and hydralazine (H-ISDN) differ between NICE and AHA/ESC. NICE guidelines recommend, under specialist supervision, that this combination may be used in patients intolerant of ACEI or ARBS but do not suggest using it in combination with ACEI/ARB. There is some evidence that patients who still have moderate to severe symptoms despite ACEI or ARB and β-blockers may benefit from the addition of hydralazine and nitrate and this is recommended in the AHA/ESC guidelines. Evidence is strongest in those of African American background.

V-HeFT-1 trial: 642 men were randomized to placebo, prazosin, or H-ISDN. No patients were on β-blocker or ACEI. With H-ISDN there was a trend to a reduction in all-cause mortality, RRR 22%. H-ISDN increased exercise capacity and LVEF compared with placebo.

A-HeFT trial: 1050 African American men and women in NYHA III or IV were randomized to either placebo or H-ISDN. Patients were already on ACEI (70%), ARB (17%) or β-blocker (74%). The trial was terminated prematurely at 10 months because of a significant reduction in mortality, 43% RRR.

The most common side effects were headache, dizziness, hypotension, and nausea.

Contraindications

Symptomatic hypotension, 'lupus syndrome' (in V-HeFT-1 and -2 there was a sustained increase in antinuclear antibody in 2–3% of patients but lupus-like syndrome was rare), and severe renal failure.

Anticoagulation in HF

RCTs have shown a reduction in the risk of stroke in patients on warfarin who have HF and AF.

There is no good evidence for warfarin in HF patients with intracardiac thrombus or an LV aneurysm but the consensus is that this group of patients probably benefits from anticoagulation.

One RCT reported no difference in the risk of death, MI, or stroke in HF patients in sinus rhythm on warfarin. The WATCH trial showed no benefit of warfarin or clopidogrel compared to aspirin.

Calcium-channel blockers in HF

Amlodipine can be used to treat hypertension and angina in patients with HF. The use of verapamil, diltiazem, or short-acting dihydropyridines can cause clinical deterioration and should be avoided.

Management of AF in HF

AF is common in patients with HF. Some people may benefit from restoration of sinus rhythm but this decision should be made on an individual basis, with specialist input.

There are no RCTs demonstrating that restoration of sinus rhythm in patients with AF and HF improves mortality.

A review of the large RCTs of β-blockers in HF showed that the benefits of these agents are the same whether the patient is in sinus rhythm or AF.

Non-pharmacological management of chronic heart failure

The description of non-pharmacological management of HF is beyond the scope of this book and the following section therefore represents just a brief summary.

Weight monitoring

Patients should weigh themselves regularly and if they have sudden weight gain (approximately 2kg in 3 days) they should know how to increase their diuretic therapy. They should also be aware of the risk of volume depletion if their weight falls rapidly.

Patients who are obese (body mass index (BMI) >30kg/m^2) should lose weight in order to improve symptoms and reduce disease progression.

Fluid restriction

Restricting volume intake to 1.5–2L fluid in patients with severe HF may be considered but does not seem to help patients with mild to moderate HF.

Sodium restriction

Reducing salt intake helps to reduce fluid retention.

Alcohol

Patients suffering with alcohol-induced cardiomyopathy should completely abstain from alcohol. All other patients should not drink excessively as alcohol has a negative inotropic effect, may increase BP, and can be cytotoxic.

Smoking

No prospective studies have evaluated the effects of smoking cessation in HF but observational studies show reduced morbidity and mortality with smoking cessation.

Vaccination

Vaccination against influenza (annual) and pneumococcus (once) should be considered.

Myocardial reperfusion

Reperfuse if there is evidence of myocardial ischaemia. Routine coronary angiography in all patients with HF is not recommended. Conduct angiography in patients with angina and perform viability studies in selected patients.

Cardiac resynchronization/implantable cardiac defibrillator (ICD)

After the CARE HF trial, NICE (in 2007) recommended cardiac resynchronization therapy–pacing (CRT-P) in patients with an EF <35% and a QRS >150ms or 120–150ms if there is evidence of dyssynchrony on the echocardiogram. The PROSPECT trial later showed that there was no single marker of dyssynchrony on echo, so now the ESC (in 2008) recommend CRT-P for those with EF <35% who are NYHA III/IV and with a QRS >120ms.

1° prevention with ICD

CRT-D (CRT with ICD) in 1° prevention. Different recommendations:
- NICE in either:
  - EF <35% if non-sustained VT and positive EP study or
  - EF <30% and QRS >120ms. Not appropriate if NYHA IV.
- AHA 2008; NYHA II/III EF <35% (based on ScDHeFT trial) or NYHA I and EF <30% (based on MADIT II trial).

2° prevention

Cardiac arrest due to VT or VF, spontaneous sustained VT causing haemodynamic compromise, sustained VT without syncope who have EF <35%.

Transplantation

Specialist assessment for transplantation should be considered for patients with severe refractory symptoms or refractory cardiogenic shock.

Indications

Objective evidence of cardiopulmonary limitation, e.g. peak $\dot{V}O_{2max}$ of <10mL/min/kg. Patient dependent on inotropes.

Contraindications/cautions

Alcohol or drug abuse, severe renal failure (creatinine clearance <50mL/min or creatinine >200μmol/L). Fixed high pulmonary vascular resistance (pulmonary artery pressure (PAP) >60mmHg), significant liver impairment.

LV assist device

Needs specialist assessment. There is not enough evidence to decide which patients should have LV assist device (LVAD) as a bridge to recovery. Do LVADs provide an alternative to transplantation in advanced HF?

Chronic heart failure with preserved LVEF (diastolic heart failure)

Definition

A simple definition of diastolic HF is that of HF with preserved LVEF. In other words, patients present with signs and symptoms of HF but the echocardiogram shows normal systolic function, with impaired filling of the LV during diastole. Under physiological circumstances, Doppler across the mitral valve during filling of the LV shows an E wave during the passive filling of the LV and an A wave during atrial contraction. In patients with diastolic dysfunction of the LV there are three types of abnormal filling patterns:

- the E/A ratio is reduced or reversed. Impaired myocardial relaxation leads to a decrease in the E wave (passive ventricular filling) and a compensatory increase in the atrial A wave component of filling
- the E/A ratio is increased. In patients with elevated left atrial (LA) pressure (due to mitral valve disease or decreased LV compliance) there may be an elevated peak E-velocity and a short E-deceleration time
- patients may have a normal E/A ratio but still have abnormal filling documented by pulmonary venous flow or tissue Doppler of the mitral plane motion.

Prevalence and prognosis

HF with preserved EF is present in up to 50% of patients presenting with HF. It is more common in elderly people and those with hypertension or diabetes. Ageing is associated with decreases in the elastic properties of the heart and great vessels. The prognosis has been shown to be similar to that of systolic HF.

Aetiology

LVH (common)
- Longstanding systemic hypertension
- Aortic valve stenosis
- Hypertrophic cardiomyopathy (with or without LV outflow tract obstruction)

Myocardial ischaemia (common)
Pericardial disease (rare)
i.e. cardiac tamponade, constrictive or effusive pericarditis.

Treatment

There is little evidence for successful treatment of HF with preserved LVEF, partly because these patients were generally excluded from many of the original HF trials.

ACEIs/ARBs are beneficial in patients with systolic HF but current evidence does not support their use in patients with diastolic HF.

Results of major trials

- *PEP-CHF trial*: among patients aged ≥70 years with clinical HF and preserved LV systolic function, treatment with perindopril did not differ from placebo in the 1° endpoint of death or unplanned hospitalizations for HF.
- *CHARM-preserved trial*: candesartan in patients with preserved LVEF did not show a significant reduction in the composite endpoint of death from cardiovascular causes or admissions with HF but did show a significant reduction in the risk of investigator-reported admissions for HF.
- *I-PRESERVE trial*: investigated patients who were mostly NYHA III (77%) with normal LVEF. The trial confirmed that angiotensin-receptor blockade with irbesartan is not associated with a reduction in cardiovascular mortality and morbidity in patients with HF and normal EF. In fact there was an increase in the incidence of observed adverse effects including hyperkalaemia.

Although there is no evidence that any of the available treatments will reduce mortality in patients with diastolic HF, the following are some useful concepts for the treatment of the condition:

- control systemic hypertension (aim for <130/80mmHg)
- relieve myocardial ischaemia, i.e. coronary revascularization
- relieve volume overload (diuretics, dialysis, nitrates)
- decrease heart rate and increase diastolic filling time (β-blockers, digoxin, and calcium-channel antagonists)
- restore atrial contraction if patient is in AF (cardioversion, antiarrhythmic drugs)
- renin–angiotensin axis blockade (ACEIs/ARBs)
- aldosterone blockade (spironolactone).

Acute heart failure

Acute HF is characterized by a rapid onset of signs and symptoms of HF requiring urgent treatment. There are several presentations possible and there can be an overlap of these presentations:

- acute pulmonary oedema with severe respiratory distress
- cardiogenic shock, defined as tissue hypoperfusion, is associated with high in-hospital mortality, i.e. 40–60%
- hypertensive HF with evidence of vasoconstriction and tachycardia. There is often a relatively normal LVEF in these patients, and in-hospital mortality is relatively low
- progressive worsening of chronic HF with gradual increase in systemic and pulmonary congestion
- isolated right HF characterized by raised venous pressure, absence of pulmonary congestion, and a low output state due to low LV filling pressures.

Aetiology

- Cardiac ischaemia:
  - MI.
  - Acute ventricular septal defect (VSD).
  - Acute mitral valve regurgitation.
- Arrhythmias.
- Heart valve dysfunction:
  - Valve stenosis.
  - Valve regurgitation.
  - Endocarditis.
- Aortic dissection.
- Pericardial disease.
- Increased vascular resistance:
  - Systemic hypertension.
  - Pulmonary hypertension.
- Circulatory failure:
  - Septicaemia.
  - Thyrotoxicosis.
  - Anaemia.
  - Pulmonary embolism.
- Decompensation of pre-existing chronic HF:
  - Lack of adherence to treatment.
  - Volume overload.
  - Infections, especially pneumonia.
  - Renal dysfunction.
  - Asthma and COPD.
  - Alcohol and drug abuse.

Treatment

In the published trials of acute HF, most agents have been shown to improve cardiovascular haemodynamics but no agent has been shown to reduce mortality. The following recommendations are from expert consensus and therefore the level of evidence is C, unless otherwise stated.

Oxygen

Administer to maintain oxygen saturation >95% (>90% in COPD if evidence of CO_2 retention has been obtained).

Non-invasive ventilation (NIV)

Early NIV with positive end-expiratory pressure (PEEP) improves LV function by reducing LV afterload. NIV should be used with caution in cardiogenic shock and RV failure. Intubation should not be delayed for a trial of NIV.

Three recent meta-analyses found that early application of NIV reduces the need for intubation and reduces short-term mortality. However, in *3CPO*, a large RCT, NIV improved clinical parameters but not mortality.

Start with a PEEP of 5–7.5cmH$_2$O and titrate up to 10cmH$_2$O. Use a fraction of inspired oxygen (FiO$_2$) >40%.

Morphine

- Good for treating restlessness, dyspnoea, anxiety, and chest pain.
- Also acts as a vasodilator.
- Use boluses of 2.5–5mg IV.
- Use anti-emetics to treat nausea.
- Use with great caution in patients with CO_2 retention due to reduced conscious level, sedated patients, hypotension. There is some evidence from the *ADHERE* study that the use of morphine is associated with a worse mortality.

Vasodilators (class I evidence B)

- IV nitrates decrease left and right filling pressures and systemic vascular resistance, i.e. glyceryl trinitrate continuous infusion of 1–10mg/h.
- They are recommended early in acute HF if SBP >110 mmHg and may be used with caution if SBP is between 90 and 110 mmHg. Particularly useful in hypertensive HF.
- Important to monitor BP levels and avoid acute drops in pressure. An arterial line would be useful but not essential.
- Use with caution in patients with aortic stenosis as they may lead to marked hypotension.

Side effects: headache, hypotension.

Loop diuretics (class I evidence B)

- Never evaluated in RCT but universally accepted to be beneficial.
- Use intravenously.
- Initial doses: furosemide 20–40mg, bumetanide 0.5–1mg.
- Higher initial doses may be needed if the patient has renal failure or is receiving chronic diuretic therapy.
- The highest dose of diuretic that should really be used is as an infusion of 240mg in 24h (in exceptional circumstances 480mg in 24h).

Concomitant use with IV vasodilators may permit a reduction in the dose of diuretic required. A combination of lower doses of different diuretics may be more effective than a higher dose of furosemide alone. Bendroflumethiazide 2.5mg, metolazone 2.5mg, or spironolactone 25mg can be added to furosemide. If diuresis cannot be restored, patients may need renal specialist treatment.

Inotropic agents
- May acutely improve haemodynamics but they increase oxygen consumption and may worsen myocardial ischaemia/necrosis. No evidence for improved mortality. Initiated as early as required but stopped as soon as no longer needed.
- Need continuous ECG telemetry. BP should be monitored invasively or non-invasively. Dose titrated up against BP and clinical condition and diuresis. When weaning off inotropes do this gradually.

Indications: low SBP in the presence of hypoperfusion if the patient has not responded to correction of preload with fluids or when there is a poor response to diuretics/nitrates due to hypotension.

Side effects: increased risk of ventricular and atrial arrhythmias. Need caution in patients with resting heart rate over 100bpm.

Additional interventions

If the measures listed earlier fail to treat cardiogenic shock, the following mechanical interventions can be considered: intra-aortic balloon pump (IABP), intubation, and LVADs as a bridge to transplantation.

If acute coronary syndrome (ACS) is the underlying cause of acute HF, then coronary reperfusion with percutaneous coronary intervention (PCI) or surgery may improve prognosis. Urgent surgery can be indicated in patients with mechanical complications after MI.

Inotropic treatment in acute HF

See Table 1.6.

Table 1.6 Inotropic treatment in acute HF

Inotrope	Dosing	Effects
Dobutamine Evidence: class IIa level B	No bolus Infusion 2–20mcg/kg/min	Stimulation of β_1 receptors Need higher doses if on β-blockers
Dopamine Evidence: class IIb level C	No bolus Infusion depends on desired effect: • <3mcg/kg/min (dopamine receptors) • 3–5mcg/kg/min (β receptors) • >5mcg/kg/min (β and α receptors)	Low dose stimulates dopaminergic receptors, can promote diuresis (may be combined with dobutamine) Medium dose has inotropic effects with β stimulation At higher dose has alpha-stimulation effect causing vasoconstriction
Milrinone Evidence: class IIb level B	Bolus 25–75mcg/kg over 10–20min Infusion 0.375–0.75mcg/kg/min	Type III phosphodiesterase inhibitor Inhibits breakdown of cAMP Increases cardiac output (CO) Reduces pulmonary vascular resistance Concomitant β-blockers do not interact
Levosimendan Evidence: class IIa level B	Bolus 12mcg/kg over 10min (if SBP <100mmHg do not use bolus) Infusion 0.05–0.2mcg/kg/min	A calcium sensitizer which binds to troponin-C improving contractility Increases CO Reduces pulmonary vascular resistance Concomitant β-blockers do not interact
Noradrenaline Evidence: class IIb level C	No bolus Infusion 0.2–1.0mcg/kg/min	Not recommended as first line in cardiogenic shock unless coexisting sepsis May be used if SBP still <90mmHg despite improvement in CO with first-line inotrope and fluids
Adrenaline Evidence: class IIb level C	1mg bolus only in context of cardiac arrest Infusion 0.05–0.5mcg/kg/min	Not recommended as first line in cardiogenic shock unless coexisting sepsis

Clinical trials

3 CPbO

Effect of Continuous Positive Airway Pressure and Noninvasive Positive Pressure Ventilation in Acute Cardiogenic Pulmonary Oedema[1]

Treating patients with acute cardiogenic pulmonary oedema with NIV was not associated with a reduction in mortality or need for intubation compared with standard oxygen therapy. There was also no difference between NIV and continuous positive airway pressure.

A-HeFT

African-American Heart Failure Trial[2]

African-American patients with advanced HF were treated with isosorbide dinitrate plus hydralazine and this resulted in a reduction in the 1° composite endpoint and in all-cause mortality compared with placebo.

AIRE

Acute Infarction Ramipril Efficacy Study[3]

Patients with signs of HF early after a MI were treated with ramipril and this reduced mortality and progression to resistant HF.

ATLAS

Assessment of Treatment with Lisinopril and Survival[4]

The use of high-dose instead of low-dose lisinopril in chronic HF patients did not result in significantly lower all-cause mortality but was associated with a reduced risk of major clinical events.

CARE-HF

Cardiac Resynchronization Heart Failure Study[5]

In patients with advanced HF and evidence of dyssynchrony despite optimal medical therapy, treatment with CRT was associated with a reduction in the 1° endpoint of all-cause mortality and hospitalization for major cardiovascular events.

CHARM

Candesartan in Heart Failure—assessment of reduction in mortality and morbidity[6]

CHARM consisted of three parallel studies looking at the effects of candesartan:

- CHARM Added—Patients with LVEF ≤40% already treated with an ACEI
- CHARM Alternative—LVEF ≤40%, ACEI intolerant
- CHARM Preserved—LVEF >40%, with or without ACEIs.

Candesartan was associated with a reduction in cardiovascular death and HF in the ALTERNATIVE trial and in the ADDED trial, but not in the PRESERVED trial.

CIBIS-II
The Cardiac Insufficiency Bisoprolol Study II
CIBIS-II was the first RCT with sufficient power to address all-cause mortality as a 1° objective. The study was stopped prematurely in March 1998 because of a highly significant mortality reduction with bisoprolol.

COMET
Carvedilol Or Metoprolol European Trial[7]
The COMET trial was the first randomized mortality trial to compare two β-blockers in patients with chronic HF. Among patients with moderate and severe chronic HF, treatment with carvedilol was associated with a significantly lower rate of all-cause mortality compared with metoprolol tartrate. This study has been criticized for using the immediate-release formulation of metoprolol tartrate which differs from the controlled-release formulation of metoprolol succinate used in the MERIT HF trial.

COPERNICUS
Effect of Carvedilol on Survival in Severe Chronic Heart Failure[8]
This trial looked at the effect of carvedilol in patients with severe HF. Results showed that beta adrenergic blockade improves survival and clinical outcome in more severe HF, when patients are not fluid overloaded or acutely decompensated. The study was terminated early due to the magnitude of benefit in the carvedilol arm.

EPHESUS
Eplerenone Post-AMI Heart Failure Efficacy and Survival Study[9]
Among patients with acute MI (AMI) complicated by HF and systolic LV dysfunction, treatment with eplerenone was associated with a reduction in all-cause mortality and the composite of death or hospitalization from cardiovascular causes.

I-PRESERVE
Irbesartan in Heart Failure With Preserved Ejection Fraction Study[10]
There was no difference between the irbesartan and placebo groups in the incidence of all-cause mortality or hospitalization for cardiovascular causes. Similarly, there was no difference between the two groups in the incidence of mortality, cardiovascular hospitalizations, worsening HF, or ventricular arrhythmias.

MADIT II
Multicenter Automatic Defibrillator Implantation Trial II[11]
ICD implantation was associated with a 31% reduction in overall mortality compared to conventional therapy.

MERIT HF
Metoprolol CR/XL Randomized Intervention Trial in Congestive Heart Failure[12]
Metoprolol provided a 34% reduction in mortality in chronic HF patients with systolic dysfunction.

PEP-CHF

Perindopril for Elderly People with Chronic Heart Failure[13]

Among patients aged ≥70 years with clinical chronic HF and preserved LV systolic function, treatment with perindopril did not differ from placebo in the 1° endpoint of death or unplanned hospitalizations for HF.

RALES

Randomized Aldactone Evaluation Study[14]

Use of spironolactone in severe HF was associated with a reduction in mortality and rehospitalization and improved symptoms of HF without increasing safety events.

SAVE

Survival and Ventricular Enlargement Trial[15]

Long-term treatment with captopril started early post-MI in patients with asymptomatic or minimally symptomatic LV dysfunction improves survival and morbidity due to major cardiovascular events.

SCDHeFT

Sudden Cardiac Death in Heart Failure Trial[16]

Among patients with NYHA class II or III chronic HF and reduced LVEF, treatment with an implantable ICD was associated with a reduction in all-cause mortality compared with placebo, but there was no difference between amiodarone and placebo.

SENIORS

Study of Effects of Nebivolol Intervention on Outcomes and Rehospitalisation in seniors with heart failure[17]

Among elderly HF patients, treatment with the β-blocker nebivolol was associated with a reduction in the 1° endpoint of all-cause mortality and admission for cardiovascular events compared with placebo.

SOLVD-Prevention

The Effects of Enalapril on Mortality and the Development of Heart failure in Asymptomatic Patients with Reduced Left Ventricular Ejection Fractions[18]

In patients with an EF <35% but who are asymptomatic, enalapril reduces the risk of development of HF and hospitalization for HF. There was a trend toward fewer cardiovascular deaths in patients receiving enalapril.

References

1 N Engl J Med 2008; **359**:142–51.
2 N Engl J Med 2004; **351**:2049–57.
3 Eur Heart J 1997; **18**:41–51.
4 Circulation 1999; **100**:2312–18.
5 N Engl J Med 2005; **352**:1539–49.
6 Lancet 2003; **362**:759–66.
7 Lancet 2003; **362**:7–13.
8 N Engl J Med 2001; **334**:1651–8.
9 N Engl J Med 2003; **348**:1309–21.
10 N Engl J Med 2008; **359**:2456–67.
11 N Engl J Med 2002; **346**:877–83.
12 Circulation 1998; **98**(Suppl I):1–364.
13 Eur Heart J 2006; **27**:2338–45.
14 N Engl J Med 1999; **341**:709–17.
15 N Engl J Med 1992; **327**:669–77.
16 N Engl J Med 2005; **352**:225–37.
17 Eur Heart J 2005; **26**:215–25.
18 N Engl J Med 1992; **327**:685–91.

Coronary artery disease

Chronic stable angina

Overview of stable angina

Background

Ischaemic heart disease is the leading cause of morbidity and mortality in the developed world. The prevalence of stable angina increases with age, affecting 10–15% of women and 10–20% of men aged 65–74 years. Below the age of 50–55 years, a more distinct discrepancy between the sexes is seen, with a higher incidence seen among middle-aged men. In fact, approximately 70% of all patients with chronic stable angina are male.

The term *angina pectoris* describes a clinical symptom: chest tightness. Chronic stable angina pectoris is defined by the presence of characteristic chest discomfort, typically occurring at a predictable and reproducible level of exertion, which is relieved by rest and with nitrates. Angina often results from an imbalance between the myocardial oxygen supply and demand. Most commonly, angina is a clinical manifestation of long-standing underlying atherosclerotic coronary artery disease, but can also result from a number of other causes, i.e. coronary artery spasm as in Prinzmetal's variant angina, coronary microcirculatory dysfunction as seen in cardiac syndrome X, hypertension, LVH, cardiomyopathy, and aortic stenosis.

Symptoms of stable angina are typically triggered by effort (e.g. uphill walking or sexual activity, emotional stress, exposure to low temperature), and present as retrosternal tightness, pain, or discomfort. Symptom severity ranges from mild pressure to severe gripping pain; however, there is often no correlation between the severity of pain and extent of underlying coronary pathology. As with all types of cardiac pain, the sensation felt may radiate along the ulnar surface of the left arm, to the neck and jaw, to the epigastrium or the interscapular region due to somatic innervation. Characteristically, the progression of pain follows a crescendo–decrescendo pattern, gradually reaching its maximal intensity within minutes and slowly dissipating after 2–5min of rest or following the administration of sublingual glyceryl trinitrate. Shortness of breath, faintness, and fatigue may represent 'angina equivalents' in the elderly. Angina pectoris can be graded according to the Canadian Cardiovascular Society functional classification system.

Differential diagnoses of chest pain can often be excluded by the clinical history. Pleuritic pain, chest wall tenderness, and pain altered by position all suggest other causes. Similarly, constant prolonged pain and sharp, fleeting submammary pain are not indicative of stable angina. Patients with exercise-induced angina may have a fixed or variable threshold for when symptoms are expected. 'Crescendo angina' occurs when symptoms increase in severity and occur at a lower threshold. A patient presenting with 'crescendo angina', angina occurring at rest, or new-onset severe angina, is likely to be suffering from unstable angina and should be investigated for ACS.

Pathophysiological bases for pharmacotherapy

Cardiac function depends on a dynamic process that matches coronary blood flow to current and changing myocardial oxygen demands.

Several types of angina exist. The underlying pathophysiology in a particular patient is important when considering antiangina therapies. Pain of angina pectoris is due to ischaemic excitation of chemosensitive and mechanoreceptive receptors in the heart.

If the coronary circulation is compromised by the presence of narrowed, stiff atheromatous vessels, and flow cannot therefore adjust to increased myocardial oxygen demand, i.e. changes in heart rate, BP, contractility, or LV end-diastolic volume during exercise or stress, the heart becomes vulnerable to ischaemia—often expressed as angina pain. Angina, however, can occur also as a result of episodic coronary vasoconstriction (i.e. coronary artery spasm) which may affect both diseased and angiographically 'normal' arteries.

Drugs effective in relieving the symptoms of angina act through different mechanisms, which reduce myocardial work, improve flow, or both. Some act primarily as systemic or coronary vasodilators, whereas others exert their efficacy mainly through reduction of heart rate and contractility. This alters the threshold at which an angina episode is triggered.

The transient ischaemia that occurs in chronic stable angina can be exacerbated by alterations in intracellular ion concentrations and microvascular hypoperfusion. Calcium overload, resulting from ischaemic-induced sodium channel dysfunction generating a late inward sodium current affecting Na^+/Ca^{2+} channels, leads to impaired diastolic relaxation and increased diastolic wall tension. This worsens the oxygen imbalance and prolongs the chest pain experienced by the patient.

Important clinical risk factors for coronary artery disease
- Age
- Male gender
- Postmenopausal status
- Smoking
- Obesity
- Hypertension
- Hyperlipidaemia
- Diabetes mellitus
- Family history of premature ischaemic heart disease (IHD) (1st-degree relative, male <55 years, or female <65 years)
- Previous IHD, peripheral vascular disease, stroke

Treatment of stable angina

Treatment of chronic stable angina aims to relieve symptoms, slow disease progression, and increase survival through prevention of future cardiac events and death. These objectives can be achieved with lifestyle modification, pharmacological intervention, and, if necessary, myocardial revascularization (📖 Fig. 2a.1 and Box 2a.1, pp.35, 36). For the treatment of refractory angina, several novel therapeutic options exist.

Lifestyle modification

Lifestyle modification plays a vital role in the management of chronic stable angina pectoris. Smoking cessation, weight loss, healthy eating, and exercise are among the most effective. In very symptomatic patients, certain physically strenuous activities and jobs may need to be avoided. Stress management and increased conditioning through modest isotonic exercise may also help.

Control of underlying medical conditions

Optimization of underlying medical conditions in patients with angina includes paying particular attention to BP control in hypertensive patients and to glycaemic control in patients with diabetes. Current guidelines suggest a target BP of ≤130/80mmHg in patients with diabetes, which may also apply to patients with renal disease and those with known coronary artery disease. A glycosylated haemoglobin (HbA_{1c}) level of <7% in patients with diabetes is recommended. Anaemia, tachyarrhythmias, fever, thyroid disease, and hypoxaemia are other comorbidities that exacerbate angina and should be addressed.

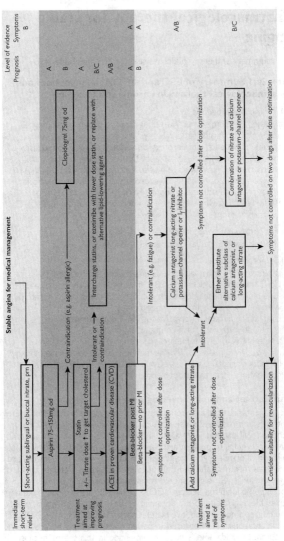

Fig. 2a.1 ESC treatment algorithm for stable angina.

Pharmacological therapy for stable angina

For a summary of therapy guidelines see Box 2a.1 and Table 2a.1.

> **Box 2a.1 Summary of ESC and ACC/AHA guidelines on pharmacological therapy in chronic stable angina**
>
> *A) To improve prognosis*
> - Aspirin, 75–150mg od or 75–325mg od in all patients; clopidogrel 75mg od if contraindication/allergy.
> - Statins, all patients with coronary disease and elevated low-density lipoprotein (LDL) cholesterol, dose titrated to target cholesterol, alternative lipid-lowering agent used if intolerance or contraindication.
> - ACEIs, if previous MI or known coronary artery disease, particularly in patients with diabetes without severe renal disease.
> - β-blockers, if previous MI or LV dysfunction present (unless contraindication).
>
> *B) For immediate symptom relief*
> - Short-acting nitrates, as required, in all patients.
>
> *C) Symptom control*
> - β-blockers, 1st-line in all patients unless contraindication
> - Calcium-channel blockers (CCBs), if intolerant or contraindication to β-blockers, or in addition to β-blockers or long-acting nitrate if symptoms are refractory to monotherapy.
> - Long-acting nitrates, alternative for 2nd-line monotherapy or combination therapy, or if contraindication to CCB or when treatment with CCB is ineffective.
> - Nicorandil, alternative for 2nd-line monotherapy or combination therapy.
> - Metabolic agents, used where available as add-on therapy or when conventional drugs are not tolerated.*

Antiplatelet and lipid-lowering drugs

These agents are used in patients with stable angina, to improve long-term prognosis and reduce the risk of ACS. Aspirin 75–150mg daily is recommended in all patients with stable angina who have no specific contraindications. It helps to prevent arterial thrombosis, and acts via irreversible inhibition of platelet cyclo-oxygenase-1 (COX-1), which reduces the production of thromboxane and thus platelet aggregation. Patients at risk of gastrointestinal (GI) bleed should receive concomitant treatment with a proton pump inhibitor. Selective COX-2 inhibitors are avoided in patients with stable angina due to the potential increased risk of coronary events. Clopidogrel, a non-competitive platelet adenosine diphosphate (ADP) receptor antagonist, is often used in patients with angina who are allergic to aspirin. Dipyridamole is not recommended in this setting because of a potential risk of worsening angina symptoms. Statins, which inhibit the enzyme HMG-CoA reductase, reduce endogenous cholesterol synthesis, and also have anti-inflammatory and antithrombotic properties that are likely to contribute to the improved survival benefits seen with the use of these drugs. Statins are indicated for all patients with documented coronary artery disease, irrespective of their plasma total cholesterol levels.

Anti-angina drugs (Table 2a.1)

Table 2a.1 Anti-angina drugs

Drug	Indications	Action	Comment
Short-acting nitrates (sublingual) Glyceryl trinitrate Isosorbide dinitrate	1st-line treatment for acute angina symptoms Prophylaxis of angina	Systemic venodilator, decreases preload, wall tension and oxygen requirements Systemic and coronary artery vasodilator, decreases afterload and improves myocardial perfusion	Usually sublingual preparations Interaction with phosphodiesterase-5 (PDE-5) inhibitors can cause life-threatening hypotension Nitrates avoided in patients with severe aortic stenosis and hypertrophic obstructive cardiomyopathy (HOCM)
Long-acting nitrates Isosorbide dinitrate Isosorbide-5-mononitrate	2nd-line treatment for angina symptoms	(As above)	Oral or chewable tablets, transdermal patch, or paste preparations Nitrate-free interval necessary to avoid tolerance Nitrates avoided in patients with aortic stenosis and HOCM Interaction with PDE-5 inhibitors
β-adrenergic receptor blockers Metoprolol Bisoprolol Atenolol (long-acting, cardioselective beta-blocker lacking intrinsic sympathomimetic activity preferred)	1st-line anti-angina drugs used in all patients unless contraindication Improves survival in patients with previous MI	Decreases myocardial oxygen demand by reducing heart rate and contractility and systemic arterial pressure	Dose titrated to achieve target resting heart rate of 50–60bpm Contraindicated in asthma and severe peripheral vascular disease (PVD) Ineffective in Prinzmetal's variant angina, and may induce coronary vasospasm Not recommended in patients with bradycardia atrioventricular (AV) block, and sinus node dysfunction

(continued)

Table 2a.1 (Contd.)

Drug	Indications	Action	Comment
Calcium-channel blockers (CCBs) Nifedipine Verapamil Diltiazem Amlodipine	2nd-line treatment for angina symptoms 1st-line treatment for Prinzmetal's variant angina	Reduce myocardial oxygen demand via systemic and coronary vasodilatation, reduced atrioventricular conduction (diltiazem and verapamil), contractility (diltiazem and verapamil), and systemic arterial pressure	Long-acting or sustained-release preparations preferred Verapamil used with caution if combined with beta-blocker because of combined effect on heart rate and contractility Short-acting dihydropyridines avoided because risk of precipitating infarction Long-acting dihydropyridine CCB used in patients with depressed LV function Dihydropyridine CCB avoided in patients with HOCM Negative chronotropic CCB avoided in patients with bradycardia, AV block, and sinus node dysfunction
Potassium-channel openers Nicorandil	2nd-line treatment for angina symptoms	Potassium-channel opener with nitrate moiety and nitrate-like effects Coronary and systemic vasodilator, decreases preload and afterload, and improves coronary flow	Vasodilatory drugs avoided in patients with aortic stenosis and HOCM Preconditions myocardium against ischaemia
Metabolic agents Trimetazidine Perhexiline	Refractory angina	Inhibition of fatty acid oxidation promotes glucose oxidation, which increases efficiency of cardiac metabolism	Perhexiline can cause hepatotoxicity and peripheral neuropathy

Table 2a.1 (*Contd.*)

Drug	Indications	Action	Comment
Inhibitors of the late sodium current Ranolazine		Ranolazine is thought to prevent Ca^{2+} overload in ischaemic myocardial cells by blocking late Na^+ influx, which prevents increased diastolic wall tension and decreases oxygen demand	Ranolazine is contraindicated in patients with pre-existing prolonged QT interval, in those taking other drugs that prolong the QT interval, in hepatic failure, and with certain drugs that inhibit liver enzymes, such as verapamil and diltiazem. It also interacts with digoxin and simvastatin
Sinus node inhibitors Ivabradine	Stable angina	Selective inhibitor of the Na^+/K^+ I_f channel that controls sino-atrial (SA) node pacing Reduces spontaneous firing of SA node pacemaker cells, slowing the heart rate	Contraindicated in patients with sick sinus syndrome Ineffective in patients with AF Drug interaction with certain liver enzyme inhibitors Shown to decrease hospital admissions for fatal and non-fatal MIs, and decrease the need for coronary revascularization in a sugroup of patients with stable angina, LV systolic dysfunction, and a resting heart rate >70bpm when compared to placebo ('BEAUTIFUL' trial)

Medications indicated in high cardiovascular risk patients

These include ACEIs, which are recommended for all patients with known coronary artery disease, a previous history of MI, and EF <40%, and in those with diabetes mellitus, hypertension, and chronic kidney disease. Spironolactone is also considered in post-MI patients who have a low EF and diabetes or heart failure. β-blockers, which are recommended as 1st-line therapy in all patients with chronic stable angina, are particularly important in those with prior MI, as they have been shown to improve survival. β-blockers are also used in patients with poor LV function. Influenza vaccination is suggested for patients with chronic stable angina who have had a previous coronary event.

Myocardial reperfusion therapies for stable angina

PCI and coronary artery bypass graft (CABG) surgery are considered in patients with severe coronary artery stenosis detected by coronary angiography whose symptoms cannot be controlled by conventional medical therapy. Revascularization improves prognosis and symptoms in appropriately selected patients. Revascularization is not indicated in patients without significant coronary artery stenosis, in those with mild or no symptoms who have not received optimal medical therapy and do not have significant proximal left anterior descending stenosis or demonstrable ischaemia seen with non-invasive imaging, and in those deemed to be at a high risk of procedure-related morbidity or mortality.

Other therapies

- Mechanical therapies, such as enhanced external counterpulsation (EECP) and spinal stimulation can be used in patients with refractory angina who are not suitable for reperfusion therapies. In EECP, pneumatic cuffs placed on the lower legs are used to increase arterial BP and retrograde aortic blood flow during diastole, which decreases cardiac work and oxygen demand, and improves coronary flow. Spinal stimulation therapy is based on the gate theory of pain, and works via an electrode placed in the epidural space at T1/T2.
- Other medical therapies under investigation for potential use in the treatment of stable angina are: bosentan, an endothelin receptor blocker; fasudil, a rho kinase inhibitor; and testosterone.

Prinzmetal's variant angina

Patients with Prinzmetal's variant angina present with angina-type pain, which occurs predominantly at rest. There is often transient ST-segment elevation. Variant angina, also called vasospastic angina, is caused by epicardial coronary artery spasm. There may be a number of triggers, including hyperventilation, smoking, and cocaine use. The diagnosis is made following demonstration of focal spasm seen during coronary angiography, which may require provocation tests using acetylcholine or ergonovine. Coronary spasm can occur in both subjects with angiographically normal coronary arteries and patients with stenotic, atherosclerotic arteries. Short-acting nitrates are usually effective in ending the episode. Long-acting nitrates and, importantly, CCBs provide the mainstay of preventative treatment.

Cardiac syndrome X

Patients with typical angina pain, a positive stress test, negative tests for coronary artery spasm, and angiographically normal coronary arteries, are referred to as cardiac syndrome X. This syndrome occurs most often in postmenopausal women. The pathogenesis of cardiac syndrome X is heterogeneous, encompassing different patient populations. Microvascular dysfunction, abnormal endothelium-dependent vasoreactivity, and altered pain perception are among the proposed pathogenic mechanisms. Treatment of cardiac syndrome X focuses on symptomatic relief, as the prognosis in terms of mortality is good. Nitrates are effective in around half of patients and can be used in the first instance. CCBs and β-blockers are helpful, and nicorandil and metabolic agents are tried in refractory cases. In patients with endothelial dysfunction, use of ACEIs and statins may be of benefit. Imipramine, aminophylline, psychological therapy, oestrogen replacement, and spinal cord stimulation are additional therapies that have shown some efficacy in the treatment of this type of chronic angina.

Further reading

Clinical guidelines

Fox K *et al.* (2006). Guidelines on the management of stable angina pectoris: executive summary: the Task Force on the Management of Stable Angina Pectoris of the European Society of Cardiology. *Eur Heart* **27**:1341–81.

Gibbons RJ *et al.*; American Heart Association Task Force on practice guidelines (Committee on the Management of Patients With Chronic Stable Angina) (2003). ACC/AHA 2002 guideline update for the management of patients with chronic stable angina–summary article: a report of the American College of Cardiology/American Heart Association Task Force on practice guidelines. *J Am Coll Cardiol* **41**:159–68.

Background reading

Morrow DA and Gersh BJ (2008). Chronic coronary artery disease. In Libby P *et al.* (eds) *Braunwald's Heart Disease: A Textbook of Cardiovascular Medicine*, 8th edn, pp. 1353–417. Saunders.

Clinical trials

SAPAT[1]

Swedish Angina Pectoris Aspirin Trial
- 2035 patients with stable angina.
- Aspirin 75mg daily showed a 34% reduction in MI and sudden death when compared to placebo.

4S[2]

Scandinavian Simvastatin Survival Study
- 4444 patients with increased cholesterol.
- Simvastatin reduced low-density lipoprotein (LDL) cholesterol by 35% and cardiac death by 42% over 4 years when compared to placebo.

TIBET[3]

Total Ischaemic Burden European Trial
- 682 patients with chronic stable angina.
- Combination therapy with nifedipine and atenolol shown to be better than monotherapy in reducing symptoms, and ambulatory and exercise ischaemia in patients with severe angina.

CAMELOT[4]

Comparison of Amlodipine vs. Enalapril to Limit Occurrences of Thrombosis
- 1991 patients with coronary artery disease and diastolic blood pressure (DBP) <100mmHg followed over 24 months.
- Treatment with amlodipine produced a 31% relative reduction in cardiovascular events, including hospitalization for angina, acute MI, and stroke, when compared to placebo.

IONA[5]

Impact Of Nicorandil in Angina
- 5126 patients followed over 1.6 years.
- Nicorandil produced a 0.83 RRR in cardiac death, non-fatal MI, and admission for cardiac pain when compared to placebo.

BEAUTIFUL[6]

Effects of Ivabradine in Patients With Stable Coronary Artery Disease and Left Ventricular Systolic Dysfunction
- 10,917 patients with coronary artery disease and LV dysfunction.
- Ivabradine decreased admission for fatal and non-fatal MI and need for coronary revascularization in a subgroup of patients with a heart rate >70bpm.

References

1 Juul-Moller S *et al.* for the Swedish Angina Pectoris Aspirin Trial (SAPAT) Group (1992). Double blind trial of aspirin in primary prevention of myocardial infarction in patients with stable chronic angina pectoris. *Lancet* **340**:1421–5.

2 Scandanavian Simvastatin Survival Study Group (1994). Randomized trial of cholesterol lowering in 4444 patients with coronary heart disease: The Scandanavian Simvastatin Survival Study (4S). *Lancet* **344**:1383–9.

3 Dargie HJ et al. (1996) Total Ischaemic Burden European Trial (TIBET). Effects of ischaemia and treatment with atenolol, nifedipine SR and their combination on outcome in patients with chronic stable angina. The TIBET Study Group. *Eur Heart J* **17**:104–12.

4 Nissen SE et al. for the CAMELOT investigators (2004). Effects of antihypertensive agents on cardiovascular events in patients with coronary artery disease and normal blood pressure: The CAMELOT study: a randomized controlled trial. *JAMA* **292**:2217–25.

5 The IONA Study Group (2002). Effect of nicorandil on coronary events in patients with stable angina: the Impact Of Nicorandil in Angina (IONA) randomised trial. *Lancet* **359**:1269–75.

6 Fox K et al. (2008). Ivabradine for patients with stable coronary artery disease and left-ventricular systolic dysfunction (BEAUTIFUL): a randomized, double-blind, placebo-controlled trial. *Lancet* **372**:807–16.

Acute coronary syndrome

Background

Acute coronary syndrome (ACS) encompasses a spectrum of disorders resulting from severe acute myocardial ischaemia. The most common pathogenic mechanism is acute intracoronary thrombosis resulting from atheromatous plaque disruption or erosion. Platelet activation, thrombosis, and coronary vasoconstriction are all important pathogenic mechanisms in ACS.

Two major clinical presentations have been identified that require urgent and effective treatment:
- unstable angina and non-ST-segment elevation myocardial infarction (NSTEMI)
- ST-segment elevation myocardial infarction (STEMI).

Despite a common pathophysiological background, differences exist between these two forms of ACS regarding treatment, mainly in relation to the need for thrombolysis and the timing of PCI.

Current global therapeutic strategy

See Fig. 2b.1.

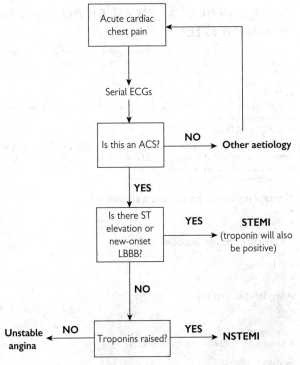

Fig. 2b.1 Diagnostic algorithm for chest pain suggestive of ACS.

Management of ST elevation myocardial infarction (STEMI)

In STEMI, myocardial necrosis is commonly caused by the complete occlusion of a coronary vessel which is often precipitated by disruption of an atherosclerotic plaque. Myocardial necrosis occurs within 15–30min of complete occlusion. ECG changes include:
- ST elevation ≥1–2mm in adjacent chest leads
- dominant R waves and ST depression in V_1 to V_3 (posterior infarction)
- new-onset LBBB
- pathological Q waves.

These ECG changes are associated with a rise in cardiac troponins but it is important to note that if suspected, STEMI should be treated immediately even before the result of cardiac troponins is available. Refer to Fig 2b.2 for treatment of STEMI.

General measures for patient stabilization
- Oxygen
- Morphine

Anti-ischaemic medications
- Nitrates
- β-blockers
- CCBs

Antiplatelet therapy
- Aspirin
- Clopidogrel
- Prasugrel
- Glycoprotein IIb/IIIa receptor inhibitors

Anticoagulants
- Heparin (unfractionated or low-molecular-weight heparin, LMWH)
- Direct thrombin inhibitors
- Fondaparinux

Thrombolytics (for STEMI only)
- Non-fibrin-specific lytics: streptokinase
- Fibrin-specific lytics: recombinant tissue plasminogen activator (rTPA)

Interventional therapy
- PCI

Prevention of further cardiovascular events
- Aspirin
- β-blockers
- ACEIs or ARBs
- Lipid-lowering drugs (statins and fibrates)
- Omacor®

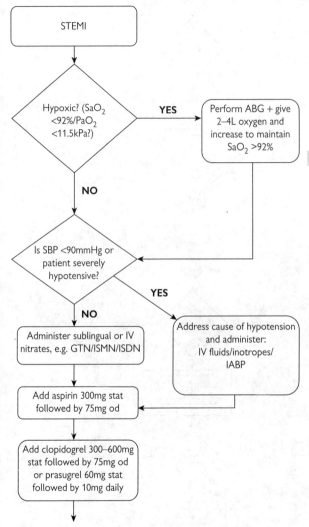

Fig. 2b.2 Algorithm for treatment of STEMI. Based on ESC guidelines for management of STEMI ACS, 2008.

ABG, arterial blood gas; GTN, glyceryl trinitrate; IABP, intra-aortic balloon pump; ISDN, isosorbide dinitrate; ISMN, isosorbide mononitrate; PaO₂, partial pressure of oxygen in arteries; SaO₂, arterial oxygen saturation; UFH, unfractionated heparin.

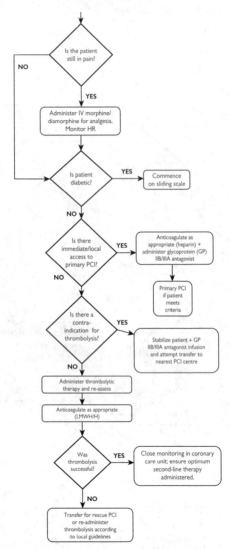

Fig. 2b.2 (*Cont'd*) Algorithm for treatment of STEMI. Based on ESC guidelines for management of STEMI ACS, 2008.

Non-ST elevation myocardial infarction (NSTEMI)

In NSTEMI, myocardial necrosis is caused by distal embolization of micro-thrombi from larger vessels or due to plaque instability. ECG changes associated with NSTEMI include:

• persistent or transient ST depression
• T-wave changes (inversion, flattening, pseudo-normalization).

Occasionally, no ST changes are present on admission, but with a convincing history and raised troponins, NSTEMI may be diagnosed. Although patients presenting with NSTEMI have lower immediate and short-term mortality than those with STEMI, long-term mortality is significantly increased in such patients and so NSTEMI should also be managed aggressively. Refer to Fig. 2b.3 for treatment of NSTEMI.

Unstable angina

• Unstable angina (UA) is diagnosed when there is new-onset severe angina, angina occurring at rest, or—in the case of previously diagnosed angina—which is increasing in frequency or with reduced exertion and lasting longer in duration. In UA, troponins are not raised but ECG changes are similar to those in NSTEMI. Refer to Fig. 2b.3 for treatment of UA.

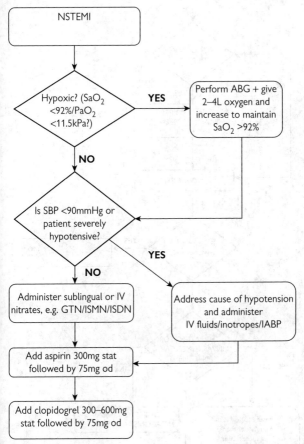

Fig. 2b.3 Algorithm for treatment of NSTEMI/UA. Based on ESC guidelines for NSTE-ACS, 2007.

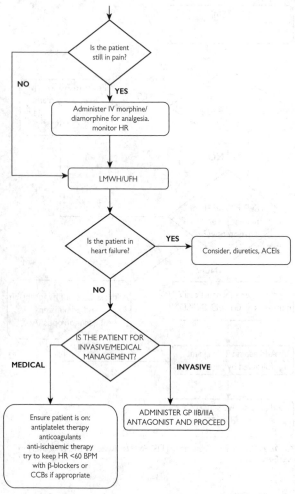

Fig. 2b.3 *Cont'd* Algorithm for treatment of NSTEMI/UA. Based on ESC guidelines for NSTE-ACS, 2007.

Therapeutic agents

This section deals with the therapeutic agents used in STEMI, NSTEMI, or UA, as described in 📖 Figs. 2b.2 and 2b.3, p.49, 53.

General measures for patient stabilization (applicable to patients with STEMI, NSTEMI, and UA)

Morphine

This agent has to be administered IV (initial dose, 4–8mg followed by an additional 2mg dose at 5–15min intervals until pain resolves)[1] to all patients with severe ischaemic chest pain and/or symptoms of heart failure. *Alleviating pain reduces sympathetic overdrive and myocardial oxygen demand thus reducing the risk of arrhythmia and, potentially, reducing infarct size.*

☻ *Side effects*

Nausea, vomiting, respiratory depression, hypotension, and bradycardia.

Practical notes
- Associate morphine administration to antiemetics, i.e. metoclopramide, 5–10mg IV.
- Watch out for respiratory depression. Naloxone may be required to reverse the effects of morphine.
- Atropine may be required for treatment of bradycardia.
- Tranquillizers may also be helpful if the patient is still in considerable pain despite maximal analgesic therapy.
- Avoid non-steroidal anti-inflammatory drug (NSAID) analgesia due to possible prothrombotic effect in the acute stage.

Oxygen

Not all patients need oxygen (see 'Indications'). All patients should undergo non-invasive oxygen monitoring, i.e. pulse oximeter. Oxygen can be given at 2–4L/min and increased as necessary.

Indications in STEMI/NSTEMI/UA
- Patients who are breathless or hypoxic (SaO_2 <90%)
- Acute pulmonary oedema

Practical notes
- In severe cases, invasive ventilation may be required.
- There is no evidence that oxygen therapy will improve patient clinical outcome or infarct size.
- Patients with COPD may be given high-flow oxygen at presentation, provided their ABGs are monitored regularly. *Remember that hypoxia will kill before hypercapnia can do so.*

Anti-ischaemic medications

Nitrates

Indications in STEMI/NSTEMI/UA

Nitrates should be used to:
- Relieve angina.
- Prevent/relieve symptoms of heart failure.

IV nitrates are recommended in the acute management of ischaemic episodes. Sublingual nitrate spray can be used for immediate relief of ischaemia/angina.

☺ *Side effects*

Headache, hypotension.

Contraindications

Concomitant use of PDE-5 inhibitors, i.e. sildenafil.

Practical notes
- Use with caution in patients with baseline SBP <90mmHg.
- Tolerance to nitrates is closely related to drug dose and duration of treatment.

β-blockers

Administration of β-adrenergic receptor blockers reduces myocardial workload and increases the duration of diastole. Early use in low-risk haemodynamically stable patients yields a modest benefit.

β-blocker therapy should be initiated as soon as possible post-MI (ideally within the first 24h), and the dose of the drug should be titrated upwards to the maximum tolerated dose. Contraindications to administration include acute decompensated heart failure, evidence of a low cardiac output state, cardiogenic shock, asthma, and severe COPD. Patients with contraindications to these agents should be re-evaluated for β-blocker therapy for 2° prevention.

NICE guidelines recommend that β-blockers should be continued indefinitely post-MI as their long-term benefit is well established.

Indications in STEMI, NSTEMI, and UA
- In the acute setting, to reduce myocardial oxygen demand
- In the 2° prevention of ACS.

☺ *Side effects*

GI disturbances, extreme bradycardia, heart failure, hypotension, conduction disturbances, peripheral artery vasoconstriction, bronchospasm, headaches, and fatigue.

Caution
- May precipitate bronchospasm in asthmatics.
- There is a risk of early-onset cardiogenic shock if given to haemodynamically unstable patients.

Calcium-channel blockers

CCBs have been shown to have similar effects to β-blockers in improving angina in patients with ACS. They are recommended as substitutes to β-blockers when the former are contraindicated.[2]

Practical notes

Diltiazem and verapamil (DAVIT and MDPIT) have been suggested to have deleterious effects in patients with LV dysfunction. Subsequent trials showed that verapamil associated with an ACEI can be beneficial in patients presenting with MI and heart failure.

Verapamil and diltiazem have negative chronotropic actions and may be used in the absence of heart failure or significant LV dysfunction.

Indications in STEMI, NSTEMI, and UA

• When negative chronotropic effect is required and β-blockers are contraindicated.

Antiplatelet agents

Aspirin

Aspirin improves patient outcome[3] and should be given to all patients with ACS as soon as possible unless specifically contraindicated. It prevents the production of thromboxane A_2, thus reducing platelet aggregation and thrombus formation.

The CURE trial showed that aspirin 300mg loading dose (followed by 75–150mg daily) combined with clopidogrel 300mg loading dose (followed by 75–150mg daily thereafter) significantly reduces cardiovascular death with benefits seen within 24h.[4] The ISIS-2 study demonstrated that aspirin saves 50 lives per 1000 MI patients treated.[5]

All patients with suspected ACS should receive 150–325mg chewable non-enteric-coated aspirin, followed by 75–100mg once daily.

Practical notes

• The patient does not necessarily need to chew the aspirin or dissolve it but can swallow it whole.
• Preferably use non-enteric-coated aspirin, due to the shorter onset of action.
• Aspirin can be given via other routes if the oral route is not appropriate.

☺ Side effects and contraindications

• GI bleeding. In patients with high-risk GI bleeding an oral proton pump inhibitor (PPI) (i.e. omeprazole, lansoprazole, esomeprazole) can be added.
• Bronchospasm in patients with asthma.
• Anaphylactic shock in hypersensitive individuals.
• Aspirin is contraindicated in patients with hypersensitivity to this agent, active GI bleeding, and severe hepatic disease.

Thienopyridines (clopidogrel, ticlopidine, prasugrel)

Clopidogrel is used in the treatment of both STEMI and NSTEMI. It antagonizes the platelet ADP receptor and thus blocks platelet aggregation.

Current ESC guidelines recommend that all patients presenting with MI should receive a loading dose of 300–600mg of clopidogrel, followed by a 75mg daily dose for 12 months.[1]

The CURE trials showed a significant reduction in the occurrence of vascular events in patients treated with aspirin and clopidogrel compared to those treated with aspirin alone, without a significant increase in life-threatening bleeds.[4]

☻ Ticlopidine is not routinely used currently in clinical practice because of its potential side effects, i.e. agranulocytosis and life-threatening neutropenia.

Prasugrel is a novel thienopyridine, which has shown to be more potent and more consistent in preventing platelet aggregation. The TRITON-TIMI38 trial has shown in patients who have had PCI following STEMI, that prasugrel was superior to clopidogrel. A loading dose of 60mg is given initially followed by a daily 10mg dose thereafter. Overall mortality did not differ between the two groups; however, prasugrel showed a net reduction in non-fatal MI with a slight increase in bleeding compared with clopidogrel.

Indications for clopidogrel
- All patients with STEMI, NSTEMI, and UA, in addition to aspirin
- Patients with a contraindication to aspirin
- After coronary stenting to aid stent patency.

☻ *Side effects of thienopyridines*
Bleeding, GI symptoms (i.e. diarrhoea and constipation).

Practical notes
- If coronary surgery is indicated, clopidogrel should be stopped for 5 days prior to the intervention to minimize the risk of excessive bleeding.
- Clopidogrel should not be used concomitantly with PPIs as these agents have been shown to reduce the anti-aggregant efficacy of clopidogrel. H_2 antagonists (i.e. ranitidine) may be used instead.

New emerging antiplatelet therapies

Data on new antiplatelet therapies that may help optimize anti-aggregant treatment and decrease morbidity and mortality in patients with ACS are emerging. Trials are now being conducted to assess the safety and efficacy of the new antiplatelet agents, *ticagrelor* and *cangrelor*. Head-to-head comparative studies of these agents versus clopidogrel and aspirin are necessary to define the true role of these emerging therapies in the management of patients with ACS. Preliminary reports appear to show promising results with these new agents in relation to both safety and efficacy.

Glycoprotein IIb/IIIa antagonists

Main agents in this drug category include abciximab, eptifibatide, and tirofiban. These agents block the final pathway of platelet aggregation by inhibiting bridging mechanism between platelets. Abciximab is a monoclonal antibody, eptifibatide a cyclic peptide, and tirofiban a peptidomimetic inhibitor. They are given in ACS patients undergoing PCI.

Abciximab: this is a GP IIb/IIIa inhibitor that is derived from the Fab fragment of immunoglobulins and is used to antagonize the GP IIb/IIIa receptor on activated platelets. It is given to patients during elective (especially in patients with diabetes or who are known to have renal insufficiency) or urgent angioplasty and infused in patients undergoing 1° PCI for STEMI. It reduces the risk of ischaemia intraprocedurally and the need for revascularization within 1 month of treatment. It has a relatively short half-life of 10min but postinfusion, its effect on platelet aggregation can linger for hours to days.

Abciximab reduces 30-day mortality if given periprocedurally in PCI.[6]

Eptifibatide and tirofiban are GP IIb/IIIa inhibitors that are recommended in high-risk patients with unstable angina or NSTEMI. This includes patients presenting within 24–48h of chest pain with dynamic ECG changes, raised troponin levels, and multiple risk factors. They reduce the risk of further cardiac ischaemia (progression to myocardial infarct) and risk of death. Tirofiban is a synthetic, non-peptide molecule that antagonizes the GP IIb/IIIa receptor. Eptifibatide is a cyclic heptapeptide.

Eptifibatide and tirofiban have been shown to reduce significantly the incidence of ischaemic events when given to patients prior to revascularization.

Current NICE guidelines recommend that GP IIb/IIIa antagonists in conjunction with aspirin and heparin should be given to patients with high-risk unstable angina or NSTEMI.

☻ All GP IIb/IIIa antagonists carry the risk of potentiating bleeding by virtue of their mode of action. They also carry the risk of inducing thrombocytopaenia, particularly abciximab, which can result in platelet levels falling from normal to zero. In such cases, the GP IIb/IIIa inhibitor infusion needs to be terminated and specialist advice sought, including platelet transfusion. The effect on thrombocytopaenia can last for up to 5 days after termination of infusion. As such, they are contraindicated in patients that are already significantly thrombocytopaenic or in those with bleeding disorders.

Indications in STEMI, NSTEMI and UA (See Fig. 2b.4)
- Prior to coronary revascularization (PCI)
- When PCI is not available and thrombolysis is contraindicated in STEMI patients
- All high-risk NSTEMI and UA patients.

Practical notes
- Use eptifibatide or tirofiban in intermediate- or high-risk NSTEMI patients (significant ST depression and/or troponin positivity).
- GP IIb/IIIa antagonists must be combined with anticoagulant therapy (heparin).
- Abciximab is given as 0.25mg/kg IV bolus followed by 0.125mcg/kg/min infusion (maximum 10mcg/min) over 12h.[1]

☻ Side effects
- Increased risk of bleeding
- Thrombocytopaenia.

Anticoagulant agents

Heparin

Heparin (LMWH and unfractionated heparin) should be administered to all patients with ACS. LMWH has more selective antithrombin and anti-factor Xa actions than unfractionated heparin. It is administered SC and does not require regular APTT (activated partial thromboplastin time) measurements and is less likely to cause heparin-induced thrombocyto-paenia (HIT) compared to unfractionated heparin.[7]

Heparin is very important in patients with STEMI given thrombolytic therapy as there is a prothrombotic effect after thrombolytic administration of rTPA. As such, all patients given rTPA should be given heparin cover for the first 48h to reduce the risk of re-infarction.

Indications in STEMI
- Prior to coronary revascularization in PCI
- With rTPA administration, for 48h
- In patients in whom fibrinolysis is contraindicated and PCI is unavailable within 2h

Indications in NSTEMI and UA

In all patients, and especially prior to PCI.

Fondaparinux

This synthetic pentasaccharide is a selective factor Xa inhibitor that binds to antithrombin III and potentiates its anticoagulant function. It is a relatively new treatment used in the management of ACS, STEMI, and NSTEMI in place of LMWH. It has the added advantage that a fixed SC dose of 2.5mg can be given daily for 3 days from hospital presentation and the dose applied does not depend on body weight. Less thrombocytopaenia is reported compared to fractionated heparin.

The OASIS 5 and OASIS 6 trials compared fondaparinux against enoxaprin in patients with unstable angina or NSTEMI and STEMI. Fondaparinux showed fewer bleeding events, at 1 and 6 months after ACS and a good preventative action regarding re-infarction and mortality in STEMI, UA, and NSTEMI patients. Recommended dose: 2.5mg daily SC.

Indications in ACS
- Same as enoxaparin
- Known history of HIT

Caution
- Not to be given before PCI, and has no role in 1° PCI
- Reduce dose in patients with renal impairment

Direct thrombin inhibitors

These drugs provide a useful alternative if there is a contraindication to heparin anticoagulation. Examples of direct thrombin inhibitors are hirudin and lepirudin.

Thrombolytic therapy
Practical notes

- This is a valid treatment option in patients with STEMI but not for those with NSTEMI or UA. Not indicated in NSTEMI/UA patients.
- Fibrinolytic therapy allows plasminogen to be converted to plasmin, which causes lysis of the fibrin-rich clot to allow coronary reperfusion.
- Time plays an important role regarding the benefit of thrombolysis. The earlier it is administered after onset of chest pain, the greater the beneficial effects. The overwhelming benefit of fibrinolytic treatment is seen in patients presenting within 12h of chest pain onset. The greatest benefit is within the first 2h and it then falls off dramatically after 4h.
- Administration after 12h from symptom onset appears to be associated with an increased incidence of serious complications such as cardiac rupture.[8]
- Importantly, PCI and stenting produce better results in STEMI patients than thrombolytic therapy.[2]
- STEMI patients in whom fibrinolytic therapy failed once, and PCI facilities are unavailable, can undergo a 2nd trial of fibrinolysis.
- Thrombolysis can be inhibited with tranexamic acid and aprotinin; both drugs can be used to treat conditions in which there is bleeding or a risk of bleeding.

Indications in STEMI
When 1° PCI is not available.

☺ *Side effects of thrombolytics*
- Haemorrhage: intracranial haemorrhage is the most serious
- Reperfusion arrhythmias may occur
- Allergic reaction, particularly with streptokinase, which may require treatment with 100mg IV hydrocortisone and 10mg IV chlorphenamine
- Hypotension

Absolute contraindications to thrombolytic therapy:[1]
- Active intracranial malignancy
- Suspected aortic dissection
- Surgery within the past 2 weeks
- Any history of haemorrhagic stroke
- History of ischaemic stroke within 1 year
- Active internal bleeding

Relative contraindications to thrombolytic therapy:[1]
- Ischaemic stroke >1 year ago
- General surgery >2 weeks ago
- Significant hepatic dysfunction
- Significant renal dysfunction
- Chronic severe hypertension

⚕ Dose

The dose depends on the fibrinolytic agent chosen. As such, always consult the BNF and your local hospital protocols. Please see 📖 p.327, Section 2 of this book for further details.

Non-fibrin-specific lytics

Streptokinase: the least effective of the fibrinolytic medications to achieve full coronary arterial reperfusion, with the lowest survival rates. However, streptokinase is also the least expensive of the thrombolytic therapies.

Practical note

Never re-administer streptokinase because of the risk of an anaphylactic reaction and the development of antibodies which can impair its activity.

⚕ Dose

1.5 million units given intravenously in 100ml of normal saline over one hour.[1]

Fibrin-specific lytic agents

Alteplase (recombinant tissue plasminogen activator)

The TIMI trial and an angiographic substudy of GUSTO showed that this was better than streptokinase in terms of myocardial reperfusion (54% coronary reperfusion vs. 31% for streptokinase at 90min).[9]

Alteplase should be given as 15mg IV as a bolus injection followed by 0.7mg/kg over half an hour (up to a maximum of 50mg), followed by 0.5mg/kg over 1h (up to a maximum of 35mg). Then IV heparin should be administered.[1]

or

3h infusion: 100mg administered as 60mg in the first hour (of which 6–10mg is administered as a bolus), 20mg over the 2nd hour, and 20mg over the 3rd hour.

Tenecteplase and reteplase

These have longer half-lives and so can be administered via a bolus injection rather than as IV infusions, allowing for more rapid drug administration. The GUSTO III trial showed similar coronary reperfusion results for alteplase and reteplase. Although they can be provided by means of a bolus, they have not been shown to confer a survival advantage over the other fibrinolytics that need to be administered by means of infusion.[10]

References

1 The task force of the management of ST segment elevation acute myocardial infarction of the European Society of Cardiology (2008). Management of acute myocardial infarction in patients presenting with persistent ST segment elevation. *Eur Heart J* **29**:2909–45.

2 Antman EM *et al.* and the writing committee to revise the 1999 guideline for the management of patients with acute MI: ACC/AHA guideline for the management of patients with STEMI (2004). A report of the American College of Cardiology/AHA task force on practice guidelines. *J Am Coll Cardiol* **44**:671–719.

3 SIGN (2007). *Acute Coronary Syndrome. A national clinical guideline.* 93. Edinburgh: SIGN.

4 Fox KA *et al.* (2004). Benefits and risks of the combination of clopidogrel and aspirin in patients undergoing surgical revascularization for non-ST-elevation acute coronary syndrome: the Clopidogrel in Unstable angina to prevent Recurrent ischemic Events (CURE) Trial. *Circulation* **110**:1202–8.

5 ISIS-2 (Second International Study of Infarct Survival) Collaborative Group (1988). Randomised trial of intravenous streptokinase, oral aspirin, both, or neither among 17,187 cases of suspected acute myocardial infarction: ISIS-2. *Lancet* **ii**:349–60.

6 De Luca G *et al.* (2005). Abciximab as adjunctive therapy to reperfusion in acute ST-segment elevation myocardial infarction: a meta-analysis of randomized trials. *JAMA*; **293**:1759–65.

7 Fox KA *et al.* (2002). Comparison of enoxaparin versus unfractionated heparin in patients with unstable angina pectoris/non-ST-segment elevation acute myocardial infarction having subsequent percutaneous coronary intervention. *Am J Cardiol* **90**:477–82.

8 Fibrinolytic Therapy Trialists' (FTT) Collaborative Group (1994). Indications for fibrinolytic therapy in suspected acute myocardial infarction: collaborative overview of early mortality and major morbidity results from all randomised trials of more than 1000 patients. *Lancet* **343**:311–22.

9 Sheehan FH *et al.* (1987). The effect of intravenous thrombolytic therapy on left ventricular function: a report on tissue-type plasminogen activator and streptokinase from the Thrombolysis in Myocardial Infarction (TIMI Phase I) trial. *Circulation* **75**:817–29.

10 The Global Use of Strategies to Open Occluded Coronary Arteries (GUSTO III) Investigators (1997). A comparsion of reteplase with alteplase for acute myocardial infarction. *N Engl J Med* **337**:1118–23.

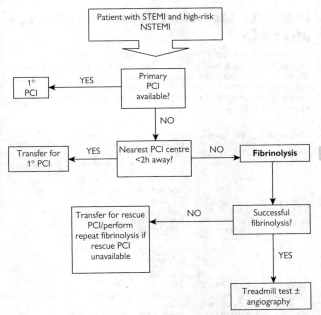

Fig. 2b.4 Algorithm: determining whether to use PCI/thrombolysis. Based on ESC guidelines for management of STEMI ACS, 2008.

Drugs for secondary prevention therapy after ACS

A variety of drugs are useful in the post-ACS episode and it is important that both the hospital and general practice ensure that the patient is on the optimum dose and variety of medications to improve morbidity and minimize mortality. Such medications are listed in Table 2b.1. Drugs used in 2° prevention of ACS not already discussed in this chapter are summarized in Table 2b.2.

Table 2b.1 Drugs used for secondary prevention after ACS

Pharma-cological agents	Mechanism of action	Side effects	Contra-indications	Trials supporting use
ACEIs (ARBs to be used if ACEIs contraindicated)	Inhibition of renin–angiotensin–aldosterone system (RAAS) and potentiation of bradykinin effect	Hypotension, dry cough, hyperkalaemia, angio-oedema	Renal artery stenosis, pregnancy, women of child-bearing potential, breastfeeding	HOPE study, EUROPA study
Statins	Inhibit HMG CoA reductase thus inhibiting cholesterol synthesis. Reduce atheromatous plaque growth and stabilize plaques	Myopathy or myalgia, rhabdo-myolysis, tiredness, headaches, GI disturbances	Myopathy, pregnancy, breastfeeding, active liver disease	4S trial, CARE study, MIRACL Study, LIPID study
Fibrates	Reduce triglyceride concentration	GI disturbances, anorexia	Severe hepatic and renal impairment, biliary cirrhosis, hypoalbumin-aemia	VA-HIT Trial

Table 2b.2 Summary of therapeutic agents in ACS

Name	Classification	Indications	Suggested dose	Caution
Oxygen	Immediate therapy	Hypoxia (SpO_2[1] <92%/PaO_2 <11.5kPa) or dyspnoea	2–4L/min progressing to high-flow O_2	COPD
Morphine	Immediate therapy/ analgesia	Ongoing ischaemic cardiac pain	3–5mg IV or SC morphine	Respiratory depression; bradycardia
Aspirin	Antiplatelet therapy	Inhibits platelet aggregation and reduces risk of further thrombosis	300mg then 75mg od	Peptic ulcer; allergy
Clopidogrel	Antiplatelet therapy	Inhibits platelet aggregation and reduces risk of further thrombosis; post-coronary stenting; contraindication to aspirin	300–600mg followed by 75mg od	Peptic ulcer; allergy; bleeding, PPIs
Prasugrel	Antiplatelet therapy	Inhibits platelet aggregation and reduces risk of further thrombosis; post-coronary stenting; contraindication to aspirin	60mg followed by 10mg od	Bleeding
Nitrates	Anti-ischaemic therapy	Hypertensive at presentation; ongoing ischaemic cardiac pain; relief of symptoms of heart failure	Sublingual GTN every 5min for 15min then IV GTN	Hypotension; concomitant use with phosphodi-esterase inhibitors not recommended
β-blocker	Anti-ischaemic therapy	To reduce heart rate and myocardial oxygen demand; 2° prevention if inappropriate initially	Bisoprolol 1.25mg then titrate upwards or use IV labetalol	Cardiogenic shock; hypotension; bradycardia; asthma

(continued)

Table 2b.2 (Contd.)

Name	Classification	Indications	Suggested dose	Caution
CCBs	Anti-ischaemic therapy	To reduce myocardial oxygen demand; contraindication to β-blockers	Diltiazem 120–360mg slow-release daily	Significant LV dysfunction; use with β-blockers
Heparin	Anticoagulant	STEMI; post rTPA for 48h	Enoxaparin 1.5mg/kg bd for 5 days	Bleeding; HIT
LMWH	Anticoagulant	Prevents further clot formation in NSTEMI	Enoxaparin 1.5mg/kg bd for 5 days	Bleeding; HIT
Insulin sliding scale	Additional therapy	Diabetes mellitus	Insulin and 5% glucose IV	Hypogly-caemia
PCI ± stenting	Coronary reperfusion therapy	STEMI/new onset LBBB (within 90min); facility available. NSTEMI: intervention for high-risk patients, ongoing chest pain and ECG changes despite optimal therapy	Clopidogrel 75mg od after stenting	Coronary artery rupture; if there will be a >90min door-to-needle time
GP IIb/IIIa antagonist	Antiplatelet therapy	Prior to PCI in patients with STEMI NSTEMI: patients prior to PCI, high-risk patients	Abciximab: bolus 250mcg/kg over 1min followed by IV infusion of 125ng/kg/min. Tirofiban: 400ng/kg/min for 30min, followed by 100ng/kg/min for at least 48h. Max 108h	Bleeding disorders
Strepto-kinase	Thrombolytic agent (coronary reperfusion therapy)	STEMI; new-onset LBBB with cardiac chest pain; facility for PCI not available	1.5 million units IV in 100mL 1M saline over 1h	STEMI only; haemorrhage; allergy; recent surgery; not to be given if previous exposure

Table 2b.2 (Contd.)

Name	Classification	Indications	Suggested dose	Caution
Alteplase	Thrombolytic agent (coronary reperfusion therapy)	STEMI; new-onset LBBB with cardiac chest pain; facility for PCI not available; previous exposure to streptokinase	15mg IV bolus then 0.75mg/kg over 30min (max 50mg) then 0.5mg/kg over 1h (max 35mg) with IV heparin	STEMI only; haemorrhage; allergy; recent surgery
ACEI	Additional therapy	Important in 2° prevention of MI and improves mortality results	Ramipril 1.25mg od then titrate upwards	Renal artery stenosis; pregnancy; breastfeeding
Statins	Additional therapy	Inhibit plaque growth and stabilize plaque; reduce cholesterol levels	Simvastatin 20–40mg daily	Myopathy; rhabdomyolysis; liver dysfunction, pregnancy

^{1}SpO$_2$, oxygen saturation measured by pulse oximetry.

Further reading

Acute coronary syndromes. (2005). In: 2005 International Consensus Conference on Cardiopulmonary Resuscitation and Emergency Cardiovascular Care Science with Treatment Recommendations. *Circulation* **112**(22 Suppl): III55–72.

Anderson JL et al. (2007). ACC/AHA 2007 Guidelines for the Management of Patients With Unstable Angina/Non ST-Elevation Myocardial Infarction: A Report of the American College of Cardiology/American Heart Association Task Force on Practice Guidelines (Writing Committee to Revise the 2002 Guidelines for the Management of Patients With Unstable Angina/Non ST-Elevation Myocardial Infarction). *J Am Coll Cardiol* **50**;e1–e157.

Gershlick AH et al. (2005). Rescue angioplasty after failed thrombolytic therapy for acute myocardial infarction. *N Engl J Med* **353**: 2758–68.

Grines CL et al. (1999). Coronary angioplasty with or without stent implantation for acute myocardial infarction. Stent Primary Angioplasty in Myocardial Infarction Study Group. *N Engl J Med* **341**:1949–56.

Gruppo Italiano per lo Studio della Sopravvivenza nell'infarto Miocardico (1994). GISSI-3. Effects of lisinopril and transdermal glyceryl trinitrate singly and together on 6-week mortality and ventricular function after acute myocardial infarction. *Lancet* **343**:1115–22.

ISIS-4 (Fourth International Study of Infarct Survival) Collaborative Group (1995). ISIS-4. A randomised factorial trial assessing early oral captopril, oral mononitrate, and intravenous magnesium in 58,050 patients with suspected acute myocardial infarction. *Lancet* **345**:669–85.

Keeley EC et al. (2003). Primary angioplasty versus intravenous thrombolytic therapy for acute myocardial infarction: a quantitative review of 23 randomised trials. *Lancet* **361**:13–20.

Montalescot G et al.; TRITON-TIMI 38 investigators (2009). Prasugrel compared with clopidogrel in patients undergoing percutaneous coronary intervention for ST-elevation myocardial infarction (TRITON-TIMI 38): double-blind, randomised controlled trial. *Lancet* **373**:723–31.

The Fifth Organization to Assess Strategies in Acute Ischemic Syndromes Investigators (2006). Comparison of fondaparinux and enoxaparin in acute coronary syndromes. *N Engl J Med* **354**:1464–76.

The OASIS-6 Trial Group (2006). Effects of fondaparinux on mortality and reinfarction in patients with acute ST-segment elevation myocardial infarction. The OASIS-6 randomized trial. *JAMA* **295**:1519–30.

The Task Force for the Diagnosis and Treatment of Non-ST-Segment Elevation Acute Coronary Syndromes of the European Society of Cardiology (2007). Guidelines for the diagnosis and treatment of non-ST-segment elevation acute coronary syndromes. *Eur Heart J* **28**:1598–660.

Prevention of cardiovascular disease

Prevention of cardiovascular disease

The aim of prevention is to improve life expectancy and quality of life by reducing cardiovascular events in high-risk patients.

Prevention is often described as *primary*, involving subjects who are at risk of developing cardiovascular disease (CVD) but are currently asymptomatic and have no evidence of CVD, or *secondary*, in those with diagnosed CVD.

Three high-risk groups require their modifiable risk factors to be treated intensively. These are:
- patients with diagnosed CVD
- individuals with ≥20% risk of developing CVD over 10 years
- patients with diabetes.

In addition, other subgroups that require aggressive 1° prevention are those whose 10-year cumulative risk of CVD is <20% but who have one risk factor which is very high, i.e.:
- hypertensive subjects with a SBP >160 mmHg or DBP >100mmHg and/or end organ damage
- subjects with total cholesterol:high-density lipoprotein (TC:HDL) ratio ≥6
- individuals with familial dyslipidaemia.

All these patient subgroups require lifestyle advice, and management of BP, lipids, and glucose. Selected groups of patients will also require additional cardioprotective measures (such as antiplatelet treatment).

Calculating CVD risk

Several charts can be used to estimate the probability of developing CVD over 10 years (see Figs. 2c.1 and 2c.2). Anyone over 35–40 years of age should have their CVD risk calculated.

CVD risk estimation is of less relevance in patients with diabetes or known CVD, as they are all at high risk and need to be treated as such.

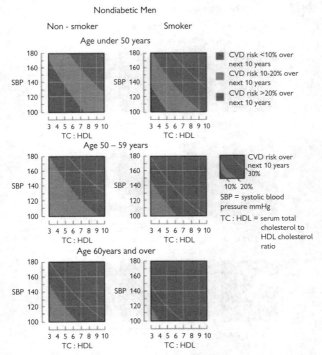

Fig. 2c.1 Charts to calculate the percentage risk of a cardiovascular event in the next 10 years in asymptomatic men. Pretreatment figures should be used but if they are not available assume SBP 160mmHg, and TC 6mmol/L. © University of Manchester.

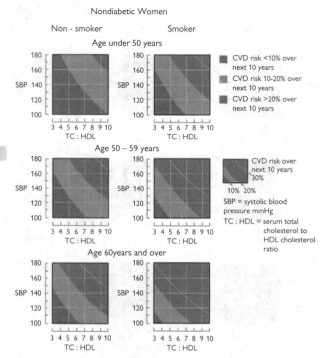

Fig. 2c.2 Charts to calculate the percentage risk of a cardiovascular event in the next 10 years in asymptomatic women. Pretreatment figures should be used but if they are not available assume SBP 160mmHg, and TC 6mmol/L. © University of Manchester.

Treatment

Lifestyle advice

- Stop smoking: in patients with known coronary heart disease (CHD) the future cardiovascular risk falls to the level of non-smokers 2–3 years after smoking cessation. In asymptomatic patients it takes 5–10 years to get the risk of future events down to the level of non-smokers. Nicotine replacement combined with smoking cessation counselling can increase cessation rates by up to 2-fold. Antidepressants, bupropion and nortriptyline may be helpful.
- Dietary advice: aim for a salt intake <100mmol/L per day. Alcohol consumption maximum 21 units per week for men and 14 units per week in women. Polyunsaturated fatty acids are inversely related to CHD risk. Plant sterols incorporated in the diet will reduce the absorption of cholesterol by 5–10%. Aim for dietary fat <30% of total energy intake.
- Physical activity: at least 30min of aerobic exercise per day.
- Optimal weight and weight distribution: aim for a BMI of 20–25kg/m^2. Avoid central obesity.

Blood pressure

Hypertension is defined as a SBP persistently ≥140mmHg *or* DBP ≥90mmHg.

Specifics of the pharmacological management of BP are discussed on 🕮 pp.95–111.

Who needs blood pressure-lowering drugs?

- Anyone with a SBP ≥160mmHg or DBP ≥100mmHg.
- If SBP 140–160mmHg or DBP 90–100mmHg then drug treatment should be started if the patient has:
  - diabetes
  - known CVD
  - CVD risk ≥20% over 10 years (1° prevention)
  - target organ damage.
- If SBP >130mmHg or DBP >80mmHg and patient is at very high risk—previous MI/cerebrovascular accident (CVA)/transient ischaemic attack (TIA)/chronic renal failure (CRF)/diabetes mellitus—then intervention should be started.

Target for treatment

Aim for SBP <140mmHg *and* DBP <85mmHg if no evidence of target organ damage. If there is evidence of target organ damage aim for SBP <130mmHg and DBP <80mmHg. Similarly, in patients with diabetes aim for <130mmHg SBP and <80mmHg DBP.

Practical notes

- Target organ damage = HF, CHD, CVA, TIA, PVD, CRF, retinopathy, LVH.
- A reduction in BP by an average of 12/6mmHg can reduce stroke by 40% and CHD by 20%.

Lipids

LDL and HDL cholesterol levels are important determinants of cardio-vascular risk. A high LDL and low HDL are associated with increased incidence of cardiovascular events. The main target for management is LDL but many people have mixed dyslipidaemia, even then the 1° target is LDL. Triglycerides (TGs) also appear to have a significant role. 2° causes of hyperlipidaemia, i.e. alcohol excess, diabetes mellitus, renal disease, liver disease, and hypothyroidism, should be identified and corrected.

Who needs lipid-lowering treatment?

- Everyone with a diagnosis of CVD (2° prevention required in these subjects regardless of cholesterol levels).
- 1° prevention in high-risk individuals (10-year CVD risk ≥20%). Recheck risk after 3–6 months of lifestyle changes before commencing drugs.
- 1° prevention if TC:HDL ratio ≥ 6.
- *Patients with type 1 and 2 diabetes should be on statins if >40 years of age or aged 18–39 and with at least 1 of the following:*
  - retinopathy
  - nephropathy
  - poor glycaemic control (HbA$_{1c}$ >9%)
  - high BP requiring medication
  - TC ≥6mmol/L
  - metabolic syndrome
  - family history of premature CVD.

Treatment options

- Statins: main effect is LDL reduction but they also increase HDL by 3–10%.
- Fibrates: increase HDL and reduce TGs but have a modest effect on LDL.
- Ezetimibe: lowers LDL by about 15–20% when added to diet modification or by 20–25% when added to diet and a statin.
- Nicotinic acid increases HDL.
- Omega-3-acid ethyl esters (Omacor®) reduce TGs.
- Bile acid sequestrants (colestyramine and colestipol): they reduce cholesterol substantially and are appropriate for patients with severe elevations in LDL such as in familial hypercholesterolaemia. However, they are generally not well tolerated (colesevelam has been reported to be better tolerated).

What to treat with?

Patients requiring drug treatment are, for cost reasons in the United Kingdom, commenced on simvastatin and titrated up to 40 or 80mg od (many would argue that the risk of 80mg outweighs the benefit and particularly should not be used for 1° prevention). If a patient does not achieve target cholesterol on simvastatin the options are to either switch to a higher-intensity statin such as atorvastatin or rosuvastatin, or add ezetimibe to simvastatin. NICE guidelines (May 2008) suggest that it is not cost-effective to switch to atorvastatin but clinicians vary in their choice.

If 2nd-line choice is to change to atorvastatin and the cholesterol is still not controlled then ezetimibe 10mg od can be added.

For 1° prevention, *powerful* statins, fibrates, or anion exchange resins should not be routinely offered.

For ACS, NICE recommends a 'high-intensity' statin and in the UK some primary care trusts will recommend simvastatin 80mg od for cost reasons. However, many physicians would prefer to use atorvastatin 40mg. In patients unable to tolerate statins, ezetimibe monotherapy may be a reasonable option.

Targets for treatment in high-risk patients
• TC <4mmol/L or 25% reduction from baseline (whichever is lower).
• LDL <2mmol/L or 30% reduction from baseline (whichever is lower).

In the CARE and LIPID studies there was no benefit of statins if the pretreatment LDL cholesterol concentration was <3.5mmol/L. However, the Heart Protection Study showed that even with pretreatment LDL levels of 2.6mmol/L, lowering LDL to 1.7mmol/L after treatment produced a similar relative risk reduction compared with higher pretreatment LDL cholesterol levels. This was confirmed by ASCOT.

The Cholesterol Trialists Collaboration showed a linear relationship between absolute reductions in LDL and proportional reductions in vascular events; a 21% reduction in major vascular events for every 1mmol LDL reduction. This is why, regardless of the pretreatment cholesterol level, the aim should be to reduce it further.

If target levels for cholesterol are not achieved on statin monotherapy then add ezetimibe or a bile acid sequestrant.

For isolated low HDL or high TG, 1st-line treatment is a fibrate; nicotinic acid can be also considered.

For management of isolated hypertryglyceridaemia, a fibrate can be used. Omega-3 fatty acids, i.e. Omacor® 1–2g od, can be added if required.

Glycaemic control
• A continuous relationship exists between glycaemia and CVD risk.
• See Fig. 2c.3 for diagnosis of diabetes, impaired glucose tolerance (IGT), and impaired fasting glucose (IFG). IFG and IGT are associated with an increased risk of type 2 diabetes. Progression to diabetes can sometimes be prevented with lifestyle changes. Other treatments that reduce the rate of progression are acarbose in patients with IGT and orlistat in obese subjects.
• Professional dietary advice, weight management, and increased physical activity are recommended for all individuals with abnormal glucose metabolism.
• Insulin is required in subjects with type I diabetes.
• In individuals with type 2 diabetes, metformin should be prescribed to obese patients. It does not cause hypoglycaemia but caution is required with renal failure.
• Gliclazide is safer in patients with renal failure but can cause hypoglycaemia.
• Glitazones are contraindicated in HF.

Targets for treatment

For people with type 1 and 2 diabetes mellitus, the targets for optimal glycaemic control are a fasting glucose of 4.0–6.0mmol/L and an HbA$_{1c}$ of ≤6.5%.

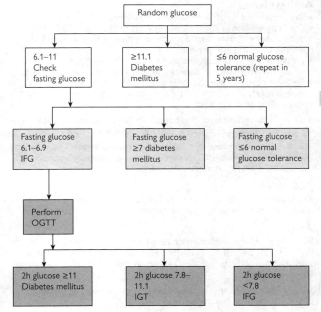

Fig. 2c.3 Oral glucose tolerance test (OGTT). After an overnight fast 75g of glucose are administered. Blood samples are taken 2h after the glucose load. All units for glucose are in mmol/L. IFG, impaired fasting glucose; IGT; impaired glucose tolerance.

Cardioprotective agents

In addition to controlling BP, lipids, and glucose, there are other interventions that are known to be cardioprotective:

Aspirin (75mg)

- Recommended for all people with atherosclerotic disease.
- For 1° prevention in anyone over 50 years of age with a CVD risk ≥20%. There is some debate after a recent meta-analysis as to the benefit of aspirin in 1° prevention.
- All patients with diabetes should be on aspirin if ≥50 years old, or younger if they have had diabetes for >10 years or are on treatment for hypertension. Note: this indication may be revised in the future in view of results of recent trials and meta-analyses that have questioned the value of aspirin in this setting.

If aspirin is contraindicated, clopidogrel can be used (shown to be marginally more effective than aspirin in CAPRIE trial, but not cost-effective).

The Antithrombotic Trialists Collaboration meta-analysis in patients with known atherosclerotic CVD showed that aspirin reduces all-cause mortality, vascular mortality, non-fatal MI, and stroke.

β-blockers

These agents are indicated for all people following MI, particularly if there is evidence of HF or ventricular arrhythmias.

ACEIs

Indicated in patients with signs or symptoms of HF at the time of MI and in those with persistent LV dysfunction post infarction (EF<40%). Consider ACEIs in subjects with CHD especially if BP >130mmHg systolic and 80mmHg diastolic.

ACEs/ARBs are indicated in diabetes when there is microalbuminuria, proteinuria, or diabetic nephropathy.

The HOPE and EUROPA trials showed that ACEIs reduced the risk of MI and CV mortality in high-risk individuals even in the absence of LV dysfunction or hypertension.

Statins

See next section for details (📖 Statins, p.81).

Treatment following acute MI

Antiplatelet

Following a NSTEMI, all patients should be on aspirin and clopidogrel for a year. Continue aspirin indefinitely thereafter. CURE showed that this strategy reduced the composite endpoint of cardiovascular death, MI, and stroke in the first year after ACS.

For patients with STEMI, NICE recommends a shorter period of time on clopidogrel, one month. For patients who undergo PCI see 📖 p.88, Antiplatelet therapy, for duration of antiplatelet therapy.

For patients with a history of aspirin-induced ulcer bleeding whose ulcers have healed and who are *Helicobacter pylori* negative, consider a full-dose PPI and low-dose aspirin.

Practical note

The cytochrome P450 system, which converts clopidogrel to its active component, is inhibited by PPIs. As such, PPIs may reduce the effectiveness of clopidogrel and it may be necessary to switch from a PPI to alternative forms of gastric protection if the patient requires clopidogrel.

For patients unable to take aspirin or clopidogrel consider warfarin (international normalized ratio (INR) 2–3). For patients unable to take clopidogrel who are at a low risk of bleeding consider aspirin and warfarin (INR 2–3).

β-blockers

For acute thrombolysed STEMI, previous guidelines recommended the use of IV β-blockers, followed by oral β-blockers. Guidelines have changed with later evidence. COMMIT/CCS-2 showed that acute IV high-dose metoprolol within 24h followed by oral metoprolol did not significantly reduce death or reinfarction. In fact, metoprolol led to more cardiogenic shock from days 0–1 in high-risk patients. Current recommendations suggest that oral β-blocker therapy should be initiated in the first 24h after STEMI and NSTEMI in patients who do not have signs of HF, evidence of a low output state, or increased risk of cardiogenic shock.

Patients with moderate or severe LV failure should receive β-blocker therapy as 2° prevention, once stable, with a gradual titration scheme.

It is reasonable to administer an IV β-blocker at the time of presentation to STEMI patients who are hypertensive and who do not have any signs of HF.

If β-blockers are contraindicated, consider diltiazem or verapamil for 2° prevention in patients without HF. The aim is to reduce the heart rate in these patients.

ACEIs

Offer ACEIs early after presentation and titrate upwards to the maximum tolerated or target dose. If intolerant to ACEI consider ARB. Continue ACEIs indefinitely regardless of LV function. After MI, ACEIs reduce the risk of death.

Statins

Start as soon as possible after MI. Either simvastatin 40mg od or atorvastatin 40mg od. NICE recommends higher doses after ACS (i.e. simvastatin 80mg od) although, as stated earlier, many prefer to start with atorvastatin 40mg od.

Practical note

Fasting lipids should be estimated at least 8 weeks after the event. Cholesterol falls during an acute event and only rises back to baseline after 2 to 3 months.

NICE recommends the use of Omacor® within 3 months of an MI when dietary intervention is insufficient to provide adequate levels of omega-3 fatty acid supplementation.

Aldosterone antagonists

For patients with symptoms and/or signs of HF, an aldosterone antagonist should be commenced. Eplerenone has been shown to benefit this group of patients in the EPHESUS trial.

Glucose control

DIGAMI-1 showed that following an acute MI if the glucose is ≥11mmol/L then an insulin infusion followed by at least 3 months of insulin treatment improved mortality

DIGAMI-2, however, did not confirm the results of DIGAMI and there was no evidence of benefit in total or coronary mortality or non-fatal CV events in this trial.

Trials supporting current recommendations

Statins

4S (Scandinavian Simvastatin Survival Study Group)[1]

- Simvastatin vs. placebo in patients with angina pectoris or previous MI and serum cholesterol 5.5–8.0mmol/L.
- Patients in the simvastatin arm had a 30% RRR in overall mortality, as well as 39% fewer non-fatal MIs, 41% fewer ischaemic heart disease deaths, and 34% fewer myocardial revascularization procedures.

HPS (Heart Protection Study)[2]

- Simvastatin vs. placebo. Simvastatin significantly reduced total mortality by 12% in patients at high risk of CHD. In terms of all major vascular events there was a 24% reduction in total CHD, total stroke, and revascularization.
- There was a significant reduction in vascular events in all groups, irrespective of their starting cholesterol level.

PROVE IT/TIMI 22[3]

- Compared pravastatin 40mg with atorvastatin 80mg in patients hospitalized for an ACS.
- Use of atorvastatin was associated with a reduction in composite of death, MI, unstable angina requiring rehospitalization, revascularization, and stroke at 2 years.

ACEIs

EUROPA (European Trial on Reduction of Cardiac Events with Perindopril in Stable Coronary Artery Disease)[4]

- Among patients with stable coronary artery disease, treatment with perindopril was associated with a reduction in the 1° endpoint of cardiovascular mortality, non-fatal MI, and cardiac arrest compared with placebo.
- Largest trial to show benefit in stable, low-risk coronary artery disease patients.

HOPE (The Heart Outcomes Prevention Evaluation Study)[5]

- Among patients at high risk for cardiovascular events but without LV dysfunction or HF, treatment with ramipril was associated with a reduction in cardiovascular death, MI, or stroke, as well as each of the individual endpoints, compared with placebo.

Antiplatelets

Antiplatelet Trialist Group[6]

- Overview of 174 randomized trials of antiplatelet agents.
- Among all high-risk patients, antiplatelet therapy was associated with reductions of 30% in non-fatal MI and non-fatal stroke, and 15% in vascular death.

- The use of aspirin for 1° prevention was associated with only a trend toward decreased vascular events. No benefit for 1° prevention in low-risk patients.

CURE (The Clopidogrel in Unstable Angina to Prevent Recurrent Events)[7]
- Patients with ACS but no ST elevation.
- Treatment with clopidogrel plus aspirin was associated with a reduction in the composite of cardiovascular death, MI, and stroke compared with aspirin alone for up to 1 year.

β-blockers

ISIS-1 (First International Study of Infarct Survival)[8]
- Atenolol 5–10mg IV over 5min, followed by 100mg/day for 7 days.
- Vascular mortality during the treatment period (days 0–7) was significantly lower in the treated group, but this 15% relative difference had wide 95% confidence limits (1–27%).
- At 1 year, overall vascular mortality was significantly lower for the atenolol group. There was a lower rate of deaths attributed to myocardial rupture or electromechanical dissociation in the atenolol group.

The COMMIT/CCS-2 (Clopidogrel and Metoprolol in Myocardial Infarction Trial/Second Chinese Cardiac Study)[9]
- Patients with a suspected MI were treated with metoprolol within 24h. Initially 3 IV doses then oral.
- Metoprolol did not reduce the composite of death, reinfarction, or cardiac arrest. In fact there was an increase in the risk of cardiogenic shock, although note that the metoprolol was at high dose.
- The excess of cardiogenic shock was seen chiefly from days 0–1 after hospitalization, whereas there were reductions in reinfarction and ventricular fibrillation appearing from day 2 onward.

Aldosterone antagonists

EPHESUS (Eplerenone Post-AMI Heart Failure Efficacy and Survival Study)[10]
- Patients with acute MI complicated by HF and systolic LV dysfunction, eplerenone was associated with reduction in all-cause mortality and death or hospitalization from cardiovascular causes.

References

1 Lancet 1994; 344:1383–9.
2 Eur Heart J 1999; **20**:725–41.
3 N Engl J Med 2004; **350**: 1495–504.
4 Lancet 2003; **362**:782–8.
5 N Engl J Med 2000; **342**: 145–53.
6 BMJ 1994; **308**:81–106.
7 N Engl J Med 2001; **345**:494–502.
8 Lancet 1986; **2**:57–66.
9 Lancet 2005; **366**:1622–32.
10 N Engl J Med 2003; **348**:1309–21.

Further reading

JBS 2 (2005): Joint British Societies' Guidelines on Prevention of Cardiovascular Disease in Clinical Practice. *Heart* **91**(Suppl 5):v1–v52.

NICE (2007). *Secondary prevention in primary and secondary care for patients following a myocardial infarction*. London: NICE.

NICE (2008). *Lipid modification: cardiovascular risk assessment and the modification of blood lipids for the primary and secondary prevention of the cardiovascular disease*. London: NICE.

Post-PCI management

Antiplatelet therapy

One of the most important measures following PCI and stenting is dual antiplatelet therapy. All patients should be prescribed aspirin 75mg and clopidogrel 75mg after loading prior to PCI.

Evidence that after PCI, treatment with aspirin plus a thienopyridine (clopidogrel and ticlodipine are both thienopyridines) is better than aspirin alone or aspirin plus anticoagulation comes from MATTIS, CREDO, and other trials.

If a patient had a NSTEMI prior to the intervention, the dual therapy should be continued for 1 year after the NSTEMI (CURE trial), followed by aspirin alone thereafter.

If intervention is carried out in the absence of a recent NSTEMI then the duration of dual therapy depends on the type of stent used. For bare-metal stents (BMSs) the duration of dual therapy is 1 month and aspirin should be continued thereafter. If a drug-eluting stent (DES) is used then dual therapy should be used for 1 year and aspirin continued alone thereafter.

The importance of dual therapy following coronary stent insertion cannot be over-emphasized. However, two scenarios when antiplatelet therapy causes consternation are: (1) a patient is bleeding and (2) an operation is to be performed and there are risks of perioperative bleeding. If a patient is bleeding then the source of the bleeding should be identified and treated. Only if the risk of life-threatening bleeding is greater than the risk from in-stent thrombosis should it be considered appropriate to stop antiplatelet agents. If a patient is due to have an elective operation then either this should be performed on dual antiplatelet therapy or the operation should be delayed until the time when dual therapy is no longer required. Planning prior to PCI includes deciding to use BMSs in patients at risk of bleeding or who are due to have an operation in the near future.

Clopidogrel non-responders: data show that approximately 4–30% of patients treated with conventional doses of clopidogrel do not display an adequate platelet response. These patients may be at higher risk for thrombotic events. Platelet aggregation studies may be considered and the dose of clopidogrel increased to 150mg per day if <50% inhibition of platelet aggregation is demonstrated. However, platelet aggregation studies do not reliably correlate with in-stent thrombosis, and genetic studies are becoming more important to identify clopidogrel non-responders.

GP IIb/IIIa antagonists and heparin may be used pre- or intra-PCI to reduce thrombosis on instruments and vessel wall/plaque.

Routine use of unfractionated heparin after an uncomplicated coronary angioplasty is no longer recommended, as it may be associated with more frequent bleeding events. Subcutaneous administration of low-molecular-weight heparin may provide a safer way of extending antithrombin therapy if there are clinical reasons, such as residual thrombus or significant residual coronary dissections.

Antiplatelet therapy in patients on warfarin

The use of dual antiplatelet therapy is more complicated in patients who also require warfarin for AF or mechanical heart valves. There is no general consensus as to the correct management of these patients. Risk versus benefit should be assessed on a patient-by-patient basis.

In patients undergoing PCI, the effect of adding aspirin and clopidogrel to those receiving warfarin has not been well studied. This regimen will decrease the incidence of stent thrombosis and ischaemic stroke 2° to embolism but will also increase the risk of bleeding. How do we balance the risk of stroke if warfarin is stopped following PCI with the risk of major bleeding if warfarin is continued? There is no consensus.

For each patient a risk assessment should be made weighing up the risk of thromboembolism versus the risk of bleeding.
- Identifiable risk factors for thromboembolism include: age >65 years, hypertension, diabetes, impaired LV function, and previous ischaemic stroke.
- Identifiable risk factors for bleeding include: age >75 years, history of stroke, serum creatinine >1.5mg/dL, diabetes mellitus, recent MI, history of GI bleed, and haematocrit <30%.

PCI and atrial fibrillation

Management of patients at low to moderate risk of thromboembolism
Because these patients are at low to moderate risk of thromboembolism it is relatively safe to hold off warfarin for the period of antiplatelet therapy required.

If the patient presented with an ACS or had a DES inserted then start dual antiplatelet therapy, which should be continued for 12 months; warfarin can be continued alone thereafter.

If the patient did not have an ACS and a BMS was used, then dual antiplatelet therapy should be continued for 1 month and warfarin alone thereafter.

If the patient is at a very low risk of bleeding, an alternative strategy would be to treat them with aspirin, clopidogrel, and warfarin (triple therapy) for the time dual antiplatelet therapy is required and warfarin alone thereafter. The INR should be carefully monitored during this time period.

Patients at high risk of thromboembolism
An example of a patient at high risk for thromboembolism would be one who has had a previous stroke, who is hypertensive, and over the age of 75 years. These patients are at a high risk of thromboembolism if warfarin is stopped. It has been shown that treatment with dual antiplatelet therapy is not as good as warfarin at preventing stroke in AF. As such, it is likely that triple therapy will be required for a period of time.

It is particularly important in this group of patients to plan on using a BMS during PCI to reduce the duration of triple therapy.

It must be stressed that there is no consensus on treatment in this group of patients and what follows is one suggested approach.

If the patient presented with an ACS or if a DES is used then the patient should be on triple therapy for 3–6 months then warfarin and clopidogrel up to month 12 and warfarin alone thereafter. The reason that aspirin is dropped rather than clopidogrel at months 3–6 is that registry data have shown significantly more stent thrombosis in patients on warfarin and aspirin compared to warfarin and clopidogrel.

If a patient has not had an ACS and a BMS is used then they should receive triple therapy for 1 month and warfarin alone thereafter.

If the patient is at a high risk for both thromboembolism and bleeding and presents with ACS or has a DES (there would need to be a very good reason for not using a BMS in these patients), it may be worth considering triple therapy for 1 month only then warfarin and clopidogrel up to month 12 and warfarin alone thereafter.

PCI and metallic heart valves

Patients with prosthetic valves are prone to valve thrombosis and systemic embolization without adequate anticoagulation. The risk of thromboembolism or valve thrombosis with the bileaflet valves without anticoagulation is 12% per year in the aortic position, and 22% per year in the mitral position.

Patients with mechanical valves undergoing PCI need to be carefully evaluated prior to the procedure.

Patients should be classified as low risk based on the absence of risk factors for bleeding, or high risk if patients are at increased risk of bleeding.

Patients at low risk of bleeding

These patients can be treated with warfarin, with the INR carefully regulated between 2 and 2.5, aspirin, and clopidogrel for 4 weeks when a BMS has been used. If DESs are inserted, the patient would require 3–6 months depending on the type of stent used. While triple therapy does place these patients at a higher risk for bleeding (4–9% per year), the benefit of reducing thromboembolism and stent thrombosis clearly exceeds the risk of bleeding.

Patients at high risk of bleeding

These patients pose a particularly difficult problem. In this subgroup, the risk of bleeding with triple therapy may exceed 50%. Optimal stent deployment is critical. The use and safety of only using clopidogrel and warfarin in this subgroup has not been assessed in large trials.

Renal impairment

Contrast-induced nephropathy is clinically defined as an increase in serum creatinine >25% from baseline that occurs within 48h of PCI.

Patients with pre-existing renal impairment, diabetes, and dehydration are at increased risk of developing contrast-induced nephropathy.

To help prevent contrast-induced nephropathy ensure the patient is well hydrated; in patients taking metformin stop this drug before PCI and do not restart treatment until 48h after PCI or even longer if renal function deteriorates. Consider withholding ACEIs/ARBs and diuretics. The administration of NAC (*N*-acetyl cysteine) (600mg to 1.2g bd PO) for 48h either side of PCI has been recommended. *Practical note: This is not a licensed indication for NAC.*

Secondary prevention

In addition to the earlier listed measures, all patients requiring coronary intervention, by definition, require intensive risk factor modification. Secondary prevention measures can be found in the cardiovascular disease prevention section of this book, (📖 pp.71–86).

Clinical trials

CREDO[1]

Clopidogrel for the Reduction of Events During Observation

A randomized, double-blind, controlled trial of early and sustained dual oral antiplatelet therapy after PCI (666). In this trial of 2116 patients undergoing PCI from 99 North American centres, the patients received either a 300-mg loading dose of clopidogrel (n=1053) or placebo (no loading dose; n=1063) 3–24h before PCI. All patients thereafter received clopidogrel 75mg daily through to day 28. For the following 12 months, patients in the loading dose group received clopidogrel and those in the control group received placebo. All patients received aspirin (325mg per day through to day 28 and 81–325mg daily thereafter) throughout the study. At 1 year, long-term clopidogrel therapy was associated with a 27% RRR in the combined risk of death, MI, or stroke for an absolute reduction of 3% (P=0.02).

MATTIS[2–4]

The Multicenter Aspirin and Ticlopidine Trial After Intracoronary Stenting

Showed that among high-risk patients undergoing PCI combined asprin and ticlodipine was superior to aspirin alone and aspirin with anticoagulation at 30 days (reduce CV death, MI or repeat revascularization).

References

1 Steinhubl SR et al. (2002). Clopidogrel for the reduction of events during observation (CREDO). JAMA 288:2411–20.
2 Urban P et al. (1998). Randomized evaluation of anticoagulation versus antiplatelet therapy after coronary stent implantation in high-risk patients: the multicenter aspirin and ticlopidine trial after intracoronary stenting (MATTIS). Circulation 98:2126–32.
3 Arab D et al. (2005). Antiplatelet therapy in anticoagulated patients requiring coronary intervention. J Invasive Cardiol 17:549–54.
4 Lip GY (2008). Managing the anticoagulated patient with atrial fibrillation at high risk of stroke who needs coronary intervention. BMJ 337:a840.

Systemic hypertension

Background

Prevalence estimates of systemic hypertension are 1 billion worldwide, contributing to 4.5% of global disease burden, 64 million DALYs (disability adjusted life-years), and 7.1 million premature deaths. Analyses by the World Health Organization (WHO) indicate that about 62% of CVD and 49% of ischaemic heart disease are attributable to suboptimal BP levels (SBP >115mmHg).[1] The prevalence of systemic hypertension increases with age,[2] and is higher in patients of African or South Asian origin, as compared to Caucasians.[3,4]

Definition and long-term complications

Systemic hypertension is defined as persistently elevated BP, i.e. systolic or diastolic pressures ≥140 and 90mmHg, respectively. Hypertension can be subdivided into degrees of severity, as shown in Table 3.1.

Table 3.1 Definitions and classification of blood pressure (BP) levels (mmHg)*

Category	Systolic		Diastolic
Optimal	<120	and	<80
Normal	120–129	and/or	80–84
High normal	130–139	and/or	85–89
Grade 1 hypertension	140–159	and/or	90–99
Grade 2 hypertension	160–179	and/or	100–109
Grade 3 hypertension	≥180	and/or	≥110
Isolated systolic hypertension	≥140	and	<90

Isolated systolic hypertension should be graded (1,2,3) according to systolic blood pressure values in the ranges indicated, provided that diastolic values are <90 mmHg. Grades 1, 2 and 3 correspond to classification in mild, moderate and severe hypertension, respectively. These terms have now been omitted to avoid confusion with quantification of total cardiovascular risk.

* Reproduced with permission from Mancia G et al. (2007). 2007 Guidelines for the management of arterial hypertension: The Task Force for the Management of Arterial Hypertension of the European Society of Hypertension (ESH) and of the European Society of Cardiology (ESC). *Eur Heart J* **28**:1462–536.

Importantly, systemic BP represents a continuum of risk, whereby cardiovascular mortality rates increase with increased BP levels, without a threshold down to at least 115/75mmHg (Fig. 3.1).[2]

Based on lifetime risk and risk of cardiovascular complications associated with BP levels, the JNC 7 report has proposed a new classification of hypertension that includes the term 'prehypertension', i.e. BP ranging from 120–139/80–89mmHg.[5]

In the long term, hypertension is a risk factor for:
- CVAs
- ischaemic heart disease
- LV hypertrophy
- cardiac failure
- peripheral vascular disease
- chronic hypertensive renal disease
- vascular complications of diabetes
- hypertensive retinopathy.

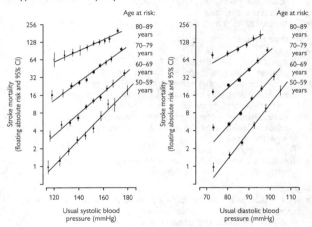

Fig. 3.1 Stroke mortality rate in each decade of age versus usual blood pressure at the start of that decade. CI, confidence interval. Reproduced from Lewington *et al.* (2002). Age-specific relevance of usual blood pressure to vascular mortality: a meta-analysis of individual data for one million adults in 61 prospective studies. *Lancet* **360**:1903–13, with permission from Elsevier.

References

1 World Health Organization (2002). *The World Health Report 2002: Risks to Health*. Geneva: World Health Organization.
2 Lewington S *et al.*; Prospective Studies Collaboration (2002). Age-specific relevance of usual blood pressure to vascular mortality: a meta-analysis of individual data for one million adults in 61 prospective studies. *Lancet* **360**:1903–13.
3 Cappuccio FP *et al.* (2002). Application of Framingham risk estimates to ethnic minorities in United Kingdom and implications for primary prevention of heart disease in general practice: cross sectional population based study. *BMJ* **325**:1271.
4 Brown MJ (2006). Hypertension and ethnic group. *BMJ* **332**:833–6.
5 Chobanian AV *et al.*; Joint National Committee on Prevention, Detection, Evaluation, and Treatment of High Blood Pressure. National Heart, Lung, and Blood Institute; National High Blood Pressure Education Program Coordinating Committee (2003). Seventh report of the Joint National Committee on Prevention, Detection, Evaluation, and Treatment of High Blood Pressure. *Hypertension* **42**:1206–52.

Causes

Hypertension is predominantly an idiopathic and multifactorial disease (in approximately 95% of cases), related to a combination of genetic and environmental factors. Important social aetiological factors that contribute to the development of hypertension include increased dietary salt intake, obesity, excessive alcohol consumption, and age.

Secondary causes of hypertension

Renal disease
- Parenchymal disease
- Renovascular disease: e.g. atherosclerotic renal artery stenosis, fibromuscular dysplasia
- Channelopathies (rare): e.g. Liddle's syndrome

Endocrine disease
- Adrenal:
  - mineralocorticoid excess, e.g. Conn's syndrome—adrenal adenoma, bilateral/congenital adrenal hyperplasia, ectopic adrenocorticotrophic hormone (ACTH), exogenous mineralocorticoid, renin-secreting tumours, glucocorticoid-remediable aldosteronism
  - corticosteroid excess: e.g. Cushing's disease, exogenous corticosteroids, apparent mineralocorticoid excess, and liquorice ingestion—see later
  - phaeochromocytoma
- Non-adrenal: acromegaly, hypo- and hyperparathyroidism, hyperthyroidism, carcinoid syndrome

Drugs
- e.g. NSAIDs, oestrogen-containing contraceptives, corticosteroids, ciclosporin, monoamine oxidase inhibitors, ergotamine, symphathomimetics, amphethamines, cocaine

Aortic coarctation

Obstructive sleep apnoea

Pregnancy-induced hypertension, pre-eclampsia and eclampsia

Monogenic disease (rare), for example:
- Liddle's syndrome: autosomal dominant, gain-of-function mutation of *ENaC* (epithelial sodium channel) expressed in the apical surface of collecting duct cell within the kidney, resulting in excess sodium retention
- glucocorticoid-remediable aldosteronism: autosomal dominant, gain-of-function mutation with crossing over and fusing of the 5' regulatory region of 11-hydroxylase and the coding region of aldosterone synthase (usually these two genes are close together on chromosome 8). This hybrid gene encodes an aldosterone synthase that is ACTH sensitive. Treatment is by suppressing ACTH with exogenous glucocorticoids

- apparent mineralocorticoid excess: autosomal recessive, inactivating mutation of 11β-hydroxysteroid dehydrogenase type 2 (which metabolizes cortisol to cortisone in renal tissue, therefore normally 'protects' mineralocorticoid receptors from cortisol stimulation). This is a similar mechanism to the effects of liquorice, which inhibits 11 β-hydroxysteroid dehydrogenase type 2
- congenital adrenal hyperplasia: autosomal recessive, 11β-hydroxylase or 17α-hydroxylase deficiency, resulting in shunting of production towards the mineralocorticoid pathway, and hence mineralocorticoid excess
- Gordon's syndrome: autosomal dominant, gain-of-function mutation of *WNK1* or *4*, inactivating the negative regulators of the sodium-chloride symporter (NCCT), resulting in excess sodium retention
- single gene mutations and phaeochromocytomas: e.g. MEN II syndrome, von Hippel–Lindau disease, neurofibromatosis type I.

Practical note

A sizeable proportion of patients with untreated borderline hypertensive measurements in clinic may have 'white-coat' hypertension. This is defined as the presence of elevated office/clinic BP values and normal out-of-office/clinic BP values. The prognostic impact of 'white-coat' hypertension is currently unclear but may carry an intermediate risk.

Clinical assessment

Following the diagnosis of hypertension, aims of clinical assessment include:
- identification of lifestyle factors, other cardiovascular risk factors, and concomitant disorders that may affect prognosis and guide treatment
- identification of potential causes of hypertension
- identification of the presence of organ damage.

History
- Contributory lifestyle factors (dietary salt intake, obesity, alcohol consumption, sedentary lifestyle and smoking)
- Suggestion of 2° hypertension (young age, sudden onset, presentation as malignant hypertension, resistant hypertension—requiring ≥3 drugs)
- Family history of hypertension and other cardiovascular risk factors
- Previous antihypertensive treatment (duration, efficacy, and adverse reactions) and concomitant drugs (e.g. corticosteroids, oral contraceptives)

Examination
- Appropriate measurement of BP, and verification in contralateral arm
- Calculation of BMI and waist circumference
- Potential evidence of hypertensive complications (carotid, abdominal, and femoral bruits, peripheral pulses in peripheral vascular disease, optic fundi in hypertensive retinopathy)
- Examination of the heart may reveal evidence of complications of hypertension
- Assessment of peripheral oedema and fluid status
- Examination of the abdomen for enlarged kidneys, renal bruits, distended urinary bladder, and abnormal aortic pulsation

Investigations
- Assess potential underlying 2° causes, i.e. renal or endocrine disease, initially with serum electrolytes, urea, and creatinine.
- Detect target organ damage, assessed by fundoscopy (hypertensive changes), electrocardiographic and echocardiographic studies (LV hypertrophy and strain), renal function tests, and urine dipstick (proteinuria). Assessment of blood vessels by ultrasound of carotid arteries (limited by availability) and ankle–brachial index is also recommended.
- Assess other cardiovascular risk factors (e.g. toTC:HDL ratio, diabetes etc.) that may require aggressive management.
- Ambulatory BP monitoring may be useful in the presence of unusual BP variability and when 'white-coat' hypertension is suspected. Other indications include the assessment of antihypertensive treatment (efficacy during the 24h, drug-resistant or nocturnal hypertension, occurrence of drug-induced symptomatic hypotension), episodic hypertension, and autonomic dysfunction.

Classification of hypertension

There is potentially a large normal variation in BP measurements within individuals (see □ Table 3.1, p.96).

Practical note: the definition of hypertension requires the documentation of persistently elevated BP, i.e. high levels in repeated readings, as opposed to a single reading.

General management principles

Practical note on general management principles: according to current guidelines, not all individuals who meet the definition of hypertension will require pharmacological antihypertensive therapy.

We identified two useful guidelines for pharmacological intervention (see Figs. 3.2 and 3.3).

Certain guidelines require full cardiovascular risk assessment of the individual based on age, gender, smoking status, SBP, and TC:HDL cholesterol ratio (see ☐ Fig. 2a.1, p.35). A discussion on the limitations of these risk-prediction charts is beyond the scope of this chapter.

These guidelines are useful but each patient should be evaluated specifically and management tailored to the specific clinical picture. However, it is important to stress that every hypertensive individual always merits careful investigation and requires lifestyle and dietary advice.

Main therapeutic options include:
- treatment and prevention of organ damage and other complications
- management of potential causes of 2° hypertension
- management of CV risk factors.

	Blood pressure (mmHg)				
Other risk factors, OD or disease	Normal SBP 120–129 or DBP 80–84	High normal SBP 130–139 or DBP 85–89	Grade 1 HT SBP 140–159 or DBP 90–99	Grade 2 HT SBP 160–179 or DBP 100–109	Grade 3 HT SBP ≥ 180 or DBP ≥ 110
No other risk factors	No BP intervention	No BP intervention	Lifestyle changes for several months then drug treatment if BP uncontrolled	Lifestyle changes for several months then drug treatment if BP uncontrolled	Lifestyle changes + immediate drug treatment
1–2 risk factors	Lifestyle changes	Lifestyle changes	Lifestyle changes for several months then drug treatment if BP uncontrolled	Lifestyle changes for several months then drug treatment if BP uncontrolled	Lifestyle changes + immediate drug treatment
≥3 risk factors, MS or OD	Lifestyle changes	Lifestyle changes and consider drug treatment	Lifestyle changes + drug treatment	Lifestyle changes + drug treatment	Lifestyle changes + immediate drug treatment
Diabetes	Lifestyle changes	Lifestyle changes + drug treatment	Lifestyle changes + drug treatment	Lifestyle changes + drug treatment	Lifestyle changes + immediate drug treatment
Established CV or renal disease	Lifestyle changes + immediate drug treatment	Lifestyle changes + immediate drug treatment	Lifestyle changes + immediate drug treatment	Lifestyle changes + immediate drug treatment	Lifestyle changes + immediate drug treatment

Fig. 3.2 ESH-ESC Guidelines for the management of arterial hypertension. Reproduced with permission from 2007 ESH-ESC Practice Guidelines for the management of arterial hypertension. Mancia G et al. (2007). *Blood Press* **16**:135–232.

MS, metabolic syndrome; OD, subclinical organ damage.

Risk factors include pulse pressure (in elderly), age (male >55 years, female >65 years), smoking, dyslipidaemia (TC >5.0mmol/L or LDL-C >3.0mmol/L or HDL-C <1.0 in male, <1.2 in females or TG >1.7mmol/L), fasting plasma glucose 5.6–6.9mmol/L, abnormal glucose tolerance, abdominal obesity (waist circumference male >102cm, female >88cm) and family history of premature CV disease (male <55 years, female <65 years).

Subclinical organ damage includes electrocardiographic or echocardiographic LVH, carotid wall thickening or plaque, carotid-femoral pulse velocity >12m/s, ankle–brachial pressure index <0.9, slight increases in plasma creatinine (male 115–133μmol/L, female 107–124μmol/L), low estimated glomerular filtration rate (eGFR) or creatinine clearance (<60ml/min/1.73m^2), and microalbuminuria or elevated albumin–creatinine ratio (male ≥22mg/g, female ≥31mg/g).

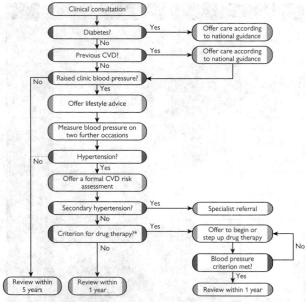

Fig. 3.3 Flowchart for management of hypertension. Adapted from NICE (CG34) Guidelines *Care pathway for hypertension*, 2006. © Crown Copyright. Reproduced under the terms of the Click-Use Licence.

* Threshold for offering drug treatment:
• BP of more than 160/100mmHg, or
• isolated systolic hypertension (SBP of ≥160mmHg), or
• BP of more than 140/90mmHg and:
  • 10-year CVD risk of at least 20%, or
  • existing CVD or target organ damage

Treatment targets

Optimum BP targets depend on the global clinical situation of the individual. The recommended BP target for patients with no cardiovascular complications or comorbidities is <140/90mmHg and <130/80mmHg for patients with diabetes and high-risk patients, such as those with a history of stroke, MI, renal dysfunction, and proteinuria. Latest NICE guidelines for chronic kidney disease recommend a target of <125/75mmHg for patients with chronic kidney disease and proteinuria.

Acute presentation of hypertension

Systemic hypertension is largely asymptomatic. However, it can—albeit rarely—present acutely as hypertensive crises.

Malignant hypertension

Defined as severely elevated BP (systolic >220mmHg and diastolic >120mmHg), associated with target organ damage—visual disturbance, hypertensive retinopathy, and papilloedema; breathlessness and cardiac failure; headaches and hypertensive encephalopathy; renal failure and proteinuria. *This is a medical emergency that requires immediate intervention and a gradual reduction of BP over hours* (see 📖 *Management of hypertension*, p.106).

Accelerated hypertension

Severely elevated BP that is associated with target organ damage (as for malignant hypertension), but without papilloedema on fundoscopic examination (flame-shaped haemorrhages or soft exudates often present). *Management is the same and as important as for malignant hypertension.*

Severe hypertension

Severely elevated BP (as for malignant hypertension), but without evidence of target organ damage.

Management of hypertension

(See letters in parentheses for the current level of evidence for each treatment and Fig. 3.4 for management algorithm.)

Non-pharmacological measures

The British Hypertension Society guidelines recommend general lifestyle measures for all patients with hypertension and for those with borderline or high-normal BP.

- Reduce dietary salt intake to less than 100mmol/day (<2.4g of sodium or <6g of sodium chloride) **(A)**.
- Weight reduction to maintain ideal BMI of 20–25kg/m^2 **(A)**.
- Regular aerobic exercise such as brisk walking for at least 30min each day.
- Reduce consumption of saturated and total fat in meals and increase intake of fruit and vegetables **(A)**.
- Moderate alcohol consumption (men <21 units per week and women <14 units per week) **(A)**.

Pharmacological therapy

Reducing BP is more important than the specific group of drugs used for the purpose. Each drug will lower the BP by about 7–8% but each drug has a wide interpatient response variability. Several classes of drugs are used for treatment of hypertension and a sizeable proportion of patients will require two or more drugs to control their BP. Age and ethnic groups are important factors in the response to pharmacological therapy—black patients respond better to thiazide diuretics and CCBs, whereas non-black patients respond better to ACEIs or β-blockers.[1]

Rationale for 'A/CD' rule:

- in younger white patients, hypertension is associated with high plasma renin activity. Therefore blocking the RAAS would be a logical start to hypertension management
- CCBs and thiazide diuretic work independently of the RAAS system. Therefore they are logical starting point in patients with low renin activity, i.e. older patients and black patients of African or Caribbean descent, not mixed-race, Asian, or Chinese individuals.

β-blockers are not the preferred drug in hypertension management, except for:

- those with intolerance or contraindications to ACEIs or ARBs
- women of child-bearing potential
- patients with increased sympathetic drive.

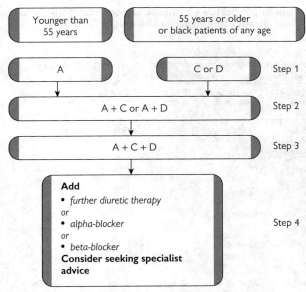

Fig. 3.4 NICE/British Hypertension Society (BHS) guidelines for management of hypertension.[2] A, ACEI (consider angiotensin-II receptor antagonist if ACE intolerant); C, calcium-channel blocker; D, thiazide-type diuretic.

Compelling indications, cautions, and contraindications to various classes of antihypertensive drugs (Table 3.2)

Table 3.2 Compelling indications, cautions, and contraindications to various classes of antihypetensive drugs. Adapted from BHS and European School of Haematology (ESH) guidelines[2,3]

Class of drug	Compelling indications	Possible indications	Caution	Compelling contra-indications
α-blockers	Benign prostatic hyperplasia(BPH)		Postural hypotension HF	Urinary incontinence
ACEIs	HF LV dysfunction LVH Post MI Established CHD Type I diabetic nephropathy 2° stroke prevention	Chronic renal disease Type II diabetic nephropathy Proteinuric renal disease AF Metabolic syndrome	Renal impairment PVD	Pregnancy Renovascular disease
ARBs	ACEI intolerance Type II diabetic nephropathy LVH Post-MI	LV dysfunction post MI Proteinuric renal disease Chronic renal disease HF	Renal impairment PVD	Pregnancy Renovascular disease
β-blockers	MI Angina Tachyarrhythmia	(Chronic) HF	(Acute) HF PVD Diabetes (except with CHD) Metabolic syndrome COPD Physically active	Asthma COPD Heart block
CCBs (dihydro-pyridine)	Elderly ISH LVH Pregnancy Blacks	Elderly Angina	Tachyar-rhythmia HF	

Table 3.2 *(Contd.)*

Class of drug	Compelling indications	Possible indications	Caution	Compelling contra-indications
CCBs (rate-limiting)	Angina SVT	MI	Combination with β-blockade	Heart block HF
Thiazide and thiazide-like diuretics	Elderly ISH HF 2° stroke prevention Blacks		Metabolic syndrome Glucose intolerance	Gout

ISH, isolated systolic hypertension

References

1 Materson BJ et al. (1995). Department of Veterans Affairs single-drug therapy of hypertension study. Revised figures and new data. Department of Veterans Affairs Cooperative Study Group on Antihypertensive Agents. Am J Hypertens **8**:189–92.
2 Parati G et al.; ESH Working Group on Blood Pressure Monitoring (2008). European Society of Hypertension guidelines for blood pressure monitoring at home: a summary report of the Second International Consensus Conference on Home Blood Pressure Monitoring. J Hypertens **26**: 1505–26.
3 Williams B et al.; British Hypertension Society (2004). Guidelines for management of hypertension: report of the fourth working party of the British Hypertension Society, 2004—BHS IV. J Hum Hypertens **18**:139–85.

Management of hypertension in specific clinical circumstances

Hypertension in chronic kidney disease

- The target treated BP (<130/80mmHg) is lower than that of the non-kidney disease group **(B)**. In patients with chronic kidney disease associated with heavy proteinuria, the target is 125/75mmHg **(C)**.
- Patients with diabetic kidney disease, with or without hypertension, should be managed with an ACEI or ARB. ACEIs are more effective than other antihypertensive agents in slowing the progression of chronic kidney disease with macroalbuminuria due to type I diabetes. Both ACEIs and ARBs are more effective than other antihypertensive agents in slowing the progression of microalbuminuria due to type I and II diabetes **(A)**.
- Higher levels of BP are associated with a more rapid progression of diabetic kidney disease.
- ACEIs and ARBs are often the antihypertensive agent of choice, but should be used with caution, close supervision, and specialist advice if there is established and significant renal impairment.
- Multiple agents are often required to achieve target BPs.
- Diuretics are often 2nd-line agents, and should be included in the antihypertensive regimen of most patients **(A)**. This is followed by either β-blockers or CCBs, depending on clinical situation.
- There is insufficient evidence to indicate a preferential class of antihypertensive agent for renal artery stenoses, but *ACEIs and ARBs should only be used with extreme caution in renal artery stenosis*, due to an increased risk of hypotension, sudden decrease in GFR, and hyperkalaemia **(C)**.

Hypertension in pregnancy

- Antihypertensive treatment is demonstrated to reduce the risk of progression to severe hypertension, but with an associated increased risk of adverse drug reactions **(A)**.
- There is not enough evidence to show benefit of antihypertensive drugs in mild to moderate hypertension in pregnancy with regard to other maternal and fetal/neonatal events **(A)**.
- Methyldopa is recommended as the 1st-line agent, whereas 2nd-line agents are often longer-acting CCBs **(C)**.
- In a meta-analysis, it has been demonstrated that β-blockers (labetalol in particular) are better than methyldopa at reducing the risk of progression to severe hypertension **(A)**. However, this is balanced with the increased risk of inhibited fetal growth **(B)**.
- *ACEIs and ARBs are contraindicated in pregnancy* **(B)**.

Accelerated/malignant hypertension

- It is common practice **to lower BP by no more than 25% in the first 2h** (due to the potential for precipitating MI or CVAs), aiming to achieve a BP of 160/100mmHg after 6h of therapy **(C)**.
- A meta-analysis was unable to demonstrate any difference in risks of cardiac or respiratory events comparing treatments and control arms. Additionally, no differences in outcomes between the different pharmacological therapies were noted. These findings are limited by a small number of studies with low number of participants as well as short-term follow-up **(B)**.
- **When there is acute, life-threatening organ damage, IV agents are used in a high-dependency setting. Sodium nitroprusside is the 1st-line drug of choice.** Other agents to be considered, particularly in specific scenarios, include: glyceryl trinitrate in the presence of LV failure or symptomatic coronary artery disease; labetalol in the presence of aortic dissection; hydralazine (arteriolar dilator) in pregnancy; and phentolamine (short-acting α-blocker) in the presence of, or suspected, phaeochromocytoma **(C)**.
- In the absence of life-threatening organ damage, oral agents are preferred. 1st-line drug is nifedipine (MR), starting at 10mg, repeated after 2h if required, and up to 20mg three times a day. 2nd-line therapy involves addition of a β-blocker (e.g. atenolol 50mg). ACEIs and diuretics are used with caution due to the potential rapid fall in BP, especially if there is volume depletion **(C)**.

Arrhythmias, conduction disturbances, and neurocardiogenic syncope

Atrial fibrillation

Background

Atrial fibrillation (AF) is the commonest cardiac arrhythmia, with an increasing incidence with age. The numerous patterns and changing aetiological factors in AF have led to an evolution in its clinical classification. Today the most widely accepted and practically useful classification system breaks AF into the following categories: first episode or new AF; paroxysmal; persistent; and permanent AF. Although catheter ablative therapies are increasingly being employed in cases where patients are highly symptomatic and refractory to pharmacotherapy, drug therapy remains the mainstay of treatment for the majority of patients with AF.

Electrophysiological basis of AF

There are several electrophysiological mechanisms underlying AF. In many patients AF is due to a focal discharge of rapid frequency (350–600bpm) and fibrillatory, heterogeneous conduction throughout the atria owing to the frequency of impulses generated by this focus. This activity can be recorded as f waves within the atria. The f waves conduct in an irregularly irregular fashion through the atrioventricular (AV) node, and the ventricular rate is thus determined by the conductivity and refractory period of the AV node. The phenomenon of 'concealed conduction' occurs, whereby some impulses arrive at the AV node during the refractory period and may render the AV node refractory for an extended period without generating a conducted ventricular beat. This further contributes to the irregularity of the ventricular rhythm.

Considerations for drug therapy

In the broadest sense, the most important decisions for pharmacotherapy in AF are firstly whether a *rhythm* or *rate* control strategy is preferred and which agent/agents are the most appropriate, and secondly whether anticoagulation is warranted for the prevention of thromboembolic complications. The merits of a rhythm or rate control strategy are discussed in turn for each of the subclassifications described here. Antithrombotic management is dealt with separately.

Table 4.1 Vaughan Williams classification of antiarrhythmic drugs*

Class	Mechanism	Examples
Ia	Sodium-channel blockers: moderate reduction in phase 0 slope; increase APD; increase ERP	Quinidine, procainamide, disopyramide
Ib	Sodium-channel blockers: small reduction in phase 0 slope; reduce APD; decrease ERP	Lidocaine, mexiletine
Ic	Sodium-channel blockers: pronounced reduction in phase 0 slope; no effect on APD or ERP	Flecainide, propafenone
II	β-blockers: blocks sympathetic activity, virtually no proarrhythmic effect	Atenolol, bisoprolol, metoprolol
III	Potassium-channel blockers: delay repolarization, prolong APD and ERP; proarrhythmic risk for acquired long QT syndrome	Sotalol, amiodarone, dronedarone
IV	Calcium-channel blockers: act on SA and AV node; virtually no proarrhythmic effect	Diltiazem, verapamil
Miscellaneous		Digoxin, magnesium sulphate, adenosine

APD, action potential duration; ERP, effective refractory period.

*In practice this classification system is not very helpful as many drugs fit multiple categories.

New (acute)-onset atrial fibrillation

The symptomatology of first presentation of AF is varied and ranges from those who are symptom free (often these patients are discovered incidentally), to those in extremis with pulmonary oedema and cardiogenic shock. Management is largely dependent on symptoms and the clinician must decide whether acute treatment is necessary.

Absent or mild symptoms

These patients generally require no acute drug therapy if resting ventricular rate is controlled (generally regarded as <90bpm). An assessment of ambulatory heart rate response and thromboembolic risk should be made and the decision to treat and anticoagulate made (Ⅲ p.128).

Intolerable symptoms or haemodynamic instability

If the patient has a ventricular rate of >150bpm, signs of circulatory collapse (hypotension or pulmonary oedema), chest pain, dyspnoea, or intolerable palpitations, they should be treated as an acute medical emergency (see Fig. 4.1). It is important to consider 2° causes of AF such as thyrotoxicosis, pulmonary embolism, and sepsis, as AF tends to respond poorly until the underlying cause is treated (see Ⅲ p.117).

Patients should undergo direct current cardioversion (DCCV) in the presence of life-threatening signs. Whilst evidence supports there being little increased thromboembolic risk with DCCV performed within 48h of acute onset of AF, in practice there is often no clear history of symptom onset and indeed patients may be asymptomatic in AF.

Key points

- Digoxin has traditionally been used as 1st-line treatment but is generally inappropriate due to its long duration of onset. It is likely to be most effective in vagally mediated AF.
- IV amiodarone (5mg/kg or 300mg in 50mL 5% glucose over 5–10min administered via a peripheral line) is usually the treatment of choice in the emergency setting in the UK. It acts to rapidly reduce ventricular rate and is effective in restoring sinus rhythm. If the initial bolus is unsuccessful, a further 900mg in 500mL is administered over the remainder of the 24h.
- Consider Wolff–Parkinson–White (WPW) syndrome in those presenting with very high ventricular rates (often >200bpm) and a broad QRS complex. *In known WPW with AF, flecainide is a useful alternative to amiodarone for cardioversion.*
- The recent ATHENA study, in which the antiarrhythmic dronedarone was added to standard therapy, has shown a significant reduction in cardiovascular hospitalizations, death, and stroke, and may become more widely used in the future although it is not yet licensed in the UK.

AV node-blocking agents (non-dihydropyridine CHBs, adenosine, and digoxin) should not be used in AF with WPW as AV nodal blockade leads to increased ventricular rates via uninhibited antegrade accessory pathway conduction.

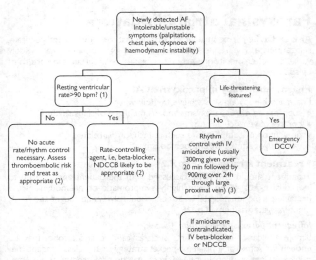

Fig. 4.1 Treatment algorithm for newly diagnosed or acute onset of AF.

Notes:

(1) Important to consider effect of exercise on ventricular rate response which should be 90–115bpm with moderate activity.

(2) If the patient is asymptomatic, i.e. the AF has been discovered incidentally, further investigations may be considered prior to pharmacotherapy to establish the pattern of AF (paroxysmal, persistent, permanent) but anticoagulation should be strongly considered in those with significant risk (see 📖 p.128).

(3) Only if structural heart disease is present, otherwise start with class Ic agent. Risk of skin necrosis from extravasation of amiodarone. Longer courses of IV amiodarone should be administered via central venous line.

NDCCB, non-dihydropyridine calcium-channel blocker.

Paroxysmal atrial fibrillation

AF is said to be paroxysmal when episodes last for <1 week and generally self-terminate. The frequency of episodes and symptomatology are widely variable. Holter monitoring may be necessary to ascertain the pattern of episodes.

Pharmacotherapy in paroxysmal AF

Pharmacotherapy aims to achieve the following:
- suppression of AF paroxysms and maintenance of sinus rhythm
- control of ventricular rate
- prevention of complications such as tachycardia-related cardiomyopathy or thromboembolism.

Treatment strategies (Fig. 4.2)

Treatment should always be discussed with the patient and tailored to individual needs. In an acute highly symptomatic or haemodynamically unstable paroxysm, hospital treatment should always be sought and treatment instigated as per 📖 p.119.

Infrequent paroxysms (less than 1 week)

Simple avoidance of precipitants such as caffeine and alcohol may be enough for some, or a *pill-in-the-pocket* strategy with a class Ic agent (flecainide 300mg or propafenone 600mg) may be preferred by those comfortable with taking the responsibility. This should only be considered in patients with a low risk of proarrhythmia, i.e. absence of structural/ischaemic heart disease, and in those in whom the chosen agent is known to be efficacious. A pill-in-the-pocket strategy can also be used as an add-in for those on low-dose maintenance therapy.

Frequent symptomatic paroxysms

- In the absence of contraindications, a standard β-blocker (e.g. atenolol, bisoprolol) should be used in the first instance. Alternatively, verapamil can be used for rate control.
- If control is not achieved, a Ic agent (Table 4.1) should be used in the absence of structural or ischaemic heart disease. Co-prescription with an AV nodal blocking drug such as a β-blocker is advised due to the risk of class Ic-induced atrial flutter and 1:1 AV conduction (see 📖 p.132, Atrial flutter).
- If a Ic agent cannot be used or is unsuccessful, sotalol should be used, progressively increasing from 80mg bd to 240mg bd. Watch for QT prolongation as there may be a high proarrhythmic risk. Special care is required in the elderly.
- If the patient remains uncontrolled symptomatically, or in the case of poor LV function where β-blockers have failed, amiodarone should then be tried and consideration given to electrophysiological intervention. Consider the latter in young, highly symptomatic patients with paroxysmal AF.

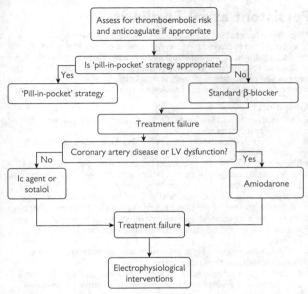

Fig. 4.2 Treatment algorithm for paroxysmal AF.

Persistent atrial fibrillation

AF is termed persistent when episodes last beyond 1 week. It commonly progresses from paroxysmal AF. As with new or paroxysmal AF, treatment should be tailored to the individual and the advantages and disadvantages of a rate or rhythm control strategy discussed with the patient. The major determinant of treatment strategy is usually the burden of symptoms. It is important to bear in mind the following evidence-based considerations.

Key points

- Overall there is no significant difference in mortality between rate- and rhythm-control strategies.
- There is no significant difference in quality of life between rate and rhythm control.
- There is no difference in likelihood between strategies of suffering MI or developing congestive cardiac failure, and the 5-year cumulative risk of thromboembolic and haemorrhagic events is similar.
- In patients older than 65 years and in those with coronary disease or HF (congestive HF or ejection fraction <50%), a *rhythm*-control strategy may confer a mortality advantage. In milder HF (up to NYHA II) there is little difference in mortality outcome between rate and rhythm control.
- A rhythm-control strategy is associated with a greater incidence of hospital admission than rate control.
- Owing to costs associated with DCCV, a greater number of hospital admissions, and generally more expensive medication, the rhythm-control strategy is more costly than rate control.
- Appropriate antithrombotic therapy should be offered based on risk, regardless of the treatment strategy (see 🕮 p.128).

Rhythm-control agents

As with treatment of acute onset and prophylaxis in paroxysmal AF, agents from classes Ic, II, and III are preferred for maintaining sinus rhythm in this group of patients. Verapamil may also be used (Table 4.1) 1st line in the absence of structural heart disease.

Pharmacological cardioversion refers to the use of an IV agent and may be chosen if the patient wishes to be admitted to hospital and does not wish to undergo electrical cardioversion. (See Fig. 4.3 for recommendations.)

In a less severe acute presentation, or if the patient does not wish to be admitted to hospital, oral treatment should be prescribed with escalation from a standard β-blocker (e.g. metoprolol or atenolol) to sotalol (up-titrated from 80mg bd to 240mg bd) or a class Ic agent, in the absence of structural heart disease. Co-prescription with an AV nodal blocking drug such as a β-blocker is advised due to the risk of class Ic-induced atrial flutter and 1:1 AV conduction (see 🕮 Atrial flutter, p.132).

If sotalol or Ic agents are contraindicated or ineffective, then amiodarone should be administered if tolerated.

See 🕮 Permanent atrial fibrillation for rate control strategies, p.122.

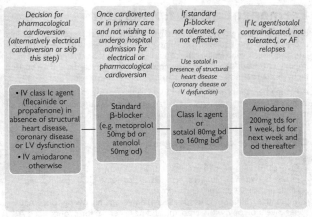

Fig. 4.3 Rhythm control algorithm for persistent AF (or unknown duration).

Notes:

Assess thromboembolic risk and anticoagulate as appropriate in the same way as for other patterns of AF.

*Sotalol is valuable if β-blocker is not effective but not valuable if β-blocker is contraindicated.

Permanent atrial fibrillation

By definition there is no role for rhythm control in this group of patients and as such, the issues in pharmacotherapy are whether to anticoagulate and which ventricular rate controlling agent (if any) is needed. This is important to reduce the risk of symptoms from tachycardia and associated tachycardia-related cardiomyopathy.

A resting heart rate <90bpm and exercise heart rate <180bpm are desirable and failure to achieve these targets requires further adjustment of medication. The level of patient activity needs to be considered in selecting which agent(s) to use.

Choice of rate controlling agent(s)

Key points

- Overall there is no difference in efficacy in ventricular rate control *at rest* between β-blockers, non-dihydropyridine CCBs (NDCCBs) (diltiazem or verapamil) and digoxin.
- In practice, diltiazem is used rather than verapamil, owing to a greater negative inotropy with verapamil and its potential for pronounced AV block and bradycardia in combination with digoxin.
- Both β-blockers and NDCCBs are more effective than digoxin at controlling ventricular rates *during exercise*. Digoxin as monotherapy is therefore only appropriate in those who are sedentary, such as the elderly.
- In the critically ill who may have excess sympathetic tone, digoxin is considered less effective than β-blockers or NDCCBs.
- If monotherapy with β-blockers or NDCCBs fails to control ventricular rate, there is proven additional benefit from adding digoxin to either a β-blocker (benefit shown only at rest) or CCB (benefit both at rest and during exercise). On this basis it may be more appropriate to instigate more active people on a NDCCB for monotherapy should they require the addition of digoxin at some stage.

See Fig. 4.4 for rate control algorithm.

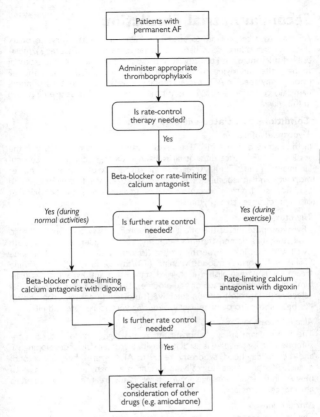

Fig. 4.4 Rate control treatment algorithm for permanent (and some cases of persistent) AF.
Reproduced from National Collaborating Centre for Chronic Conditions (2006). *Atrial Fibrillation: National guidelines for management in primary and secondary care.* London: Royal College of Physicians. Copyright © 2006 Royal College of Physicians of London.

Secondary atrial fibrillation

AF may arise secondarily to structural heart disease, surgery, coronary disease, heart failure (see Chapter 1), hypertension (see Chapter 3), metabolic disturbances, and toxicity from drugs including alcohol. It is essential to treat the underlying condition, which may in itself terminate the AF prior to any specific AF-directed therapy, unless the patient is haemodynamically compromised. Where not mentioned here, these are discussed in the relevant chapters.

Conditions associated with AF

Myocardial infarction

In the setting of acute MI, AF is usually transient. It is more likely in the setting of LVF, pericarditis, atrial ischaemic damage, and right ventricular infarction. In STEMI, AF carries increased risk of stroke and higher mortality, and anticoagulation is advised. β-blockers, with well-established benefit post-MI, are important to inhibit the excess sympathetic tone that often predisposes to arrhythmias.

Thyrotoxicosis

Thyroxine potentiates the effect of the adrenergic system on the heart. One study has demonstrated a 5-fold increased incidence of AF in both overt and subclinical hyperthyroidism (low thyroid-stimulating hormone (TSH) with normal triiodothyronine (T3)/thyroxine (T4)). The 1st-line treatment is to establish a euthyroid state using antithyroid drugs (carbimazole, propylthiouracil or radioiodine). β-blockade with either a β1-selective (bisoprolol) or non-selective β-blocker (atenolol, propranolol) has been shown to be beneficial in reducing ventricular rate and HF.

Alcohol excess

The Framingham study demonstrated that a high level of alcohol consumption (>36g per day) is associated with a greater risk of developing AF and the 'holiday heart' syndrome refers to AF triggered by acute alcohol excess. Alcohol is aetiologically important in as many as 63% of cases of new AF in the <65 years age group. Rarely is any treatment, in addition to abstinence, necessary.

Mitral stenosis

Termed rheumatic or valvular AF, this was a common cause of AF and remains so in the developing world. The pathological mechanism is elevated left atrial pressure with associated atrial dilation. Exercise capacity may be increased with AV nodal blocking drugs (β-blockers or NDCCBs). Acute treatment involves anticoagulating with IV heparin followed by warfarin. IV digoxin and a β-blocker or negatively chronotropic CCB are preferred to control the ventricular response. The decision on whether to attempt cardioversion is determined by the clinical pattern of AF.

Sepsis

Excess sympathetic tone in the systemic inflammatory response lowers the threshold for arrhythmias.

Other causes
- Pulmonary embolism. Consider in all cases of new onset AF
- Perioperative (see 📖 Chapter 8, p.257)
- Hypertrophic cardiomyopathy
- Congenital heart disease
- Muscular dystrophy
- Myotonic dystrophy
- COPD
- Tall stature
- Diabetes mellitus
- Sleep apnoea
- Metabolic syndrome

Drugs used in electrical and chemical cardioversion

There are several aspects to drug therapy in cardioversion for AF; antithrombotic medication, pre- and post-cardioversion antiarrhythmic therapy, and sedation/anaesthesia during the procedure.

Antithrombotic therapy

- If there is no clear history of time of onset, or symptoms have persisted for >48h, cardioversion should either be deferred and the patient adequately anticoagulated with warfarin(INR 2.0–3.0) for a minimum of 3 weeks, or transoesophageal echocardiography utilized to exclude left atrial and atrial appendage thrombus prior to DCCV.
- Following cardioversion attempt, whether successful or not, the patient should remain on warfarin for a minimum of 4 weeks.
- Those in whom there is a high risk of AF recurrence or high thromboembolic risk should remain anticoagulated for the long term.

Antiarrhythmic therapy

Studies have suggested that amiodarone or sotalol (gradually uptitrated from 80mg bd to 160mg bd), given at least 4 weeks in advance of electrical cardioversion, increases the success rate but in view of potential side effects this may only be appropriate in patients with a higher likelihood of procedure failure or in whom an attempt has already failed. Use is therefore not recommended routinely.

Although unlicensed in the UK, ibutilide has been shown to facilitate electrical cardioversion from AF to sinus rhythm in resistant AF but increases the risk of torsades de pointes.

Whilst there is no need to withdraw digoxin prior to the cardioversion attempt, if digoxin toxicity is suspected, this should be reversed in advance of cardioversion.

Sedation or anaesthesia

Drugs used for sedation/anaesthesia in DCCV must provide adequate sedation and analgesia, and minimal cardiovascular compromise whilst enabling rapid recovery. Traditionally, general anaesthetic agents such as propofol, sevoflurane, and etomidate have been used safely with rapid recovery the main advantage, whilst dependence of these regimens on anaesthetic department input has led others to use IV midazolam at the expense of prolonged sedation and resedation.

Antithrombotic treatment

The largest studies of AF treatment so far have concluded that oral anticoagulation in those at most risk of thromboembolic complications is more important than any rate- or rhythm-controlling treatment, offering approximately 60% risk reduction in stroke compared with 20% offered by antiplatelet agents. Furthermore, oral anticoagulation should be given to those at high risk of thromboembolic complications regardless of the duration or pattern of AF. The CHADS2 score is widely used in the UK to guide treatment but there are several thromboembolic risk-stratification systems (Box 4.1).

Box 4.1 CHADS2 score

- Congestive heart failure   1
- Hypertension (systolic >160mmHg)   1
- Age >75 years   1
- Diabetes mellitus   1
- Stroke or TIA previously   2

A score >2 indicates high risk of thromboembolism, and benefits of anticoagulation outweigh the risks. Intermediate-risk patients (1 or 2) should be assessed on an individual basis and those considered low risk should have aspirin 75–150mg od.

Special considerations for anticoagulation in AF

- Hypertension should be controlled prior to anticoagulation.
- Following cerebral infarction, anticoagulation should be delayed for 2 weeks or longer if a large infarct.
- Anticoagulation should not be given in the case of intracranial haemorrhage.
- Following a TIA, anticoagulation should begin as soon as possible once intracerebral haemorrhage is excluded radiologically.
- The following factors have been shown to be associated with an increased risk of bleeding:
  - age >75 years
  - concomitant antiplatelet drug use
  - uncontrolled hypertension
  - history of bleeding or intracerebral haemorrhage
  - anaemia
  - polypharmacy.

Anticoagulant agents

The vitamin K antagonist warfarin is by far the most widely used anticoagulant and requires therapeutic INR monitoring to achieve target anticoagulation safely, because of a narrow therapeutic range and widely variable individual dose requirements. Alternative coumarol anticoagulants such as phenindione and acenocoumarol are used in cases of warfarin intolerance.

The recently published RELY study[1] compared the direct thrombin inhibitor dabigatran with warfarin for anticoagulation of patients in AF.

The findings were a similar rate of stroke and a reduced rate of major haemorrhage in those treated with dabigatran 110mg bd vs. adjusted-dose warfarin, and a lower rate of stroke with a similar rate of major haemorrhage in those treated with 150mg bd dabigatran vs. adjusted-dose warfarin.[1] This study shows promise for a future of safe anticoagulation without therapeutic INR monitoring.

Initiating anticoagulation

Undue delay puts the patient at increased risk of stroke and therefore prompt treatment is advisable. A target INR of 2.5 (range 2–3) offers the best ratio of protection from the risk of thromboembolic bleeding events.

Slow-loading regimens for warfarin are usually safe and the majority reach target INR within 4 weeks (Table 4.2). They often result in lower rates of over-anticoagulation than rapid-loading regimens.

Reference

1 ℗ http://clinicaltrials.gov/ ClinicalTrials.gov number, NCT00262600.

Table 4.2 Examples of a slow warfarin loading regimen

Day 1: start warfarin 3mg daily after obtaining baseline INR

Table 4.2a Day 8: check INR

INR	Continuing dose	
<1.4	6mg	See Table 4.2b
1.4–1.5	5mg	Check INR day 15:
1.6–1.8	4mg	INR 2–3—continue dose Otherwise see Table 4.2c
1.9–2.1	3mg	
2.2–2.5	2.5mg	
2.6–2.7	2mg	
2.8–3	Omit for 2 days then 1mg	
>3	Stop	Restart in 3–5 days at 1mg

Table 4.2b Day 15: check INR

INR		
<1.4	10mg	Check compliance
1.4–1.5	7mg	Check INR day 22:
1.6–1.8	6mg	INR 2–3 -continue dose
		Otherwise
1.9–2.4	5mg	see Table 4.2c
2.5–2.9	4mg	
3.0–4.0	Omit for 2 days then restart at 3mg	
4.1–5.0	Omit for 2 days then restart at 2mg	
>5	Omit for 3 days then recheck INR	Recheck INR day 19

Table 4.2c Day 22: check INR

INR	
<1–1.2	Increase dose by 30%
1.3–1.5	Increase dose by 25%
1.6–1.9	Increase dose by 20%
3.1–3.5	Decrease dose by 15%
3.6–4.0	Decrease dose by 20%
4.1–6.0	Omit for 1 day or until INR <5 and decrease dose by 25%
6.1–7.9	Omit for 2–3 days or until INR <5 and decrease dose by 33%
>8	Reduce dose by 50% once INR <5

NB: Always consider underlying cause for high or low INR. Significant variation in diet may give rise to unpredictable INR.

If a dose adjustment gives a fraction, round up to nearest 0.5mg.

Source: Janes et al. (2004). Safe introduction of warfarin for thrombotic prophylaxis in atrial fibrillation requiring only a weekly INR. *Clin Lab Haematol* **26**(1):43–7.

Atrial flutter

Introduction

Atrial flutter is caused by a macro-re-entrant circuit in the atria. Typical (classical or type I) atrial flutter is the most common form of atrial flutter, and the macro-re-entrant circuit is right atrial with an anticlockwise direction. It is dependent upon a region of slow conduction in the isthmus between the tricuspid valve and the inferior vena cava. Less commonly, the circuit conducts in the clockwise direction. Clockwise flutter gives rise to a regular sawtooth wave (250–350bpm) seen most clearly in the inferior leads and V1 on 12-lead ECG. Other forms of atrial flutter usually arise from structural abnormalities and myocardial scarring. Those prone to atrial flutter may also have episodes of AF.

Diagnosis

It may not be possible to discern the flutter wave without slowing the ventricular rate through vagal manoeuvres or administration of adenosine (see 🕮 p.133). Atrial flutter often presents with a ventricular rate of 150bpm, which represents 2:1 conduction through the AV node with an atrial rate around 300bpm. The ventricular rate may be slower in the presence of AV nodal-blocking drugs.

Pharmacological cardioversion

Whilst longstanding atrial flutter is increasingly treated with ablative therapy, acute atrial flutter is often poorly tolerated and requires cardioversion, either electrically or pharmacologically, usually with class III agents (Table 4.1). If there is 1:1 AV conduction, then there is a high chance of haemodynamic instability and precipitation of ventricular arrhythmia.

- *Amiodarone* is usually 1st-line treatment of acute atrial flutter in the UK. One suggested regimen is 5mg/kg or 300mg IV in 50mL 5% glucose over 10min followed by 900mg in 500mL 5% glucose over 23h. It is important to use a large proximal vein to reduce the risk of venous thrombophlebitis and tissue necrosis. It is effective in both cardioversion and ventricular rate reduction.
- *Sotalol* 1mg/kg IV in 10min has been shown to be equally efficacious.
- *Ibutilide* and *dofetilide* have been shown to be effective in cardioverting atrial flutter but are not licensed in the UK.

Maintenance of sinus rhythm

In recurrent atrial flutter, isthmus ablation is the treatment of choice. Class Ia or c agents may be used for long-term maintenance of sinus rhythm. These work by preventing atrial ectopic beats which trigger the onset of atrial flutter. Amiodarone is an alternative in the presence of structural heart disease (often only a low dose of amiodarone is required, i.e. 200mg od). The most important long-term treatment is ablation (Table 4.1).

Important note: class I agents usually slow the flutter rate, thus increasing the chance that the AV node may not be refractory when flutter waves attempt to conduct to the ventricle. This may result in 1:1 AV conduction, which may be life threatening. Class I agents should always therefore be co-prescribed with AV nodal blockers in atrial flutter. Commonly, typical flutter may be induced by a class Ic agent given for AF, and co-prescription of an AV nodal blocking drug is similarly advised.

Ventricular rate control

Ventricular rate control is harder to achieve in atrial flutter because the modest increase in AV node refractory period generated by the AV blocking agents is less likely to generate a higher degree of AV conduction block. Agents used are as for AF:

- β-blockers
- NDCCBs
- digoxin
- amiodarone.

Antithrombotic treatment

No trials have been conducted looking specifically at anticoagulation in atrial flutter and as such, recommendations have been largely extrapolated from AF data. In paroxysmal and persistent atrial flutter, anticoagulation is recommended. As atrial function has been shown to be compromised following cardioversion, there is a greater thromboembolic risk which continues for some time. It is therefore recommended that anticoagulation is continued for 4 weeks after cardioversion or for 4–6 weeks following catheter ablation.

Supraventricular (narrow complex) tachycardias

Diagnosis

It may not be easy to determine the nature of a regular narrow complex tachycardia (NCT) on presentation. Fig. 4.5 shows an algorithm indicating the use of IV adenosine in the diagnosis of underlying rhythm in NCT.

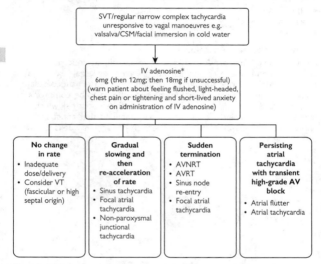

Fig. 4.5 Guide to diagnosis of supraventricular tachycardia/regular narrow complex tachycardia.

Notes:

*Continuous ECG recording should commence on administration.

Adenosine should be given as push IV injection through antecubital fossa vein (adenosine is more likely to induce AF if given via central venous line).

Adenosine is contraindicated in the severely asthmatic owing to bronchiolar constriction.

Adenosine effects are potentiated by dipyridamole.

Higher rates of AV block seen if concomitantly administered with carbamazepine.

Verapamil IV can be used as alternative AV-blocking agent for diagnosis/arrhythmia/termination but is only recommended to be used by experienced cardiologists.

AVNRT, atrioventricular nodal reciprocating tachycardia; AVRT, atrioventricular reciprocating tachycardia.

Pharmacotherapy

See Tables 4.3–4.5.

Table 4.3 Pharmacological options for NCT originating in the sinoatrial node

Type of NCT	Acute treatment	Long-term treatment
Physiological sinus tachycardia	Vagal manoeuvres	β-blockers NDCCBs
Inappropriate sinus tachycardia	As above	β-blockers NDCCBs Ivabradine (anecdotal evidence, no approved indication) Ablation
Paroxysmal orthostatic tachycardia syndrome (POTS)	As above	β-blockers Fludrocortisone ± bisoprolol SSRIs Other agents; midodrine, clonidine, octreotide, erythropoietin
Sinus node re-entry tachycardia	As above, plus IV amiodarone, NDCCBs, β-blockers or digoxin	Little scope for pharmacotherapy–ablation is mainstay if poorly tolerated symptoms present

Table 4.4 Pharmacotherapy for atrial (non-sinus node)-origin NCT

Type of NCT	Acute treatment	Long-term treatment
Focal atrial tachycardia	Reverse digitoxicity/hypokalaemia Vagal manoeuvres IV; adenosine, β-blockers, NDCCBs, procainamide, flecainide, propafenone, amiodarone, sotalol	β-blockers, NDCCBs Disopyramide, flecainide, propafenone (in absence of structural/ischaemic heart disease) Sotalol, amiodarone (NB class I agents should not be used without AV nodal-blocking agent)
Multifocal atrial tachycardia (irregular rhythm often mistaken for AF)	Correct pulmonary disease or electrolyte disturbances	NDCCBs β-blockers often contraindicated due to pulmonary disease. No role for antiarrhythmics

Table 4.5 Pharmacotherapy for junctional/AV nodal rhythms (NB ablative therapies have become the mainstay treatment of these rhythms)

Type of NCT	Acute management	Chronic management
AV nodal reciprocating tachycardia (AVNRT)	Vagal manoeuvres IV adenosine IV amiodarone	NDCCBs, β-blockers, digoxin, Flecainide or propafenone if no ischaemic or structural heart disease. 'Pill-in-the-pocket' treatment for infrequent and well-tolerated episodes (further evidence required). Diltiazem 120mg + propranolol 80mg more effective than flecainide.
AV reciprocating tachycardia (AVRT)—including WPW syndrome	Vagal manoeuvres IV adenosine (contraindicated in preexcited AF owing to risk of rapid ventricular response deteriorating into VF)	NDCCBs, β-blockers, digoxin (should not be used as monotherapy in those with accessory pathway that may be capable of rapid conduction during AF) Propafenone, flecainide, sotalol, amiodarone. 'Pill-in-the-pocket'—as above
Focal junctional tachycardia	As above IV flecainide	Variable responsiveness to β-blockers, flecainide
Non-paroxysmal junctional tachycardia May be precipitated by: myocardial ischaemia/myocarditis cardiac surgery COPD hypokalaemia digitoxicity	Correct underlying abnormality, i.e. correct digitoxicity or hypokalaemia	Usually not required but persisting tachycardia can be suppressed by β-blockers or NDCCBs

Landmark trials for atrial arrhythmias

AFFIRM (Atrial Fibrillation Follow-up Investigation of Rhythm Management)[1]
- Comparison of rate versus rhythm control strategies.
- Randomized multicentre study involving 4060 patients, mean age 70 years.
- Outcomes: at 5 years 356 deaths in rhythm control group and 310 in rate control group (P=0.08, i.e. not statistically significant).
- Fewer hospital admissions and adverse drug effects in rate-control group.
- Overall it was observed that the majority of strokes occurred when warfarin was either withdrawn or INR subtherapeutic.

CAST (Cardiac Arrhythmia Suppression Trial)[2]
Although this study investigated post-MI ventricular arrhythmia suppression, its conclusion has been extrapolated to recommend against the use of class Ic antiarrhythmics for atrial arrhythmias in structural heart disease. There were a significantly larger number of fatal and non-fatal cardiac arrests in the group treated with flecainide or encainide compared with placebo (trial stopped at 10 months).

BAFTA (Birmingham AF Treatment of the Aged) 2007[3]
- Comparison of stroke rate in over 75s treated with warfarin (INR 2–3) and aspirin 75mg; 973 patients recruited prospectively from general practices in the UK.
- Outcomes: warfarin group had half the number of strokes (1.8% vs. 3.8%).
- No significant difference in rates of extracranial haemorrhagic complications.
- This study selected only those in whom best treatment option was not known, i.e. those at high risk would have been anticoagulated.

ACTIVE-W (Atrial fibrillation Clopidogrel Trial with Irbesartan for prevention of Vascular Events)[4]
- 6700 patients randomized to oral anticoagulation (OAC) (INR 2–3) or aspirin 75mg plus clopidogrel 75mg.
- Outcomes: OAC is superior to clopidogrel plus aspirin for prevention of vascular events.
- The rates of major bleeding complications are similar in both groups.

References
1 *N Engl J Med* 2002; **347**:1825–33.
2 *N Engl J Med* 1989; **321**:406–12.
3 *Lancet* 2007; **370**:493–503.
4 *Lancet* 2006; **367**:1903–12.

Further reading

Aguilar MI, Hart R, Pearce LA (2007). Oral anticoagulants versus antiplatelet therapy for preventing stroke in patients with non-valvular atrial fibrillation and no history of stroke or transient ischaemic attacks. Cochrane Database Syst Rev 2007; (**3**):CD006186. 'Adjusted-dose warfarin and related oral anticoagulants reduce stroke, disabling stroke and other major vascular events for those with non-valvular AF by about one-third when compared with antiplatelet therapy.'

Blomström-Lundqvist C et al. (2003). Management of patients with supraventricular arrhythmias. ACC/AHA/ESC guidelines. *J Am Coll Cardiol* **42**:1493–531.

Cordina J, Mead C (2005). Pharmacological cardioversion for atrial fibrillation and flutter. Cochrane Database Syst Rev (**2**):CD003713. This review looks at results of AFFIRM and PIAF trials and concludes that there is no evidence that pharmacological cardioversion to sinus rhythm is superior to rate control although most patients studied were over 60 and cannot be extrapolated to younger people.

Fuster V et al. (2006). ACC/AHA/ESC 2006 guidelines for the management of patients with atrial fibrillation. *Europace* **8**:651–745.

The National Collaborating Centre for Chronic Conditions (2006). *Atrial Fibrillation: National Guidelines for Management in Primary and Secondary Care.* London: Royal College of Physicians.

Ventricular arrhythmias

Background

Ventricular arrhythmias are abnormal rhythms that originate from below the AV node. They include premature ventricular complexes, VT, and ventricular fibrillation (VF). Premature ventricular complexes (PVCs) are ectopic beats that occur independently of normal cardiac rhythm. They may be single or repetitive. VTs are divided into non-sustained and sustained VT. By definition, non-sustained ventricular tachycardias (NSVTs) last >6 consecutive beats and <30s. VT can also be divided according to the morphology of the QRS complexes into monomorphic VT and polymorphic VT. VF refers to irregular uncoordinated ventricular contraction resulting from disorganized electrical activity.

Ventricular arrhythmias may occur in patients with structural heart disease or in patients with structurally normal hearts. Potential underlying causes include:
- patients with structural heart disease:
  - ischaemic heart disease
  - cardiomyopathies: dilated cardiomyopathy (DCM), hypertrophic cardiomyopathy (HCM), arrhythmogenic right ventricular cardiomyopathy (ARVC)
  - valvular heart disease, e.g. mitral regurgitation
- patients with structurally normal hearts:
  - genetic arrhythmia syndromes: long QT syndrome (LQTS), Brugada syndrome, catecholaminergic polymorphic ventricular tachycardia (CPVT)
  - idiopathic VT: right ventricular outflow tract VT (RVOT VT), left ventricular outflow tract VT (LVOT VT).

Some causes of ventricular arrhythmias may affect patients with structural heart disease and patients with structurally normal hearts:
- drugs: including antiarrhythmics with pro-arrhythmogenic potential
- metabolic abnormalities: electrolyte abnormalities, acidosis, hypoxia.

Symptoms associated with ventricular arrhythmias depend on the frequency, duration, and haemodynamic effects of the arrhythmia. PVCs and non-compromising VT may be asymptomatic or may cause symptoms such as palpitations, shortness of breath, chest discomfort, or dizziness. VT with more profound haemodynamic effects may present with syncope or cardiac arrest. VF rapidly results in collapse and cardiac arrest due to total ventricular chaos.

Management of ventricular arrhythmias

The focus of this chapter is on the role of antiarrhythmic drugs in the management of ventricular arrhythmias. For practical purposes, the discussion is divided into management of acute ventricular arrhythmias and management of ventricular arrhythmias in the chronic setting. The recommendations for antiarrhythmic drug therapy are based on the ACC/AHA/ESC 2006 guidelines for management of patients with ventricular arrhythmias.[1] Where possible, the level of evidence and class of indication for the use of an antiarrhythmic drug for a given situation has been specified.

The antiarrhythmic drugs listed in Tables 4.6–4.13 are classified according to their mechanism of action using the Vaughan Williams classification (see 📖 Table 4.1, p.115). Most of the drugs routinely used for the treatment of ventricular arrhythmias are included in the Vaughan Williams classification system. One of the limitations of using this system, however, is that some antiarrhythmics do not fit just one of the categories.

Reference

1 Zipes DP *et al.* (2006). ACC/AHA/ESC 2006 guidelines for management of patients with ventricular arrhythmias and the prevention of sudden cardiac death: a report of the American College of Cardiology/American Heart Association Task Force and the European Society of Cardiology Committee for Practice Guidelines (Writing Committee to Develop Guidelines for Management of Patients With Ventricular Arrhythmias and the Prevention of Sudden Cardiac Death). *J Am Coll Cardiol* **48**(5):e247–346.

Acute management of ventricular arrhythmias

The management of acute ventricular arrhythmias depends on the haemodynamic effect of the arrhythmia. The following section outlines guidelines for management of cardiac arrest and guidelines for management of stable VT.

Management of cardiac arrest

Cardiac arrest refers to an abrupt loss of cardiac output. Cardiac arrest may arise due to ventricular arrhythmias (VF, pulseless VT), pulseless electrical activity (PEA), or asystole. Patients with cardiac arrest due to ventricular arrhythmia require urgent defibrillation.

Antiarrhythmic drug therapy is recommended in patients with cardiac arrest and recurrent shock refractory ventricular arrhythmias (VT/VF). Amiodarone is generally recommended as 1st line for shock refractory VT/VF. Lidocaine may be used as an alternative, particularly in patients with evidence of underlying coronary ischaemia. Recommendations for antiarrhythmic drug therapy are summarized in Table 4.6.

The cardiac arrest algorithm (Fig. 4.6) is based on the 2005 European Resuscitation Council guidelines.[1]

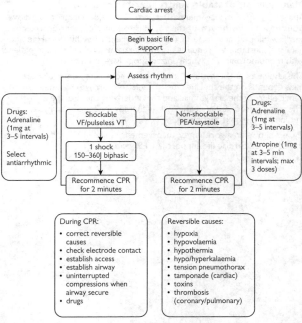

Fig. 4.6 Algorithm for management of cardiac arrest (based on the 2005 European Resuscitation Council guidelines).

Management of stable ventricular tachycardia

The options for management of stable VT include electrical cardioversion and antiarrhythmic drug therapy. It is reasonable to perform electrical cardioversion at any stage in the management of stable VT. Haemodynamically unstable VT requires urgent electrical cardioversion. In patients with monomorphic VT, synchronized shock is recommended.

The choice of antiarrhythmic drug therapy for acute ventricular arrhythmias depends on the specific type of ventricular arrhythmia, the haemodynamic effect of the arrhythmia, and the underlying cause of the arrhythmia. The guidelines for antiarrhythmic drug therapy for specific arrhythmias are outlined in the next section.

Fig. 4.7 shows an algorithm for management of stable VT and is based on the advanced cardiac life support (ACLS) guidelines.[2]

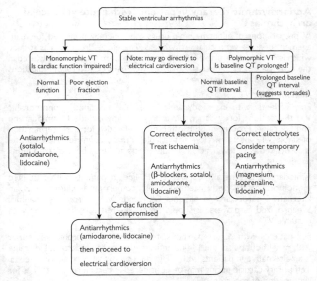

Fig. 4.7 Treatment algorithm guide to management of ventricular tachycardia with pulse.

Antiarrhythmic therapy in patients with acute ventricular arrhythmias

IV preparations of antiarrhythmic drugs are generally preferred for management of acute ventricular arrhythmias. Therefore, drugs such as sotalol, which is not widely available in an IV preparation, are less commonly used in the acute setting. Table 4.6 summarizes ACC/AHA/ESC (2006) indications for antiarrhythmic drug therapy.

Monomorphic VT

For patients with haemodynamically stable sustained monomorphic VT, the options for antiarrhythmic drug therapy include IV amiodarone and lidocaine. Procainamide is often more effective for early termination of stable VT, but it is no longer available in many countries. Amiodarone is associated with fewer adverse side effects and may be preferred in HF patients.

Amiodarone is generally considered 1st line in patients with sustained monomorphic VT with haemodynamic compromise. Lidocaine is an alternative, particularly in patients with underlying coronary ischaemia. Synchronized cardioversion should be considered early in patients with unstable VT.

For patients with recurrent shock, refractory monomorphic VT, either with or without pulse, the 1st-line antiarrhythmic is amiodarone. Lidocaine is an alternative in patients with VT in the context of coronary ischaemia. Temporary cardiac pacing may be considered in certain circumstances for suppression of recurrent VT.

Polymorphic VT (with normal QT interval)
Unstable polymorphic VT generally requires urgent cardioversion.
High-energy defibrillation is recommended. In patients with recurrent polymorphic VT who have a normal baseline QT interval, the options for antiarrhythmic drug therapy include IV β-blockers, amiodarone and lidocaine.

Polymorphic VT with normal repolarization is commonly caused by acute coronary ischaemia. IV β-blockers are particularly useful in this setting. Urgent coronary angiography should be considered in patients with suspected ischaemia-driven polymorphic VT. CPVT, a genetic arrhythmia syndrome, may also respond well to β-blockade.

Torsades de pointes
Torsades de pointes refers to polymorphic VT in patients with LQTS. QT prolongation may be congenital or acquired. Acquired QT prolongation may be drug induced or may occur in the context of bradycardia due to conduction block. Drugs that prolong QT interval include:
- class Ia drugs: procainamide, quinidine, disopyramide
- class Ic drugs: flecainide, encainide, propafenone
- class III drugs: amiodarone, sotalol.

A variety of non-cardiac drugs prolong QT interval. For a list of drugs refer to 📖 Section 2, p.327.

Management of torsades de pointes often depends on the underlying cause of abnormal repolarization. General measures include withdrawal of QT-prolonging drugs and correction of electrolyte abnormalities. Serum potassium should be maintained between 4.5 and 5mEq/L. IV magnesium sulphate may be effective for acute suppression of torsades de pointes (even when serum magnesium is normal).

In patients with torsades de pointes 2° to bradycardia, temporary pacing is recommended. IV β-blockers may be used in combination with temporary pacing. In patients with drug-induced torsades de pointes, if temporary pacing is not available, IV isoprenaline may be used as an alternative.

Ventricular arrhythmias secondary to acute coronary ischaemia

PVC and NSVT are common in patients with ACSs. Apart from β-blockers, antiarrhythmic drug therapy for suppression of PVC and NSVT is not indicated. β-blockers are indicated as standard treatment of patients with ACSs. In addition to reducing myocardial oxygen demand, β-blockers are effective for suppression of ventricular arrhythmias.

For patients with sustained ventricular arrhythmias, the choice of antiarrhythmic depends on LV function. In patients with preserved LV function, options include IV procainamide, amiodarone, and lidocaine. Sotalol may also be considered but is not widely available in an IV preparation. In patients with impaired systolic function, amiodarone or lidocaine is recommended. Lidocaine is an effective alternative to amiodarone in patients with underlying coronary ischaemia.

Ventricular arrhythmias are common in the first 48h following acute MI. While sustained ventricular arrhythmias in the peri-infarct period are associated with a higher in-hospital mortality, they are not associated with an increased long-term risk. In patients with recurrent ischaemia-driven ventricular arrhythmias, urgent coronary angiography and revascularization should be considered.

Idioventricular rhythms are also common in patients with acute MI, particularly following reperfusion. In the absence of haemodynamic compromise, idioventricular rhythms do not require antiarrhythmic drug therapy apart from β-blockers.

Table 4.6 Acute ventricular arrhythmias—indications for antiarrhythmic drug therapy

Type of arrhythmia	Drug	Comments
Cardiac arrest with shock-resistant VF/VT	Amiodarone (IV) (class III antiarrhythmic)	Amiodarone generally considered 1st line (class I recommendation/level of evidence B)
	Lidocaine (IV) (class Ib antiarrhythmic)	Lidocaine may be considered as an alternative to amiodarone in ischaemia-driven VF/VT (class of recommendation indeterminate)
Sustained monomorphic VT	Amiodarone (IV) (class III antiarrhythmic)	Indications for IV amiodarone include: haemodynamically unstable sustained VT recurrent sustained monomorphic VT despite cardioversion recurrent sustained monomorphic VT despite therapy with other antiarrhythmics (class IIa recommendation/level of evidence C) in patients with HF, the use of amiodarone for acute management of haemodynamically unstable VT and shock-refractory VT is a class I indication (level of evidence B)
	Lidocaine (IV) (class Ib antiarrhythmic)	Lidocaine may be used for treatment of ischaemia-driven stable monomorphic VT (class IIb recommendation/level of evidence C)
Polymorphic VT with normal QT interval	β-blockers (IV) (class II antiarrhythmic)	IV β-blockers are effective for suppression of polymorphic VT with normal QT interval (class I recommendation/level of evidence B)
	Amiodarone (IV) (class III antiarrhythmic)	IV amiodarone loading is effective for suppression of polymorphic VT with normal QT interval (class I recommendation/level of evidence C)
	Lidocaine (IV) (class Ib antiarrhythmic)	Lidocaine may be effective for management of ischaemia-driven polymorphic VT with normal QT interval (class IIb recommendation/level of evidence C)

Table 4.6 *(Contd.)*

Type of arrhythmia	Drug	Comments
Torsades de pointes	Magnesium sulphate (IV)	IV magnesium sulphate may be considered in patients with LQTS and torsades de pointes (class IIa recommendation/level of evidence B)
	β-blockers (IV (class II antiarrhythmic)	Patients with bradycardia and torsades de pointes may be treated with β-blockers and pacing (class IIa recommendation/level of evidence C)
	Isoprenaline (IV)	Indicated in recurrent torsades de pointes associated with significant pauses in patients who do not have congenital LQTS (class IIa recommendation/level of evidence B)
	Lidocaine (IV) (class Ib antiarrhythmic)	May be indicated in patients with LQT3 and torsades de pointes (class IIa recommendation/level of evidence B)

References

1 Nolan JP et al. (2005). European Resuscitation Council Guidelines for Resuscitation 2005. *Resuscitation* **67**(Suppl 1):S39–S86.
2 The American Heart Association in collaboration with the International Liaison Committee on Resuscitation (2000). Guidelines 2000 for Cardiopulmonary Resuscitation and Emergency Cardiovascular Care. Part 6: advanced cardiovascular life support: section 7: algorithm approach to ACLS emergencies: section 7A: principles and practice of ACLS. *Circulation* **102**(Suppl 8):I136–9.

Management of ventricular arrhythmias in the chronic setting

The longer-term treatment goals for patients with ventricular arrhythmias are prevention of sudden cardiac death and suppression of symptomatic ventricular arrhythmias. Treatment options include implantation of a cardiac defibrillator (ICD), pharmacological therapy, and radiofrequency ablation. Implantation of an ICD is the main strategy for prevention of sudden cardiac death, either for 1° or 2° prevention. Indications for ICD include:

- abortive cardiac arrest 2° to VF or VT with no identifiable cause
- spontaneous sustained VT in patients with structural heart disease
- unexplained syncope with sustained VT/VF on electrophysiological (EP) studies or high probability of ventricular arrhythmias
- ischaemic heart disease with impaired LV function (ejection fraction <40%), spontaneous NSVT and sustained monomorphic VT on EP studies
- ischaemic heart disease with severe LV dysfunction (ejection fraction <30%) and NYHA class II or III HF on optimal medical therapy
- dilated cardiomyopathy (non-ischaemic) with severe LV dysfunction (ejection fraction <30–35%) and NYHA class II or III HF on optimal medical therapy
- inherited conditions associated with life-threatening ventricular arrhythmias e.g. LQTS, ARVC, HCM, Brugada syndrome.

Apart from β-blockers, antiarrhythmic drugs have not been demonstrated to reduce the incidence of sudden cardiac death. Chronic antiarrhythmic drug therapy is aimed mainly at suppression of ventricular arrhythmias in order to reduce the symptom burden. Antiarrhythmic drugs can be used in isolation or in combination with ICD therapy. In patients with ICDs, antiarrhythmic drug therapy may reduce the number of shocks and anti-tachycardia pacing episodes delivered by the device.

In addition to the antiarrhythmic action, a number of drugs have pro-arrhythmic potential and therefore have to be used with caution. The choice of antiarrhythmic agent often depends on the underlying cause of the ventricular arrhythmia.

An emerging treatment for patients with ventricular arrhythmias is radio-frequency ablation. Catheter ablation is particularly useful in patients who are unable to tolerate pharmacological therapy or have arrhythmias that are resistant to antiarrhythmic drug therapy. Catheter ablation is also used in patients with ICDs and recurrent arrhythmias that are refractory to drug therapy.

Drug therapy for ventricular arrhythmias in specific patient populations

Patients with impaired LV function due to previous MI and patients with symptomatic HF

The following section outlines guidelines for chronic management of ventricular arrhythmias in patients with impaired LV function due to pre-vious MI and patients with symptomatic HF (irrespective of aetiology).

There is significant overlap between the two patient groups and therefore not surprisingly, the guidelines for antiarrhythmic drug therapy are very similar (Tables 4.7 and 4.8). There are, however, some differences relating to level of evidence and class of indication for some drugs, which have been highlighted in Table 4.7.

Chronic antiarrhythmic drug therapy in these two patient groups is indicated for suppression of symptomatic ventricular arrhythmias, adjunctive therapy in patients with ICD, and alternative therapy in patients who cannot have or refuse ICD therapy. Routine suppression of asymptomatic PVC and NSVT is not recommended.

The options for chronic antiarrhythmic drug therapy include β-blockers, amiodarone, and sotalol. β-blockers should be commenced as standard therapy in patients with impaired LV function unless specifically contraindicated. In patients with persistent ventricular arrhythmias despite β-blocker therapy, amiodarone may be effective, often in combination with β-blockers. Sotalol may be used as an alternative to amiodarone; however, it is not recommended in patients with severely depressed LV function due to adverse haemodynamic effects.

Class Ia drugs (e.g. procainamide, quinidine, disopyramide) and class Ic drugs (e.g. flecainide, encainide, propafenone) are associated with pro-arrhythmic effects in patients with ischaemic heart disease and patients with impaired ventricular function and are therefore contraindicated. CCBs are also particularly contraindicated in patients with severely depressed LV function due to their negative inotropic effects.

In patients with impaired LV function, irrespective of aetiology, optimization of pharmacological HF therapy, and, where appropriate, cardiac resynchronization therapy, has been demonstrated to reduce the risk of sudden cardiac death. Guidelines for management of HF are discussed in Chapter 1, p.3.

The indications for ICD therapy, either for 1° or 2° prevention of sudden cardiac death, are listed on pp.18–19. In patients with underlying ischaemic heart disease in whom ventricular arrhythmias are precipitated by recurrent coronary ischaemia, coronary revascularization is an important consideration.

Table 4.7 Antiarrhythmic drug therapy in patients with impaired LV function due to previous MI

Drug	Indications	Comments
β-blockers (class II antiarrhythmic)	1st-line therapy All patients should routinely be commenced on β-blockers unless specifically contraindicated	Prognostic benefit in patients with impaired LV function due to previous MI May be used as an adjunct to ICD therapy May also be considered as an alternative in patients who refuse or cannot have ICD
Amiodarone (class III antiarrhythmic)	Chronic suppression of symptomatic ventricular arrhythmias unresponsive to β-blockers (class IIa indication/ level of evidence B) Adjunct to ICD therapy—decreases risk of inappropriate shocks (class IIa indication/level of evidence C) Patients with an indication for ICD who refuse ICD or cannot have ICD implantation (class IIa indication/level of evidence C) In patients with symptomatic HF: adjunct to ICD therapy—decreases risk of inappropriate shocks (class I indication/level of evidence C): In patients with symptomatic HF: pharmacological alternative to ICD therapy (class IIb indication/level of evidence C)	Well tolerated in patients with impaired LV function Often used in combination with β-blockers No clear prognostic benefit
Sotalol (class III antiarrhythmic)	Chronic suppression of symptomatic ventricular arrhythmias unresponsive to β-blockers (class IIa indication/ level of evidence C) Adjunct to ICD therapy—decreases risk of inappropriate shocks (class IIa indication/level of evidence C)	Greater proarrhythmic potential than amiodarone. Amiodarone therefore generally preferred Not recommended in patients with prolonged QT interval Not recommended in patients with severely depressed LV function No clear prognostic benefit

Table 4.8 Antiarrhythmic therapy in patients with HF

Drug	Indications	Comments
β-blockers (class II antiarrhythmic)	1st-line therapy All patients should routinely be commenced on β-blockers unless specifically contraindicated	Prognostic benefit. β-blockers reduce overall risk of sudden cardiac death
Amiodarone (class III antiarrhythmic)	Adjunct to ICD therapy—decreases the risk of inappropriate shocks (class I indication/level of evidence C) Pharmacological alternative to ICD therapy (class IIb indication/level of evidence C)	Safe and well tolerated in patients with severely impaired ventricular function
Sotalol (class III antiarrhythmic)	Adjunct to ICD therapy—decreases risk of inappropriate shocks (class I indication/level of evidence C) Pharmacological alternative to ICD therapy (class IIb indication/level of evidence C)	Greater proarrhythmic potential than amiodarone. Amiodarone therefore generally preferred.

Patients with hypertrophic cardiomyopathy (HCM)

Patients with HCM who have a high risk of sudden cardiac death require ICD therapy, for either 1° or 2° prevention. Major risk factors for sudden cardiac death in HCM patients include: cardiac arrest (VF), spontaneous sustained VT, family history of sudden cardiac death, unexplained syncope, abnormal exercise BP, spontaneous NSVT, and LV wall thickness >30mm.

In patients with a high risk of sudden cardiac death who cannot have an ICD, amiodarone may be used as an alternative. β-blockers, which are often used as standard therapy in patients with HCM to improve diastolic filling, may have the added benefit of suppressing symptomatic ventricular arrhythmias but are not thought to have the same potential mortality benefit as amiodarone (Table 4.9).

Table 4.9 Antiarrhythmic therapy in patients with HCM

Drug	Indications	Comments
Amiodarone (class III antiarrhythmic)	Chronic therapy for patients with previous sustained VT/VF when ICD is not feasible (class IIa indication/level of evidence C) Chronic therapy for 1° prevention in HCM patients with a high risk of sudden cardiac death when ICD is not feasible(class IIb indication/ level of evidence C)	Considered the most effective antiarrhythmic in patients with HCM Useful in prevention of sudden cardiac death in non-randomized studies
β-blockers (class II antiarrhythmic)	Standard therapy in patients with HCM—improve diastolic filling	No clear evidence for reduction of sudden cardiac death

Patients with arrhythmogenic right ventricular cardiomyopathy (ARVC)
ARVC is a condition characterized by fibrofatty infiltration of the RV myocardium, and is associated with ventricular arrhythmias and sudden cardiac death. The impact of ICD therapy or antiarrhythmic drug therapy on mortality in patients with ARVC is not established. ICD therapy is indicated in patients with a history of sustained haemodynamically unstable VT or cardiac arrest due to VT/VF. ICD may also be considered for 1° prevention in ARVC patients with unexplained syncope. In patients with a high risk of sudden cardiac death who are not candidates for ICD, or have well-tolerated VT, antiarrhythmic drug therapy with amiodarone and sotalol may be considered (Table 4.10).

Table 4.10 Antiarrhythmic drug therapy in patients with ARVC

Drug	Indications	Comments
Amiodarone (class III antiarrhythmic)	Chronic therapy in patients with sustained VF or VT when ICD implantation is not feasible (class IIa indication/level of evidence C)	Impact on mortality not established
Sotalol (class III antiarrhythmic)	Chronic therapy in patients with sustained VF or VT when ICD implantation is not feasible (class IIa indication/level of evidence C)	Impact on mortality not established

Patients with congenital LQTS
β-blockers represent the mainstay of chronic antiarrhythmic drug therapy in patients with congenital LQTS. In patients who have a high risk of sudden cardiac death, i.e. patients with a history of cardiac arrest, patients with syncope or VT while receiving β-blockers, ICD therapy is recommended in combination with β-blockers. The use of β-blockers is not recommended in patients who have significant bradycardia associated with LQTS (unless used in combination with permanent pacing) (Table 4.11).

Table 4.11 Antiarrhythmic drug therapy in patients with congenital LQTS

Drug	Indications	Comments
β-blockers (class II antiarrhythmic)	Chronic therapy for suppression of torsades de pointes in patients with a clinical diagnosis of LQTS (class 1 indication/level of evidence B)	Not recommended in LQTS associated with prominent bradycardia (unless used in combination with permanent pacing)
	Chronic therapy for suppression of torsades de pointes in patients with a molecular diagnosis of LQTS who have a normal QT interval (class IIa indication/level of evidence B)	

Patients with Brugada syndrome

Brugada syndrome is a genetic condition associated with a high risk of ventricular arrhythmias and sudden cardiac death. Diagnosis is based on characteristic ECG features associated with a history of aborted sudden cardiac death or a family history of sudden cardiac death. ECG abnormalities include right bundle branch block and ST segment elevation in leads V1–V3. The ECG changes may not be evident until unmasked by provocative tests using flecainide, procainamide, or ajmaline. β-blockers may also augment the ECG changes.

No effective chronic antiarrhythmic drugs are available for treatment of Brugada syndrome. The mainstay of treatment is ICD therapy. Isoprenaline and quinidine can be used acutely in patients with arrhythmia storm (even in the presence of an ICD). Quinidine has also been shown to reduce the frequency of ICD shocks long term.

Patients with catecholaminergic polymorphic ventricular tachycardia

CPVT is an inherited disorder characterized by stress-related polymorphic VT. Patients have structurally normal hearts and normal QT intervals. β-blockers counteract sympathetic stimulation and are highly effective for suppression of ventricular arrhythmias in patients with CPVT (see Table 4.12). β-blockers should be commenced in all patients with a diagnosis of CPVT and documented stress-induced ventricular arrhythmias. β-blockers may also be used as prophylactic therapy in patients who are diagnosed with CPVT on the basis of genetic testing with no previous documented arrhythmias. β-blockers are used in combination with ICD therapy in patients with CPVT who have had previous cardiac arrest.

Table 4.12 Antiarrhythmic drug therapy in patients with CPVT

Drug	Indications	Comments
β-blockers (class II antiarrhythmic)	CPVT with documented stress-induced ventricular arrhythmias (class I indication/level of evidence C)	May be used in combination with ICD in patients with high risk of sudden cardiac death
	Prophylactic therapy in patients with a diagnosis of CPVT based on genetic analysis with no previous episodes of ventricular arrhythmia (class IIa indication/level of evidence C)	

Patients with structurally normal hearts (idiopathic VT)
Idiopathic VT may arise in the right ventricular outflow tract (RVOT VT) or
the left ventricular outflow tract (LVOT VT). RVOT VT is by far the most
common type of idiopathic VT. Chronic therapy with β-blockers and CCBs
may be effective for suppression of RVOT VT and LVOT VT. Class Ic drugs
may also be used for management of RVOT VT (see Table 4.13). Catheter
ablation is useful in patients with symptomatic drug-refractory VT or in
those who are drug intolerant (class I indication/level of evidence C).

Table 4.13 Antiarrhythmic drug therapy in patients with
idiopathic VT

Drug	Indications	Comments
β-blockers (class II antiarrhythmic)	RVOT VT (class IIa recommendation/level of evidence C) LVOT VT	May be used for acute termination or chronic suppression of idiopathic VT
CCBs (class IV antiarrhythmic)	RVOT VT (class IIa recommendation/level of evidence C) LVOT VT	May be used for acute termination or chronic suppression of idiopathic VT
Flecainide, encainide, propafenone (class Ic drugs)	RVOT VT (class IIa recommendation/level of evidence C)	β-blockers and CCBs usually preferred for RVOT VT
Adenosine	Acute termination of RVOT VT	RVOT VT is typically adenosine sensitive

Landmark trials for ventricular arrhythmias

β-blockers

MUSTT (Multicenter UnSustained Tachycardia Trial)[1]

- Prospective RCT.
- Demonstrated that in patients with coronary artery disease, ejection fraction ≤40% and asymptomatic NSVT, β-blockers have beneficial effects on survival (5-year mortality 50% with β-blockers vs. 66% without β-blockers; adjusted $P=0.0001$).
- There was no significant effect of β-blocker therapy on the rate of arrhythmic death or cardiac arrest (adjusted $P=0.2344$).

Note: multiple studies have demonstrated beneficial effects of β-blockers in patients with coronary artery disease and HF (see ☐ Chapters 2 and 3, p.29, p.95)

Amiodarone

EMIAT (European Myocardial Infarction Amiodarone Trial)[2]

- Randomized placebo controlled trial.
- Demonstrated that in high-risk patients post MI, there was no significant reduction in overall mortality in patients treated with amiodarone compared with placebo.
- Post hoc analysis demonstrated that a combination of amiodarone and β-blocker had a significant mortality benefit (unadjusted all-cause mortality reduction of 30%).

CAMIAT (Canadian Amiodarone Myocardial Infarction Arrhythmia Trial)[3]

- Randomized placebo-controlled trial.
- Demonstrated that in high-risk patients post MI, there was no significant reduction in incidence of arrhythmic death in patients treated with amiodarone compared with placebo.
- Post hoc analysis demonstrated that a combination of amiodarone and β-blocker had a significant mortality benefit (unadjusted all-cause mortality reduction of 60–72%).

SCD-HeFT (Sudden Cardiac Death in Heart Failure Trial)[4]

- Randomized placebo-controlled trial.
- Demonstrated that in patients with NYHA class II or III HF and LV ejection fraction ≤35% on optimal medical therapy, while ICD therapy reduced all-cause mortality, amiodarone had no favourable effect.

Sotalol

SWORD (Survival With Oral D-Sotalol)[5]

- Randomized placebo-controlled trial.
- Demonstrated that in patients with LV ejection fraction of ≤40% and either a recent MI or symptomatic HF with a remote MI, sotalol was associated with an increased mortality, presumed 2° to arrhythmias (5.0% mortality in sotalol group compared with 3.1% in placebo group).

Class I antiarrhythmics

CAST I (The Cardiac Arrhythmia Suppression Trial)[6]

- Randomized placebo-controlled trial.
- Demonstrated that in post-MI patients with ventricular premature depolarizations, encainide and flecainide were associated with increased mortality and non-fatal cardiac arrests compared to placebo (encainide and flecainide-treated patients had a 3.6-fold excessive risk of arrhythmic death compared with placebo-treated patients).

References

1 *Circulation* 2002; **106**:2694–9.
2 *Lancet* 1997; **349**:667–74.
3 *Lancet* 1997; **349**:675–82.
4 *N Engl J Med* 2005; **352**:225–37.
5 *Lancet* 1996; **348**:7–12.
6 *N Engl J Med* 1989; **321**:406–12.

Bradycardia

Background

Bradycardia is defined as a heart rate of <60bpm. However, patients do not usually develop symptoms until the heart rate falls to <50bpm. Bradycardias can broadly be divided into sinus bradycardia and bradycardia due to AV conduction block.

Sinus bradycardia

Sinus bradycardia may be physiological or pathological. Examples of physiological sinus bradycardia include nocturnal sinus bradycardia and bradycardia in trained athletes. Pathological sinus bradycardia may arise due to extrinsic causes (e.g. drugs, metabolic disorders) or intrinsic sinus node dysfunction i.e. sick sinus syndrome. Sick sinus syndrome is characterized by failure to generate or transmit impulses at the sinus node. Most patients with sinus bradycardia who have normal sinus node function are asymptomatic. Symptoms, e.g. dizziness, syncope, and dyspnoea, are more common in patients with sinus node dysfunction.

Bradycardia due to AV conduction block

AV conduction block can be classified into 1st-degree, 2nd-degree, or 3rd-degree heart block, according to the part of the conduction system affected and the appearance on the surface ECG as follows:

1st-degree heart block
- Majority of cases are due to conduction delay at the level of the AV node.
- ECG is characterized by a prolonged PR interval (PR interval >200ms).

2nd-degree heart block
- Mobitz I:
  - majority of cases are due to conduction delay at the level of the AV node
  - ECG is characterized by progressive prolongation of the PR interval followed by failure to conduct a beat.
- Mobitz II:
  - majority of cases are due to dysfunction of the conduction system distal to the AV node (His–Purkinje system)
  - ECG: constant PR interval with intermittent failure to conduct beats.

3rd-degree heart block
- Majority of cases are due to dysfunction of the conduction system distal to the AV node (His–Purkinje system).
- ECG: complete AV dissociation.

1st-degree and Mobitz I 2nd-degree heart block are generally considered to be benign conditions and may be physiological (e.g. in patients with high vagal tone) or pathological. Mobitz II 2nd-degree AV block and 3rd-degree AV block are almost always pathological and may arise due to degeneration or injury to conduction tissue. Mobitz II 2nd-degree AV block is associated with a higher risk of developing symptomatic bradycardias and progressing to 3rd-degree AV block. In patients with 3rd-degree AV block, atrial impulses are not conducted to the ventricles and an escape rhythm is generated from an accessory pacemaker distal to the AV node. The escape rhythm may originate from the bundle of His or the distal ventricular conduction system. Patients with more distal ventricular pacemakers have a broad complex escape rhythm on the surface ECG.

In patients with partial AV block, i.e. bundle branch block and fascicular block, AV conduction is maintained and therefore bradycardia is rare. There is, however, a risk of progression to complete heart block and hence symptomatic bradycardia. In isolated bundle branch or fascicular block, progression to complete heart block is rare. In patients with bifascicular and trifascicular block, the risk of development of complete heart block is higher; however, the overall incidence is still low.

In patients with AV block, symptoms are more common with higher degrees of block. Most patients with 1st-degree and Mobitz I 2nd-degree AV block are asymptomatic. Patients with higher degrees of AV block may present with symptoms such as dizziness, syncope, shortness of breath, fatigue, and chest pain. Patients with complete heart block, especially those with a broad complex escape rhythm, are at risk of developing haemodynamic compromise due to severe bradycardia or asystolic cardiac arrest. Those with QT prolongation are also at risk of torsades de pointes.

Management of bradycardias

The following section is divided into management of acute bradycardias and management of bradycardias in the chronic setting. The role of pharmacological agents is restricted to management of acute bradycardia, which is the main focus of this chapter.

Acute management of bradycardias

The management of acute bradycardia depends on the severity of the bradycardia, the haemodynamic effect of the bradycardia, and the underlying cause of the bradycardia. Principles of management of symptomatic bradycardias in the acute setting include correction of reversible underlying causes and, where appropriate, the use of drugs to increase heart rate or temporary cardiac pacing.

The algorithm in Fig. 4.8 outlines the 2005 European Resuscitation Council guidelines[1] for management of acute bradycardia. The next section contains a discussion on the role of drugs for management of acute bradycardia and guidelines for specific management of drug-induced bradycardia.

Drugs for acute management of bradycardias

Atropine is considered the 1st-line pharmacological agent for acute management of severe or haemodynamically compromising bradycardia. In patients who do not respond to initial treatment with atropine, transcutaneous pacing is usually the next step. Alternatively, 2nd-line drugs such as adrenaline and dopamine may be used. Pharmacological therapy and transcutaneous pacing are often used as temporizing measures until transvenous pacing is initiated. Table 4.14 outlines guidelines for pharmacological therapy for acute bradycardias which are based on the 2005 American Heart Association Guidelines for Cardiopulmonary Resuscitation and Emergency Cardiovascular Care.[2]

In addition to the drugs listed in Table 4.14, drugs such as isoprenaline and glycopyrronium bromide may be used in certain circumstances for management of acute bradycardias. IV isoprenaline has been used as a 2nd-line agent for management of acute symptomatic bradycardia; however, it has fallen out of favour due to adverse side effects such as hypotension and arrhythmias. Glycopyrronium bromide is commonly used during anaesthesia to block vagal inhibitory reflexes.

References

1 Nolan JP *et al.* (2005). European Resuscitation Council Guidelines for Resuscitation 2005. *Resuscitation* **67**(Suppl 1):S39–S86.

2 AHA (2005). 2005 American Heart Association Guidelines for Cardiopulmonary Resuscitation and Emergency Cardiovascular Care. *Circulation* **112**:IV-67–IV-77.

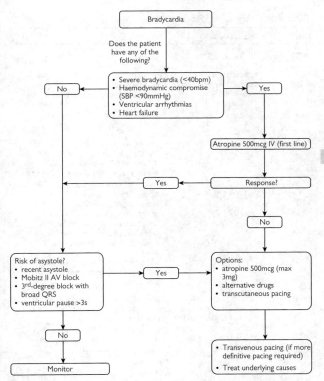

Fig. 4.8 Treatment algorithm for acute bradycardia. Data from Brignole M et al. (2004). Guidelines on management (diagnosis and treatment) of syncope–update 2004. *Europace* **6**:467–537.[1]

Table 4.14 Drugs to increase heart rate

Drug	Indications	Comments
Atropine	1st-line drug for treatment of acute symptomatic bradycardia (level of evidence IIa)	Initial dose 0.5mg IV (repeat to a maximum dose of 3mg) More useful in patients with: • sinus bradycardia • Mobitz I 2nd-degree heart block • 3rd-degree heart block with high Purkinje or AV nodal escape rhythm Ineffective or less effective in patients with: • sick sinus syndrome • Mobitz II 2nd-degree heart block • 3rd-degree heart block with low Purkinje or ventricular escape rhythm Use with caution in patients with coronary ischaemia: • can precipitate ventricular arrhythmias • in ischaemia-induced conduction block atropine may increase oxygen demand of AV node and worsen block • increase in heart rate may worsen ischaemia or increase the zone of infarction
Adrenaline	2nd-line agent—may be used for persistent severe bradycardia if atropine or temporary pacing fails (level of evidence IIb)	Can be used as a temporary measure until definitive pacing is instituted or if pacing is not available Particularly useful if hypotension is an issue (due to vasoconstricting effect) Infusion 2–10mcg/min (titrate against response) Use with caution in patients with coronary ischaemia—can exacerbate ischaemia
Dopamine	2nd-line agent—may be used for persistent severe bradycardia if atropine or temporary pacing fails (level of evidence IIb)	Can be used as temporary measure until definitive pacing instituted or if pacing is not available Infusion 5–20mcg/kg/min (titrate against response) Can be administered alone or added to adrenaline Use with caution in patients with coronary ischaemia—can exacerbate ischaemia

Management of drug-induced bradycardias

In the majority of patients with drug-induced bradycardia, the only treatment required is withdrawal of the offending drug. Common cardiac drugs that may cause bradycardia include β-blockers, CCBs, digoxin, class I antiarrhythmics, and class III antiarrhythmics. Non-cardiac drugs that may induce bradycardia are covered in 📖 Non-cardiac drugs affecting the heart, p.637.

In patients with bradycardia 2° to toxic levels of rate-slowing drugs, in addition to the drugs listed in Table 4.15, specific antidotes may be used in certain circumstances. Such measures are often reserved for patients with profound bradycardia with evidence of end-organ hypoperfusion or a high likelihood of clinical deterioration.

Table 4.15 Specific treatment options for bradycardia 2° to drug toxicity

Drug causing bradycardia	Treatment	Comments
β-blocker	Glucagon	1st-line antidote
		Inotropic effect not mediated by β-receptors; therefore more effective for β-blocker toxicity
		2–10mg bolus followed by 2–5mg/h infusion
	Inotropes: adrenaline, dobutamine, isoprenaline	Competitive β-receptor agonists
		High doses often required to overcome the effect of β-blockade
	Phosphodiesterase inhibitors: amrinone, milrinone	Inotropic; however, causes peripheral vasodilatation which exacerbates hypotension—therefore not commonly used
		Can be used in combination with vasoconstricting inotropes
	High-dose insulin	Evidence restricted to case reports
		Infusion in combination with dextrose— monitor glucose and potassium
CCBs	IV calcium	1st-line antidote
		Partially overcomes calcium blockade
		Calcium chloride or calcium gluconate can be given as boluses or infusion—monitor levels
	Glucagon	Can be used as bolus or infusion: 2–10mg bolus followed by 2–5mg/h infusion
	High-dose insulin	As with β-blocker, toxicity evidence restricted to case reports
Digoxin	Digoxin-specific antibodies (digibind)	1st-line antidote
		Digoxin-specific antibodies (Fab fragments)
		Also indicated for haemodynamically unstable arrhythmias induced by digoxin toxicity

Management of bradycardias in the chronic setting

The management of patients with bradycardias in the chronic setting depends on the presence of symptoms, the correlation of symptoms to the bradycardia, and the underlying cause of the bradycardia. Patients with physiological bradycardia are usually asymptomatic and do not require specific treatment. The management of symptomatic bradycardias due to extrinsic causes involves correction of potential underlying causes, e.g. withdrawal of rate-limiting drugs. Pacemaker implantation represents the mainstay of treatment of patients with intrinsic conduction disease who have symptomatic bradycardia. Pacemaker implantation may also be indicated in asymptomatic patients with high-degree AV block and patients with incomplete AV block (bundle block and fascicular block) who are deemed to have a high risk of developing high-degree AV block.

The following section summarizes the ACC/AHA/HRS (2008) indications for permanent cardiac pacing in patients with sinus bradycardia, bradycardia due to AV conduction block, or incomplete AV block.

Indications for permanent pacing in patients with sinus node dysfunction (SND)

Class I indications

- Sinus bradycardia (<40bpm) with symptoms clearly related to the bradycardia
- Sinus node dysfunction with symptomatic chronotropic incompetence
- Symptomatic sinus bradycardia induced by drug therapy which is required for other medical conditions

Class II indications

- Sinus bradycardia (<40bpm) with symptoms; however, no clear association demonstrated between symptoms and bradycardia
- SND (on EP studies) and unexplained syncope
- Sinus bradycardia with rates <40bpm whilst awake with minimal symptoms

Indications for permanent pacing in patients with AV block

Class I indications

- Complete (3rd-degree) heart block
- Advanced 2nd-degree heart block
- Mobitz I or Mobitz II 2nd-degree AV block with symptoms

Class II indications

- 1st-degree heart block with adverse haemodynamic effects due to a prolonged AV delay
- Asymptomatic Mobitz II 2nd-degree AV block with narrow QRS (type II 2nd-degree AV block with a wide QRS is a class I recommendation)

Indications for permanent pacing in patients with incomplete AV block

Class I indications
- Advanced 2nd-degree AV block or intermittent 3rd-degree AV block
- Type II AV block
- Alternating bundle branch block

Class IIa indications
- Syncope not demonstrated to be due to AV block when other likely causes have been excluded, specifically VT

Neurocardiogenic syncope

Background

Neurocardiogenic syncope, also known as vasovagal syncope, is an example of a neurally mediated syncope. It is the most common cause of syncope and is usually associated with a benign prognosis. Some patients, however, experience recurrent episodes of syncope, which can be severely disabling.

The pathophysiology of neurocardiogenic syncope is incompletely understood. It is believed to be due to triggering of a paradoxical reflex. Under normal circumstances, when peripheral blood pooling occurs (e.g. on standing), decreased venous return results in sympathetic activation which increases heart rate and causes peripheral vasoconstriction. In patients with neurocardiogenic syncope, vigorous cardiac contraction due to sympathetic activation is thought to activate a paradoxical reflex. The reflex results in suppression of the sympathetic nervous system and paradoxical activation of the parasympathetic nervous system. This results in a cardio-inhibitory (bradycardia) or a vasodepressor (peripheral vasodilatation) response, or a mixture of both. The overall effect is hypotension, which results in cerebral hypoperfusion and transient syncope.

A wide variety of stimuli can trigger an episode of syncope. Typical triggers include:
- prolonged periods of standing
- prolonged exposure to heat
- dehydration
- emotional distress
- painful stimuli
- urination
- defecation
- coughing

Syncope almost always occurs when the patient is in the upright position. The onset of syncope may be abrupt or, more commonly, may be preceded by prodromal symptoms such as light-headedness, diaphoresis, nausea, and visual disturbances. Loss of consciousness is usually brief and recovery rapid.

Diagnosis of neurocardiogenic syncope requires a detailed assessment for exclusion of other potential causes of syncope, e.g. cardiac arrhythmias. The investigation of choice is the head-up tilt test—a provocative test aimed at inducing syncope under controlled circumstances. A tilt test is considered positive if syncope is reproduced with a significant cardio-inhibitory or vasodepressor response, or a combination of both.

Management of neurocardiogenic syncope

In the majority of patients presenting with neurocardiogenic syncope, management involves reassurance and patient education. General measures for avoidance of recurrent syncope include:

• recognition and avoidance of triggers
• recognition of prodromal symptoms and use of physical manoeuvres to avoid syncope
• increased intake of salt and water
• manoeuvres to reduce peripheral blood pooling, e.g. orthostatic training, graded support stockings, etc
• withdrawal of vasodilator drugs.

In a small proportion of cases, i.e. patients with recurrent syncope who do not respond to the lifestyle measures, pharmacological therapy and permanent pacing may be considered. However, evidence to demonstrate efficacy of either strategy is limited. This section contains a discussion on pharmacological therapy for management of neurocardiogenic syncope and indications for permanent pacing.

Drug therapy for treatment of neurocardiogenic syncope

A variety of different drugs have been used for treatment of recurrent neurocardiogenic syncope. However, most of the evidence is limited to non-randomized studies or short-term RCTs. The majority of large long-term randomized trials have failed to demonstrate benefit. Table 4.16 contains a list of drugs and summarizes the evidence for their use in treatment of neurocardiogenic syncope. Where available, the level of evidence and class of indication from the 2004 ESC guidelines for management of syncope has been specified.[1] For the majority of drugs, however, there are no recommendations due to a lack of evidence.

Table 4.16 Drugs for management of neurocardiogenic syncope

Drug	Comments
β-blockers	Most commonly used drugs for treatment of neurocardiogenic syncope
	Majority of large RCTs have failed to demonstrate efficacy[2–4] (class III indication/level of evidence A)
	Exact mechanism of action unclear. Thought to suppress catecholinergic surge, which in turn suppresses the paradoxical reflex
	Use with caution in patients with marked cardioinhibitory response—negative chronotropy may enhance cardioinhibitory response
α-blockers (midodrine, etilefrine)	Commonly used for treatment of neurocardiogenic syncope
	Midodrine has been shown to be effective in a number of small trials. Evidence from large randomized trials lacking[5–7]
	Etilefrine failed to demonstrate efficacy in a randomized controlled trial[8] (class III indication/level of evidence B)
	Mechanism of action: increases arterial tone, which counters vasodepressor response. Also increases venous tone which reduces peripheral pooling of blood.
	Potential harmful side effect: hypertension
Fludrocortisone	Insufficient evidence to support its use
	Mechanism of action: volume expansion by salt and water retention
	Potential harmful side effects in elderly patients: hypertension oedema, cardiac failure
Disopyramide	Not generally recommended as 1st line due to potential side effects
	Has been used in cases resistant to conventional 1st-line drugs
	Potential harmful side effects: proarrhythmic effect (class I antiarrhythmic) negatively inotropic
	One RCT failed to show efficacy—insufficient evidence to prove efficacy[9]
	Mechanism of action: not clearly understood. Anticholinergic effect may counteract excessive vagal activity and suppress cardioinhibitory response.
SSRIs (e.g. paroxetine)	Not generally recommended as 1st line
	Have been used in cases resistant to conventional medical treatment
	Evidence limited to one small RCT—insufficient evidence to prove efficacy[10]
	Mechanism of action: unclear. Thought to modify the baroreflex response centrally. Central serotonergic neuronal pathways involved in neural regulation of cardiovascular function.

Table 4.16 *(Contd.)*

Drug	Comments
Theophylline	Not generally recommended as 1st line due to potential side effects
	Evidence limited to uncontrolled reports—insufficient evidence to prove efficacy[11]
	Has been used in cases resistant to conventional medical treatment (rarely)
	Mechanism of action: non-selective and competitive PDE-3 and -5 inhibitor adenosine receptor antagonist

Permanent pacing for treatment of neurocardiogenic syncope

Implantation of permanent pacemakers in patients with neurocardiogenic syncope is controversial. Overall, pacing plays a minor role and is indicated in selected patients, i.e. patients with predominantly cardioinhibitory syncope. The 2008 ACC/AHA/HRS indications for pacemaker implantation in patients with neurocardiogenic syncope are listed here:[12]

Class IIa indication
• Permanent pacing is reasonable for syncope without clear, provocative events and with a hypersensitive cardioinhibitory response of ≥3s or longer.

Class IIb indication
• Permanent pacing may be considered for significantly symptomatic neurocardiogenic syncope associated with bradycardia documented spontaneously or at the time of tilt-table testing.

References

1 Brignole M et al. (2004). Guidelines on management (diagnosis and treatment) of syncope – update 2004. *Europace* 6:467–537.

2 Sheldon R et al.; POST Investigators (2006). Prevention of Syncope Trial (POST). A randomized, placebo-controlled study of metoprolol in the prevention of vasovagal syncope. *Circulation* 113:1164–70.

3 Flevari P et al. (2002). Vasovagal syncope: a prospective, randomized, crossover evaluation of the effect of propranolol, nadolol and placebo on syncope recurrence and patients' well-being. *J Am Coll Cordial* 40:499–504.

4 Madrid AH et al. (2001). Lack of efficacy of atenolol for the prevention of neurally mediated syncope in a highly symptomatic population: a prospective, double-blind, randomized and placebo-controlled study. *J Am Coll Cardiol* 37:554–9.

5 Perez-Lugones A et al. (2001). Usefulness of midodrine in patients with severely symptomatic neurocardiogenic syncope: a randomized control study. *J Cardiovasc Electrophysiol* 12:935–8.

6 Ward CR et al. (1998). Midodrine: a role in the management of neurocardiogenic syncope. *Heart* 79:45–9.

7 Kaufmann H et al. (2002). Midodrine in neurally mediated syncope: a double-blind, randomized, crossover study. *Ann Neurol* 52:342–5.

8 Raviele A et al. (1999). Effect of etilefrine in preventing syncopal recurrence in patients with vasovagal syncope: a double-blind, randomized, placebo-controlled trial. The Vasovagal Syncope International Study. *Circulation* 99:1452–7.

9 Morillo CA *et al.* (1993). A placebo-controlled trial of intravenous and oral disopyramide for prevention of neurally mediated syncope induced by head-up tilt. *J Am Coll Cardiol* **22**:1843–8.

10 Di Girolamo E *et al.* (1999). Effects of paroxetine hydrochloride, a selective serotonin reuptake inhibitor, on refractory vasovagal syncope: a randomized, double-blind, placebo-controlled study. *J Am Coll Cardiol* **33**:1227–30.

11 Nelson SD *et al.* (1991). The autonomic and hemodynamic effects of oral theophylline in patients with vasodepressor syncope. *Arch Intern Med* **151**:2425–9.

12 Epstein AE *et al.* (2008). ACC/AHA/HRS 2008 Guidelines for Device-Based Therapy of Cardiac Rhythm Abnormalities: a report of the American College of Cardiology/American Heart Association Task Force on Practice Guidelines (Writing Committee to Revise the ACC/AHA/NASPE 2002 Guideline Update for Implantation of Cardiac Pacemakers and Antiarrhythmia Devices) developed in collaboration with the American Association for Thoracic Surgery and Society of Thoracic Surgeons. *J Am Coll Cardiol* **51**:e1–62.

Structural heart disease

Valvular heart disease

The most common causes of 1° structural defects in the heart are valvular heart disease, heart muscle disease (cardiomyopathy), and congenital structural heart diseases. Less commonly, 2° heart damage may be caused by infection.

Any of the four valves of the heart can be affected, although left-sided valvular disease is far more common than right-sided disease.

Mitral stenosis

Mitral stenosis (MS) has become much less prevalent in developed countries, as the main aetiological factor, rheumatic fever, is now rare. Whilst physical examination, chest X-ray (CXR), and ECG can lead to diagnosis, echocardiography has become the mainstay in the assessment of the severity of MS. It detects coexisting mitral regurgitation (MR), enables measurement of LA dimensions, and is used to monitor the outcomes of surgical or percutaneous valvotomy.

Symptoms may not develop for many years but most frequently include exertional dyspnoea.

Medical management

Dyspnoea can be helped by *diuretics* or *long-acting nitrates*. *β-blockers* and NDCCBs improve exercise tolerance by prolonging diastole and increasing LV filling time hence improving cardiac output. Patients in AF require *anticoagulation* with INR in the range 2–3. Class Ic or III antiarrhythmics can postpone the development of AF but are seldom helpful once AF is established. In patients in sinus rhythm, anticoagulation should take place when there is LA thrombus or a history of thromboembolism. It is also recommended when LA diameter is >5cm or spontaneous echo contrast is seen on trans-oesophageal echo.

Surgery is indicated in symptomatic patients or in those with a mitral valve area <1.5cm^2 (1.7–1.8cm^2 if the patient is large).

Mitral regurgitation

MR can be divided into organic (valve leaflet abnormality), ischaemic, and functional.

Organic MR

As with MS, echocardiography is the principal investigation to establish the diagnosis and severity of regurgitation and to monitor progress before and after surgery. Echo should generally be performed every 2 years in moderate MR and yearly in severe MR.

Medical management

- *Nitrates* and *diuretics* reduce filling pressures and *sodium nitroprusside* reduces afterload and hence the degree of regurgitation.
- *Inotropes* are required in cases of cardiogenic shock.
- *Anticoagulation* is required in the presence of AF (either permanent or paroxysmal) or when there is a history of thromboembolism or LA thrombus and *for 3 months after MV repair.*
- *ACEIs* are indicated when there is evidence of LV dysfunction.
- *β-blockers* and *spironolactone* should also be used in the setting of LV dysfunction.
- *Endocarditis prophylaxis* should also be used as appropriate (see 📖 p.218).

Ischaemic MR

This can be chronic, due to tethering by the subvalvular apparatus in LV dilatation, or acute, due to papillary muscle rupture, presenting with acute shock usually in the setting of acute MI. Surgery is often indicated but operative mortality is higher than in organic MR. Acute papillary muscle rupture requires urgent surgery once haemodynamically stabilized by means of IABP and vasodilators. Coronary bypass is usually conducted at the same time as valve replacement/repair.

Functional MR

In this situation, the valve structure is normal but affected by distorted LV architecture as with LV impairment or cardiomyopathy. MR in this setting may be exacerbated by dyssynchrony of the ventricles, and resynchronization therapy may be beneficial.

Medical management

Drug therapy is usually the preferred treatment prior to considering surgical correction of the regurgitant MV.

- *ACEIs* and *β-blockers* may reduce MR by progressive inverse remodelling of the LV.
- *Nitrates* and *diuretics* are useful for treating acute breathlessness.

Mitral valve prolapse

Also known as 'Barlow syndrome', mitral valve prolapse (MVP) is due to abnormal mitral valve apparatus such as excessively large valve leaflets, enlarged annulus, long chordae tendinae, or disordered papillary muscle contraction. Although more common in young women, the disease tends to be more severe in men aged 50 years or over. It is the most common cardiac condition that predisposes to infective endocarditis. Normally, the mitral valve billows slightly into the LA, and mild mitral prolapse is so common that it may be regarded as a normal variant. MVP usually occurs as a 1° condition; however, it may be associated with a variety of conditions such as connective tissue disorders.

Medical management

- *β-blockers* may be helpful if palpitations 2° to arrhythmia are severe. They are also effective for atypical chest pain which may occur in patients with MVP. If the arrhythmias are uncontrollable with β-blockers, then other antiarrhythmic drugs may be utilized.
- *Antiplatelet therapy*, such as aspirin or clopidogrel, is indicated in those patients with a history of TIA or stroke in whom no other cause is apparent. Some recommend prophylaxis with antiplatelet agents in all patients with MVP and a murmur because of a small but significant increase in risk of stroke (10%) in these individuals.
- There is no evidence to support the use of *ACEIs* to halt the progression of MVP to MR. However, these medications may improve the MR in the setting of hypertension.

Mitral valve repair is indicated in patients with MVP and severe MR as this condition is associated with a high risk of sudden cardiac death.

- For infective endocarditis prophylaxis, see 📖 p.218.

Aortic stenosis

Aortic stenosis (AS) has three main causes:
- congenital AS develops due to turbulent flow across a congenitally abnormal aortic valve which may be uni-, bi-, or tricuspid
- rheumatic fever—usually with coexistent mitral valve disease
- degenerative AS is 2° to calcification of the aortic valve and is the commonest cause of AS.

While AS progresses, there are usually no symptoms until the aortic orifice is reduced to about 1.0–1.5cm². At this stage, the usual triad of symptoms consists of angina, syncope, and dyspnoea, progressing to HF. Patients with congenital or rheumatic AS usually present in their 50s and 60s. Those with degenerative AS usually present in their 70s and 80s.

Medical management

Asymptomatic patients should be regularly followed-up with echocardiography, and asked to report any new symptom development. Symptoms of AS are a good marker of severity, and all patients with symptoms should undergo an aortic valve replacement, as medical therapy has little to offer. If the patient is deemed inoperable, then medical intervention has a role.
- *Antibiotic prophylaxis* for infective endocarditis should be considered, and risks/benefits discussed on an individual basis. Good oral hygiene should be encouraged.
- *Cardiac glycosides* can be used as inotropic agents and also to control the ventricular rate in associated AF, which usually occurs late. Treatment of atrial arrhythmia is beneficial as its presence leads to loss of the atrial contribution to ventricular filling.
- *Diuretics* may be used for management of pulmonary and peripheral oedema.
- *ACEIs* may be used for HF and hypertension.
- In selected patients with pulmonary oedema, *sodium nitroprusside* may be used under close supervision.

Practical note: diuretics and ACEIs should be used with caution to avoid critically reducing preload in those with significant AS and a hypertrophic non-compliant LV. β-blockers and CCBs can depress myocardial function thereby precipitating HF and should be avoided.

The progression of degenerative AS is an active process, sharing many similarities with atherosclerosis. Therefore, modification of atherosclerotic risk factors must be recommended following the guidelines for 2° prevention. Recently, several small observational studies suggested that HMG-CoA reductase inhibitors (statins) can reduce aortic valve calcification and delay the progression of AS severity. Although these retrospective studies are promising for a potential role of these drugs in the management of calcific/degenerative aortic valve disease, data are conflicting and the only randomized trial assessing the effect of statin therapy is negative. Therefore, the ESC guidelines state that it is currently too early to provide a recommendation. In similar observational studies, use of ACEIs was associated with slower calcium accumulation in the aortic valve; however, no haemodynamic benefit was seen during the same period.

Aortic regurgitation

Aortic regurgitation (AR) may be caused by 1° disease of the aortic valve leaflets or by disease of the aortic root (see Table 5.1).

Table 5.1 Causes of aortic regurgitation

Valve disease	Aortic root disease
• Rheumatic fever—may result in combined AR and AS • Infective endocarditis • Rheumatoid arthritis • Systemic lupus erythematosus (SLE) • Drugs, e.g. appetite suppressants • Iatrogenic—following aortic valvotomy or deterioration of a prosthetic valve	• Hypertension • Degenerative aortic dilatation • Trauma • Aortic dissection • Seronegative spondyloarthritides e.g. ankylosing spondylitis • Marfan syndrome (cystic medial necrosis) • Osteogenesis imperfecta • Syphilis

History

The main symptoms—dyspnoea, palpitations, and angina—occur late, developing once LV failure has occurred. This is because the LV gradually enlarges while the patient is asymptomatic. 'Pounding' of the heart is particularly troublesome and occurs due to premature ventricular contraction. Arrhythmias, however, are uncommon.

Management

• The risks vs. benefits of antibiotic prophylaxis should be discussed and good oral hygiene recommended (see 🕮 Chapter 6, p.191).
• Asymptomatic patients require no specific treatment; however, regular echocardiographic monitoring of LV function and dimensions is prudent, and may need to be as often as every 6 months in patients with severe AR.
• Some physicians advocate the use of vasodilators in asymptomatic patients to retard LV enlargement and dysfunction and delay the need for surgery; however, the ESC guidelines state that this is unproven.
• Vasodilator therapy is useful in preparing patients for surgery. In hypertensive asymptomatic patients, treatment with *ACEIs* or *dihydropyridine CCBs* is recommended (ESC guideline). Symptomatic patients usually require surgical intervention, and this should be performed before significant symptoms occur.
• Those patients who are unsuitable for surgery should commence treatment with *ACEIs*, *diuretics*, *digoxin*, and salt restriction.
• *β-blockers* should be used with extreme caution as they lengthen diastole, thereby increasing the regurgitant volume. However, they are useful for patients with Marfan syndrome as they slow the progression of aortic dilatation.

- Acute AR is a medical emergency, rapidly leading to LV failure and cardiogenic shock. The treatment of choice is aortic valve replacement. Medical therapy can be used as a bridge to surgery but should not replace it. Inotropic agents such as *dobutamine* or *dopamine* reduce afterload and thus assist with outflow. Afterload reduction with *sodium nitroprusside* improves cardiac performance, greatly decreases LV preload, and reduces aortic regurgitant volume.

Tricuspid disease

Tricuspid stenosis

Tricuspid stenosis (TS) is now rare in the Western world as it is almost always 2° to rheumatic fever. Rarer causes of TS include carcinoid syndrome, endomyocardial fibrosis, SLE, tumours of the RA, and congenital tricuspid atresia. Frequently, TS is associated with other valve pathology especially mitral stenosis.

Medical management

- This should be focused on management of the underlying cause.
- Any arrhythmias should be addressed.
- Endocarditis prophylaxis should be given as appropriate.
- Sodium restriction and *diuretic* therapy may eliminate fluid overload and its associated symptoms, as well as improving hepatic function.

TS is largely a surgical condition and requires either commissurotomy or replacement of the valve if right heart failure or low cardiac output has resulted. As TS is rarely an isolated lesion, surgery usually involves multiple valves.

Tricuspid regurgitation

Causes of tricuspid regurgitation (TR) are either organic or, more commonly, functional. Functional TR occurs whenever the RV dilates, i.e. with any cause of RV failure. The most common cause is mitral valve disease (see Table 5.2).

Table 5.2 Causes of tricuspid regurgitation

Functional causes (normal valve)	Organic causes (abnormal valve)
<ul><li>Cor pulmonale</li><li>MI</li><li>Pulmonary hypertension</li><li>Congenital heart disease, e.g. pulmonary stenosis and Eisenmenger syndrome</li><li>Dilated cardiomyopathy</li></ul>	<ul><li>Rheumatic heart disease</li><li>Infective endocarditis (particularly *Staphylococcus* from IV drug misuse)</li><li>Carcinoid syndrome</li><li>Ebstein anomaly</li><li>Tricuspid valve prolapse (occurs in 20% of patients with MVP)</li><li>Connective tissue disorders e.g.:<ul><li>Marfan syndrome</li><li>Ehler–Danlos syndrome</li><li>Osteogenesis imperfecta</li></ul></li></ul>

Treatment is again determined largely by the underlying cause.
- If the TR is 2° to left heart failure, then medical management centres on the control of fluid overload and symptoms of HF and *diuretic* therapy may be required.
- Other medications include *cardiac glycosides* and *ACEIs*.

Surgical treatment is required in the presence of the following:
- structural deformity of the valve
- infective endocarditis
- TR uncontrolled with medical therapy.

Pulmonary valve disease

Medical options for management are limited for disease of the pulmonary valve.

Pulmonary stenosis

Pulmonary stenosis (PS) is commonly congenital and is associated with Turner syndrome, Noonan syndrome, Williams syndrome, congenital rubella infection, and tetralogy of Fallot. The rare acquired causes include rheumatic fever and carcinoid syndrome (in association with tricuspid valve disease).

Management

Infective endocarditis prophylaxis is administered as necessary. In neonates, prostaglandins are administered if there is duct-dependent circulation. In adults, treatment is indicated if the patient is symptomatic, or asymptomatic with RVOT gradient >50mmHg. Balloon dilatation of the pulmonary valve performed during cardiac catheterization has replaced surgical pulmonary valvotomy as the treatment of choice.

Pulmonary regurgitation

Pulmonary regurgitation (PR) is caused by any condition that causes pulmonary hypertension. Other causes include Marfan syndrome, Takayasu arteritis, rheumatic heart disease (rare), infective endocarditis, carcinoid syndrome, and iatrogenic damage.

Management

Specific treatment of PR is rarely necessary. This is because the RV normally adapts to low-pressure volume overload without difficulty. However, treatment of the underlying condition is warranted in severe PR. *Cardiac glycosides* may be helpful if right heart failure exists.

Antithrombotic management in valve heart disease

Approximately 75% of complications after valve replacement relate to thromboembolism or bleeding from over-anticoagulation.

Indications for oral anticoagulation:
- lifelong in patients with mechanical heart valves (INR 2.5–4 depending on thrombogenicity of mechanical valve, site of valve, and presence of patient risk factors for thromboembolism)
- for first 3 months in patients with bioprostheses (INR target 2.5) although aspirin 75–100mg can be considered as alternative
- lifelong in patients with bioprostheses with other conditions requiring anticoagulation, e.g. AF, LVEF <30%.

Oral anticoagulation is usually initiated in the first few postoperative days and heparin is used as a bridge to attaining therapeutic INR. The first post-operative month represents the highest risk of valve thrombosis and INR should be regularly checked to avoid subtherapy.

Type of valve and target INR

Patient factors that predispose to thromboembolism are non-aortic position, concurrent LA enlargement, AF, previous thromboembolism or dense spontaneous echo contrast, LVEF <35%, and hypercoagulable state.

Excessive anticoagulation

INR >6 requires reversal of anticoagulation—in this case the patient requires admission to hospital to allow temporary withdrawal of the anti-coagulant and close monitoring of the falling INR. If INR is >10 it is likely that fresh frozen plasma will be required. More active reversal is required with the use of vitamin K if spontaneous bleeding occurs.

Interruption of anticoagulation

Some minor surgical procedures do not require complete reversal of anti-coagulation and if possible INR reduced to 2. If major surgery is needed, prior admission is necessary to switch the patient to IV unfractionated heparin. This should be stopped 6h prior to operation and recommenced 6–12h postoperatively.

Prosthetic valve thrombosis

This requires treatment and reversal of provoking factors. Thrombolytic agents should be infused for 24–72h with heparin and aspirin co-administered. If no response, or in the case of large or mobile thrombi, surgery is required.

Further reading

Hering D et al. (2001). Management of prosthetic valve thrombosis. Eur Heart J Suppl **3**:Q22–6.

Cardiomyopathy

Disease of the heart muscle is referred to as cardiomyopathy. Broadly there are three main types of functional impairment in cardiomyopathy although often there is some overlap:

- hypertrophic cardiomyopathy (HCM)
- dilated cardiomyopathy (DCM)
- restrictive cardiomyopathy.

Hypertrophic cardiomyopathy

HCM affects 1 in 500 people. It can occur at any age and is character-ized by asymmetrical ventricular septal hypertrophy in the absence of an obvious cause for the hypertrophy. Many cases of HCM are familial, with autosomal dominant inheritance; 50% of cases are sporadic. HCM can cause clinical symptoms at all ages; dyspnoea (usually 2° to diastolic dysfunction), angina (due to increased myocardial oxygen demand and abnormal microvasculature), palpitations (AF commonest associated arrhythmia), syncope, and sudden death.

Management

The priority in the management of HCM is prevention of sudden death. Otherwise, it is directed towards minimizing symptoms and reducing complications. The use of prophylactic drug therapy in asymptomatic or minimally symptomatic patients to prevent or delay disease progression remains unfounded. The majority of patients only require medical therapy, with 5–10% requiring surgical intervention. Approximately half of patients treated medically will experience symptomatic benefit. Medical therapy involves the use of β-blockers, CCBs, and disopyramide. Infective endo-carditis prophylaxis tends to be needed only for those with an outflow gradient. AF should be treated accordingly, as loss of the atrial contribu-tion to ventricular filling leads to deterioration.

- *β-blockers:* reduce myocardial oxygen demand and improve LV filling via their negative chronotropic effect. As such, they may alleviate angina, as well as dyspnoea and syncope. Patient responses to drugs are highly variable in terms of magnitude and duration of benefit, and the selection of medications has not achieved widespread standardization and has been dependent, in part, on the experiences of individual practitioners, investigators, and centres.[1] As there is little evidence suggesting that β-blocking agents consistently reduce outflow obstruction under resting conditions, they are preferred for symptomatic patients with outflow gradients present only with exertion.

- *Calcium-channel blockers (up to 480mg verapamil daily sustained release):* often utilized in symptomatic patients who are unresponsive to β-blockers, or suffer from asthma. There is no evidence that the combined medical therapy of β-blockers and CCBs is more advantageous than the use of either drug alone. The benefit of CCBs is thought to derive from their ability to address the hypercontractile systolic function while improving diastolic relaxation and filling of the LV. Caution is needed when administering these drugs, especially in those with high LV filling pressure, as their vasodilator property may exaggerate the LV outflow gradient, causing cardiac failure and sudden death.

- *Disopyramide:* this class Ia antiarrhythmic drug is used as 2nd-line therapy in patients with an outflow gradient who are non-responsive to either β-blockers or calcium-channel antagonists. Disopyramide may cause accelerated AV node conduction, thus leading to increased ventricular rate during AF; therefore, concomitant therapy with low-dose β-blockers is recommended to achieve normal resting heart rate.[1]

Cardiac glycosides may be utilized if there is AF, or if systolic dysfunction is present. The latter may also be an indication for diuretic therapy. In patients with a high risk of sudden cardiac death (those with non-sustained ventricular tachycardia on Holter monitoring or recurrent syncope), ICD therapy is indicated. For those with a lower risk, amiodarone is a suitable alternative.

Other therapeutic options include DDD (dual chamber) pacing, alcohol septal ablation therapy, and resection of the hypertrophied myocardium. 'End stage' or 'dilated' HCM requires treatment with ACEIs, diuretics, cardiac glycosides, β-blockers, or spironolactone, in a bid to reduce afterload. Eventually, cardiac transplantation may be needed.

Dilated cardiomyopathy

Myocardial damage can be caused by a variety of infective metabolic, cytotoxic inherited, and immunological mechanisms. As the cause is often neither known nor reversible, treatment is symptomatic and largely as in standard treatment of HF, i.e. diuretics, ACE inhibition, β-blockade, aldosterone antagonism (spironolactone), and digoxin (see 📖 Chapter 1, p.3). If ACE inhibition is not tolerated, vasodilatation with hydralazine and nitrate therapy can be considered.

As an autoimmune process has been implicated in the pathophysiology of DCM, immunosuppressants have been used but results have been disappointing.

Supraventricular arrhythmias in DCM can be treated/prevented with use of class III agents such as amiodarone, but there is little evidence to support their use in suppression of ventricular arrhythmias, and ICD therapy or definitive surgical treatment (i.e. cardiac transplant) is often required.

Restrictive cardiomyopathy

See 📖 Chapter 10, p.297.

Marfan syndrome

Marfan syndrome is a congenital connective tissue disorder demonstrating autosomal dominant inheritance. It has a worldwide prevalence of 2–3 per 10,000 subjects. Diagnosis largely depends on identifying the cardinal manifestations in the eye, skeleton, and cardiovascular system. Other systems involved include the integument, pulmonary, and central nervous systems. Cardiovascular disease (primarily aortic root dilatation and dissection) is the major cause of morbidity and mortality.

Manifestations of Marfan syndrome in the cardiovascular system

- Aortic root dilatation (aneurysm)
- Aortic dissection
- AR
- MVR
- MR
- Arrhythmia
- Tricuspid valve prolapse

Medical management

Regular patient monitoring with echocardiography is required. Antibiotic prophylaxis for infective endocarditis is generally recommended for medical procedures likely to cause significant bacteraemia.

β-blocker therapy is the mainstay of medical treatment. β-blockers work by reducing aortic root expansion and therefore delay progression to aortic root dissection. The patient should be counselled regarding the requirement of long-term β-blocker therapy, avoiding exertion (because of ocular, cardiac, and skeletal involvement) and the risk of passing the condition to their children.

Management in pregnancy

Of importance: if the aortic root diameter is >4.2cm in the sinus of Valsalva at commencement of pregnancy, the risk of dissection is at least 10% during pregnancy. β-blocker therapy should be commenced, serial echocardiograms performed, and delivery by Caesarean section considered if the aortic root enlarges significantly during pregnancy.

Reference

1 Maron BJ et al. (2003). American College of Cardiology/European Society of Cardiology Clinical Expert Consensus Document on Hypertrophic Cardiomyopathy. *Eur Heart J* **24**:1965–91.

Further reading

Elliott P (2000). Diagnosis and management of dilated cardiomyopathy. *Heart* **84**:106–12.
Vahanian A et al.; Task Force on the Management of Valvular Heart Disease of the European Society of Cardiology (2007). Guidelines on the management of valvular heart disease. *Eur Heart J* **28**:230–68.

Infective and inflammatory cardiac conditions

Infective endocarditis

Infective endocarditis is an infection of the endocardium which usually involves the heart valves. In current clinical practice, endocarditis encompasses a heterogeneous collection of infections that may involve native cardiac tissues, prosthetic valves, pacing systems, and a variety of intra-cardiac implants. Endocarditis is mainly caused by bacteria, but fungi are occasionally implicated.

Causes of endocarditis

- *Streptococcus* species: oral streptococci, *Strep. bovis*, *Strep. pneumoniae*, β-haemolytic streptococci
- *Staphylococcus* species: *Staph. aureus*, *Staph. epidermidis*
- *Enterococcus* species: *E. faecalis*, *E. faecium*
- HACEK organisms: *Haemophilus*, *Actinobacillus*, *Cardiobacterium*, *Eikenella*, and *Kingella* spp.
- Other rare bacterial causes: *Coxiella burnetii*, *Bartonella* spp., *Listeria* spp., *Corynebacterium* spp., *Brucella* spp., *Mycobacterium* spp., *Tropheryma* spp., *Pseudomonas* spp., *Enterobacteriaceae*, *Neisseria* spp., *Chlamydia* spp., *Mycoplasma* spp.
- Fungal endocarditis: *Candida*, *Aspergillus*

In a proportion of cases, no organism is identified, so-called culture negative endocarditis.

The risk of developing endocarditis is significantly higher in patients with structurally abnormal hearts. Conditions associated with increased risk include:
- prosthetic heart valves
- degenerative valve disease (with stenosis or regurgitation)
- rheumatic valve disease
- congenital heart disease, especially complex cyanotic congenital heart disease
- previous history of endocarditis.

Certain patient groups, such as haemodialysis patients or IV drug users, also have a higher risk of developing endocarditis.

Diagnosis of endocarditis

The clinical presentation of endocarditis is variable. Patients may present with an insidious onset of symptoms such as fever, weight loss, night sweats, and malaise. Patients with a more fulminant infection may present with congestive heart failure due to valve destruction. Other cardiac complications include arrhythmias and AV block due to abscess formation. In some cases, patients may present with extra-cardiac complications due to pulmonary and systemic embolization of infected material.

Investigations for suspected endocarditis include:
- blood cultures (3 sets at different times)
- echocardiogram (transthoracic ± transoesophageal)
- ECG
- urinalysis
- blood tests: FBC, inflammatory markers
- serology
- valve culture ± molecular diagnostics (e.g. 16S rDNA gene polymerase chain reaction (PCR)).

Criteria for diagnosis

The modified Dukes' classification is the most widely accepted system for diagnosis of infective endocarditis. It relies upon either pathological diagnosis (i.e. on autopsy or surgical samples) or clinical diagnosis. The clinical criteria are listed in Box 6.1.

Box 6.1 Modified Dukes' classification

Major criteria
- Positive blood cultures (two separate cultures of a typical infective endocarditis micro-organism e.g. oral streptococcus; persistently positive blood cultures; or serological evidence of infection with *Coxiella burnetii*)
- Positive echocardiographic findings (e.g. oscillating mass and/or vegetation, paravalvular abscess, or dehiscence of a prosthetic valve)
- New or changing murmur

Minor criteria
- Predisposition (e.g. history of IV drug use or congenital heart disease)
- Fever (temperature >38°C)
- Vascular phenomena (arterial emboli, septic pulmonary infarcts, intracranial haemorrhage, conjunctival haemorrhage, Janeway lesions)
- Immunologic phenomena (glomerulonephritis, Osler nodes, Roth spots, positive result for rheumatoid factor)
- Positive blood cultures without meeting the criteria already listed, or serological evidence of active infection consistent with endocarditis

---

Using the criteria in Box 6.1, suspected cases of endocarditis are classified as definite, possible, or rejected as follows:

Definite endocarditis
- 2 major clinical criteria
- 1 major and three minor criteria
- 5 minor criteria

Possible endocarditis
- 1 major and 1 or 2 minor criteria
- 3 minor criteria

Diagnosis of endocarditis rejected if:
- clinical criteria for definite or possible endocarditis are not met
- a firm alternative diagnosis is made
- there is resolution of clinical manifestations after ≤4 days of antimicrobial therapy.

Treatment of endocarditis

The mainstay of treatment for infective endocarditis is antimicrobial therapy. In a proportion of patients, valve surgery may be required in addition to antimicrobials. The indications for surgical intervention include:

- severe heart failure secondary to acute valvular regurgitation
- severe persisting infection despite adequate antimicrobial therapy
- perivalvular extension of infection with complications such as abscess formation, development of abnormal communications, e.g. fistulas
- treatment of endocarditis caused by organisms resistant to antimicrobial therapy, e.g. fungal endocarditis
- surgery may be considered in patients with large vegetations and recurrent embolic events.

Antimicrobial therapy for treatment of endocarditis is generally administered parenterally. This practice is largely determined by the poor oral bioavailability of the predominant agents used to treat endocarditis, such as benzylpenicillin and vancomycin, rather than clear evidence that IV therapy is superior. 'High-dose' regimens are usually recommended, again without a clear evidence base. When antimicrobial agents with good oral bioavailability are chosen and there are no other factors that would preclude oral therapy, there is no reason why oral agents cannot be used.

Antimicrobial agents that kill bacteria rather than merely inhibit their growth are known as *bactericidal* agents. Those that inhibit growth without killing them are known as *bacteristatic* agents. Traditional teaching requires the use of bactericidal agents in the treatment of endocarditis and there is clear evidence of treatment failure with bacteristatic agents such as clindamycin.

A related microbiological phenomenon is *tolerance*. Bacteria are said to be tolerant if the minimum amount of antibiotic that will kill them (minimum bactericidal concentration, MBC) is much greater than the minimum amount of antibiotic that will inhibit their growth (minimum inhibitory concentration, MIC).

Prolonged antimicrobial therapy, often with high doses in patients with endocarditis, may be associated with a variety of adverse drug reactions. Examples of common adverse reactions include hypersensitivity reactions, *Clostridium difficile* infection associated with prolonged beta lactam therapy, and nephrotoxicity and ototoxicity associated with vancomycin and gentamicin therapy. The risk of adverse reactions is particularly high when combinations of potentially toxic drugs are used. In patients who develop adverse drug reactions, options include adjusting the dose of antimicrobial or, where appropriate, selecting an alternative antimicrobial. Where possible, laboratory measurement of drug levels may be used to monitor for toxicity and to guide dose adjustment.

The following section outlines the AHA,[1] ESC,[2] and British Society of Antimicrobial Chemotherapy (BSAC)[3] guidelines for antimicrobial therapy for infective endocarditis. For the majority of types of endocarditis, the three working groups have produced similar treatment recommendations. There are, however, marked differences in some areas which have been highlighted. The differences between the guidelines exist mainly due to a lack of large RCTs to evaluate efficacy of different antimicrobials for treatment of endocarditis.

Streptococcal endocarditis

Oral streptococci (e.g. *Strep. sanguinis*, *Strep. oralis*) account for the majority of cases of streptococcal endocarditis. They are a common cause of native valve endocarditis in patients who do not have a history of IV drug abuse. Other less common causes of streptococcal endocarditis include *Strep. bovis*, *Strep. pneumoniae*, *Strep. pyogenes*, Lancefield group B, C, and G streptococci.

The following section focuses on antimicrobial therapy for endocarditis caused by oral streptococci which is identical to therapy for *Strep. bovis*. Group B, C, and G streptococci, *Strep. pyogenes*, and *Strep. pneumoniae* are uncommon causes of endocarditis and are not discussed here.

Oral streptococci and *Strep. bovis* are usually highly penicillin sensitive. A small proportion have intermediate sensitivity and resistance is rare. Treatment is guided by the type of valve (i.e. native or prosthetic) and the organism sensitivity. The guidelines in this section are divided according to the MIC for the causative streptococcal species and the valve type.

The AHA, ESC, and BSAC guidelines for antimicrobial therapy for endocarditis caused by oral streptococci and *Strep. bovis* are very similar. All three working groups recommend therapy with beta lactams or, in patients with penicillin allergy, vancomycin. The main difference between the guidelines relates to whether concomitant use of gentamicin is recommended. There are also subtle differences in antimicrobial dosage, frequency, and duration which are detailed in Tables 6.1 and 6.2.

Native valve endocarditis due to highly penicillin sensitive oral streptococci and Strep. bovis (MIC ≤0.12mg/L)

The AHA, ESC and BSAC guidelines all recommend 4 weeks of monotherapy with either penicillin or ceftriaxone. For patients who are intolerant of penicillin, 4 weeks of vancomycin monotherapy is recommended.

In selected patients who do not have intracardiac complications or extracardiac emboli, 2 weeks of either penicillin (or amoxicillin, ESC) or ceftriaxone in combination with gentamicin (or neticmicin, ESC) is considered adequate therapy by the AHA, ESC and BSAC.

Native valve endocarditis due to oral streptococci and **Strep. bovis** *with reduced susceptibility to penicillin (MIC >0.12mg/L to ≤0.5mg/L)*

The AHA, ESC, and BSAC guidelines recommend 4 weeks of high-dose penicillin in combination with gentamicin for the first 2 weeks (AHA recommend ceftriaxone as an alternative to penicillin while ESC recommend amoxicillin). In patients with a high risk of toxicity associated with gentamicin, e.g. patients with renal impairment, the BSAC guidelines recommend a trial of monotherapy with penicillin at a higher dose (adjusted for renal function). NB: ESC define the upper limit of resistance in this category as 2 mg/L.

In patients who are intolerant of penicillin, AHA recommend 4 weeks of vancomycin monotherapy. The ESC and BSAC guidelines recommend the addition of gentamicin to vancomycin for the first 2 weeks if there are no contraindications to aminoglycoside therapy.

Prosthetic valve endocarditis (PVE) due to oral streptococci and **Strep. bovis**

The AHA and BSAC guidelines recommend 6 weeks of either penicillin or ceftriaxone with the addition of gentamicin for the first 2 weeks in patients with PVE caused by highly sensitive oral streptococci and *Strep. bovis*. In patients with PVE caused by organisms with intermediate sensitivity, a full 6-week course of combination therapy with either penicillin or ceftriaxone and gentamicin is recommended. ESC recommends penicillin (or amoxicillin) or ceftriaxone monotherapy for 6 weeks for highly sensitive organisms. The addition of gentamicin for the first 2 weeks is recommended for organisms with intermediate sensitivity.

In patients who are intolerant of penicillin, AHA recommend vancomycin monotherapy for 6 weeks (irrespective of organism sensitivity). ESC also recommend vancomycin monotherapy for fully sensitive organisms. However, for organisms with intermediate sensitivity the addition of gentamicin for the first 2 weeks is advised. The BSAC guidelines recommend vancomycin for 6 weeks in combination with gentamicin for the first 2 weeks in patients with PVE caused by fully sensitive organisms. For organisms with intermediate sensitivity, a full 6 weeks of combination therapy with vancomycin and gentamicin is recommended.

Endocarditis due to penicillin-resistant oral streptococci and **Strep. bovis**

The antibiotics for management of penicillin-resistant streptococci are the same as those used for management of enterococcal endocarditis.

Table 6.1a Summary of AHA,[1] ESC,[2] and BSAC[3] guidelines for treatment of native valve endocarditis (NVE) caused by oral streptococci and *Strep. bovis*

Indication	AHA	ESC	BSAC	Duration
NVE: organism with high penicillin sensitivity (MIC ≤0.12 mg/L)	Benzylpenicillin	Benzylpenicillin or amoxicillin	Benzylpenicillin	2 weeks
No cardiac, extracardiac, renal complications	+ gentamicin	+ gentamicin or netilmicin	+ gentamicin	2 weeks
NVE: organism with high penicillin sensitivity (MIC ≤0.12 mg/L)	Benzylpenicillin or ceftriaxone	Benzylpenicillin or amoxicillin or ceftriaxone	Benzylpenicillin or ceftriaxone	4 weeks
Reliable therapy required in patients with complications				4 weeks
NVE: organism with reduced susceptibility to penicillin (MIC >0.12mg/L to ≤0.5 mg/L)	Benzylpenicillin* or ceftriaxone + gentamicin	Benzylpenicillin* or amoxicillin + gentamicin	Benzylpenicillin + gentamicin	4 weeks / 4 weeks / 2 weeks
ESC definition: MIC 0.125–2mg/L				
Penicillin/ceftriaxone allergic patients with NVE and organism with high penicillin sensitivity	Vancomycin	Vancomycin	Vancomycin	4 weeks
Penicillin/ceftriaxone allergic patients with NVE: reduced susceptibility to penicillin (MIC >0.12mg/L to ≤0.5 mg/L)	Vancomycin	Vancomycin + gentamicin	Vancomycin + gentamicin	4 weeks / 2 weeks

Antibiotic dosage and frequency

Benzylpenicillin AHA/ESC: 12–18 million units/24h, 4–6 divided doses (IV); BSAC: 1.2–2.4g every 4h (IV).

*Benzylpenicillin** (high dose) AHA/ESC: 24 million units/24h, 4–6 divided doses (IV); BSAC: 14.4g/24h, 6 divided doses (IV).

Ceftriaxone AHA/ESC: 2g/24h, single dose (IV).

Gentamicin AHA/ESC: 3mg/kg/24h, single dose (IV); BSAC: 1mg/kg, every 8–12h (IV).

Vancomycin AHA/ESC: 30mg/kg every 24h, 2 divided doses (IV); BSAC: 1g every 12h (IV).

Table 6.1b Summary of AHA,[1] ESC,[2] and BSAC[3] guidelines for treatment of prosthetic valve endocarditis caused by oral streptococci and *Strep. bovis*

Indication	AHA	ESC	BSAC	Duration	Comments
PVE: organism with high penicillin sensitivity (MIC ≤0.12mcg/mL)	Benzylpenicillin* or ceftriaxone + gentamicin	Benzylpenicillin or amoxicillin or cefriaxone	Benzylpenicillin	Benzylpenicillin 6 weeks / 4–6 weeks / 2 weeks gentamicin	
PVE: organism with reduced susceptibility to penicillin (MIC >0.12mg/L to ≤0.5 mg/L)	Benzylpenicillin* or cefriaxone + gentamicin	Benzylpenicillin or amoxicillin + gentamicin	Benzylpenicillin + gentamicin	Benzylpenicillin 6 weeks / 6 weeks / 2–6 weeks gentamicin	ESC recommend 2 weeks of gentamicin while AHA and BSAC recommend 6 weeks
Penicillin/cefriaxone allergic patients with: PVE: organism with high susceptibility (MIC ≤0.12mcg/mL)	Vancomycin	Vancomycin + gentamicin	Vancomycin + gentamicin	6 weeks / 2 weeks gentamicin	
Penicillin/cefriaxone allergic patients with PVE: organism with: reduced susceptibility to penicillin (MIC >0.12mg/L to ≤0.5 mg/L)	Vancomycin	Vancomycin + gentamicin	Vancomycin + gentamicin	6 weeks / 2 weeks (ESC), 6 weeks (BSAC) gentamicin	

Antibiotic dosage and frequency

Benzylpenicillin BSAC: 1.2–2.4g every 4h (IV).

Benzylpenicillin * (high dose) AHA/ESC: 24 million units/24h, 4–6 divided doses (IV).

Cefriaxone AHA/ESC: 2g/24h, single dose (IV).

Gentamicin AHA/ESC: 3mg/kg/24h; single dose (IV); BSAC: 1mg/kg, every 8–12h (IV).

Vancomycin AHA/ESC: 30mg/kg every 24h, 2 divided doses (IV); BSAC: 1g every 12h (IV).

Staphylococcal endocarditis

Causes of staphylococcal endocarditis include *Staph. aureus* and coagulase-negative staphylococci (CoNS) (e.g. *Staph. epidermidis, Staph. lugdunensis*). *Staph. aureus* is a common cause of both native and prosthetic valve endocarditis. CoNS are more frequently associated with PVE, especially within the 1st year after valve-replacement surgery (early PVE).

In patients who do not have a history of IV drug use, native valve endocarditis (NVE) caused by *Staph. aureus* typically affects the left side of the heart. IV drug users commonly present with right-sided (tricuspid valve) endocarditis. Left-sided NVE is associated with a more fulminant course and a higher mortality. PVE caused by either *Staph. aureus* or CoNS is also associated with a more severe infection. In addition to antimicrobial therapy, many patients with PVE require removal of the infected valve.

Antimicrobial therapy for staphylococcal endocarditis depends on the sensitivity of the organism and the type of valve (prosthetic or native). The majority of staphylococci are penicillin resistant, and therefore, unless sensitivity is conclusively demonstrated, penicillin is not recommended for treatment of staphylococcal endocarditis. The main question when deciding upon antibiotic therapy is sensitivity to meticillin. The AHA, ESC, and BSAC guidelines all recommend penicillinase-resistant penicillin (AHA recommend nafcillin or oxacillin; ESC recommend oxacillin or flucloxacillin; BSAC recommends flucloxacillin) for treatment of meticillin-sensitive staphylococci. Vancomycin is recommended for meticillin-resistant strains and patients with hypersensitivity reactions to penicillin.

In patients with PVE, the AHA, ESC, and BSAC recommend the use of combination antimicrobial therapy. The AHA and ESC guidelines recommend the addition of gentamicin and rifampicin to either a penicillinase-resistant penicillin or vancomycin. The BSAC recommend the addition of two agents from gentamicin, rifampicin and sodium fusidate. Combination therapy may also be used in specific circumstances for management of NVE (see following guidelines).

For practical purposes, the guidelines in the following section are divided into management of meticillin-sensitive *Staph. aureus* and CoNS and meticillin-resistant *Staph. aureus* and CoNS. However, in practice, most strains of CoNS, especially those causing PVE, are oxacillin/meticillin resistant.

Staphylococcal endocarditis in the absence of prosthetic materials

Meticillin-sensitive Staph. aureus/CoNS

The AHA, ESC, and BSAC guidelines recommend 4 weeks of therapy with a penicillinase-resistant penicillin (nafcillin, oxacillin, or flucloxacillin). The AHA guidelines recommend more prolonged therapy (6 weeks) in the presence of complications associated with endocarditis. If there are no contraindications to aminoglycoside therapy, the AHA and ESC guidelines also recommend the addition of gentamicin for the first 3–5 days of treatment.

In patients with hypersensitivity-type reactions to penicillin, 6 weeks of vancomycin monotherapy is recommended by the AHA. In patients with a suboptimal response to vancomycin, the guidelines go further to recommend desensitization to penicillin. In patients with a non-anaphylactoid reaction, therapy with cefazolin and gentamicin may be tried. The BSAC and ESC guidelines recommend addition of a 2nd anti-microbial to vancomycin in penicillin-allergic patients. ESC recommend addition of gentamicin while options for a 2nd antimicrobial from BSAC include gentamicin, rifampicin or sodium fusidate.

In IV drug users who have uncomplicated right-sided endocarditis, an abbreviated course of 2 weeks of therapy with penicillinase-resistant penicillin (with or without gentamicin) is recommended by AHA. A shorter course of therapy is, however, not recommended for patients on vancomycin therapy.

Meticillin-resistant Staph. aureus/CoNS
The AHA and ESC guidelines recommend 4–6 weeks of vancomycin ther-apy with the addition of gentamicin for the first 3–5 days only if the organ-ism is sensitive to aminoglycosides. BSAC recommend at least 4 weeks of vancomycin in combination with either rifampicin, sodium fusidate, or gentamicin for the duration of therapy.

The options for treatment of patients with meticillin-resistant strains who are intolerant to vancomycin are limited. Consultation with an experi-enced microbiologist is recommended

Staphylococcal endocarditis patients with prosthetic valves
Meticillin-sensitive Staph. aureus/CoNS
The AHA and ESC guidelines recommend a minimum of 6 weeks of com-bination therapy with penicillinase-resistant penicillin (oxacillin/nafcillin) and rifampicin, with the addition of gentamicin for the first 2 weeks. BSAC recommend 6 weeks of penicillinase-resistant penicillin (flucloxacillin) in combination with either rifampicin, sodium fusidate, or gentamicin for the duration of therapy. Rifampicin is the preferred adjunct to flucloxacillin.

The guidelines for management of patients with penicillin allergy are the same as those for patients with PVE due to meticillin-resistant strains, which are outlined next.

Meticillin-resistant Staph. aureus/CoNS
Early PVE is frequently caused by CoNS that tend to be meticillin resistant. Therefore early PVE is only treated with penicillinase-resistant penicillin if susceptibility has been conclusively proven. A significant pro-portion of CoNS are also resistant to gentamicin.

The AHA and ESC guidelines recommend 6 weeks of combination therapy with vancomycin and rifampicin, with the addition of gentami-cin for the first 2 weeks. The BSAC guidelines recommend 6 weeks of vancomycin therapy in combination with either rifampicin, sodium fusidate, or gentamicin for the duration of therapy. Rifampicin is the preferred alternative.

Table 6.2 Summary of AHA,[1] ESC[2] and BSAC[3] guidelines for treatment of staphylococcal endocarditis

Indication	AHA	ESC	BSAC	Duration
NVE: oxacillin/ meticillin-susceptible *Staphylococcus*	Nafcillin/ oxacillin + gentamicin (optional)	(Flu)cloxacillin/ oxacillin + gentamicin (optional)	Flucloxacillin	4–6 weeks 3–5 days
NVE: oxacillin/ meticillin-susceptible *Staphylococcus* – patients with penicillin allergy	Vancomycin or cefazolin (non-anaphylactoid) + gentamicin	Vancomycin + gentamicin (optional)	Vancomycin + rifampicin/ gentamicin/ sodium fusidate	4–6 weeks 4–6 weeks 3–5 days
NVE: oxacillin/ meticillin-resistant *Staphylococcus*	Vancomycin + gentamicin	Vancomycin + gentamicin	Vancomycin + rifampicin/ gentamicin/ sodium fusidate	4–6 weeks 3–5 days 4–6 weeks
PVE: oxacillin/ meticillin susceptible *Staphylococcus*	Nafcillin/ oxacillin + rifampicin + gentamicin	(Flu)cloxacillin/ oxacillin + rifampicin + gentamicin	Flucloxacillin + rifampicin/ gentamicin/ sodium fusidate	≥6 weeks ≥6 weeks 2 weeks
PVE: oxacillin/ meticillin-resistant *Staphylococcus*	Vancomycin + rifampicin + gentamicin	Vancomycin + rifampicin + gentamicin	Vancomycin + rifampicin/ gentamicin/ sodium fusidate	6–8 weeks 6–8 weeks 2 weeks

Antibiotic dosage and frequency

Oxacillin AHA: 12g/24h, 4–6 divided doses (IV); ESC: 8–12g/24h, 4 divided doses (IV).
Flucloxacillin BSAC/ESC: 2g every 4–6h (IV).
Gentamicin AHA/ESC: 3mg/kg/24h, single dose (IV); BSAC: 1mg/kg, every 8–12h (IV).
Vancomycin AHA/ESC: 30mg/kg every 24h, 2 divided doses (IV); BSAC: 1g every 12h (IV).
Rifampicin AHA/ESC: 900mg/24h, 3 divided doses (IV/PO); BSAC: 300–600mg every 12h (PO).
Sodium fusidate BSAC: 500mg every 8h (PO).

References

1 Baddour LM et al. (2005). Infective endocarditis: diagnosis, antimicrobial therapy, and management of complications: a statement for healthcare professionals from the Committee on Rheumatic Fever, Endocarditis, and Kawasaki Disease, Council on Cardiovascular Disease in the Young, and the Councils on Clinical Cardiology, Stroke, and Cardiovascular Surgery and Anaesthesia, American Heart Association: endorsed by the Infectious Diseases Society of America. *Circulation* **111**:e394–434.

2 Habib G et al. (2009). Guidelines on the prevention, diagnosis, and treatment of infective endocarditis. (new version 2009): The Task Force on the Prevention, Diagnosis, and Treatment of Infective Endocarditis of the European Society of Cardiology(ESC). *Eur Heart J* **25**:267–76.

3 Elliott TS et al. (2004). Guidelines for the antibiotic treatment of endocarditis in adults: report of the Working Party of the British Society for Antimicrobial Chemotherapy. *J Antimicrob Chemother* **54**:971–81.

Enterococcal endocarditis

Causes of enterococcal endocarditis include *Enterococcus faecalis* and *Enterococcus faecium*. *Enterococcus faecalis* is responsible for the majority of cases (approx 90%). The management of enterococcal endocarditis is challenging, as enterococcal species are typically resistant to a range of antibiotics. Increased resistance necessitates the use of combination antibiotic therapy. The recommendations for treatment of enterococcal endocarditis depend on the sensitivity of the isolate to penicillin, gentamicin, and vancomycin. The guidelines in the following section are divided accordingly.

There is general agreement between the AHA, ESC, and BSAC guidelines regarding management of endocarditis caused by enterococcal species that are sensitive to the aforementioned antibiotics.[1–3] However, there are significant differences in guidelines for management of resistant enterococci. Indeed, the ESC and BSAC have not produced guidelines for management of endocarditis caused by enterococci that are resistant to penicillin, gentamicin, and vancomycin. Liaison with an experienced microbiologist is recommended. While AHA has produced guidelines for treatment of multiresistant enterococci, the evidence to support the recommendations is limited. The guidelines are discussed in detail in this section and summarized in Table 6.3.

Enterococcus susceptible to penicillin, gentamicin, and vancomycin

β-lactams and aminoglycosides act synergistically to kill enterococci. The AHA and ESC guidelines recommend combination therapy with either penicillin or ampicillin with gentamicin or streptomycin. Gentamicin is generally preferred over streptomycin if the isolate is susceptible to both, as assays to measure gentamicin levels are more readily available in most laboratories. BSAC recommends either penicillin or ampicillin with gentamicin as the only option for aminoglycoside therapy.

Four weeks of antimicrobial therapy is recommended for NVE. In patients with PVE, a minimum of 6 weeks of therapy is recommended. The AHA and ESC guidelines also recommend 6 weeks of therapy in patients with symptoms persisting for >3 months.

For penicillin-allergic patients, AHA and ESC recommend vancomycin and gentamicin for 6 weeks irrespective of the type of valve. BSAC recommend either vancomycin or teicoplanin in combination with gentamicin for a minimum of 4 weeks.

Enterococcus susceptible to penicillin, streptomycin, and vancomycin and resistant to gentamicin

Enterococci with high-level resistance to gentamicin may be sensitive to streptomycin. The AHA, ESC and BSAC guidelines recommend streptomycin as an alternative to gentamicin if the isolate is streptomycin sensitive. Four weeks of therapy with either penicillin or ampicillin in combination with streptomycin is recommended for NVE and 6 weeks for PVE. AHA also recommend 6 weeks' therapy for patients with symptoms persisting for >3 months

Practical notes

If the isolate is streptomycin resistant or streptomycin is considered inappropriate, BSAC recommend continuing ampicillin or penicillin for a minimum of 8 weeks.

For patients who are intolerant to penicillin, AHA and ESC guidelines recommend 6 weeks of combination therapy with vancomycin and streptomycin for NVE and PVE. BSAC recommend either vancomycin or teicoplanin in combination with streptomycin for 4 weeks for NVE and 6 weeks for PVE.

Enterococcus resistant to penicillin and susceptible to aminoglycoside and vancomycin

The AHA and ESC guidelines recommend 6 weeks of combination therapy with vancomycin and gentamicin in patients with intrinsic penicillin resistance. However, for β-lactamase-producing strains, AHA and ESC recommend 6 weeks of ampicillin-sulbactam or amoxicillin clavulanic acid as an alternative to vancomycin. The BSAC guidelines recommend either vancomycin or teicoplanin in combination with gentamicin for a minimum of 4 weeks.

Enterococcus resistant to penicillin, aminoglycoside, and vancomycin

Vancomycin-resistant enterococci are often resistant to multiple drugs and therefore options for antimicrobial therapy are limited. BSAC recommend consultation with experienced microbiologists and infectious disease specialists.

The AHA and ESC guidelines recommend a minimum of 8 weeks of linezolid or quinupristin-dalfopristin for treatment of multiresistant *E. faecium*. Combination therapy with either imipenem or ceftriaxone with ampicillin is recommended for *E. faecalis*. The evidence for antimicrobial treatment of vancomycin-resistant strains is limited to small numbers of patients. If antimicrobial therapy fails, valve replacement should be considered early.

Table 6.3 Summary of AHA,[1] ESC,[2] and BSAC[3] guidelines for management of enterococcal endocarditis

Indication	AHA	ESC	BSAC	Duration
NVE and PVE: *Enterococcus* susceptible to penicillin, gentamicin, and vancomycin	Benzylpenicillin or ampicillin + gentamicin or streptomycin	Benzylpenicillin or ampicillin + gentamicin or streptomycin	Benzylpenicillin or ampicillin + gentamicin	≥4 weeks ≥4 weeks ≥4 weeks ≥4 weeks
Penicillin-allergic patients NVE and PVE: *Enterococcus* susceptible to penicillin, gentamicin, and vancomycin	Vancomycin + gentamicin	Vancomycin + gentamicin	Vancomycin or teicoplanin + gentamicin	6 weeks 6 weeks
NVE and PVE: *Enterococcus* susceptible to penicillin, streptomycin, and vancomycin and resistant to gentamicin	Ampicillin or benzylpenicillin + streptomycin	Ampicillin or benzylpenicillin + streptomycin	Ampicillin or benzylpenicillin + streptomycin	≥4 weeks ≥4 weeks ≥4 weeks
Penicillin-allergic patients NVE and PVE: *Enterococcus* susceptible to penicillin, streptomycin, and vancomycin and resistant to gentamicin	Vancomycin + streptomycin	Vancomycin + streptomycin	Vancomycin or teicoplanin + streptomycin	≥4 weeks ≥4 weeks
NVE and PVE: *Enterococcus* resistant to penicillin and susceptible to aminoglycoside and vancomycin	Ampicillin-sulbactam or vancomycin + gentamicin	Ampicillin-sulbactam or vancomycin + gentamicin	Teicoplanin or vancomycin + gentamicin	≥4 weeks ≥4 weeks ≥4 weeks

Table 6.3 (Contd.)

Indication	AHA	ESC	BSAC	Duration
PVE and NVE: *Enterococcus faecium* resistant to penicillin, aminoglycoside and vancomycin	Linezolid or quinupristin-dalfopristin	Linezolid or quinupristin-dalfopristin		≥8 weeks ≥8 weeks
PVE and NVE: *Enterococcus faecalis* resistant to penicillin, aminoglycoside and vancomycin	Imipenem/cilastatin or ceftriaxone + ampicillin	Imipenem/cilastatin or ceftriaxone + ampicillin		≥8 weeks ≥8 weeks ≥8 weeks

Antibiotic dosage and frequency

Benzylpenicillin AHA: 18–30million units/24h, 6 divided doses (IV); ESC: 16–20million units/24h, 4–6 divided doses (IV); BSAC: 2.4g every 4h (IV).

Ampicillin AHA: 12g/24h, 6 divided doses (IV), BSAC: 2g every 4h (IV).

Ampicillin-sulbactam AHA: 12g/24h, 4 divided doses (IV).

Gentamicin AHA: 3mg/kg/24h, 3 divided doses (IV); ESC: 3mg/kg/24h,2 divided doses (IV). BSAC: 1mg/kg, every 8–12h (IV).

Vancomycin AHA/ESC: 30mg/kg every 24h, 2 divided doses (IV); BSAC: 1g every 12h (IV).

Teicoplanin BSAC: 10mg/kg every 24h (IV).

Streptomycin AHA/BSAC: 15mg/kg/24h, 2 divided doses (IV).

Ceftriaxone AHA: 2g/24h, single dose (IV).

Linezolid AHA/ESC: 1.2g/24h, 2 divided doses (IV/PO).

Quinupristin-dalfopristin AHA/ESC: 22.5mg/kg/24h, 3 divided doses (IV).

Imipenem/cilastatin 2g/24h, 4 divided doses (IV).

References

1 Baddour LM *et al.* (2005). Infective endocarditis: diagnosis, antimicrobial therapy, and management of complications: a statement for healthcare professionals from the Committee on Rheumatic Fever, Endocarditis, and Kawasaki Disease, Council on Cardiovascular Disease in the Young, and the Councils on Clinical Cardiology, Stroke, and Cardiovascular Surgery and Anaesthesia, American Heart Association: endorsed by the Infectious Diseases Society of America. *Circulation* **111**:e394–434.

2 Habib G *et al.* (2004). Guidelines on prevention, diagnosis and treatment of infective endocarditis (new version 2009): The Task Force on the Prevention, Diagnosis, and Treatment of Infective Endocarditis of the European Society of Cardiology(ESC). *Eur Heart J* **25**:267–76.

3 Elliott TS *et al.* (2004). Guidelines for the antibiotic treatment of endocarditis in adults: report of the Working Party of the British Society for Antimicrobial Chemotherapy. *J Antimicrob Chemother* **54**:971–81.

Endocarditis caused by HACEK organisms

HACEK organisms (*Haemophilus, Actinobacillus, Cardiobacterium, Eikenella,* and *Kingella* species) are a group of Gram-negative bacilli that account for 5–10% of all cases of infective endocarditis. **Prolonged incubation may be required to detect growth of HACEK organisms and therefore identification of the causative organism and information regarding antibiotic sensitivity is delayed. As a consequence, endocarditis caused by HACEK organisms can be wrongly labelled 'culture negative' during the prolonged culture period.**

The guidelines from ESC[1] and BSAC[2] for management of endocarditis caused by HACEK organisms are similar. For patients with NVE, 4 weeks of therapy with either ampicillin or ceftriaxone in combination with gentamicin for the first 2 weeks is recommended. In patients with PVE, ampicillin, or ceftriaxone therapy is extended to 6 weeks. Ceftriaxone is recommended for treatment of ampicillin-resistant strains (β-lactamase-producing strains) and for empirical therapy when antibiotic sensitivity of the organism is not known.

Due to the emergence of ampicillin-resistant strains and difficulty in performing antibiotic susceptibility testing, the AHA[3] do not recommend use of ampicillin for treatment of endocarditis caused by HACEK organisms. Monotherapy with either ampicillin-sulbactam or ceftriaxone is recommended for 4 weeks in NVE and 6 weeks in PVE. Concomitant use of gentamicin is not recommended.

Guidelines for antimicrobial therapy for HACEK organisms are summarized in Table 6.4.

References
1 Habib G et al. (2004). Guidelines on prevention, diagnosis and treatment of infective endocarditis (new version 2009): The Task Force on the Prevention, Diagnosis, and Treatment of Infective Endocarditis of the European Society of Cardiology(ESC). *Eur Heart J* **25**:267–76.
2 Elliott TS et al. (2004). Guidelines for the antibiotic treatment of endocarditis in adults: report of the Working Party of the British Society for Antimicrobial Chemotherapy. *J Antimicrob Chemother* **54**:971–81.
3 Baddour LM et al. (2005). Infective endocarditis: diagnosis, antimicrobial therapy, and management of complications: a statement for healthcare professionals from the Committee on Rheumatic Fever, Endocarditis, and Kawasaki Disease, Council on Cardiovascular Disease in the Young, and the Councils on Clinical Cardiology, Stroke, and Cardiovascular Surgery and Anaesthesia, American Heart Association: endorsed by the Infectious Diseases Society of America. *Circulation* **111**:e394–434.

Table 6.4 Summary of AHA,[3] ESC,[1] and BSAC[2] guidelines for management of endocarditis caused by HACEK organisms

Indication	AHA	ESC	BSAC	Duration
PVE or NVE caused by HACEK organisms	Ampicillin-sulbactam or	Ampicillin or	Ampicillin or	4 weeks
	ceftriaxone	ceftriaxone +	ceftriaxone +	4 weeks
		gentamicin	gentamicin	2 weeks

Antibiotic dosage and frequency

Ampicillin-sulbactam AHA: 12g/24h, 4 divided doses (IV).

Ampicillin ESC: 12g/24h, 4 divided doses (IV); BSAC: 2g every 4h (IV).

Ceftriaxone AHA/ESC/BSAC: 2g/24h, single dose (IV).

Gentamicin ESC: 3mg/kg/24h, 3 divided doses (IV); BSAC: 1mg/kg, every 8h (IV).

Ciprofloxacillin AHA: 1g or 800mg/24h, 2 divided doses (IV).

Fungal endocarditis

Fungi are an unusual cause of endocarditis. Fungal endocarditis is more common in patients with prosthetic valves, patients with a history of IV drug use, and immunocompromised patients. *Candida* spp. and *Aspergillus* spp. account for the majority of cases of fungal endocarditis.

Mortality rates associated with fungal endocarditis are high. Antimicrobial therapy alone is rarely effective and most patients require valve-replacement surgery. Valve replacement is considered by many to be mandatory in patients with PVE caused by fungi.

The guidelines for antimicrobial therapy for fungal endocarditis are limited due to a lack of trial evidence. AHA and ESC have not produced specific guidelines. BSAC[2] have produced more comprehensive guidelines. For patients with fungal endocarditis caused by *Candida* species, BSAC recommend amphotericin B in combination with flucytosine or fluconazole or caspofungin. Options for endocarditis caused by *Aspergillus* spp. include amphotericin B and voriconazole. A minimum of 6 weeks of therapy is recommended.

The guidelines for management of fungal endocarditis are summarized in Table 6.5.

References

1 Habib G *et al.* (2004). Guidelines on prevention, diagnosis and treatment of infective endocarditis (new version 2009): The Task Force on the Prevention, Diagnosis, and Treatment of Infective Endocarditis of the European Society of Cardiology(ESC). *Eur Heart J* **25**:267–76.
2 Elliott TS *et al.* (2004). Guidelines for the antibiotic treatment of endocarditis in adults: report of the Working Party of the British Society for Antimicrobial Chemotherapy. *J Antimicrob Chemother* **54**:971–81.

Table 6.5 Summary of guidelines for management of fungal endocarditis

Indication	AHA	ESC	BSAC	Duration
Fungal endocarditis caused by *Candida* spp.			Ampho-tericin B + flucytosine	≥6 weeks
			or fluconazole	≥6 weeks
			or caspofungin	≥6 weeks
				≥6 weeks
Fungal endocarditis caused by *Aspergillus* spp.			Ampho-tericin B or voriconazole	≥6 weeks
				≥6 weeks

Antibiotic dosage and frequency

Amphotericin B BSAC: 1mg/kg/24h—adjust to renal function.

Flucytosine BSAC: 100mg/kg/24h, 4 divided doses (IV).

Fluconazole BSAC: 400mg every 12h (PO).

Caspofungin BSAC: 70mg loading dose followed by 50mg/24h.

Voriconazole BSAC: 6mg/kg 12-hourly (loading for 2 doses) followed by 4mg/kg or 400mg 12-hourly for 24h followed by 200mg 12-hourly (PO).

Culture-negative endocarditis

Culture-negative endocarditis (CNE) is defined as endocarditis with three negative cultures using standard blood culture systems. The most common cause of CNE is previous antimicrobial therapy. Less commonly, CNE may be due to infection with fastidious bacteria which do not grow easily under standard blood culture conditions, e.g. *Bartonella* spp., *Chlamydia* spp., *Coxiella burnetii*, *Brucella* spp., *Legionella* spp., *Tropheryma whippleii*, and non-*Candida* fungi.

The choice of antimicrobial for treatment of CNE depends on the type of valve affected (native or prosthetic) and the likely underlying organism. For patients who present with acute NVE, antimicrobial therapy is directed against *Staph. aureus*. For patients who present with a more indolent course, antimicrobial therapy to cover viridans group streptococci and enterococci is recommended. In cases of culture-negative PVE, especially early PVE, empirical therapy should cover meticillin-resistant staphylococci. The duration of antibiotic treatment for CNE is 4–6 weeks depending on response to treatment.

In cases of CNE that are suspected to be due to fastidious organisms which do not grow easily under standard blood culture conditions, e.g. *Bartonella* spp., *Chlamydia* spp., *Coxiella burnetii*, *Brucella* spp., *Legionella* spp., *Tropheryma whippleii*, and non-*Candida* fungi, the management strategy should be decided after consultation with an experienced microbiologist or infectious disease specialist.

Empirical antimicrobial therapy may also be considered in acutely unwell patients with suspected endocarditis before the results for blood cultures are available. Examples of conditions in which acute empirical therapy is indicated include patients with heart failure due to valvular dysfunction, patients with severe sepsis/septic shock, and patients with cardiovascular instability. The guidelines for antimicrobial therapy in such patients are the same as those for patients with CNE who present acutely.

The following section outlines the AHA,[1] ESC,[2] and BSAC[3] guidelines for empirical antimicrobial therapy for suspected endocarditis. The guidelines are summarized in Table 6.6.

Empirical therapy for native valve endocarditis

For patients with NVE who present acutely, the AHA and BSAC guidelines recommend penicillinase-resistant penicillin (nafcillin, oxacillin, or flucloxacillin) in combination with gentamicin. In cases where patients present with a more indolent course, the AHA guidelines recommend combination therapy with ampicillin-sulbactam and gentamicin. BSAC recommend either penicillin or ampicillin in combination with gentamicin. ESC recommend ampicillin-sulbactam or amoxicillin clavulanic acid in combination with gentamicin for acute or indolent NVE.

In patients with penicillin allergy, the guidelines are the same irrespective of whether clinical presentation is acute or indolent. The AHA and ESC guidelines recommend combination therapy with vancomycin, ciprofloxacin, and gentamicin. The BSAC guidelines recommend vancomycin, rifampicin, and gentamicin.

Empirical therapy for prosthetic valve endocarditis

For patients with PVE within 1 year of valve-replacement surgery, the AHA and ESC guidelines recommend combination therapy with vancomycin, rifampicin, and gentamicin. If the infection occurs within 2 months of valve replacement, AHA recommend the addition of cefepime to cover Gram-negative bacilli. For patients with late PVE, AHA recommend combination therapy with vancomycin, rifampicin, and gentamicin while ESC recommendations are the same as those for NVE (outlined above).

The BSAC guidelines recommend vancomycin, rifampicin, and gentamicin, irrespective of the timing of endocarditis relative to valve surgery.

References

1 Baddour LM *et al.* (2005). Infective endocarditis: diagnosis, antimicrobial therapy, and management of complications: a statement for healthcare professionals from the Committee on Rheumatic Fever, Endocarditis, and Kawasaki Disease, Council on Cardiovascular Disease in the Young, and the Councils on Clinical Cardiology, Stroke, and Cardiovascular Surgery and Anaesthesia, American Heart Association: endorsed by the Infectious Diseases Society of America. *Circulation* **111**:e394–434.

2 Habib G *et al.* (2004). Guidelines on prevention, diagnosis and treatment of infective endocarditis (new version 2009): The Task Force on the Prevention, Diagnosis, and Treatment of Infective Endocarditis of the European Society of Cardiology(ESC). *Eur Heart J* **25**:267–76.

3 Elliott TS *et al.* (2004). Guidelines for the antibiotic treatment of endocarditis in adults: report of the Working Party of the British Society for Antimicrobial Chemotherapy. *J Antimicrob Chemother* **54**:971–81.

Table 6.6 Summary of guidelines for treatment of culture-negative endocarditis

Indication	AHA	ESC	BSAC
NVE (acute presentation)	Nafcillin/oxacillin	Ampicillin-sulbactam or amoxicillin-clavulanate	Flucloxacillin
	+	+	+
	gentamicin (optional)	gentamicin	gentamicin
NVE (subacute presentation)	Ampicillin-sulbactam	Ampicillin-sulbactam or amoxicillin-clavulanate	Penicillin or ampicillin
	+	+	+
	gentamicin	gentamicin	gentamicin
NVE (penicillin-allergic patients)	Vancomycin + ciprofloxacin + gentamicin	Vancomycin + ciprofloxacin + gentamicin	Vancomycin + rifampicin + gentamicin
Prosthetic valve infection (early)	Vancomycin + rifampicin + gentamicin + cefepime	Vancomycin + rifampicin + gentamicin	Vancomycin + rifampicin + gentamicin
Prosthetic valve infection (late)	Ampicillin-sulbactam or vancomycin + gentamicin + rifampcin	Ampicillin-sulbactam or amoxicillin-clavulanate + gentamicin	Vancomycin + rifampicin + gentamicin

Antibiotic dosage and frequency

Ampicillin AHA/ESC: 12g/24h, 4 divided doses (IV); BSAC: 2g every 6h (IV).

Flucloxacillin BSAC: 8–12g/24h, 4–6 divided doses (IV).

Penicillin BSAC: 7.2g/24h, 6 divided doses (IV).

Vancomycin AHA/ESC: 30mg/kg every 24h, 2 divided doses (IV); BSAC: 1g every 12h (IV).

Cefepime AHA: 6g/24h, 3 divided doses (IV).

Gentamicin AHA/ESC/BSAC: 3mg/kg/24h, 3 divided doses (IV);.

Rifampicin AHA: 900mg/24h, 3 divided doses (PO/IV); ESC: 1200 mg/day in 2 divided doses (PO); BSAC: 300–600mg 12-hourly (PO).

Ciprofloxacin AHA: 1g/24h or 800mg/24h, 2 divided doses (IV); ESC: 1000mg/day in 2 divided doses (PO) or 800mg/day in 2 divided doses (IV).

Amoxicillin clavulanic acid ESC: 12g/day (IV) in 4 divided doses.

Antimicrobial prophylaxis

Traditionally, the AHA, ESC, and BSAC guidelines have advocated the use of prophylactic antibiotics for patients with valvular heart disease undergoing dental procedures and procedures involving instrumentation of the genitourinary (GU) and gastrointestinal (GI) tracts. However, owing to a lack of evidence to support efficacy and cost-effectiveness of prophylactic antibiotics for prevention of endocarditis and potential adverse effects associated with routine antibiotic prophylaxis, the guidelines have undergone a radical revision. The issue of antibiotic prophylaxis for infective endocarditis has generated considerable controversy and confusion in recent years. The following section provides a summary of the latest guidelines.

In contrast to previous guidelines, the updated AHA guidelines[1] have restricted the use of prophylactic antibiotics to high-risk patients undergoing high-risk procedures. Prophylactic antibiotics are now only recommended for dental procedures involving manipulation of the gingival or peri-apical region of teeth or perforation of the oral mucosa in patients with conditions associated with the highest risk of adverse outcome from endocarditis. High-risk conditions include:

- prosthetic cardiac valves
- previous infective endocarditis
- certain types of congenital heart disease
- cardiac transplantation with valvulopathy.

For the majority of routine dental procedures, the emphasis of the AHA guidelines has shifted away from antibiotic prophylaxis towards maintenance of good dental and oral health. Similarly, for patients undergoing GI or GU tract procedures, antibiotic prophylaxis solely to prevent endocarditis is not recommended. Overall, based on the updated guidelines, far fewer patients will receive antibiotic prophylaxis.

For high-risk cases where antibiotic prophylaxis is indicated, the AHA guidelines recommend oral amoxicillin as first line. Alternatives in patients with non-anaphylactoid reactions to penicillin include 1st-generation cephalosporins, clindamycin, azithromycin, or clarithromycin. 1st-generation cephalosporins are not recommended in patients with anaphylactoid reactions to penicillin due to the potential for cross-reactions. IV preparations of antibiotics may be used in patients who are unable to tolerate oral preparations. Antibiotic doses are provided in Table 6.7.

In 2008, NICE[2,3] in the UK went one step further and recommended that, irrespective of risk, patients with valvular heart disease undergoing interventional procedures should no longer receive antibiotic prophylaxis against endocarditis. The only exception to this recommendation is at-risk patients undergoing GI and GU procedures who have active infection at the site of the procedure. Such patients should still receive antibiotics to cover organisms that cause endocarditis.

The BSAC guidelines for antibiotic prophylaxis have been revised on two occasions in recent years. The 2006 guideline update advised restricting the use of prophylactic antibiotics to patients with the highest risk of endocarditis, i.e. patients with a prior history of endocarditis, prosthetic cardiac valves, and surgically constructed pulmonary or system shunts/conduits.

However, in response to the aforementioned NICE recommendations, the BSAC guidelines[4] were revised for a second time. In line with NICE, the latest BSAC guidelines[3] recommend a nil prophylaxis strategy.

Updated ESC guidelines no longer recommend prophylaxis for respiratory tract, gastrointestinal, urological or skin and soft tissue procedures but continue to recommend prophylaxis in high-risk patients for selected dental procedures.

Table 6.7 Summary of AHA guidelines for antimicrobial prophylaxis for infective endocarditis

Source	Antimicrobial	Dose (single dose)	Comments
AHA	Amoxicillin	2g (PO)	Standard treatment: • patients with no penicillin allergy • able to swallow
	Amoxicillin	2g (IM/IV)	Recommended for patients unable to take oral antibiotics No allergy to penicillin
	Cefazolin or ceftriaxone or cephalexin or clindamycin or azithromycin/ clarithromycin	1g (IM/IV) 1g (IM/IV) 2g (PO) 600mg (PO) 500mg (PO)	Recommended for patients with allergy to penicillin/ampicillin Note: cephalosporins should not be used in patients with anaphylaxis/ angio-oedema/urticaria due to penicillin/ampicillin use
	Cefazolin or ceftriaxone or clindamycin	1g (IM/IV) 1g (IM/IV) 600mg (IV)	Recommended for patients with allergy to penicillin/ampicillin Patients unable to take oral antimicrobials Note: cephalosporins should not be used in patients with anaphylaxis/ angio-oedema/urticaria due to penicillin/ampicillin use

References

1 Nishimura RA et al. (2008). ACC/AHA 2008 Guideline update on valvular heart disease: focused update on infective endocarditis: a report of the American College of Cardiology/American Heart Association Task Force on Practice Guidelines endorsed by the Society of Cardiovascular Anesthesiologists, Society for Cardiovascular Angiography and Interventions, and Society of Thoracic Surgeons. J Am Coll Cardiol **52**:676–85.

2 NICE (2008). Prophylaxis against infective endocarditis. Antimicrobial prophylaxis against infective endocarditis. London:NICE.

3 Watkin RW et al. (2008). New guidance from NICE regarding antibiotic prophylaxis for infective endocarditis – response by the BSAC working party. J Antimicrob Chemother **62**:1477–8.

4 Habib G et al. (2009). Guidelines on the prevention, diagnosis, and treatment of infective endocarditis (new version 2009): The Task Force on the Prevention, Diagnosis, and Treatment of Infective Endocarditis of the European Society of Cardiology (ESC). Eur Heart J **25**: 267–76.

Pericarditis

Pericarditis is defined as an inflammation of the pericardium. In the majority of cases, pericarditis is an acute, self-limiting condition. Chronic or relapsing forms of pericarditis are less common. In a small proportion of cases, pericarditis is associated with complications such as pericardial effusion, pericardial tamponade, and constrictive pericarditis.

Causes of pericarditis

- Viral infection: coxsackie virus, echo viruses, adenoviruses, mumps virus
- Bacterial infection: *Mycobacterium tuberculosis, Staphylococcus aureus, Streptococcus pneumoniae, Neisseria meningitidis, Salmonella species*
- Connective tissue diseases: rheumatoid arthritis, SLE, sarcoidosis
- Uraemia
- Radiation
- Inflammation following myocardial infarction: Dressler's syndrome
- Drugs: hydralazine, procainamide, penicillin, isoniazid, phenytoin, ciclosporin, tetracyclines, doxorubicin, cyclophosphamide, methyldopa, mesalazine, reserpine, dantrolene, minoxidil
- Cardiac surgery: post-pericardiotomy syndrome
- Primary and metastatic neoplasms

In a proportion of cases, no cause is found, i.e. idiopathic pericarditis. The majority of cases of pericarditis are either idiopathic or due to viral infection.

Chest pain is the most common symptom associated with pericarditis. The pain is typically exacerbated by lying flat and deep inspiration. Physical examination may reveal a low-grade pyrexia and a pericardial friction rub. The presence of a significant pericardial effusion causing tamponade may be associated with hypotension, tachycardia, and pulsus paradoxus.

Management of pericarditis

The management of pericarditis depends on the pattern of disease, the underlying cause, and the presence or absence of complications. The following section outlines the ESC guidelines[1] for treatment of pericarditis.

Acute uncomplicated pericarditis

Most cases of pericarditis, particularly idiopathic and viral pericarditis, are uncomplicated and are associated with self-limiting symptoms. The only treatment required in such cases is NSAIDs (Table 6.8).

Relapsing pericarditis

Medical management options for relapsing pericarditis are outlined in Table 6.9. For patients with severe symptomatic recurrences that are refractory to medical therapy, pericardectomy should be considered.

Table 6.8 NSAIDs

Drug	Comments
Ibuprofen	Indication: acute pericarditis (class I indication/level of evidence B) Dose: 300–600mg every 8h (PO) Duration ≥4 weeks Few adverse side effects
Indometacin	Indication: acute pericarditis (class I indication/level of evidence B) Dose: 400–800mg every 4–8h (PO) Duration ≥ 4weeks Reduces coronary blood flow—avoid in elderly patients and patients with ischaemic heart disease
Colchicine	May be used as initial treatment for acute pericarditis (in combination with NSAIDs or as monotherapy in patients intolerant to NSAIDs)—class IIa indication/level of evidence B Dose: 0.5mg every 12h (PO) Duration ≥4 weeks Well tolerated—fewer side effects than NSAIDs

Table 6.9 Treatment of relapsing pericarditis

Drug	Comments
Colchicine	Effective as prophylactic therapy to prevent recurrent episodes of pericarditis—class I indication/level of evidence B Dose: 2mg/day for 1–2 days followed by 1mg/day
Steroids	Use of corticosteroids reserved for: • severe pericarditis which does not respond to initial therapy • recurrent pericarditis with frequent relapses which does not respond to 1st-line therapy • pericarditis due to underlying conditions which respond to steroid therapy, e.g. autoimmune inflammatory conditions Corticosteroids have been reported to exacerbate pericarditis in certain circumstances—therefore not recommended as initial therapy

Treatment of the underlying cause of pericarditis

Treatment directed at the underlying cause of pericarditis is indicated in the following situations:

• pericarditis due to bacterial infection:
  • without appropriate antibiotic therapy, purulent bacterial pericarditis is usually fatal
  • empirical antibiotic therapy may be commenced pending culture results. The choice of antibiotic is then tailored based on the sensitivity of the causative organism
  • pericardial drainage is necessary for purulent pericarditis
• tuberculous pericarditis:
  • in the absence of anti-tuberculous chemotherapy, tuberculous pericarditis is associated with a high mortality
  • steroids may be considered as an adjunct to antituberculous therapy (level of evidence A/class IIb indication)
• uraemic pericarditis:
  • most patients with uraemic pericarditis respond to renal replacement therapy
  • additional systemic or intrapericardial corticosteroids therapy may be effective
  • NSAIDs and corticosteroids are unlikely to be effective in patients with pericarditis which persists despite dialysis
• pericarditis due to autoimmune inflammatory conditions:
  • treatment with steroids and other immunomodulating drugs may be effective.

Management of complications associated with pericarditis

• In patients with a significant pericardial effusion complicated by pericardial tamponade, urgent pericardiocentesis is essential. Patients with recurrent pericardial effusions may require a subxiphoid pericardiotomy.
• Patients with constrictive pericarditis may require a pericardiectomy.

Reference

1 Maisch B et al. (2004). Guidelines on the diagnosis and management of pericardial diseases executive summary; The Task Force on the Diagnosis and Management of Pericardial Diseases of the European Society of Cardiology. *Eur Heart J* **25**:587–610.

Myocarditis

Myocarditis is defined as inflammation of the myocardium. The clinical manifestations of myocarditis vary from a mild, self-limiting disease to severe inflammation, irreversible myocyte necrosis, and development of a dilated cardiomyopathy.

Causes of myocarditis

- Viral infection: coxsackie B, HIV, echovirus, Epstein–Barr virus, rubella, varicella
- Bacterial infections: *Staphylococcus aureus*, diphtheria, Lyme disease, Chagas disease
- Autoimmune inflammatory conditions: Churg–Strauss syndrome, Wegener's granulomatosis, SLE
- Rejection in heart transplant patients
- Drugs: acetazolamide, amitriptyline, cefaclor, clozapine, colchicine, doxorubicin, furosemide, isoniazid, lidocaine, methyldopa, penicillin, phenytoin, reserpine, streptomycin, tetracycline, thiazides
- Toxins

In a proportion of cases, no cause is identified, i.e. idiopathic myocarditis.

The clinical presentation of myocarditis is variable. Patients with mild disease may be asymptomatic or may present with non-specific symptoms such as fever and myalgia. Patients with more severe myocarditis may present with fulminant HF due to acute LV dysfunction. Arrhythmias are commonly associated with severe myocarditis and may be the cause of sudden cardiac death.

Management of myocarditis

Treatment of myocarditis is largely supportive. In patients with significant impairment of LV function and congestive HF, treatment with ACEIs, β-blockers, and diuretics is indicated (see 📖 Chapter 1, p.3).

Antiarrhythmic drug therapy should be used with caution in patients with severe myocarditis due to their negative inotropic effect (see 📖 Chapter 4, p.113)

In patients with severe LV dysfunction, inotropic support and mechanical ventricular assist devices may be necessary. In a proportion of such cases, cardiac transplantation is the only treatment option.

Immunosuppression is not routinely used in the treatment of myocarditis. A subset of patients in whom immunosuppression may be effective are patients with myocarditis due to systemic inflammatory conditions.

Cardiovascular drugs in pregnancy and breastfeeding

Cardiac disease in pregnancy

Cardiac disease is the leading cause of mortality in pregnancy, although overall only small numbers of women are affected. *Pregnant women with known cardiac disease should be managed in specialist clinics by a multidisciplinary team involving cardiologists, obstetricians, obstetric physicians, and anaesthetists.*

The physiological changes of pregnancy affect drug absorption, distribution, metabolism, and elimination, and these vary in each trimester.

Physiological changes in pregnancy

- Blood volume and cardiac output increase by 30–50%.
- Protein levels fall and there is a reduction in drug protein binding.
- Changes in GI motility and secretions as well as hormonal effects on liver enzymes alter drug metabolism.
- Renal excretion of drugs is increased, as glomerular filtration rate (GFR) rises.

Close drug monitoring is important and doses may often need modifying. Haemodynamic changes mostly return to normal within a few days after delivery, but it takes up to 6 weeks before the hormones of pregnancy are back to normal.

Unlike the majority of treatments in cardiovascular medicine, the evidence base during pregnancy is limited due to the lack of trial data in this patient group. There are, however, guidelines to aid management but these are often based on observational data and, in some instances, the lack of consensus is apparent.

The use of drugs in breastfeeding women is dependent upon the concentration of drug excreted in the breast milk; however, adequate information is not always available, particularly with the newer agents. *As such, women may have drugs withheld or be advised not to breastfeed because of the lack of evidence rather than known neonatal concerns.*

The US Food and Drug Administration (FDA) categorizes drugs that may be used in pregnancy according to risk to the fetus from exposure. However, data are limited in pregnancy for most drugs, so evidence for many drugs falls into category C (see Table 7.1), which limits the usefulness of this grading system.

Table 7.1 Current FDA categories for drug use in pregnancy

Category	Description
A	Adequate, well-controlled studies in pregnant women have not shown an increased risk of fetal abnormalities
B	Animal studies have revealed no evidence of harm to the fetus; however, there are no adequate and well-controlled studies in pregnant women *or* Animal studies have shown an adverse effect, but adequate and well-controlled studies in pregnant women have failed to demonstrate a risk to the fetus
C	Animal studies have shown an adverse effect and there are no adequate and well-controlled studies in pregnant women *or* No animal studies have been conducted and there are no adequate and well-controlled studies in pregnant women
D	Studies, adequate well-controlled or observational, in pregnant women have demonstrated a risk to the fetus. However, the benefits of therapy may outweigh the potential risk
X	Studies, adequate well-controlled or observational, in animals or pregnant women have demonstrated positive evidence of fetal abnormalities. The use of this product is contraindicated in women who are or may become pregnant

Hypertension

Hypertension (BP >140/90mmHg) in pregnancy is common, affecting approximately 1 in 10 pregnancies. It is classified into three main groups:

1. Chronic hypertension is defined as hypertension diagnosed prior to or during the first 20 weeks' gestation, or persisting for >3 months postpartum. Women with chronic hypertension are considered to be at higher risk of developing superimposed pre-eclampsia (see discussion of aspirin therapy in point 3).

The risk of developing severe hypertension seems to be reduced with antihypertensive medications. Prior to conception, women with a history of hypertension should be reviewed by a specialist. For women with 'low-risk' chronic hypertension (BP 140–160/90–110mmHg, normal examination, no proteinuria, and normal ECG and echocardiogram) it may be appropriate to discontinue antihypertensive drugs or reduce the dose of these drugs. If treatment does need to be continued, consideration should be given to switching to drugs that are safer in pregnancy.

2. Pregnancy-induced hypertension is hypertension arising for the first time after the 20th week of pregnancy. The systemic features of pre-eclampsia are absent and BP falls to normal levels postpartum. These women are also at increased risk of developing pre-eclampsia and should be closely monitored.

3. Pre-eclampsia–eclampsia syndrome Pre-eclampsia is hypertension with proteinuria (++ in 2 urine samples or >300mg over 24h) occurring after 20 weeks' gestation. It is a multisystem disorder with varying degrees of thrombocytopenia, haemolytic anaemia, abnormal LFTs, impaired renal function, and hyperuricaemia. The hypertension may be new or there may be a rise in BP in someone with chronic hypertension. Eclampsia is the occurrence of one or more seizures in the presence of pre-eclampsia. Magnesium sulphate still remains a key therapy in the treatment of severe pre-eclampsia and eclampsia, although the only definitive treatment for pre-eclampsia is delivery of the fetus.

The 2007 Cochrane review[1] concluded that antiplatelet agents (almost exclusively aspirin) confer a moderate reduction (approximately 15%) in the risk of pre-eclampsia and pre-term (before 34 weeks) birth without an increased risk of haemorrhage. However, they could not identify which subgroup of women would benefit from treatment from the data available. In general, it is accepted practice that aspirin (<75mg) may be used in high-risk patients (e.g. previous pre-eclampsia in >1 pregnancy), but may also be considered for women with a modestly increased risk of developing pre-eclampsia (e.g. pre-eclampsia in one previous pregnancy, or chronic hypertension) after discussion with the mother of the risks and benefits of treatment.

Categories of blood pressure in pregnancy

- BP ≤140/90mmHg: normal/acceptable in pregnancy
- BP 140–159/90–109mmHg: mild to moderate hypertension
- BP ≥160/110mmHg: severe hypertension

There is limited evidence on which to base guidance for the threshold at which to start treatment or indeed the target BP once treatment has been initiated. Suggested guidelines vary in different countries. A Cochrane review in 2007 of 46 trials involving 4282 women concluded that it remains unclear whether therapy is worthwhile in mild to moderate hypertension in pregnancy (in this review this was SBP 140–169mmHg or DBP 90–109 mmHg or both), and that there is insufficient evidence that any antihypertensive is better than another.[2] However, in practice it is appropriate to consider starting antihypertensive treatment once SBP reaches 150mmHg or DBP is 90–100mmHg, with an aim to reduce BP to 140/90mmHg. For patients with mild–moderate chronic hypertension who may have had medications stopped prior to or early in pregnancy, treatment should be restarted if SBP rises to 140–150mmHg or DBP is 90–100mmHg.

Drug treatment of hypertension in pregnancy depends on whether the patient has mild to moderate hypertension or if treatment is required for severe hypertension. Table 7.2 displays the drug treatments typically used and a suggested order for their introduction. It should be noted that the choice of drug may be largely dependent on the clinician's experience of its use and may vary between institutions.

Reference

1 Duley L et al. (2007). Antihypertensive drug therapy for mild to moderate hypertension during pregnancy. Cochrane Database Syst Rev (1):CD002252.
2 Abalos E et al. (2007). Antihypertensive drug therapy for mild to moderate hypertension during pregnancy. Cochrane Database Syst Rev (1):CD002252.

Table 7.2 Drug treatment of mild to moderate hypertension in pregnancy

Drug/drug class	FDA category	Risk profile and use	Side effects	Dose	Compatible with breast-feeding?
1st line/preferred					
Methyldopa	B	Drug of choice in the months before conception or 1st-line during pregnancy Limited efficacy compared to newer agents when used in isolation Considered safe throughout pregnancy despite crossing placenta	Frequently causes xerostomia Associated with maternal depression, therefore consider replacing in postnatal period and avoid use if there is a significant risk of maternal depression Can cause elevated liver enzymes, hepatitis, and hepatic necrosis; stop drug and seek advice Chronic use can be associated with a positive Coombs' test and a haemolytic anaemia Monitor FBC and LFTs before treatment and every 2–3 weeks for the first 6–12 weeks	500mg–3g/day PO in 2–3 divided doses	Yes Excreted in small amounts in breast milk
Labetalol (see below)	C	Can be used 1st-line in 3rd trimester			
2nd line					
Nifedipine (**only** long-acting/slow-release preparations—but NB unlicensed indication)	C	Short-acting formulations and sublingual administration are **not** recommended Used alone or in combination with methyldopa or labetalol	Risk of tachycardia, palpitations, headaches, facial flushing, and peripheral oedema May inhibit labour	30–120 mg PO/day (slow-release preparation)	Yes But excreted in breast milk

Table 7.2 (Contd.)

Drug/drug class	FDA category	Risk profile and use	Side effects	Dose	Compatible with breast-feeding?
Hydralazine	C	Has been used in 2nd and 3rd trimesters but poor efficacy compared to other drugs. Use generally reserved for IV treatment in severe hypertension	May cause thrombocytopenia in neonate. Risk of headache, nausea, flushing, and palpitations so may be poorly tolerated. Chronic use may be associated with drug-induced lupus and pyridoxine-responsive polyneuropathy (rare)	50–300mg PO/day in 2–4 divided doses	Yes. But excreted in breast milk

3rd line

Drug/drug class	FDA category	Risk profile and use	Side effects	Dose	Compatible with breast-feeding?
Doxazosin	C	Inadequate studies in humans	High doses in animal studies show delayed postnatal development	1mg PO/day for 1–2 weeks, increasing to 2–4mg/day as necessary	No. Accumulated in breast milk. Consider switch to alternative, e.g. enalapril
Labetalol (see below for other β-blockers)		Do not use in asthmatics. Avoid use in severe peripheral vascular disease, diabetes, or liver disease. No effect on fetal heart rate. More effective in BP lowering than methyldopa	Previous concern about risk of intrauterine growth retardation (IUGR) but less concern after review and not if started after 1st trimester. May cause neonatal hypoglycaemia at high doses. Risk of lethargy and fatigue, reduced exercise tolerance, peripheral vasoconstriction, sleep disorders, and broncho-constriction. Severe hepato-cellular damage has been reported	200mg–1.2g PO/day in 2–3 doses	Yes, but observe fetus for signs of β-blockade. Excreted in breast milk

(continued)

Table 7.2 (Contd.)

Drug/drug class	FDA category	Risk profile and use	Side effects	Dose	Compatible with breast-feeding?
Limited use/additional agents in refractory hypertension					
β-blockers		All cross placenta Some extensively used in pregnancy None are associated with teratogenicity in any trimester Safety profile likely to be variable for individual drug due to lipid solubility and receptor specificity Fetal growth should be monitored regularly	The risk of IUGR appears to be small, predominantly with atenolol at high doses and only if this drug is started before conception or after the 1st trimester Risk of lethargy and fatigue, reduced exercise tolerance, peripheral vasoconstriction, sleep disorders, and broncho-constriction		
Atenolol	D	Avoid in isolated hypertension until after 1st trimester Avoid high doses	Increased risk of IUGR in 1st trimester exposure Fetal bradycardia		No Concentrated in breast milk
Propranolol	C D in 2nd/3rd trimester	Limited data in 1st trimester use	Chronic high doses in 2nd and 3rd trimesters can cause IUGR, fetal bradycardia, respiratory depression, and hypoglycaemia Unknown long-term effects on exposed infants	160–320mg PO/day in two divided doses	Yes Excreted in breast milk Observe fetus for signs of beta-blockade
Metoprolol	C D in 2nd/3rd trimester	Limited data in 1st trimester use	Chronic high doses in 2nd and 3rd trimesters can cause IUGR, fetal bradycardia, respiratory depression, and hypoglycaemia	100–200mg/day PO in 1–2 divided doses	No Excreted in breast milk

Table 7.2 (Contd.)

Drug/drug class	FDA category	Risk profile and use	Side effects	Dose	Compatible with breast-feeding?
Bisoprolol	C D in 2nd/3rd trimester	Use in pregnancy not studied			No data available
Clonidine	C	Mainly used in 3rd trimester as additional drug in refractory hypertension Probably no increased risk of congenital anomalies but suggested cardiovascular defects in 1st-trimester exposure	Sudden withdrawal may cause a hypertensive crisis	0.1–1.2mg/day in divided doses	No long-term data available Excreted in breast milk
α-blockers		Indicated in suspected phaeochromo-cytoma Often used with β-blocker			
Doxazosin	B	(see above)			
Prazosin	C		No adverse effects reported		No data available Excreted in milk in low concentrations
Calcium-channel antagonists		Avoid sublingual or rapid IV administration due to risk of precipitous BP reduction			

(continued)

Table 7.2 (Contd.)

Drug/drug class	FDA category	Risk profile and use	Side effects	Dose	Compatible with breast-feeding?
Verapamil	C	Crosses placenta No adequate human data	Maternal hypotension and fetal hypoxia with rapid IV administration otherwise safe and especially if given as oral preparation		Compatible with breastfeeding but is excreted in milk
Diltiazem	C	No adequate human data, but possible association with cardiovascular defects in 1st-trimester exposure			Compatible with breastfeeding but is excreted in milk
Nimodipine	C	Mainly used in SAH No adequate studies in humans			Unknown excretion in breast milk
Amlodipine	C	No human data			No data available
Diuretics		Relatively contraindicated except in pulmonary oedema Poor efficacy Use only in combination with other antihypertensives such as vasodilators for fluid retention Contraindicated in pre-eclampsia	Potential risk of pre-eclampsia as reduce intravascular volume Increase serum urate (used to monitor pre-eclampsia)		Avoid in breastfeeding as reduce milk volume
Furosemide	C	Used mainly for pulmonary congestion	For exposure after 1st trimester no adverse effects reported		Excreted in breast milk No adverse effects reported

Table 7.2 (Contd.)

Drug/drug class	FDA category	Risk profile and use	Side effects	Dose	Compatible with breast-feeding?
Spirono-lactone	D	Not recommended due to anti-androgenic effects	Association with mild IUGR with use throughout pregnancy		Excreted in breast milk
ACEIs	D	Contraindicated in 2nd and 3rd trimesters Change to alternative antihyper-tensive if possible, ideally before conception 1st-trimester exposure poses an increased risk of major congenital defects (e.g. cardiovascular and central nervous system)	Can cause marked fetal renal hypoperfusion, failure, and dysgenesis		Enalapril/captopril are compatible No data for ramipril or lisinopril in breastfeeding
Angiotensin II receptor blockers	D	Limited data in pregnancy but generally accepted that have similar risk as ACEIs in 2nd and 3rd trimesters			

Acute severe hypertension (Table 7.3)

Severe hypertension with hypertensive encephalopathy, haemorrhage or eclampsia requires immediate treatment with parenteral antihypertensives.

The aim of management is to reduce and maintain BP within a safe range, with a gradual reduction while maintaining placental perfusion. SBP should be maintained between 140 and 160mmHg and DBP between 90 and 110mmHg. A Cochrane review in 2006 of the treatment of very high BP in pregnancy considered 24 trials (2949 women) and found that there is currently insufficient evidence that any antihypertensive is superior.[1] Most commonly, BP reduction is achieved with the administration of slow IV bolus doses of labetalol, hydralazine, or oral nifedipine. *Diuretics should not be used due to increased risk of pre-eclampsia. Sodium nitroprusside is relatively contraindicated.*

Table 7.3 Drug treatment of acute severe hypertension in pregnancy

Drug	FDA category	Risk profile/side effects	Dose and route
Labetalol	C	Suggested lower incidence of maternal hypotension than hydralazine **Do not use in asthmatics or women with congestive cardiac failure**	200mg PO first Then (if no response to oral therapy): 20–40mg IV every 20–30min as needed Max 300mg Infusion: 40–160mg/h
Hydralazine	C	**Long experience of safety and efficacy** Side effects mimic symptoms of deteriorating pre-eclampsia	5–10mg IV/IM (over 10–20min) every 20–40min as needed Repeat every 3h once BP is controlled Consider alternative drug if no or minimal BP reduction with 20mg IV or 30mg IM Infusion: 0.5–10mg/h
Nifedipine	C	**Unlicensed for use in pregnancy** Suggested lower incidence of maternal hypotension than hydralazine **Sublingual administration is not recommended**	Nifedipine (standard-release formulation): 10–20mg PO every 30min (max 50mg/h)

Postpartum and lactation

Most antihypertensive medications are excreted in breast milk but there is little information of the effects on the neonate.

Safety of cardiovascular drugs during lactation

- Labetalol and propranolol appear to be safe in breastfeeding mothers.
- Captopril and enalapril are the only ACEIs with enough safety data to be considered compatible with use in breastfeeding.
- Diuretics should be avoided as they reduce milk volume.

Atenolol and metoprolol should be used with caution as they are concentrated in breast milk.

Reference

1 Duley L (2006). Drugs for treatment of very high blood pressure during pregnancy. *Cochrane Database Syst Rev* (**3**):CD001449.

Arrhythmias

Palpitations are a common symptom in pregnancy, and arrhythmias and ectopic beats are also frequent. The acute management of arrhythmias is similar to that outside pregnancy, but chronic drug treatment should be reserved for frequent symptomatic or haemodynamically compromising arrhythmias, to minimize fetal exposure to drugs.

It should be noted that all commonly used antiarrhythmics cross the placenta and are excreted in breast milk; however, most are considered to be compatible with breastfeeding (see Table 7.4).

Supraventricular tachycardia

The 2003 ACC/AHA/ESC practice guidelines for the management of patients with supraventricular arrhythmias recommends that women with known symptomatic supraventricular tachycardia (SVT) should be advised to undergo a curative catheter ablation prior to conception as recurrence during pregnancy is common and, where possible, all potentially teratogenic drugs should be avoided.[1] However, clinicians with experience in the field may find that SVT is often well tolerated during pregnancy and easily controlled with antiarrhythmics. If, however, SVT is poorly tolerated and refractory to drug treatment, catheter ablation can be performed in the 2nd trimester.

Treatment to terminate SVT

1. Vagal manoeuvres can be attempted in the first instance.
2. IV boluses of adenosine can be given up to a maximum of 24mg as a single dose.
3. If adenosine fails, IV metoprolol or propranolol can be used in non-asthmatic women as 2nd-line choices. In known WPW, β-blockers are the drug of choice.
4. IV verapamil can be used but may increase the risk of prolonged maternal hypotension, particularly with rapid administration. However, if the mother is well hydrated the risk of significant hypotension is small.
5. If chemical cardioversion fails or the mother is haemodynamically compromised, electrical cardioversion should be performed and is considered reasonably safe in all trimesters. Special precautions should be followed, however, compared to the non-pregnant woman (i.e. patient should be laid on left lateral side to prevent IVC obstruction with the gravid uterus, intubation should be early, as gastric stasis is increased in the pregnant woman, and if cardioverting in the 3rd trimester, the fetus should be monitored). **Specialist multidisciplinary management is required.**

Treatment as prophylaxis to prevent SVT

- 1st-line agents are digoxin and β-blockers (metoprolol or propranolol). However, close monitoring is required with digoxin and its efficacy is unknown. β-blockers should be avoided in the 1st trimester if possible.

- Verapamil can be used as an alternative.
- The choice of other alternative agents is difficult as experience is limited; however, suggested drugs are sotalol or flecainide (in the absence of structural heart disease). Beyond this, quinidine, propafenone, and procainamide may be considered but experience with these drugs is even more limited.
- **Amiodarone is an FDA category D drug and the only antiarrhythmic with known teratogenicity**; it should only be used when there are no other therapeutic options.

Atrial fibrillation and flutter

Both of these conditions are uncommon in pregnancy, but their occur-rence is often associated with congenital heart disease, rheumatic valve disease, thyrotoxicosis, or electrolyte disturbance. The aim of treatment is to terminate the arrhythmia within 24h of onset, to avoid the need for anticoagulation, particularly as pregnancy itself is a pro-thrombotic state.

The joint ACC/AHA/ESC guidelines of 2006[2] advise the following for atrial fibrillation in pregnancy:

Rhythm control
Chemical cardioversion
- Consider chemical cardioversion for new haemodynamically stable AF, with quinidine or procainamide.
- Quinidine has the longest safety record in pregnant women. However, there is increasing experience with sotalol and flecainide and some clinicians may favour the use of these drugs as alternatives. There is limited experience with amiodarone.

Electrical cardioversion
If haemodynamically unstable, direct-current cardioversion is recom-mended.

Rate control
Ventricular rate control can be attempted with digoxin, a β-blocker, or non-dihydropyridine calcium-channel antagonist.

Anticoagulation
- For all patients with AF (with the exception of lone AF and/or low thromboembolic risk), protection against thromboembolic risk is recommended throughout pregnancy. Treatment with either anticoagulation or aspirin should be selected according to the stage of pregnancy.
- For the 1st trimester and the last month of pregnancy in patients with AF and risk factors for thromboembolism:
  - consider treatment with heparin (UFH) by continuous infusion to prolong APTT to 1.5–2.0 times control value, or UFH by SC injection twice daily to prolong the mid-interval APTT to 1.5 times control.
  - Alternatively, although data are limited, consider treatment with SC LMWH.
- Consider an oral anticoagulant (usually warfarin) during the 2nd trimester.

In clinical practice however, the risk of thromboembolism associated with AF in the context of pregnancy (including those with lone AF) may be considered sufficiently significant to anticoagulate all those affected. The Royal College of Obstetricians and Gynaecologists (RCOG) recommends the use of LMWH in the treatment of DVT/PE rather than UFH.

If warfarin is used during the 2nd trimester, counselling should be given about the risk of intraventricular haemorrhage in the fetus, and monthly fetal brain scans should be performed.

If LMWH is used, the dose given is the same as that used to treat acute coronary syndromes (i.e. 1mg/kg twice daily), and if used long term, monitored with factor Xa assays. Advice should be given to stop the treatment after the onset of labour, and consideration given to the use of IV heparin after assessment.

Ventricular tachycardia

The most common VT during pregnancy is idiopathic RVOT VT (ECG shows a monomorphic VT, LBBB pattern, with an inferior axis). This stable rhythm rarely degenerates and β-blockers are the drug of choice.

VT in the presence of structural heart disease is a risk for sudden cardiac death. In this case, antiarrhythmic therapy as well as an ICD may be necessary. Drug therapy may include a cardioselective β-blocker alone, amiodarone alone (but note that the risk of birth defects with amiodarone may be unacceptable), or both. Pregnant women who develop haemodynamically unstable VT should be electrically cardioverted. The development of stable non-long QT-related VT can be treated with intravenous lidocaine in the first instance and procainamide long term. Prophylaxis with a cardioselective β-blocker may be effective and sotalol can be considered if this is unsuccessful.

For women with symptomatic LQTS, β-blockers should be continued during pregnancy, delivery, and the postpartum unless there are definite contraindications as there are data to suggest a significant increase in the risk of cardiac events in the postpartum period.

References

1 Blomström-Lundqvist C et al. (2003). ACC/AHA/ESC guidelines for the management of patients with supraventricular arrhythmias. *J Am Coll Cardiol* **42**:1493–1531.

2 Fuster V et al. (2006). ACC/AHA/ESC 2006 guidelines for the management of patients with atrial fibrillation: a report of the American College of Cardiology/American Heart Association Task Force on Practice Guidelines and the European Society of Cardiology Committee for Practice Guidelines. *J Am Coll Cardiol* **48**:e149–e246.

3 Bonow RO et al. (2006). ACC/AHA 2006 guidelines for the management of patients with valvular heart disease. *Circulation* **48**:e1–e148.

Table 7.4 Antiarrhythmics in pregnancy

Drug	FDA category	Risk profile/side effects	Dose and route	Compatibility with breast-feeding?
Adenosine	C	Insufficient data for use in 1st trimester Safe in 2nd and 3rd trimesters Fetal heart monitor to detect possible bradycardia	6–12mg IV over 1–3s, then 20ml 0.9% sodium chloride flush Max 24mg	Yes Not excreted in breast milk
Amiodarone	D	Not used 1st line due to risk of congenital goitre, and hyper- or hypothyroidism in the neonate	5mg/kg IV over 3min, then 10mg/kg IV per day	No
Atenolol	D	Use advocated in 2006 ACC/AHA guidelines for valvular heart disease[3] Recommended for aortopathy, e.g. Marfan syndrome and may be required in severe MS to prevent decompensation due to tachycardia If possible, avoid use in 1st trimester as concerns over IUGR	50–100mg PO/day for arrhythmias (and mitral stenosis)	Avoid use
Digoxin	C	At therapeutic doses, no adverse effects on fetus Monitor closely for toxicity as maternal toxicity can be fatal to the fetus Renal clearance increases as pregnancy progresses, therefore may need increased doses	Loading : 500mcg PO Then 500mcg PO after 6h Maintenance: 125–375mcg PO daily	Yes
Diltiazem	C	(See 🕮 Table 7.2, p.234)	20mg IV bolus over 2min, repeat after 15min	Yes

(continued)

Table 7.4 (Contd.)

Drug	FDA category	Risk profile/side effects	Dose and route	Compatibility with breastfeeding?
Flecainide	C	Not teratogenic or fetotoxic Do not use in structural heart disease	100–300mg PO/day in 2 divided doses or Slow IV dose with ECG monitoring; 2mg/kg over 10–30min (max 150mg) followed (if required) by Infusion: 1.5mg/kg/h for up to 1h, then 100–250mcg/kg/h for up to 24h Then transfer to oral treatment as above	Yes
Lidocaine	B	Not teratogenic but can cause toxicity (e.g. hypothermia) Reduce dose with liver dysfunction or cardiac failure	With ECG monitoring: 1mg/kg IV bolus; repeat ½ bolus every 10min up to 4× immediately then, Infusion: 1–4mg/min; total 3mg/kg/day for 1st day If continued beyond 24h, reduce concentration further (i.e. <1mg/min)	Yes
Metoprolol	C	(See Table 7.2, p.232)	5mg IV over 5min; repeat at 10min 50–300mg/day PO 2–3 divided doses	Avoid use
Procainamide	C	Not teratogenic, but note high-dose procainamide can cause miscarriage	100mg IV over 30min, then infusion: 2–6mg/min, max 1g	Yes
Propafenone	C	Limited data in pregnancy		Not recommended

Table 7.4 *(Contd.)*

Drug	FDA category	Risk profile/side effects	Dose and route	Compatibility with breast-feeding?
Propranolol	C	(See 📖 Table 7.2, p.232)	1mg IV every 2min as required 40–160mg PO/day in 3–4 divided doses	Yes
Quinidine	C	Risk of neonatal thrombocytopenia Long safety record in pregnancy Premature labour at toxic doses Needs monitoring of serum levels	15mg/kg over 60min, then Infusion: 0.02mg/kg/min	Yes
Sotalol	B D in 2nd/3rd trimesters	Risk of IUGR (consider serial ultrasound scans) Risk in 2nd/3rd trimesters as for other β-blockers Monitor ECG	80–360mg PO/day in 2 divided doses or 20–120mg IV over 10min, repeat 6-hourly (ECG monitoring)	Yes
Verapamil	C	(See 📖 Table 7.2, p.234)	120–360mg PO/day in 3 divided doses	Yes

Prosthetic heart valves

Anticoagulation (see Table 7.5)

The physiological changes in pregnancy increase thromboembolic risk. This is of particular importance in women with a mechanical valve prosthesis. There is a lack of consensus about which anticoagulant should be used in pregnancy due to conflict between the best interests of the mother and the fetus. The concerns are related to teratogenicity and fetal anticoagulation with warfarin, efficacy and difficulties with monitoring for UFH, and safety and efficacy of LMWH.

There is a general consensus that vitamin K antagonists can be used in the 2nd and 3rd trimesters in women with mechanical valve prosthesis, with the recommendation that if this is used it should be replaced with SC heparin or IV heparin at 36 weeks to reduce the risk of neonatal intracranial haemorrhage during delivery and permit the use of epidural analgesia.

During the 1st trimester, however, there is no universally accepted 1st-choice anticoagulant. The use of warfarin in the 1st trimester (between weeks 6 and 12) is associated with an approximately 5% risk of teratogenicity. However, there are data that suggest warfarin doses <5mg/day are associated with very low risk.

Unfractionated SC heparin is an acceptable treatment option as an alternative to warfarin throughout pregnancy for most women, but has been associated with a higher incidence of thromboembolic complications, valve thrombosis, and mortality, and requires close monitoring.

The 2008 recommendations in the 8th American College of Chest Physicians (ACCP) guidelines[1] suggest three possible regimens, which are applicable in most cases (Box 7.1).

Box 7.1 The 2008 recommendations in the ACCP 8th edition guidelines[1]

1. LMWH SC twice daily throughout pregnancy in doses adjusted to achieve the manufacturer's 4-h post-injection anti-Xa level or
2. UFH twice daily throughout pregnancy administered in doses adjusted to keep the mid-interval APPT at least twice control or anti-Xa level 0.35–0.70U/mL or
3. UFH or LMWH (as in points 1. and 2.) until the 13th week, and after the 35th week, with warfarin between the 13th and 35th weeks

---

However, for women known to be at very high risk of valve thrombosis, the recommended treatment is warfarin throughout pregnancy with substitution with UFH or LMWH after 35 weeks. In addition, high-risk patients should also receive 75–100mg aspirin od throughout pregnancy.

Women considered to be at high risk are those with:
- 1st-generation prosthetic valves (such as Starr Edwards, Bjork–Shiley)
- mechanical valve in the mitral position
- multiple mechanical valves
- previous venous thromboembolism.

However, in the latest ESC guidelines (2007),[2] doubt persists about the use of LMWH for anticoagulation in these patients. This is largely because there have been some study data to suggest worse outcomes (prosthetic valve thrombosis and death) when LMWH was used. Therefore in these guidelines, warfarin remains the recommended anticoagulant until the 36th week, particularly if the dose required is <5mg.

The *Consensus views arising from the 51st Study Group: Heart Disease and Pregnancy* (RCOG guidelines)[3] acknowledge that there is currently no ideal regimen of anticoagulation in women with mechanical heart valves in pregnancy and advise that in women who elect to use SC LMWH, regular monitoring of factor Xa levels (at least monthly) should be performed and doses adjusted to achieve a peak (3–4-h post-dose) level of at least 1.0IU/mL and a trough level of at least 0.5IU/mL. In clinical practice in the UK and Europe, LMWH beginning at a dose of 1mg/kg/twice daily (with dose adjustment to factor Xa levels) is a widely accepted method of anti-coagulation for valvular prostheses in pregnancy.

Given the lack of consensus on the best anticoagulant during pregnancy, it is important that the relative benefits and disadvantages are discussed with the patient in a specialist clinic, so that a joint decision about the most appropriate option can be reached.

References

1 Bates SM et al. (2008). Venous thromboembolism, thrombophilia, antithrombotic therapy, and pregnancy: American College of Chest Physicians evidence-based clinical practice guidelines (8th edition). *Chest* **133**:844S–886S.
2 Vahanian A et al. (2007). Guidelines on the management of valvular heart disease: The Task Force on the Management of Valvular Heart Disease of the European Society of Cardiology. *Eur Heart J* **28**:230–68.
3 Steer PJ et al. (2006). *Consensus views arising from the 51st Study Group: Heart Disease and Pregnancy*. London: RCOG.

Table 7.5 Anticoagulants in pregnancy

Drug	FDA category	Risk profile and use	Side effects	Compatible with breast-feeding?
Warfarin	X	Crosses placenta causing fetus to be anticoagulated Fetal exposure is higher than in the mother, particularly in the 1st trimester Possible dose-related teratogenicity Increased incidence of abortion and stillbirths in the 1st trimester	Associated with congenital malformations (nasal hypoplasia, epiphyseal calcification, CNS abnormalities) with use in 1st trimester—possibly dose related Increased risk of miscarriage and stillbirth Risk of fetal intracranial haemorrhage	Yes Excreted in breast milk but no adverse effects have been reported
LMWH Enoxaparin	B	Efficacy in thromboembolism but limited experience of use in valve prosthesis Does not cross placenta No bleeding complications in the fetus or mother Use as anticoagulant for mechanical valve prostheses is not recommended by manufacturer For elective deliveries, withdraw LMWH 18–24h and substitute with IV UFH to prevent spinal or epidural haematoma with anaesthesia		Yes Minimal excretion in breast milk

Table 7.5 *(Contd.)*

Drug	FDA category	Risk profile and use	Side effects	Compatible with breast-feeding?
Heparin sodium	B	Does not cross placenta Long-term use in the setting of mechanical valve prosthesis may be associated with increased risk of maternal haemorrhagic and thromboembolic complications compared to warfarin Possible risk of increased incidence of spontaneous abortions, prematurity, and still-birth 1st-trimester exposure may be associated with cardiovascular defects Titrate dose to APPT or anti-factor Xa level	Hypocalcaemia in the fetus due to mode of action (calcium chelation) Increased risk of maternal osteopenia and immune-mediated thrombocytopenia	Yes

Valvular heart disease

Regurgitant valvular heart disease is generally well tolerated in pregnancy because the fall in systemic vascular resistance reduces the degree of regurgitant flow. However, if HF develops, diuretics and vasodilators (nitrates and dihydropyridine calcium channel antagonists) are the only medical treatment options.

Stenotic valvular heart disease is often poorly tolerated in pregnancy with deterioration most commonly occurring in the 2nd trimester.

Mitral stenosis

All pregnant patients with severe mitral stenosis (valve area <1.5cm^2) need regular assessment throughout pregnancy. It is advised that Doppler echocardiography measurement of mean transmitral gradient and PAP should be made at 3 and 5 months, and monthly subsequently. Cardio-specific β-blocker therapy should be initiated and uptitrated if the patient becomes symptomatic or estimated systolic PAP >50mmHg. Diuretics should be considered for persisting pulmonary congestion. As a last resort, closed mitral valvotomy may be undertaken at specialist centres, and open heart surgery reserved for cases where maternal life is threatened with delivery of a viable fetus before surgery.

Aortic stenosis

Severe aortic stenosis is uncommon in pregnancy. Conservative management consists of bed rest, oxygen, and β-blockers. Severe symptoms may be relieved by percutaneous balloon valvotomy in specialist centres.

Congenital heart disease

Pregnancy is not recommended in women with the highest risk of decompensation, or those in functional NYHA class III or IV.

High-risk patients are those with:
- pulmonary hypertension
- severe LVOT obstruction
- cyanotic heart disease.

Termination of pregnancy is advisable for these patients. If pregnancy is continued, symptomatic management with bed rest and oxygen may be necessary, with hospitalization by the end of the 2nd trimester and prophylactic treatment with SC LMWH to prevent thromboembolism.

Drug treatment for congenital heart disease in pregnancy is discussed in Chapter 9, pp.277–296.

Antibiotic prophylaxis peripartum

The risk of endocarditis following normal vaginal delivery is low. NICE guidelines (March 2008)[1] advise against the routine administration of antibiotics as prophylaxis during childbirth as well as gynaecological and obstetric procedures. Although it is acknowledged that patients with structural heart disease (acquired valvular disease, complex congenital cyanotic heart disease, surgically constructed shunts, valve replacement, HCM) and previous infective endocarditis are at risk of developing infective endocarditis, there are few data to show that antibiotic prophylaxis is effective or that there is clear association between episodes of infective endocarditis and interventional procedures. The NICE guidelines place emphasis on patient education and prevention by maintaining good oral hygiene.

However, the 2008 ACC/AHA adult congenital heart disease guidelines[2] include a recommendation that it is reasonable to consider antibiotic prophylaxis against infective endocarditis before vaginal delivery at the time of membrane rupture in selected patients with the highest risk of adverse outcomes. This includes patients with prosthetic cardiac valves or prosthetic material used for cardiac valve repair, and patients with unrepaired or palliated cyanotic heart disease, including surgically constructed palliative shunts and conduits.

References

1 NICE (2008). *Prophylaxis against infective endocarditis.* Clinical guideline 64. London: NICE.
2 Warnes CA et al. (2008). ACC/AHA 2008 Guidelines for the Management of Adults With Congenital Heart Disease. A Report of the American College of Cardiology/American Heart Association Task Force on Practice Guidelines (Writing Committee to Develop Guidelines on the Management of Adults With Congenital Heart Disease): Developed in Collaboration With the American Society of Echocardiography, Heart Rhythm Society, International Society for Adult Congenital Heart Disease, Society for Cardiovascular Angiography and Interventions, and Society of Thoracic Surgeons. *Circulation* 118:e714–e833.

Cardiomyopathy

Peripartum cardiomyopathy

Peripartum cardiomyopathy is the development of unexplained LV systolic dysfunction in the period from the last month of pregnancy to the 5th month postnatally. Echocardiography is advised before conception for women with a family history of peripartum cardiomyopathy.

Hypertensive heart failure is treated in a similar way to non-pregnant patients; however, ACEIs and ARBs are contraindicated in pregnancy. The aim of management is to reduce pre-load with diuretics (e.g. furosemide, amiloride; but avoid use of spironolactone, FDA category D) and reduce afterload with vasodilators (e.g. hydralazine and nitrates). Digoxin may be used if AF develops. β-blockers can be initiated to reduce myocardial oxygen demand but this must be done cautiously. As thromboembolic risk increases, these patients should be started on anticoagulation with UFH before delivery and warfarin postpartum. Postpartum ACEIs are the mainstay of treatment even in breastfeeding women.

More severe cases may require a ventricular assist device or cardiac transplantation. Cardiac function does recover in the majority of cases, although this may take some time. There are data to suggest that the risk of relapse in subsequent pregnancies is high.

Dilated cardiomyopathy

The 2003 expert consensus document on management of cardiovascular diseases during pregnancy[1] advises that women with known DCM should be advised against pregnancy as the likelihood of deterioration in cardiac function is high. Additionally, termination of pregnancy should be discussed if pregnancy does occur and the ejection fraction is <50% or the LV dimensions are above normal. In clinical practice, each case must be considered individually with specialist input, and if pregnancy is continued, close follow-up is necessary with regular assessment of LV function with echocardiography. Hospital admission should be arranged early if there is evidence of deterioration as the options for treatment are limited in pregnancy, particularly as ACEIs and ARBs are contraindicated.

Hypertrophic cardiomyopathy

Pregnancy is usually well tolerated and reassurance can be given that it is likely to be completed successfully *in women who are asymptomatic without a family history of sudden death*.

In the presence of severe diastolic dysfunction, it is advised that β-blockers (to prevent tachycardia) be continued, and the addition of a low-dose diuretic may be required for symptomatic pulmonary congestion. The addition of low-dose heparin is advisable if there is severe diastolic dysfunction.

AF may develop and is generally poorly tolerated. β-blockade or digoxin may be used to control ventricular rate, and a β-blocker may also prevent recurrence. Anticoagulation with LMWH is important for AF, and attempts should be made to restore sinus rhythm with DC cardioversion if necessary, after transoesophageal echocardiography excludes LA thrombus.

In the presence of persistent symptomatic ventricular arrhythmias, the use of amiodarone with a β-blocker may become necessary although this is unsuitable given the known risks to the fetus with amiodarone.

Reference

1 The Task Force on the Management of Cardiovascular Diseases During Pregnancy of the European Society of Cardiology (2003). Expert consensus document on management of cardiovascular diseases during pregnancy. *Eur Heart J* **24**:761–81.

Ischaemic heart disease

Ischaemic heart disease in pregnancy is uncommon but increasing with increasing maternal age. Patients with known ischaemic heart disease require review and optimization prior to conception. Assessment with exercise testing can be useful. The expert consensus document from the ESC in 2003[1] suggests that if angina during pregnancy is refractory to medical therapy (such as β-blockers or calcium-channel antagonists), PCI may be required and is best carried out in the 2nd trimester. There is no specific advice as to the use of drugs in pregnancy normally used for 1° or 2° prevention of cardiovascular disease; therefore the use of these drugs should be considered on an individual basis. (Note: 3-hydroxy-3-methyl-glutaryl coenzyme (HMG CoA) reductase inhibitors in common use are FDA category 'X'—the drug is contraindicated in women who are or may become pregnant.) (See Table 7.6.)

Acute severe chest pain in a woman with an abnormal ECG may be caused by MI; however, the underlying mechanism for this in pregnancy is more commonly coronary artery dissection than thrombosis. MI is more common late in pregnancy or during the postpartum period and immediate coronary angiogram with the potential to perform stenting is the preferred strategy, although thrombolytics can be given if necessary.

MI due to coronary artery vasospasm has been reported to occur when ergometrine has been administered to induce uterine contraction after delivery. This is of particular concern in women with pre-existing ischaemic heart disease and its use in this situation should be avoided. If vasospasm is suspected, the administration of IV or sublingual glyceryl trinitrate may be effective but if this fails, immediate coronary angiography may be necessary.

Reference

1 The Task Force on the Management of Cardiovascular Diseases During Pregnancy of the European Society of Cardiology (2003). Expert consensus document on management of cardiovascular diseases during pregnancy. *Eur Heart J* **24**:761–81.

Table 7.6 Drugs used in ischaemic heart disease

Drug	FDA category	Safety profile/side effects	Compatible with breastfeeding?
Antiplatelets			
Aspirin	C (if low dose used; up to 150mg) D (if full dose used in 3rd trimester)	May cause maternal antepartum or postpartum haemorrhage, prolonged gestation or labour High doses in the last weeks of pregnancy can cause premature closure of the ductus arteriosus, pulmonary hypertension, stillbirth, IUGR, and bleeding disorders in the newborn May be used in pre-eclampsia, SLE, and antiphospholipid syndrome	Cautious use only Excreted in small amounts in breast milk with possible platelet function changes in the exposed neonate
Clopidogrel	B	No adequate human data	Avoid use Unknown excretion in breast milk
Thrombolytics			
Tissue plasminogen activator (tPA)	No classification available	No human data available	No data available
Alteplase	C	Risk of placental abruption in first 18 weeks of pregnancy Inadequate human studies	Unknown excretion in breast milk
Antianginals			
β-blockers		See ☐ Table 7.2, p.232	
Calcium-channel antagonists		See ☐ Table 7.2, p.233	
Glyceryl trinitrate (GTN)	C	Nitrates previously used as tocolytics Appear safe providing they are not used in such high doses they cause maternal hypotension, which may lead to reduced placental perfusion Inadequate human studies Used in ACS and significant pulmonary oedema	Yes Unknown excretion in breast milk—no problems recorded

Table 7.6 (Contd.)

Drug	FDA category	Safety profile/side effects	Compatible with breastfeeding?
Isosorbide mononitrate	C	Stillbirth and neonatal death when used in high doses in animals; see 'GTN'	Unknown excretion in breast milk
Isosorbide dinitrate	C	Inadequate human studies See 'GTN' Prolongs gestation in animals	Unknown excretion in breast milk
Lipid-lowering drugs			
Simvastatin	X	Limited human studies Contraindicated but inadvertent use during gestation caused no fetal harm Animal studies show possible dose-related testicular atrophy and impaired spermatogenesis	No data available
Atorvastatin	X	As above	Contraindicated in breastfeeding due to potential serious side effects Unknown excretion in breast milk
Bezafibrate	X	No human data	No
Clofibrate	C	Crosses placenta in animals and excreted into milk in animals No human data	No human data available
Gemfibrozil	C	Teratogenic in animals Exposure in 1st trimester can cause structural brain defects	Unknown excretion in breast milk No problems reported
Niacin	A C (if doses above recommended daily amount (RDA))		Actively excreted in breast milk RDA during lactation is 8–20mg

(Continued)

Table 7.6 *(Contd.)*

Drug	FDA category	Safety profile/side effects	Compatible with breastfeeding?
Colestyra-mine	B	Some human data in 1st trimester with no teratogenic effects As binds fat-soluble vitamins, may cause vitamin deficiency in 2nd and 3rd trimester. Fetal vitamin K deficiency may result in haemorrhagic complication in utero (subdural haematomas, hydrocephalus)	No data available May cause deficiency of fat-soluble vitamins with prolonged use

Further reading

ACC/AHA/ESC 2006 guidelines for management of patients with ventricular arrhythmias and the prevention of sudden cardiac death: a report of the American College of Cardiology/American Heart Association Task Force and the European Society of Cardiology Committee for Practice Guidelines. *J Am Coll Cardiol* 2006; **48**:247–346.

Adamson D, Nelson-Piercy C (2007). Managing palpitations and arrhythmias during pregnancy. *Heart* **93**:1630–6.

Askie LM et al. (2007). Antiplatelet agents for prevention of pre-eclampsia: a meta-analysis of individual patient data. *Lancet* **369**:1791–8.

Dajani AS et al. (1997). Prevention of bacterial endocarditis: recommendations by the American Heart Association. *JAMA* **25**:1448–58.

Oakley C, Warnes CA (eds). *Heart disease in pregnancy* (2nd edn.). Oxford: Blackwell Publishing.

Podymow T, August P (2008). Update on the use of antihpertensive drugs in pregnancy. *Hypertension* **51**:960–9.

RCOG (2006). *The management of severe pre-eclampsia/eclampsia*. Guideline No. 10(A). London: RCOG.

Report of the National High Blood Pressure Education Program Working Group on High Blood Pressure in Pregnancy. *Am J Obstet Gynaecol* 2000; **183**:S1–S22.

Tan HL, Lie KI (2001). Treatment of tachyarrhythmias during pregnancy and lactation. *Eur Heart J* **22**:458–64.

Perioperative cardiothoracic surgical management

Perioperative management of cardiac patients undergoing non-cardiac surgery

Pre-existing CVD is associated with a significant increase in morbidity and mortality in patients undergoing non-cardiac surgery. Coronary artery disease accounts for the vast majority of adverse cardiac events associated with non-cardiac surgery. Other conditions associated with increased perioperative risk include HF, valvular heart disease, and cardiac arrhythmias.

This chapter outlines guidelines for preoperative risk assessment of cardiac patients and therapy to minimize perioperative risk. The discussion focuses mainly on the role of cardiac drugs in the perioperative setting. The recommendations are based on the updated 2007 ACC/AHA guidelines for risk stratification and management of cardiac patients undergoing non-cardiac surgery.[1]

Reference

1 Fleisher LA et al. (2007). ACC/AHA 2007 guidelines on perioperative cardiovascular evaluation and care for noncardiac surgery: a report of the American College of Cardiology/American Heart Association Task Force on Practice Guidelines (Writing Committee to Revise the 2002 Guidelines on Perioperative Cardiovascular Evaluation for Noncardiac Surgery) developed in collaboration with the American Society of Echocardiography, American Society of Nuclear Cardiology, Heart Rhythm Society, Society of Cardiovascular Anesthesiologists, Society for Cardiovascular Angiography and Interventions, Society for Vascular Medicine and Biology, and Society for Vascular Surgery. J Am Coll Cardiol **50**:e159–242.

Risk stratification of cardiac patients undergoing non-cardiac surgery

The 1st step in estimating perioperative risk of cardiac patients scheduled to undergo non-cardiac surgery involves taking a detailed history, physical examination, and assessment of the baseline ECG. The aim of the initial assessment is to determine patient-specific risk, which is influenced by the functional capacity of the patient and presence of cardiac risk factors.

Previous AHA guidelines classified cardiac risk factors into major, intermediate, and minor risk factors.[1,2] The updated AHA guidelines specify active conditions associated with major risk of adverse outcome and other conditions that contribute to overall risk. The classification system for risk factors outlined in this section is based on the updated 2007 AHA guidelines.[3]

Active cardiac conditions associated with major risk of adverse outcome

Unstable coronary syndromes
- Recent MI
- Unstable angina
- Severe angina (Canadian Cardiac Society class III or IV)

Decompensated heart failure
- NYHA class IV HF
- New-onset or deteriorating HF

Significant arrhythmias
- Symptomatic ventricular arrhythmias
- Supraventricular tachycardias with uncontrolled ventricular rate
- Symptomatic bradycardia
- Conduction abnormalities: complete heart block, high-grade AV block, Mobitz II AV block

Severe valvular heart disease
- Severe AS (aortic valve gradient >40mmHg, valve area <1cm^2)
- Symptomatic MS

Other conditions that are associated with a relatively lower risk of adverse outcome also contribute to overall risk:
- history of stable coronary artery disease
- history of compensated HF
- history of CVD
- diabetes mellitus
- renal impairment.

In addition to patient-specific factors, the type of surgery also influences the risk of cardiac complications. Surgical procedures can be classified as high, intermediate, or low risk as follows:
- high-risk procedures: vascular surgery, e.g. aortic and major peripheral vascular surgery

- intermediate-risk procedures: intraperitoneal surgery, intrathoracic surgery, head and neck surgery, orthopaedic surgery, urological surgery
- low-risk procedures: endoscopic procedures, superficial surgical procedures, breast surgery, cataract surgery.

The overall risk of non-cardiac surgery is estimated by combining surgery-specific and patient-specific risk factors. A number of multivariable risk indices have been developed in the past that take account of risk factors to calculate risk scores; however, they are not discussed here.

References

1 Eagle KA et al. (1996). Guidelines for perioperative cardiovascular evaluation for noncardiac surgery. Report of the American College of Cardiology/American Heart Association Task Force on Practice Guidelines. Committee on Perioperative Cardiovascular Evaluation for Noncardiac Surgery. *Circulation* **93**:1278–317.
2 Eagle KA et al. (2002). ACC/AHA Guideline Update for Perioperative Cardiovascular Evaluation for Noncardiac Surgery–Executive Summary. A report of the American College of Cardiology/American Heart Association Task Force on Practice Guidelines (Committee to Update the 1996 Guidelines on Perioperative Cardiovascular Evaluation for Noncardiac Surgery). *Circulation* 2002 **105**:1257.
3 Fleisher LA et al. (2007). ACC/AHA 2007 guidelines on perioperative cardiovascular evaluation and care for noncardiac surgery. *J Am Coll Cardiol* **50**:e159–242.

Management of cardiac conditions associated with increased perioperative risk

Patients who have major risk factors for adverse perioperative cardiac events (i.e. patients with unstable coronary syndromes, decompensated HF, significant arrhythmias, severe valvular disease) should undergo further investigation and treatment before proceeding with elective noncardiac surgery. Patients with poor functional capacity who have multiple other risk factors (e.g. stable coronary artery disease, compensated HF, CVD, diabetes mellitus, and renal impairment) may also require further preoperative assessment and therapy. In high-risk cases, surgery may have to be deferred until therapeutic measures to minimize perioperative risk have been instituted. In certain circumstances, non-essential surgery may be cancelled altogether.

Patients with low perioperative risk, i.e. patients with good functional capacity who do not have significant risk factors, should proceed to planned surgery without further cardiac investigations. Patients who require emergency surgery should also proceed with surgery following a limited preoperative assessment. Detailed cardiac assessment of such patients is often deferred until after the emergency procedure.

The algorithm in Fig. 8.1, which is based on the ACC/AHA cardiac evaluation and care algorithm,[1] provides a general framework to guide decision making following initial preoperative risk stratification. The class of recommendation and level of evidence for the recommendations has been included in the algorithm.

The next section outlines the guidelines for management of specific cardiac conditions associated with increased perioperative risk. The discussion focuses on issues related to the perioperative period. Detailed discussion of the general management of the conditions can be found in the relevant chapters.

Reference

1 Fleisher LA et al. (2007). ACC/AHA 2007 guidelines on perioperative cardiovascular evaluation and care for noncardiac surgery. *J Am Coll Cardiol* **50**:e159–242.

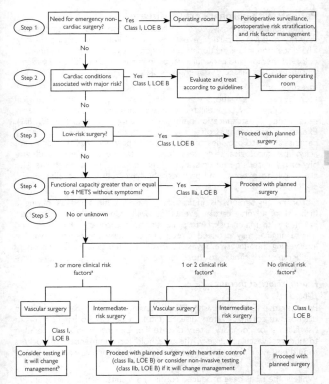

ᵃClinical risk factors: stable coronary artery disease, compensated HF, CVD, diabetes mellitus, renal impairment.

ᵇConsider perioperative β-blockade.

Fig. 8.1 Cardiac evaluation and care algorithm for non-cardiac surgery. LOE, level of evidence; METS, metabolic equivalent.

Patients with coronary artery disease

As mentioned previously, coronary artery disease accounts for the vast majority of adverse cardiac events associated with non-cardiac surgery. The discussion in this section covers preoperative investigations, pharmacological therapy, and revascularization in coronary artery disease patients who have an increased perioperative risk.

Investigations

Non-invasive investigations, e.g. exercise stress testing or pharmacological stress testing, may be indicated in intermediate-risk patients who warrant further risk stratification before proceeding to surgery (see Fig. 8.1). Exercise stress testing is often the 1st-choice investigation in ambulatory patients as it also provides an assessment of preoperative functional capacity. Pharmacological stress tests (e.g. dobutamine stress echocardiography or myocardial perfusion scanning) may be considered in patients who are unable to exercise and patients who have abnormal baseline ECGs, e.g. LBBB.

Coronary angiography is indicated in patients identified as having a high risk of adverse cardiac events following non-invasive investigations. Patients with major risk factors, i.e. unstable coronary syndromes and severe angina, may proceed directly to coronary angiography without intervening non-invasive investigations. The indications for coronary angiography are similar to those for patients who are not awaiting non-cardiac surgery.

Pharmacological therapy

β-blockers

Perioperative β-blockers should be considered in all patients with a diagnosis of coronary artery disease and in patients who have significant risk factors for coronary artery disease. For patients who are scheduled to undergo vascular surgery, the threshold for commencing β-blockers should be lower as the incidence of undiagnosed coronary artery disease in such patients is higher.

While some trials have produced conflicting results, overall, perioperative β-blockade appears to be beneficial in coronary artery disease patients, especially in high-risk patients. There is also evidence to suggest that withdrawal of β-blockers in the perioperative period increases the risk of adverse cardiac events.[1]

Questions remain over when to commence β-blockers, the optimum target heart rate, and whether long-acting β-blockers are superior to short-acting preparations. There is some evidence to support commencing β-blockers days to weeks before the operation, with a target heart rate of 60–65bpm.[2]

Based on the available evidence, the ACC/AHA recommend perioperative β-blockers in the situations listed in Table 8.1 (the level of evidence and class of indication have been specified).

Table 8.1 Perioperative use of β-blockers

Situation	Class of indication/level of evidence
Patients undergoing vascular surgery previously taking β-blockers for hypertension, arrhythmias, angina	Class I indication/level of evidence B
Patients undergoing intermediate or low-risk surgery previously taking β-blockers for hypertension, arrhythmias, angina	Class I indication/level of evidence C
Patients undergoing vascular surgery who have evidence of myocardial ischaemia on preoperative testing	Class I indication/level of evidence B
Patients with coronary artery disease undergoing vascular surgery or intermediate-risk surgery—without evidence of ischaemia or no preoperative testing	Class IIa indication/level of evidence B
One or more cardiovascular risk factors in patients undergoing vascular surgery	Class IIa indication/level of evidence B
One or more cardiovascular risk factors in patients undergoing intermediate risk surgery	Class IIb indication/level of evidence C
Patients with a single risk factor who are undergoing vascular surgery or intermediate-risk surgery	Class IIb indication/level of evidence C
Patients with no risk factors undergoing vascular surgery	Class IIb indication/level of evidence B

Statins
There is some evidence to suggest that perioperative statins may have a protective effect against adverse events such as MI, unstable angina, and death in patients undergoing non-cardiac surgery. However, evidence from RCTs to support routine statin therapy in the perioperaitve setting is limited.[3]

ACC/AHA indications for perioperative statin therapy are outlined in Table 8.2.

Table 8.2 Indicators for perioperative statin use

Situation	Class of indication/level of evidence
For patients currently taking statins and scheduled for non-cardiac surgery, statins should be continued	Class I indication, level of evidence B
For patients undergoing vascular surgery with or without clinical risk factors, statin use is reasonable	Class IIa indication, level of evidence B
For patients with at least one clinical risk factor who are undergoing intermediate-risk procedures, statins may be considered	Class IIb indication, level of evidence C

α-blockers
The efficacy of the α_2 agonists mivazerol and clonidine in reducing perioperative adverse cardiac events in patients with coronary artery disease has been evaluated in a series of randomized trials. While some trials have demonstrated a reduction in perioperative coronary ischaemia with the use of α-blockers, a mortality benefit has not consistently been demonstrated.[4–6]

The AHA guidelines recommend that α_2 blockers may be considered for perioperative control of hypertension in patients with coronary artery disease (class IIb indication/level of evidence B).

Calcium-channel blockers
Some studies suggest reduction in perioperative ischaemia with a trend towards reduced MIs and mortality in patients taking CCBs.[7] However, there is insufficient evidence to recommend the routine use of CCBs in the perioperative setting.

Revascularization
The indications for coronary revascularization, either CABG or PCI, are the same as those for patients who are not scheduled to undergo non-cardiac surgery (see p.260).

For patients who require preoperative PCI and have a high risk of intra-operative bleeding, the timing of surgery and duration of antiplatelet therapy are important considerations. For patients scheduled for non-urgent surgery, the operation may be deferred for the duration of the recommended post-PCI dual antiplatelet therapy, e.g. following PCI with a bare metal stent, surgery may be deferred for 4–6 weeks after which clopidogrel may be stopped.

Conversely, the PCI strategy may depend on the urgency of the surgery, e.g. for patients requiring urgent surgery, PCI with balloon angioplasty only may be preferable, as post-PCI dual antiplatelet therapy is not necessary.

The algorithm in Fig. 8.2 summarizes recommendations for the timing of surgery following PCI in patients who have a high risk of perioperative bleeding. The algorithm in Fig. 8.3 summarizes recommendations for PCI strategy in patients who are awaiting non-cardiac surgery. The algorithms are derived from the ACC/AHA 2007 guidelines on perioperative cardiovascular evaluation and care for noncardiac surgery.[8]

References

1 Shammash JB et al. (2001). Perioperative beta-blocker withdrawal and mortality in vascular surgical patients. Am Heart J **141**:148–53.

2 Poldermans D et al. (2006). Should major vascular surgery be delayed because of preoperative cardiac testing in intermediate-risk patients receiving beta-blocker therapy with tight heart rate control? J Am Coll Cardiol **48**:964–9.

3 Durazzo AE et al. (2004). Reduction in cardiovascular events after vascular surgery with atorvastatin: a randomized trial. J Vasc Surg **39**:967–75.

4 Oliver MF et al. (1999). Effect of mivazerol on perioperative cardiac complications during non-cardiac surgery in patients with coronary heart disease: the European Mivazerol Trial (EMIT). Anesthesiology **91**:951–61.

5 Mangano DT et al. (1997). Perioperative sympatholysis: beneficial effects of the alpha 2-adrenoceptor agonist mivazerol on hemodynamic stability and myocardial ischemia. Anesthesiology **86**:346–63.

6 Wallace AW et al. (2004). Effect of clonidine on cardiovascular morbidity and mortality after noncardiac surgery. Anesthesiology **101**:84–93.

7 Wijeysundera DN, Beattie WS (2003). Calcium channel blockers for reducing cardiac morbidity after noncardiac surgery: a meta-analysis. Anesth Analg **97**:634–41.

8 Fleisher LA et al. (2007). ACC/AHA 2007 guidelines on perioperative cardiovascular evaluation and care for noncardiac surgery: a report of the American College of Cardiology/American Heart Association Task Force on Practice Guidelines (Writing Committee to Revise the 2002 Guidelines on Perioperative Cardiovascular Evaluation for Noncardiac Surgery) developed in collaboration with the American Society of Echocardiography, American Society of Nuclear Cardiology, Heart Rhythm Society, Society of Cardiovascular Anesthesiologists, Society for Cardiovascular Angiography and Interventions, Society for Vascular Medicine and Biology, and Society for Vascular Surgery. J Am Coll Cardiol **50**:e159–242.

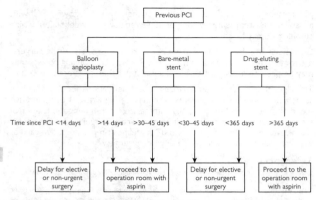

Fig. 8.2 Algorithm for management of patients with previous PCI who require non-cardiac surgery.[8]

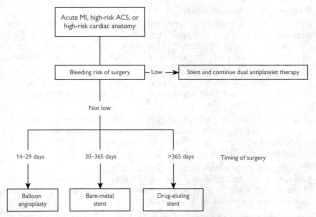

Fig. 8.3 Algorithm for management of patients requiring PCI who need subsequent surgery.[8]

Patients with heart failure

HF substantially increases the perioperative risk of adverse cardiac events and mortality in patients undergoing non-cardiac surgery. Decompensated HF is associated with a particularly high risk of adverse outcome. Patients with HF often have coexisting coronary artery disease or valvular disease, which accentuates the perioperative risk.

Patients with a new onset of symptoms suggestive of HF or established HF with a deterioration of symptoms should have non-invasive investigations to assess LV function.

In the preoperative setting, decompensated HF should be treated with diuretics to reduce preload. β-blockers may not be appropriate for management of decompensated HF acutely. Aim to optimize HF therapy with β-blockers and ACEIs in such patients at a later stage.

For patients with compensated HF who are already established on β-blockers, aim to continue β-blockade in the perioperative period. As discussed in the previous section, preoperative withdrawal of β-blockers may increase the risk of adverse cardiac events.

For guidelines on management of HF, refer to ⏀ Chapter 1, p.3.

Patients with valvular heart disease
Aortic stenosis

Severe AS, defined as a valve area of <1cm^2, is a major risk factor for adverse cardiac events in patients undergoing non-cardiac surgery. The mortality risk of non-cardiac surgery in patients with uncorrected severe AS is estimated at 10%.

Patients with symptomatic severe AS should be considered for aortic valve replacement before proceeding with non-cardiac surgery. For patients who decline surgery or who are not considered suitable candidates for aortic valve surgery, aortic balloon valvuloplasty, or, in certain circumstances, percutaneous aortic valve replacement may be alternatives. The options for pharmacological therapy in patients with AS are limited.

Mitral stenosis

MS is a relatively rare valvular lesion in developed countries. The perioperative risk is high in patients with severe stenosis with associated pulmonary hypertension (PH). Mitral valve surgery solely to facilitate non-cardiac surgery is not routinely recommended. Mitral valve surgery before elective non-cardiac surgery may be considered in patients in whom valve surgery confers a prognostic benefit unrelated to the non-cardiac surgery. If such patients are not considered suitable candidates for valve surgery, mitral balloon valvuloplasty as a bridge to non-cardiac surgery may be an alternative.

Pharmacological therapy for patients with MS consists of rate-slowing drugs for associated AF. Control of ventricular rate in patients with AF is important to optimize diastolic filling in the perioperative period. Patients with mitral valve disease who have coexisting AF are at high risk of thromboembolic complications; therefore, anticoagulation in the perioperative period is an important consideration. Refer to ⏀ Chapter 4 for guidelines on management of atrial fibrillation, p.113.

Mitral regurgitation and aortic regurgitation

Careful monitoring of volume status in patients with MR or AR in the perioperative period is important. For patients with evidence of fluid overload, preoperative diuretic therapy may be necessary. Afterload reduction with vasodilators may also be necessary intraoperatively to reduce the regurgitant volume.

Mitral or aortic valve surgery is rarely indicated prior to elective non-cardiac surgery.

Prosthetic heart valves

Management of anticoagulation in patients with prosthetic heart valves undergoing non-cardiac surgery can be challenging. Decisions regarding perioperative anticoagulation depend on the risk of thromboembolism and the risk of intraoperative bleeding.

In patients with a high risk of thromboembolic complications (i.e. prosthetic valve in mitral area, associated AF, previous embolic events) who also have a high risk of intraoperative bleeding, discontinue oral anticoagulation and commence IV UFH to cover the perioperative period.

In lower-risk patients who are undergoing minimally invasive procedures, oral anticoagulation may be transiently reduced over the perioperative period without heparin cover.

For patients who fall between the two extremes, the risks of intraoperative bleeding have to be weighed against the risk of thromboembolism on an individual basis before deciding the anticoagulation strategy.

Arrhythmias and conduction abnormalities

Ventricular arrhythmias

Isolated ventricular ectopics, couplets, and non-sustained VT are not associated with increased perioperative risk and therefore do not require specific therapy. In patients with frequent ectopics or non-sustained VT who are considered to have a high risk of developing sustained ventricular arrhythmias, prophylactic β-blocker therapy may be commenced.

Haemodynamically compromising, sustained ventricular arrhythmias may be treated with electrical cardioversion or antiarrhythmic drugs such as IV amiodarone and lidocaine. For guidelines on management of ventricular arrhythmias refer to ☐ Chapter 4, p.113.

Supraventricular arrhythmias

Sustained haemodynamically compromising SVTs in the perioperative setting may require electrical or pharmacological cardioversion. For more stable patients in whom a rate-control strategy is preferred, β-blockers, CCBs, or digoxin may be effective. For guidelines on management of patients with SVTs, refer to Supraventricular (narrow complex) tachycardias, ☐ p.134.

Bradycardias and conduction abnormalities

The principles of management of bradycardias are the same as those for patients who are not undergoing non-cardiac surgery (see ☐ Chapter 5, p.175).

Perioperative management of patients undergoing cardiac surgery

Cardiac surgery is associated with cardiovascular, pulmonary, neurological, renal, and haematological complications. Postoperative cardiac complications include:

- arrhythmias: atrial arrhythmias, ventricular arrhythmias, bradyarrhythmias
- MI: especially in patients undergoing CABG surgery
- low cardiac output syndrome.

The following section outlines guidelines for management of perioperative cardiac complications associated with cardiac surgery.

Management of arrhythmias associated with cardiac surgery

Atrial arrhythmias

AF is by far the most common atrial arrhythmia following cardiac surgery. The incidence of AF following CABG is up to 30%. The incidence in patients undergoing valve surgery is significantly higher. Other forms of postoperative atrial arrhythmias include atrial flutter, atrial tachycardia, and re-entry tachycardias.

The following section focuses on the management of AF. The recommendations are based on the ACC/AHA/ESC (2006) guidelines for management of perioperative AF,[1] and are divided into:

- prophylactic therapy for prevention of postoperative AF
- treatment of postoperative AF.

Prophylactic therapy for prevention of AF in patients undergoing cardiac surgery

β-blockers are considered standard therapy for prevention of postoperative AF. Amiodarone or sotalol may be used as alternatives in patients in whom β-blockers are contraindicated and who have a high risk of developing postoperative AF. High-risk groups include patients undergoing mitral valve surgery, elderly patients, and patients with a previous history of AF. The guidelines for prophylactic therapy for prevention of postoperative AF are summarized in Table 8.3.

Postoperative management of AF

In the majority of cases, postoperative AF is a self-limiting condition and the only treatment required is control of ventricular rate with AV-blocking drugs, i.e. β-blockers, CCBs, digoxin, and amiodarone. The guidelines for pharmacotherapy for postoperative AF are summarized in Table 8.4.

In patients with persistent postoperative AF, particularly patients in whom anticoagulation is not desirable, restoration of sinus rhythm with pharmacological cardioversion may be attempted. Options for pharmacological cardioversion include amiodarone, ibutilide, procainamide, and sotalol (class IIa indication/level of evidence B). IV amiodarone has the added benefit of slowing ventricular rate. In patients with AF with evidence of haemodynamic compromise, electrical or pharmacological cardioversion is necessary.

Table 8.3 Prophylactic drugs for prevention of postoperative AF

Drug	Comments
β-blockers	Standard prophylactic therapy to prevent postoperative AF unless specifically contraindicated (class I indication/level of evidence A)
	Aim to commence preoperatively or early in the postoperative period
Amiodarone	Alternative prophylaxis to β-blockers in patients at high risk of developing postoperative AF (class IIa indication/level of evidence B)
	IV amiodarone: aim to commence early in the postoperative period
	Oral amiodarone: aim to commence oral loading 7 days before surgery
Sotalol	Alternative prophylaxis to β-blockers in patients at high risk of developing postoperative AF (class IIa indication/level of evidence B)
	β-blocking and class III antiarrhythmic activity

Table 8.4 AV-blocking drugs for rate control of postoperative AF

Drug	Comments
β-blockers	Class I indication/level of evidence A
	Particularly effective in patients with postoperative AF as they counteract high adrenergic tone
	Use with caution in patients with haemodynamic compromise due to negative inotropic effect. Short-acting β-blockers preferred in this setting
CCBs	Class I indication/level of evidence A
	Alternative rate-controlling drug to β-blockers. As with β-blockers use with caution in patients with haemodynamic compromise due to negative inotropic effect
Digoxin	Class I indication/level of evidence A
	Less effective than β-blockers in patients with high adrenergic tone
Amiodarone	Class I indication/level of evidence A
	Less negatively inotropic compared to β-blockers and CCBs—more favourable in haemodynamically unstable patients

AF is associated with an increased risk of thromboembolic complications. In patients with AF that persists for >48h, anticoagulation with heparin or warfarin should be considered (class IIa indication/level of evidence B). The risk of perioperative bleeding has to be taken into account when deciding whether anticoagulation is appropriate. Indications for anticoagulation in patients with AF are discussed in detail in 📖 Chapter 4, p.113.

Ventricular arrhythmias

Premature ventricular ectopics and episodes of NSVT are common following cardiac surgery. They are typically benign and do not require specific therapy. Prophylactic therapy with IV magnesium has been reported in some studies to reduce the incidence of ventricular arrhythmias after cardiac surgery and may be considered in high-risk patients with frequent ventricular ectopy.[2]

Malignant ventricular arrhythmias (sustained monomorphic VT, polymorphic VT, or VF) are uncommon and are associated with a significantly higher risk of perioperative mortality. General principles of management of perioperative ventricular arrhythmias include treatment of hypoxia and correction of electrolyte abnormalities, e.g. hypokalaemia, hypomagnesaemia. Patients with evidence of haemodynamic compromise require urgent electrical cardioversion. In patients with haemodynamically tolerable sustained ventricular arrhythmias, antiarrhythmic drugs, e.g. amiodarone or lidocaine, may be used as 1st-line therapy. In certain circumstances, slow VT may be terminated with ramp or burst pacing via an epicardial or endocardial ventricular pacing lead.

The principles of management of perioperative ventricular arrhythmias are discussed in detail in 📖 Chapter 4, p.113.

Bradyarrhythmias

Conduction disturbances are a common complication following cardiac surgery. The risk of developing postoperative conduction disturbances is higher in elderly patients, patients with pre-existing conduction block (LBBB, RBBB, prolonged PR interval) and patients undergoing multivalve surgery.

Postoperative bradycardias following cardiac surgery are commonly managed with temporary pacing, through either epicardial or endocardial leads. In patients with significant impairment of LV function, AV sequential pacing may be preferable for improved haemodynamics. In the absence of temporary pacing, symptomatic bradycardias may be managed with atropine, dopamine, or adrenaline. Pharmacological management of bradycardias is discussed in detail in 📖 Chapter 4, p.113.

Permanent pacing is indicated in patients with persistent symptomatic bradycardias or patients with a high risk of developing advanced AV block.

Management of perioperative myocardial infarction in patients undergoing CABG

Perioperative MI in patients undergoing CABG is associated with increased short- and long-term mortality. Causes of postoperative MI include:
- graft-related complications: early thrombotic occlusion of venous grafts, poor distal perfusion due to anastomotic stenosis, or graft spasm
- non-graft-related complications: inadequate cardioprotection during bypass and embolization of atheromatous material following coronary manipulation.

Acute and subacute thrombotic occlusion of bypass grafts is a major cause of MI following CABG. Perioperative antiplatelet therapy is therefore an important consideration. Treatment with aspirin is associated with a significantly reduced incidence of saphenous vein graft occlusion and a lower in-hospital mortality in patients undergoing CABG.

The recommendations on perioperative antiplatelet therapy in Table 8.5 are based on the ACC/AHA (2007) guidelines on management of ST elevation MI which were initially produced in 2004[3] and updated in 2007.[4]

Table 8.5 Guidelines for antiplatelet therapy in patients undergoing CABG

Drug	Comments
Aspirin	Aspirin should not be discontinued before elective or acute CABG (class I indication/level of evidence C)
	In patients not already on aspirin therapy, aim to commence aspirin (75–325mg od) within 24h after CABG unless contraindicated (class I indication/level of evidence B)
	Bleeding may prevent use of aspirin in the immediate postoperative period. Aim to commence as soon as possible after bleeding risk is reduced
	PPIs and antacids are commonly used in the perioperative period to reduce the risk of perioperative gastric bleeding
Clopidogrel	Clopidogrel may be used as an alternative in patients who are intolerant of aspirin
	For patients who are on dual antiplatelet therapy, clopidogrel should be discontinued 5–7 days before CABG due to an increased risk of major bleeding complications (class I indication/level of evidence B)

Patients with postoperative myocardial ischaemia or infarction following CABG may require repeat coronary angiography. In those patients with early graft occlusion, a revascularization procedure with either repeat CABG or PCI may be necessary. In patients who require PCI and who have a high risk of major perioperative bleeding complications, balloon angioplasty only may be preferable, thus avoiding the need for dual antiplatelet therapy.

Management of postoperative low cardiac output

Postoperative low cardiac output is a common complication following cardiac surgery. Risk factors for a low cardiac output syndrome include pre-existing impairment of LV function, advancing age, female sex, re-operation, and emergency operation. In addition to the haemodynamic parameters from invasive monitoring, e.g. Swan–Ganz catheter, indicators of postoperative low cardiac output include oliguria, metabolic acidosis, a rising lactate level, and low mixed venous oxygen saturations.

The initial step in management of patients with compromised cardiac output is to exclude mechanical causes of compromised cardiac output. Examples of mechanical causes of impaired cardiac output include pericardial tamponade, acute valvular or paravalvular regurgitation, and saphenous vein graft occlusion resulting in MI. Patients with acute mechanical complications may require urgent surgical intervention.

General principles of management of low cardiac output include optimization of preload with volume replacement. In patients with persistently impaired cardiac output despite adequate filling and correction of reversible underlying causes, the use of inotropes (e.g. adrenaline, dopamine, dobutamine, phosphodiesterase inhibitors) may be necessary. However, vasoconstrictors such as adrenaline may cause excessive increases in afterload and compromise cardiac output. Other potential reversible causes of compromised cardiac output such as cardiac arrhythmias should also be addressed.

Persistent low cardiac output states despite inotropic drug therapy may necessitate the use of mechanical assist devices and IABP.

References

1 Fuster V *et al.* (2006). ACC/AHA/ESC 2006 Guidelines for the Management of Patients with Atrial Fibrillation: a report of the American College of Cardiology/American Heart Association Task Force on Practice Guidelines and the European Society of Cardiology Committee for Practice Guidelines (Writing Committee to Revise the 2001 Guidelines for the Management of Patients With Atrial Fibrillation): developed in collaboration with the European Heart Rhythm Association and the Heart Rhythm Society. *Circulation* **114**:e257–354. Erratum in: *Circulation* 2007; **116**:e138.

2 Shiga T *et al.* (2004). Magnesium prophylaxis for arrhythmias after cardiac surgery: a meta-analysis of randomized controlled trials. *Am J Med* **117**:325–33.

3 Antman EM *et al.* (2004). ACC/AHA guidelines for the management of patients with ST-elevation myocardial infarction; A report of the American College of Cardiology/American Heart Association Task Force on Practice Guidelines (Committee to Revise the 1999 Guidelines for the Management of Patients with Acute Myocardial Infarction). *J Am Coll Cardiol* **44**:E1–E211.

4 Antman EM *et al.* (2008). 2007 focused update of the ACC/AHA 2004 guidelines for the management of patients with ST-elevation myocardial infarction: a report of the American College of Cardiology/American Heart Association Task Force on Practice Guidelines. *J Am Coll Cardiol* **51**:210–47. Erratum in: *J Am Coll Cardiol* 2008 **51**:977.

Drugs in adult congenital heart disease

Introduction

This chapter has been subdivided into: *Part 1*, which contains general information for the management of adult patients with congenital heart disease (ACHD), and *Part 2*, which contains information specific to each type of congenital heart disease.

The key groups of ACHD are discussed separately, and management problems associated with the condition are discussed where appropriate. Subsections summarize how medical and surgical therapies should be used, and there is guidance for endocarditis prophylaxis (see separate section as indicated) and pregnancy. Where appropriate, the level of evidence on which advice is based is indicated.

The information presented is predominantly from the 2003 ESC guidelines[1] for the management of grown up congenital heart disease, and the ACC/AHA 2008 guidelines[2] for the management of adults with congenital heart disease.

References

1 ESC (2003), Management of grown up congenital heart disease. The Task Force on the Management of Grown Up Congenital Heart Disease of the European Society of Cardiology. *Eur Heart J* **24**:1035–84.
2 ACC/AHA (2008), Guidelines for the Management of Adults With Congenital Heart Disease. A Report of the American College of Cardiology/American Heart Association Task Force on Practice Guidelines. *Circulation* 2008;**118**:e714–e833.

Part 1: General information for the management of patients with congenital heart disease

Arrhythmias

Cardiac arrhythmias are a common problem in adult patients with congenital heart disease. Management can be particularly difficult, especially in patients who have undergone previous cardiac reparative surgery. There is limited research in this area.

The treatments (medical or interventional) discussed in Part 2 are similar to those used in patients without congenital heart disease but drug therapy in particular is often unsuccessful. The rapid developments in interventional electrophysiology have widened the scope of its use.

Table 9.1 lists some of the common rhythm disturbances encountered.

Table 9.1 Common rhythm disturbances affecting patients with congenital heart disease

Rhythm disturbance	Defect
WPW	Ebstein's anomaly
Intra-atrial re-entrant tachycardia/atrial flutter	Mustard, Senning, Fontan operations
AF	Congenital AS, mitral valve disease, palliated single ventricle
VT	Repair of tetralogy of Fallot (TOF), congenital AS, transposition of the great arteries (TGA), Ebstein's anomaly, single ventricle
Sinoatrial node dysfunction	Mustard, Senning, Glenn, Fontan operations
AV block	Congenitally corrected transposition of the great arteries, AVSD

Pregnancy

Women of reproductive age should receive appropriate counselling about contraception and risks associated with pregnancy. The choice of contraceptive is particularly important in women with congenital heart disease because the risks of unplanned pregnancy may be very high. Additionally, some contraceptives may have deleterious effects in congenital heart disease.

Despite its efficacy, the combined oral contraceptive pill (OCP) is not recommended for ACHD patients who are at increased risk of thromboembolism, such as those with cyanosis related to an intracardiac shunt, severe PAH, or Fontan repair (class II; level of evidence C). An additional problem with the OCP, of relevance in congenital heart disease, is its effect on anticoagulation control.

Progestogens can exacerbate fluid accumulation and should be used cautiously in patients with ventricular dysfunction.

Intrauterine contraceptive devices may be used in these patients. However, there is a risk of bradycardia and hypotension at the time of insertion and so it may be advisable for these to be inserted in well-supported specialist units.

Some conditions are associated with specific problems related to drug treatments in pregnancy (these are discussed further in 📖 Part 2 of this chapter, p.284):

- TOF: vasodilators worsen right-to left shunt.
- Coarctation of the aorta: persistent hypertension.
- TGA: risk of thromboembolism with impaired systemic ventricular function.
- Marfan syndrome: risk of worsening aortic dilatation.
- Eisenmenger syndrome: treatment may include anticoagulation.

Drugs normally used during labour in pregnancy may have major haemodynamic consequences in women with congenital heart disease. For example, ergometrine increases BP markedly and causes reflex tachycardia, and oxytocin reduces BP. Therefore, the use of these drugs needs particularly close monitoring in women with ACHD.

Heart failure

The accepted medical therapy (ACEI and β-blockers) used to treat patients with acquired HF has only been studied in very small numbers of patients with congenital heart disease. Without larger trials in these particular patients it is prudent to be cautious about their use.

Prophylaxis of infective endocarditis

Patients with congenital heart disease have increased susceptibility to infective endocarditis (IE). This risk is particularly high for patients with previously repaired disease involving the use of prosthetic or bioprosthetic material.

Despite this, the use of prophylactic antibiotics to prevent infective endocarditis remains controversial. This reflects the lack of adequate prospective trial evidence on which to inform practice. The recent 2006 guidance from the Working Party of the British Society for the Antimicrobial Chemotherapy and subsequently the 2007 guidance from the AHA is more restrictive than previously; however, many clinicians continue to advocate the use of antibiotics based on the previous Joint British Cardiac Society/Royal College of Physicians guidelines from 2004.

Although the writing committee of the 2008 AHA guidelines recognizes the reluctance to change clinical practice, it continues to give the following advice:

Antibiotic prophylaxis should be given for dental procedures that involve manipulation of gingival tissue or the peri-apical region of teeth or perforation of the oral mucosa in patients with CHD with the highest risk for adverse outcome from infective endocarditis:

Prosthetic cardiac valve or prosthetic material used for cardiac valve repair	Class IIa; level of evidence B
Previous IE	Class IIa; level of evidence B
Unrepaired and palliated cyanotic CHD, including surgically constructed palliative shunts and conduits	Class IIa; level of evidence B
Completely repaired CHD with prosthetic materials, whether placed by surgery or by catheter intervention, during the first 6 months after the procedure	Class IIa; level of evidence B
Repaired CHD with residual defects at the site or adjacent to the site of a prosthetic patch or prosthetic device that inhibits endothelialization	Class IIa; level of evidence B
Non-dental procedures; 2008 AHA guidelines suggest prophylaxis against IE is not recommended for non-dental procedures (such as oesophagogastroduodenoscopy or colonoscopy) in the absence of active infection	Class III; level of evidence: C However, in the BCS 2004 guidelines prophylaxis is advised for moderate- to high-risk patients (as listed earlier) for numerous procedures involving these systems

Vaginal delivery; it is considered reasonable to offer antibiotic prophylaxis against IE before vaginal delivery at the time of membrane rupture in selected patients with the highest risk of adverse outcomes. This includes patients with the following indications:

prosthetic cardiac valve or prosthetic material used for cardiac valve repair	Class IIa; level of evidence C
unrepaired and palliated cyanotic CHD, including surgically constructed palliative shunts and conduits	Class IIa; level of evidence C

Part 2: Information specific to each type of congenital heart disease

This section deals with the management of specific congenital heart disease diagnoses.

Atrial septal defect (ASD)

Medical therapy

- If AF occurs, anticoagulation and antiarrhythmic therapy to restore sinus rhythm should be recommended (class I; level of evidence A).
- Patients with PAH and a net left-to-right shunt should have the ASD closed. Medical management is only appropriate for irreversible PAH.
- If sinus rhythm cannot be maintained with medication or interventional means, anticoagulation and rate control is recommended (class I; level of evidence A).

Catheter/surgical therapy

- Most secundum defects can be closed with a percutaneous catheter procedure. In contrast, sinus venosus, coronary sinus, and primum defects require surgical closure.
- An ASD with RA and RV enlargement should be closed even in the absence of symptoms (class I; level of evidence B).
- Sinus venosus, coronary sinus, or primum ASD should be repaired surgically (class I; level of evidence B).
- Patients with severe irreversible PAH and no evidence of a left-to-right shunt should not undergo ASD closure (class III; level of evidence B).
- Small ASDs (diameter <5mm) without associated evidence of RV volume overload do not generally affect prognosis and do not require closure unless associated with paradoxical emboli (class IIa; level of evidence C) or orthodeoxia-platypnea (class IIa; level of evidence B).

Pregnancy

Pregnancy in patients with isolated ASDs is generally tolerated well with no significant adverse outcomes. However, pregnancy in women with an ASD and Eisenmenger syndrome is associated with increased maternal and fetal mortality and should be discouraged (class III; level of evidence A).

Endocarditis prophylaxis

Endocarditis prophylaxis is not indicated for isolated ASDs except for the first 6 months after closure. However, endocarditis may be associated with concomitant valvular pathology so this should be sought out.

Ventricular septal defect (VSD)

VSDs are often isolated lesions but may also be associated with complex cardiac abnormalities such as TOF and TGA, or obstructive left-sided lesions such as subvalvular AS or coarctation of the aorta. As such, patients may be asymptomatic, or present with signs and symptoms of LV overload or Eisenmenger syndrome.

Medical therapy
There is no specific advice with regard to medical therapy in these patients. However, consideration should be given to the use of pulmonary vasodilator therapy for patients with VSDs and progressive or severe pulmonary vascular disease (class IIb; level of evidence B)

Surgical/interventional therapy
- Closure of a VSD is indicated when there is a Q_p/Q_s (pulmonary-to-systemic blood flow ratio) of 2.0 or more and clinical evidence of LV volume overload (class I; level of evidence B).
- Closure of a VSD is indicated when the patient has a history of infective endocarditis (class I; level of evidence C).
- Closure of a VSD is reasonable when net left-to-right shunting is present at a Q_p/Q_s >1.5 in the presence of LV systolic or diastolic failure (class IIa; level of evidence B).
- VSD closure is not recommended in patients with severe irreversible PAH (class III; level of evidence B).

Pregnancy
Pregnancy in women with isolated, small VSDs and no PAH is well tolerated. However, pregnancy in women with a VSD and Eisenmenger syndrome is associated with increased maternal and fetal mortality (class III; level of evidence A).

Endocarditis prophylaxis
See 📖 Part 1, p.280, and p.218.

Atrioventricular septal defect (AVSD)

Medical therapy
In general, patients without specific problems do not require any medical treatment. In the presence of AV valve regurgitation or symptomatic heart failure, ACEIs and diuretics can be used. In patients with PAH who are considered too high risk for surgical repair, it may be appropriate to consider vasodilator therapy as long as there is no significant left-to-right shunt, as this may produce a significant right-to-left shunt.

Surgical therapy
1° surgical repair in adults is rarely advised as there is generally coexistent fixed PAH. However, re-operation may be required if deterioration occurs.

Endocarditis prophylaxis
This should be as per guidelines in 📖 Part 1, p.280, and p.218.

Pregnancy
Pregnancy is usually well tolerated in women with previous successful repair and asymptomatic women with a primum defect. Pregnancy is not recommended if there is PAH.

Patent ductus arteriosus

This may occur as an isolated lesion or in association with other congenital heart defects such as ASDs or VSDs.

Medical therapy

In the recent 2008 AHA guidelines, endocarditis prophylaxis is not recommended for repaired patent ductus arteriosus (PDA) in the absence of residual shunt (class III; level of evidence C) and in most cases can be discontinued 6 months after PDA closure. However, practice may differ from this (see 📖 Part 1 for further explanation, p.280, and p.218).

Surgical/interventional therapy

- Surgical closure of PDA in an adult is rarely indicated, and indeed percutaneous closure is the preferred option particularly in view of the calcification and friability of the tissue in this area beyond the childhood years.
- Closure of a PDA is indicated in the presence of LA/LV enlargement, PAH or left-to-right intracardiac shunting (class I; level of evidence C).
- It is reasonable to close an asymptomatic small PDA by catheter device (class IIa; level of evidence C).
- PDA closure is reasonable for patients with PAH with a left-to-right shunt (class IIa; level of evidence C).
- PDA closure is not indicated for patients with PAH and right-to-left shunt (class III; level of evidence C).

Left-sided obstructive lesions

This includes aortic valve disease/bicuspid aortic valve (BAV), subvalvular and supravalvular aortic stenosis, and coarctation of the aorta.

Bicuspid aortic valve

BAV gradually progresses to aortic stenosis (AS) or AR, and there is increased risk of aneurysm of the ascending aorta and aortic dissection.

Medical therapy

No specific drug treatment is advised to treat systemic hypertension in patients with AS but treatment is considered reasonable with monitoring of DBP to avoid reducing coronary perfusion (class IIa; level of evidence C).

Pregnancy

Patient referral to a paediatric cardiologist experienced in fetal echocardiography is indicated in the 2nd trimester of pregnancy to search for cardiac defects in the fetus (class I; level of evidence C).

Women with BAV and ascending aorta diameter >4.5cm should be counselled about the high risks of pregnancy (class I; level of evidence C).

In general, vaginal delivery is preferable to caesarean section unless there is a specific contraindication to this, such as critical aortic stenosis, aortic aneurysm, or dissection. Despite the most recent AHA guidelines which do not recommend the administration of prophylactic antibiotics for vaginal or caesarean section, many obstetricians may still administer antibiotics to women with aortic valve disease at the time of membrane rupture.

Subaortic and supravalvular stenosis

There is no specific medical therapy advised but it may be prudent to offer endocarditis prophylaxis.

Coarctation of the aorta

Adults with previous surgical repair of coarctation are more likely to also have BAV, subvalvular AS, VSD, and aortic arch hypoplasia. Patients with unoperated disease have problems with hypertension and congestive cardiac failure, and are at increased risk of aortic dissection, MI, infective endocarditis, and intracerebral haemorrhage.

Medical therapy

1st-line medications to control hypertension in these patients should be with β-blockers, ACEIs, or ARBs.

Endocarditis prophylaxis

This is not required in uncomplicated native coarctation or successfully repaired coarctation unless there is a history of endocarditis or a conduit has been inserted, or the patient is within 6 months of surgical repair or stenting (see 📖 Part 1, p.280).

Right ventricular outflow tract obstruction

This includes valvular, subvalvular, and supravalvular obstruction.

Medical therapy

There is no specific medical treatment for PS; however, symptomatic right HF may be treated with diuretics, and arrhythmias may be treated medically with antiarrhythmic drugs. Catheter ablation may be required for some arrhythmias.

Intervention/surgical therapy

Significant PS requires percutaneous balloon valvuloplasty or surgery.

Endocarditis prophylaxis

Pulmonary valve endocarditis is rare and therefore prophylaxis is not routinely recommended.

Pregnancy

Pregnancy is generally well tolerated unless the lesion is very severe.

Pulmonary hypertension/Eisenmenger physiology

There are a number of congenital heart defects that may lead to PAH, including:
- ASD
- VSD
- AVSD
- PDA
- partial/total anomalous pulmonary venous return
- truncus arteriosus
- TGA
- single ventricle
- pulmonary vein stenosis.

In these conditions, vascular changes develop over time and hypoxaemia that is unresponsive to oxygen therapy results from large vascular shunts, or bidirectional or predominantly right-to-left shunts; this is Eisenmenger physiology.

The prognosis of Eisenmenger physiology is more favourable than that of 1° PH and ventricular function is better preserved long term.

Medical therapy

The medical strategies used in 1° PH have been used in Eisenmenger physiology. These include anticoagulation, calcium-channel antagonists, IV epoprostenol, oral prostacyclin analogues, inhaled nitric oxide, oral endothelin antagonists (e.g. bosentan), and oral phosphodiesterse inhibitors (e.g. sildenafil, tadalafil). However, only very small numbers of Eisenmenger patients have been the subjects of clinical trials and so data are limited.

The use of anticoagulation in 1° PH is an established treatment that improves survival in these patients. However, there is limited data for Eisenmenger patients and with the known coagulation abnormalities of these patients, and their tendency to spontaneous mucosal bleeding which may include massive haemoptysis, the decision to anticoagulate is not a straightforward one and is not routinely recommended.

Small studies in Eisenmenger patients have shown some benefit with phosphodiesterase inhibitors, prostacyclin analogues, and endothelin receptor antagonists. The recent BREATH-5 study showed that bosentan improved exercise capacity and haemodynamics. However, systemic vasodilators such as calcium-channel antagonists should only be used cautiously as afterload reduction can worsen right-to-left shunting. In small studies however, nifedipine has been shown to improve exercise tolerance and reduce pulmonary vascular resistance.

Recommendations for medical therapy include:

- all medications given to patients with Eisenmenger physiology should undergo rigorous review for the potential to change systemic BP, loading conditions, intravascular shunting, and renal or hepatic flow or function (class IIa; level of evidence C)
- pulmonary vasodilator therapy can be beneficial for patients with Eisenmenger physiology because of the potential for improved quality of life (class IIa; level of evidence C).

Pregnancy

There is a significant risk of maternal mortality and fetal loss associated with Eisenmenger physiology and as such pregnancy is contraindicated in these patients. The following advice should be noted:

- women with Eisenmenger physiology, and their partner should be counselled about the absolute avoidance of pregnancy in view of the high risk of maternal death, and they should be educated regarding safe and appropriate methods of contraception (class I; level of evidence B)
- the use of single-barrier contraception alone in women with CHD-PAH is not recommended, due to the frequency of failure (class III; level of evidence C)
- oestrogen-containing contraceptives should be avoided (class III; level of evidence C) due to the increased risk of thrombosis.

Endocarditis prophylaxis
Patients with Eisenmenger physiology should receive endocarditis prophylaxis (see 📖 Part 1, p.280).

Tetralogy of Fallot

TOF consists of:
- subpulmonary infundibular stenosis
- VSD
- over-riding aorta (aorta over-riding the VSD by >50% of its diameter)
- RV hypertrophy.

Most patients will have had reparative surgery and will have no symptoms for some time postoperatively. Others may only have had a palliative shunt procedure such as a Blalock–Taussig shunt. Most longer-term problems are related to PR or residual RVOT obstruction.

Medical therapy
Most patients without significant haemodynamic abnormalities do not require specific medical treatment. However, right or left HF may require appropriate treatment.

Arrhythmias
Long-term follow-up of these patients shows a significant risk of sudden cardiac death associated with VT, rapidly conducted atrial flutter, or AV block. However, there is no universally agreed method for risk stratification or treatment if a deterioration is detected in patients with repaired tetralogy.

In addition to regular assessment including careful history taking, examination, and ECG, other investigations such as Holter monitoring or exercise testing to search for frequent ventricular ectopics, and echocardiograms or MRI to monitor RV function may also be utilized regularly. Management of asymptomatic non-sustained VT varies according to each institution but may include further investigation with electrophysiological studies, initiation of antiarrhythmic therapy, implantation of an ICD as 1° prevention, or no further treatment in the absence of symptoms, as many of these patients have VT but this does not reliably risk stratify them in isolation. Similarly, in the presence of deteriorating RV function and PR, pulmonary valve replacement may be recommended.

Symptoms such as dizziness, syncope, or palpitations warrant further investigation with catheterization and electrophysiology studies. Serious symptoms (i.e. non-sustained VT or cardiac arrest) are managed with an ICD.

Surgical therapy
This is indicated for symptomatic patients with severe PR, and asymptomatic patients with severe PS or PR and progressive or severe RV enlargement or dilatation.

Endocarditis prophylaxis
Prophylaxis for endocarditis is recommended (see 📖 Part 1, p.280).

Pregnancy

Patients with unrepaired TOF should be advised against pregnancy. However, the outcome of pregnancy in women with repaired tetralogy, good functional capacity, and favourable haemodynamics is promising. Even in the presence of marked PR, pregnancy appears to be well tolerated if sinus rhythm is maintained and RV function is only minimally reduced. All women should have a thorough review prior to any pregnancy.

Women with substantially impaired systemic ventricular function may be at increased risk of thromboembolism and in these patients some clinicians may consider prophylactic treatment with SC LMWH. There are no specific guidelines for this treatment.

Women should be counselled appropriately about the increased risk of fetal loss and congenital abnormalities. Genetic screening of the women before pregnancy should be considered, in particular to identify the 22q11.2 microdeletion, which further increases the risk of congenital abnormalities. Fetal echocardiography should be offered in the 2nd trimester.

Transposition of the great arteries

(More accurately dextro-TGA (DTGA)—see later.)

TGA is AV concordance and ventriculoarterial discordance and implies that the two great arteries arise from the incorrect ventricle. DTGA describes the aorta arising rightward and anterior to pulmonary artery from the systemic RV and is a more accurate way of describing the abnormality. Frequently these patients have other cardiac abnormalities such as VSDs, LVOT obstruction, and coarctation.

TGA is incompatible with life in the absence of admixture of blood. In surviving neonates this occurs naturally in the atria but many require catheter intervention to enlarge this connection (atrial septostomy) and allow greater mixing before complex surgery. In early life, these patients may have had either an arterial switch operation, pulmonary artery banding (to prepare the RV), or atrial shunt (baffle) procedure. Others may have had a Rastelli procedure in the presence of a large VSD (redirecting LV outflow to the aorta with VSD closure with a baffle within the RV; a valved conduit is then connected between the RV and pulmonary artery). Before the 1980s, patients will have had a Mustard or Senning procedure (atrial switch operations for complete TGA, where venous return is directed to the contralateral ventricle by an atrial baffle, and the RV supports the systemic circulation).

Medical therapy

There are few trial data on which to base medical treatment for ventricular dysfunction in patients with repaired TGA. The role for ACEIs and β-blockers is unclear. β-blockers in particular should be used with caution as they may worsen existing sinus node disease after previous baffle procedures, and precipitate AV block.

Interventional/electrophysiological therapy

Patients who have had a previous atrial baffle procedure are at particular risk of sudden cardiac death due to VT or intra-atrial re-entrant tachycardia (IART), and also the tachy–brady syndrome. Treatment with a pacemaker, catheter ablation, atrial antitachycardia pacemaker, or ICD may become necessary.

Endocarditis prophylaxis

Patients should receive antibiotic prophylaxis (see 🕮 Part 1, p.280).

Pregnancy

All women should be evaluated at an appropriate expert ACHD centre prior to pregnancy. There is a small risk of cardiovascular complications during pregnancy after atrial baffle procedures, and a risk of potentially irreversible RV dysfunction has been suggested after a Mustard procedure. A few reports after pregnancy in women with previous arterial switch operations suggest it is well tolerated in the absence of major haemodynamic abnormalities.

Congenitally corrected TGA (l-transposition)

This consists of AV discordance and ventricular-arterial discordance. Therefore, in these patients the morphological RV functions as the systemic ventricle, and the morphological LV as the pulmonary ventricle, and the physiological direction of blood flow is maintained. The aorta is generally anterior to and to the left of the pulmonary artery.

Congenitally corrected transposition of the great arteries (CCTGA) is frequently associated with other cardiac abnormalities including VSD, PS, and an abnormally placed systemic AV valve. Conduction abnormalities are also common, as the AV node and bundle of His are abnormally positioned and an accessory AV node is often present. The development of complete heart block is not uncommon, occurring either spontaneously or after surgery involving a VSD or systemic AV valve.

Medical therapy

It is important to maintain sinus rhythm where possible. However, anti-arrhythmic therapy should be introduced cautiously as the risk of complete AV may be high and, as always, these drugs can be pro-arrhythmogenic and negatively inotropic.

There are few data to support the use of drugs used to treat acquired LV dysfunction (i.e. ACEIs, ARBs, and β-blockers) in the context of systemic ventricle dysfunction, and in particular β-blockers should be administered with particular caution as there is a risk of complete AV block.

Surgical therapy

Some of the indications for surgical intervention in adults are listed in the following sections. In general terms, surgery in adults is indicated for the onset of symptoms due to systemic AV valve regurgitation, or systemic ventricle dysfunction. Surgery is generally limited to systemic AV valve replacement and should be performed before ejection fraction is <45%. Rarely, restoring the LV to a systemic valve may be considered in adult patients but this is associated with a higher mortality in this patient group.

Arrhythmias
Patients with CCTGA are at risk of tachyarrhythmias associated with accessory pathways. It is important to maintain sinus rhythm where possible. Additionally, they often develop spontaneous complete heart block as the AV node can be displaced and suboptimal in function.

Endocarditis prophylaxis
Patients should receive antibiotic prophylaxis (See 📖 Part 1, p.280).

Pregnancy
Women should be counselled before pregnancy by clinicians with appropriate expertise in ACHD. Pregnancy is unlikely to be well tolerated in women with a compromised systemic ventricle (ejection fraction <40%) and systemic AV regurgitation that is more than mild in severity. The risk of miscarriage is also increased.

Ebstein's anomaly

This describes abnormalities of the morphological tricuspid valve and RV. There may be associated ASDs or patent foramen ovale and hence cyanosis, and there is a risk of sudden death from supraventricular arrhythmias associated with accessory pathways.

The age of presentation depends of the haemodynamic consequences of the abnormality. Presentation in neonates and early childhood has a poor prognosis. In contrast, some adult patients may be asymptomatic.

Medical therapy
Patients frequently develop supraventricular arrhythmias requiring antiarrhythmic therapy or EP intervention. Diuretics may reduce the peripheral oedema associated with deteriorating RV function.

Anticoagulation with warfarin is recommended for patients with Ebstein's anomaly with a history of paradoxical embolus or AF (class I; level of evidence C).

Electrophysiological therapy
Supraventricular tachycardia associated with the accessory pathways that often accompany Ebstein's anomaly are amenable to catheter ablation. However, this may be challenging as multiple accessory pathways are frequently present.

Catheter ablation can be beneficial for treatment of recurrent supraventricular tachycardia in some patients with Ebstein's anomaly (class IIa; level of evidence B).

Surgical therapy
Surgery to repair or replace the tricuspid valve, with concomitant closure of an ASD, when present, is indicated for patients with Ebstein's anomaly and the following:
- symptoms of deteriorating exercise capacity (class I; level of evidence B)
- cyanosis (oxygen saturation <90%) (class I; level of evidence B)
- paradoxical embolism (class I; level of evidence: B)

- progressive cardiomegaly on CXR (class I; level of evidence B)
- progressive RV dilation or reduction of RV systolic function (class I; level of evidence B).

Pregnancy

Women considering pregnancy should be appropriately counselled. In most cases, however, pregnancy can have a successful outcome but significant cyanosis is associated with miscarriage of the fetus and low birth weight. Additionally there is a risk of CHD in the child.

Endocarditis prophylaxis

This is appropriate in cyanotic patients and postoperatively in patients with prosthetic cardiac valves (see 📖 Part 1, p.280).

Single ventricle

The conditions considered here include various types of cardiac abnormality that are not amenable to biventricular repair. This includes: tricuspid atresia, mitral atresia, double-inlet LV, hypoplastic RV, and hypoplastic LV. These conditions are often associated with a wide range of other cardiac abnormalities.

The clinical course in these patients is variable. Adult patients may have had a variety of surgical procedures.

Protein-losing enteropathy (PLE) is an incompletely understood problem that seems to affects patients after a Fontan procedure but has been reported in association with high SVC pressure with an obstructed Mustard baffle and after a Glenn procedure. In the presence of persistent oedema, pleural effusions, and ascites, a diagnosis of PLE should be sought with low serum albumin and elevated α_1 antitrypsin in the stool.

Medical therapy

- This may be required for arrhythmias, ventricular dysfunction, thromboembolism, and oedema.
- Warfarin should be given for patients who have a documented atrial shunt, atrial thrombus, atrial arrhythmias, or a thromboembolic event (class I; level of evidence C).
- It is reasonable to treat SV dysfunction with ACEIs and diuretics (class IIa; level of evidence C).
- Medical treatment for PLE is difficult and specific treatment is advised. Cardiac transplantation may be considered. One small study in Fontan patients in 2003 has shown some improvement in PLE after treatment with spironolactone. Other suggested treatments have included corticosteroid and heparin therapy to modulate intestinal mucosa.

Arrhythmias

Patients who have undergone the Fontan procedure are often troubled by recurrent IART, particularly if they have undergone an atriopulmonary connection and subsequently developed RA dilatation and scarring. The episodes of tachycardia can result in significant haemodynamic compromise and, if prolonged, clot formation.

Antiarrhythmic drugs may be used but negatively inotropic drugs should be used with particular caution in these patients. In addition, sinus node dysfunction is common and if AV block occurs with drug therapy, the Fontan anatomy may not be amenable to transvenous pacing.

Acute episodes of IART can be terminated with DCCV, over-drive pacing, and some class I or III antiarrhythmics. Prevention is difficult and no single option is applicable in all cases. If IART episodes occur only rarely (e.g. once a year), can be recognized promptly, and are well tolerated, it may be appropriate to perform only periodic cardioversion. In this case, a long-term AV nodal blocking drug such as digoxin, a β-blocker, or calcium-channel antagonist in conjunction with anticoagulation can be used to lessen the risk of a rapid ventricular response should a similar episode recur. However, in all other cases one or more of the following more aggressive strategies should be used:

- implantation of an antibradycardia pacemaker (if significant sinoatrial node dysfunction is present)
- implantation of an atrial antitachycardia pacemaker
- catheter ablation
- surgical revision of the atriopulmonary connection to the lateral tunnel or extracardiac conduit, combined with atrial Maze operation.

Endocarditis prophylaxis
Endocarditis prophylaxis is indicated (see ▢ Part 1, p.280).

Pregnancy
All women considering pregnancy who have had a previous Fontan operation should be counselled and reviewed by an appropriate ACHD specialist. Potential maternal complications include arrhythmias, ventricular dysfunction, oedema, and ascites. In addition to the increased risk of miscarriage and premature birth, there are side effects and complications as a result of anticoagulation therapy, which require careful consideration.

Marfan syndrome

This results from an abnormal fibrillin gene on chromosome 15q. Inheritance is autosomal dominant. These patients should have regular follow-up with at least annual assessment of aortic root diameter (transthoracic echocardiogram (TTE), transoesophageal echocardiogram (TOE), MRI, or computed tomography (CT) are considered acceptable) and monitoring for aortic and mitral valve insufficiency.

Medical therapy
The use of β-blockers to reduce the rate of aortic dilatation and the risk of aortic dissection in these individuals is widely practised. Treatment should begin when the aortic root diameter is >40mm but may be considered before this stage.

ACEIs or calcium-channel antagonists are suggested alternatives in patients who cannot take β-blockers.

Surgical therapy
Surgical management depends on symptoms and the diameter of the aortic root as well as the speed of dilatation and a family history of dissection, with the knowledge that the risk of dissection and sudden death increases with increasing aortic root size.

Elective replacement in all patients should be advised with aortic root diameter >55mm. However, even after surgery the risk of dilatation and dissection of the aortic arch and descending aorta remains, and annual review is appropriate.

Endocarditis prophylaxis

Prophylaxis against endocarditis is recommended after aortic valve and aortic root replacement, and in patients with mitral valve prolapse and consequent mitral incompetence (see 📖 Part 1, p.280).

Pregnancy

Pregnancy is associated with risk of further aortic root dilatation for the mother, and each child has a 50% chance of inheritance. Patients should be appropriately counselled. Dissection is rare at an aortic root diameter of <40mm, and pregnancy is relatively safe. With a diameter >45mm, pregnancy is extremely hazardous and elective surgical intervention should be considered. Aortic size should be carefully monitored during pregnancy.

β-blocker therapy should continue throughout pregnancy.

Hypertrophic obstructive cardiomyopathy

These patients have a variable clinical course. Some patients may be severely affected by symptoms whereas others are not. A key aim of management is prevention of sudden cardiac death.

Medical therapy

Commonly used drugs for symptomatic relief are β-blockers and verapamil. High doses are often required. The negative chronotropic and inotropic effects of these drugs allow greater ventricular filling. Verapamil should be used with caution in patients with severe LVOT obstruction as there is a risk of marked vasodilatation which may worsen the gradient here. Peripheral vasodilators such as nifedipine should also be avoided.

Usual HF treatments (e.g. ACEIs, diuretics) should be used once LV dilatation occurs.

Neither β-blockers nor verapamil have been demonstrated to prevent sudden cardiac death, so the use of these drugs in asymptomatic cases is unclear.

Supraventricular tachyarrhythmias (AF in particular) can cause marked haemodynamic compromise. Amiodarone is appropriate for paroxysmal AF. Oral anticoagulation should be advised for chronic or paroxysmal AF.

Interventional/surgical therapy

Septal myomectomy is the usual treatment for patients with symptomatic LVOT obstruction. Another possible option is percutaneous transcoronary septal myocardial ablation.

Some patients may benefit from dual-chamber pacing for LVOT obstruction, although this is not universal.

Risk of sudden cardiac death should be assessed to guide decisions about ICD insertion. Low-dose (200mg/day) amiodarone is an option for sudden cardiac death prevention but this is based on only one non-randomized study.

It should be noted that there are no randomized prospective studies available for ICD insertion to prevent sudden cardiac death in patients with HOCM.

The major risk factors include:
- prior cardiac arrest
- spontaneous sustained VT
- spontaneous non-sustained VT
- family history of sudden cardiac death
- syncope
- LV thickness ≥30mm
- abnormal BP response to exercise.

Endocarditis prophylaxis

Endocarditis prophylaxis is recommended for LVOT obstruction (see 📖 Part 1, p.280).

Pregnancy
- Women should receive appropriate counselling before pregnancy, particularly with respect to disease transmission.
- Pregnancy is generally well tolerated.
- β-blockers or verapamil should be continued throughout.

Further reading

ACC/AHA 2008 Guidelines for the Management of Adults With Congenital Heart Disease. A Report of the American College of Cardiology/American Heart Association Task Force on Practice Guidelines. *Circulation* 2008; **118**:e714–e833.

Galiè N et al. (2006). Bosentan therapy in patients with Eisenmenger syndrome. A multicenter, double-blind, randomized, placebo-controlled study. *Circulation* **114**:48–54.

Gatzoulis MA et al. (2003). *Diagnosis and Management of Adult Congenital Heart Disease.* Churchill Livingstone.

Gatzoulis MA et al. (2005). *Adult Congenital Heart Disease: A Practical Guide.* Oxford: Blackwell.

Head CEG, Thorne SA (2005). Congenital heart disease in pregnancy. *Postgrad Med J* **81**:292–8.

Management of grown up congenital heart disease. The Task Force on the Management of Grown Up Congenital Heart Disease of the European Society of Cardiology. *Eur Heart J* 2003; **24**: 1035–84.

Cardiac manifestations of inborn errors of metabolism and infiltrative cardiac disease

Introduction

Inherited metabolic disorders cause heart disease through the accumulation or infiltration of abnormal metabolic products. They generally cause diastolic impairment, with different degrees of systolic impairment and arrhythmias. The particular importance of these conditions is that some cases can be treated with enzyme-replacement therapy.

Table 10.1 Cardiac manifestations of inborn errors of metabolism

	Genetics/enzyme deficiency	Cardiac features	Treatment
Anderson–Fabry disease	X-linked Alpha galactosidase deficiency leads to accumulation of glycosphingolipids in lysosomes	Angina: multifactorial, predominantly microvascular dysfunction Myocardial infiltration leads to LVH with diastolic dysfunction Valve infiltration (esp. mitral) leads to regurgitation CCF	Recombinant A-galactosidase A (subtypes α and β) IV infusion. Reduces amount of glycosphingolipids in the heart and other tissues leading to symptomatic and echocardiographic improvement • α-galactosidase A β (Fabrazyme®) 1mg/kg every 2 weeks • α-galactosidase A α (Replagal®) 200mcg/kg every 2 weeks Side effects: • Infusion-related reactions very common. Manage by slowing infusion rate or pretreat with antihistamines, antipyretic, or steroids • GI disturbances, taste disturbances; tachycardia, bradycardia, palpitation, hypertension, hypotension, chest pain, oedema, flushing; dyspnoea, cough, wheezing, hoarseness, rhinorrhoea; headache, fatigue, dizziness, asthenia, paraesthesia, syncope, neuropathic pain, tremor, sleep disturbances; influenza-like symptoms, nasopharyngitis; pain in extremities; eye irritation; tinnitus, vertigo; hypersensitivity reactions, pruritus, urticaria, rash, acne; less commonly, bronchospasm, angio-oedema, cold extremities, parosmia, ear pain and swelling, skin discolouration, and injection-site reactions

(continued)

Table 10.1 (Contd.)

	Genetics/enzyme deficiency	Cardiac features	Treatment
Gaucher disease	β-glucosidase deficiency leads to accumulation of cerebrosides in the spleen, liver, bone marrow, lymph nodes, brain, and heart	Little evidence for cardiac involvement Valvular and aortic calcification, HF and pericarditis are reported Pulmonary hypertension occurs in up to 30% of untreated patients	Enzyme replacement with imiglucerase or miglustat reduces cerebrosides with variable clinical improvement. In extreme cases hepatic transplantation Imiglucerase: enzyme produced by recombinant DNA technology. For neurological manifestations of type I or III Gaucher disease. Initially IV infusion 60units/kg every 2 weeks. Maintenance dose depends on response. Lower doses may improve haematological parameters and organomegaly but not blood parameters Side effects: • Hypersensitivity, nausea and vomiting, diarrhoea, abdominal cramps, headache • Monitor for imiglucerase antibodies Miglustat: inhibitor of glucosylceramide synthase. For mild to moderate type I Gaucher disease in patients in whom imiglucerase is unsuitable. Oral 100mg tds Caution with hepatic/renal impairment. Monitor cognitive and neurological function. Men should not father a child during or within 3 months of treatment Side effects: • Hypersensitivity reactions (including urticaria, angio-oedema, hypotension, flushing, tachycardia) • Less commonly, nausea, vomiting, diarrhoea, abdominal cramps, headache, dizziness, paraesthesia, fatigue, fever, arthralgia, injection-site reactions

| Muco-polysaccharidosis MPS I (Hurler syndrome) | Autosomal recessive α-L-iduronidase deficiency leads to accumulation of heparin sulphate and dermatan sulphate | Children with Hurler syndrome often die before the age of 10 years, from respiratory or cardiac complications

Valvular lesions:
• Mitral thickening/MS/MR
• Aortic thickening/AR

Arterial hypertension ~30%:
• Associated with aortic stenosis and renal artery stenosis

ECG:
• ↑PQ, ↑QTc

Myocardial changes:
• Interstitial infiltration/fibrosis (collagen-like fibres)
• LVH (septal, non-obstructive)

Endomyocardial infiltration (fibroelastosis) | Laronidase (enzyme produced by recombinant DNA) IV infusion

For symptomatic improvement in non-neurological manifestations of Hurler

Caution—monitor for the development of antibodies

Dose: 100 units/kg once weekly

Side effects:
• Nausea, vomiting, diarrhoea, abdominal pain; cold extremities, pallor, flushing, tachycardia, BP changes; dyspnoea, cough, angio-oedema, anaphylaxis; headache, paraesthesia, dizziness, fatigue, restlessness; influenza-like symptoms; musculoskeletal pain, pain in extremities; rash, pruritus, urticaria, alopecia, infusion-site reactions; bronchospasm and respiratory arrest also reported

Bone marrow transplantation and umbilical cord blood transplantation can be used but are associated with high rates of morbidity and mortality |
| MPS II (Hunter syndrome) | X-linked

Deficiency of iduronate-L-sulfatase | Death from upper airways disease or cardiovascular failure usually occurs by age 15 years (MPS IIA)

MPS IIB is a less severe form and patients may survive into their 50s | Idursulfase (enzyme produced by recombinant DNA)

Dose: 500mcg/kg weekly

Caution—severe respiratory distress, acute febrile respiratory illness (consider delaying treatment) |

(continued)

Table 10.1 (Contd.)

	Genetics/enzyme deficiency	Cardiac features	Treatment
			Side effects:
			• Infusion-related reactions very common. Manage by slowing infusion rate or pretreat with antihistamines, antipyretic, or steroids
			• GI disturbances, swollen tongue; arrhythmia, chest pain, cyanosis, peripheral oedema, hypertension, hypotension, flushing, pulmonary embolism; bronchospasm, cough, wheezing, tachypnoea, dyspnoea; headache, dizziness, tremor; pyrexia; arthralgia; increased lacrimation; facial oedema, urticaria, pruritus, rash, infusion-site swelling, erythema, and eczema; anaphylaxis also reported
MPS VI (Maroteaux–Lamy syndrome)	N-acetylgalactosamine-4-sulfatase deficiency	Nearly all children have some form of heart disease, usually involving valve dysfunction	Galsulfase (enzyme produced by recombinant DNA) IV infusion Dose: 1mg/kg weekly Caution—respiratory distress, acute febrile illness (consider delaying treatment) Side effects:
			• Infusion-related reactions very common. Manage by slowing infusion rate or pretreat with antihistamines, antipyretic, or steroids
			• Abdominal pain, umbilical hernia, gastroenteritis; chest pain, hypertension; dyspnoea, apnoea, nasal congestion; rigors, malaise, areflexia; pharyngitis; conjunctivitis, corneal opacity; ear pain; facial oedema

Pompe disease	Glycogen storage disease type II. Autosomal recessive. A lysosomal storage disorder caused by the deficiency of acid alpha-glucosidase	Inability to break down glycogen leads to its accumulation in heart, skeletal muscles, liver, and nervous system	Alglucosidase alfa is an enzyme produced by recombinant DNA technology and licensed for the treatment of Pompe disease. Recommended dose is 20mg/kg every 2 weeks as an IV infusion. The infusion is given over 4h. Initial rates should not exceed 1mg/kg/h but can be increased by 2mg/kg/h every 30min to a maximum rate of 7mg/kg/h if the patient's observations are stable
Haemochroma-tosis	Hereditary form (autosomal recessive *HFE* gene chromosome 6) or idiopathic aetiology. Iron overload may occur as a consequence of repeated transfusion as with thalassaemia	Iron deposition in tissues including myocardium. Gives rise to mixed dilated and restrictive cardiomyopathy often with arrhythmias. Severity dependent on quantity of iron present in myocardium	Treatment with repeated venesection to maintain ferritin <50ng/mL. Iron chelation therapy with desferrioxamine (deferoxamine) 20–50mg/kg daily given SC over 8–12h 3–7 days a week. Oral iron chelators (deferasirox and deferiprone) are not licensed for haemochromatosis but can be used to treat iron overload 2° to multiple blood transfusions
Sarcoidosis	Granulomatous multisystem inflammatory disorder of unknown cause	Right-sided HF often ensues following pulmonary fibrosis. Less commonly, 1° cardiac involvement occurs causing congestive HF, heart block, ventricular arrhythmias, and sudden death. Cardiac aneurysm formation from scar tissue. May involve smaller coronary vessels	Arrhythmias often do not respond to antiarrhythmic drugs. Corticosteroids (prednisolone 1mg/kg daily for 4 weeks followed by tapering dose) may have some benefit in managing myocardial dysfunction, arrhythmias, and conduction system disturbance, and possibly improve survival. Possibility of role for hydroxychloroquine, cyclophosphamide, and methotrexate, although anecdotal evidence only. Initiated during taper of corticosteroids, i.e. steroid-sparing effect

(continued)

Table 10.1 (Contd.)

	Genetics/enzyme deficiency	Cardiac features	Treatment
Carcinoid heart disease	Caused by metastasizing carcinoid tumour. Carcinoid syndrome (flushing diarrhoea, bronchoconstriction, and fibrous endocardial plaque formation)	Right heart failure 2° to pulmonary and tricuspid regurgitation. Small percentage have LV dysfunction. Cardiac infiltration rare, symptoms caused by high concentrations of serotonin and other vasoactive substances secreted by the tumour	Digoxin and loop/thiazide diuretics to treat congestive HF Symptomatic benefit seen with somatostatin analogues/chemotherapy but do not improve survival; octreotide is started at 50mcg od or bd increasing to 200mcg tds—rarely, higher doses are needed. Should be stopped after 1 week if no improvement. BP and glucose monitoring required during treatment. Abrupt withdrawal can lead to biliary colic and pancreatitis. Predisposes to gallstones. Lanreotide (30mg SC every 14 days increasing frequency to every 7–10 days according to response) may be preferable as less frequent administration
Cardiac amyloidosis	1° amyloidosis (AL): immunoglobulin-related amyloid protein associated with myeloma 2° amyloidosis (AA): non-immunoglobulin protein	More common in men than women and rare before 40 years of age. Cardiac involvement common in 1° amyloidosis. Clinical manifestations rare in 2° amyloidosis. Approx ¼ cases of familial form develop cardiac disease, usually affecting conducting system	<5% patients survive >5 years Alkylating agents such as cyclophosphamide may be used in 1° amyloidosis. Oral melphalan (100–200mg/m²) and prednisolone have also been used in 1° amyloidosis with some success.

Familial amyloidosis: autosomal dominant—production of abnormal serum carrier protein transthyretin

Senile systemic amyloidosis: age-associated production of atrial natriuretic type protein or transthyretin

Amyloid is deposited between the myocardial fibres with predilection for papillary muscles. Causes ventricular walls to become thickened and non-compliant

4 general presentations with varying degree of overlap:

- Restrictive cardiomyopathy (right heart more commonly affected)
- Congestive heart failure/systolic dysfunction
- Orthostatic hypotension and syncope
- Arrhythmias and conduction disturbance

Caution with use of digitalis glycosides as patients tend to be sensitive, although may be cautiously used in associated AF

Caution also with CCBs as negative inotropic effect is more profound in cardiac amyloidosis

Low-dose diuretics and vasodilators may offer symptomatic benefit but patients are more prone to postural hypotension

Anticoagulation is often required owing to atrial dilatation and atrial blood stasis

Pulmonary hypertension

Introduction

Pulmonary hypertension (PH) is characterized by an increase in BP in the lung vasculature that leads to shortness of breath, dizziness, syncope, chest pain, and other symptoms, all of which are exacerbated by exertion. PH can be a severe condition with a markedly reduced exercise tolerance and lead to heart failure and death.

Clinical suspicion

Patients in whom the diagnosis of PH should be considered are:
- patients with breathlessness of unknown cause in whom cardiac and respiratory disease have been excluded
- patients with known cardiac or respiratory disease whose symptoms are greater than expected for their disease severity
- patients with a diagnosis that is known to be associated with the development of PH such as connective tissue diseases
- patients who have an echocardiogram for a different indication that coincidentally suggests PH.

Investigations/diagnosis

Doppler echocardiography
- Best screening tool for PH; it shows an elevated pulmonary artery systolic pressure (PASP).
- PASP in the range of 36–50mmHg is considered to represent mild PH.
- This definition will, however, result in a number of false positives, particularly in elderly patients in whom a right heart catheter (RHC) may be necessary to confirm diagnosis.

Right heart catheter
- Definitive investigation for diagnosis and assessment of PH.
- Diagnostic criteria:
  - mean pulmonary arterial pressure (PAP) of 25mmHg at rest or 30mmHg on exercise
  - pulmonary capillary wedge pressure (PCWP) ≤15mmHg
  - pulmonary vascular resistance (PVR) >240dynes/s/cm^2.
- In addition, at the time of RHC the response of the pulmonary vasculature to vasodilators is assessed in order to aid choice of treatment (as will be seen later).

Some investigations to diagnose any underlying cause or associated conditions
- Autoimmune screen for connective tissue diseases (CTDs)
- CT pulmonary angiogram for pulmonary embolism
- Pulmonary function tests
- ABG
- CXR
- High-resolution CT for lung disease

Classification/prognosis

After the diagnosis of PH it is important to classify the patient based on the Venice classification (see Table 11.1). This classification groups together diseases with similar pathophysiology and response to treatment.

NYHA and 6min walk time (6MWT) help stratify prognosis and response to treatment. 6MWT is simple to perform and is predictive of survival in idiopathic pulmonary arterial hypertension (IPAH). It is also useful for measuring the response to treatment. Baseline plasma N-terminal prohormone brain natriuretic peptide (NT-proBNP) is a useful prognostic marker in PAH patients without significant renal or left ventricular impairment.

Table 11.1 Clinical classification of pulmonary hypertension and its influence on treatment (Venice 2003). This classification is based upon groups of diseases causing PH that demonstrate similarities in clinical presentation, pathophysiology, and treatment options. Note that there is a distinction between pulmonary hypertension as a generic diagnosis and pulmonary arterial hypertension. In bold are those situations when treatment is directly aimed at treating pulmonary hypertension (see Fig. 11.1)

Classification	Treatment

Pulmonary arterial hypertension (PAH)
• Idiopathic (IPAH) (previously 1° PH) familial (FPAH)
• Associated with (APAH):
  • connective tissue disease (CTD)
  • anorexigens
  • portal hypertension
  • HIV infection
  • systemic to pulmonary shunts
	Treatment to target PH

PH associated with left heart disease Left ventricular, atrial, or valvular disease	Treatment of chronic heart failure, coronary artery disease, valve disease, and pericardial disease
PH associated with lung diseases and/or hypoxaemia • COPD • Interstitial lung disease • Sleep-disordered breathing	Treat the lung disease. May include oxygen **Treatment to target PH** if it is out of proportion to the lung disease
PH due to chronic thrombotic and/or embolic disease	Pulmonary thromboendarterectomy for proximal disease **Treatment to target PH** for distal disease
Miscellaneous, e.g. sarcoidosis, histiocytosis X, lymphangiomatosis, compression of pulmonary vessels	Specific to the individual diseases although not specifically targeting PH

Treatment

As can be seen from Table 11.1, p.309, treatment is either directed at the underlying cause in conditions such as COPD and left heart diseases, or directed specifically at PH. The following discussion and algorithm in Fig. 11.1 only relates to treatment directed to PH.

Vasoreactivity

As can be seen in Fig. 11.1, there is an important distinction to be made between patients with pulmonary vasculature that responds to vasodilators and those who do not respond. A vasoreactivity study should be performed in patients with IPAH, FPAH, and APAH (excluding scleroderma APAH).

The vasoreactivity test is done at the time of RHC. A short-acting vasodilator such as epoprostenol or nitric oxide is given, and the change in PAP measured. A patient is considered to have a positive result if the PAP decreases by ≥10mmHg to an absolute value of mean PAP ≤40mmHg. Those who do respond to vasodilators should be given a trial of a CCB. Only 10–15% of patients with IPAH will have a positive result, and of those only half will respond to CCBs. Patients are considered non-responders if there is no improvement after 1 month or patients are unable to achieve WHO class I or II with associated improvement in haemodynamics after 3 months.

The algorithm in Fig. 11.1 shows the treatment of IPAH, FPAH, and APAH. The algorithm needs to be adjusted for the case of APAH associated with CTD as follows:

- patients with scleroderma should not have a vasoreactivity study and should be treated as negative responders at WHO III classification in the algorithm
- all other groups with CTD should be immunosuppressed if their disease is active and if they are negative responders at the time of vasoreactivity testing, they should all be treated as if they were WHO III.

As can be seen from Fig. 11.1, all patients with PAH can be considered for background measures of oxygen, diuretics, anticoagulation, and digoxin (the level of evidence for each treatment is shown in brackets in the following sections).

Oxygen (IIa C)

- Acute administration of oxygen reduces PVR in hypoxic and non-hypoxic patients with PAH.
- All patients should have nocturnal oxygen saturation monitoring at initial assessment and thereafter when clinically indicated.
- No consistent data are available on the effects of long-term oxygen treatment on PAH.
- Long-term oxygen therapy (LTOT) if partial pressure of oxygen (pO_2) <8mmHg on air when well and should be prescribed for at least 15h per day.

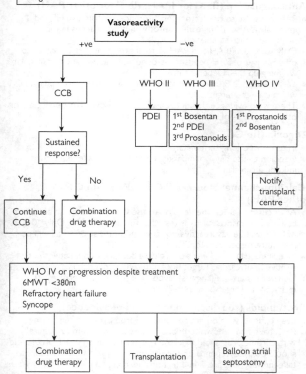

Fig. 11.1 Algorithm for treatment directed to PH. CCB, calcium-channel blocker; PDEI, phosphodiesterase inhibitor. The prefixes 1st, 2nd, and 3rd indicate preferred and alternative drugs. See text for vasoreactivity testing and the meaning of sustained response.

Diuretics (I C)

- Diuretics are of symptomatic benefit in patients with right HF.
- There are no specific RCTs and the choice of diuretic, as well as the dose, depends on the experience of the physician.

Anticoagulation (IIa C for IPAH, IIb C for other PAH)

- PAH gives rise to risk factors for thromboembolism like HF and immobility. Also, PAH leads to prothrombotic changes in the pulmonary microcirculation.
- Only studied in IPAH and PAH 2° to anorexigens. Extrapolation to other causes of PAH needs to be done with caution and in particular weighing up the risk:benefit ratio.
- Target INR is 2–3 unless the patient has risk factors for bleeding, in which case the target is 1.5–2.5.
- There is no evidence that anticoagulation improves functional class or other measures of severity.

Digoxin (IIb C)

- There are no long-term data.
- Decision to use digoxin in patients with right HF is left with the individual clinician.

Calcium-channel blockers (I C for IPAH, IIb C for other PAH)

- As discussed earlier, the decision to use CCBs depends on a positive result when vasoreactivity is tested at the time of RHC. Only 10–15% of IPAH will be vasoreactive positive, and of those only half will be persistent responders to CCBs.
- Nifedipine (start at 30mg slow-release bd) favoured if patient has relative bradycardia. Target dose 120–240mg/day.
- Diltiazem (start at 60mg tds) favoured if patient has relative tachycardia. Target dose 240–720mg/day.

Prostanoids (see discussion for level of evidence)

- Even patients who do not respond to vasodilators acutely during RHC have been shown to improve clinically and haemodynamically with chronic prostanoid therapy. The decision as to which prostanoid should be used depends on the patient and physician, and factors to take into account are side-effect profile, complexity of delivery system, and patient acceptability.
- Modes of administration (problem with IV is access and infection):
  - continuous IV epoprostenol is the only treatment to be shown in RCTs to improve survival in IPAH. For IPAH and PAH associated with CTD, grade of recommendation is I and level of evidence is A. For other PAH conditions, grade of recommendation is IIa and level of evidence is C
  - inhaled iloprost has been evaluated in one RCT. For IPAH the grade of recommendation is IIa and level of evidence B. Advantage over IV treatment is that local effect has fewer systemic side effects.

- Continuous IV iloprost appears to be as effective as epoprostenol in a small series. The advantage it has over epoprostenol is that it is stable at room temperature and does not need to be reconstituted and refrigerated.
- Sodium beraprost is the first oral prostacyclin analogue. Development is currently on hold.

Bosentan (I A for NYHA III IPAH and PAH associated with scleroderma. IIa B for the same group but NYHA IV. Scleroderma should not be associated with significant lung fibrosis)

- Endothelin receptor antagonist.
- Bosentan improves exercise capacity and haemodynamics in IPAH. Slows disease progression in patients with PAH associated with scleroderma.

Type 5 phosphodiesterase inhibitors (I A)

These are the newest class of drugs for disease-targeted therapy in PAH and there is less long-term experience than with prostanoids and endothelin-receptor antagonists. Only sildenafil is currently available for use in PAH. There are other agents available, some of which may come into clinical use soon.

Sildenafil improves exercise capacity and haemodynamics in PAH.

Combination therapy (IIb C)

Individuals who demonstrate an inadequate response to monotherapy should be considered for a combination of two or more disease-targeted therapies. Where combination therapy is to be used, patients should be entered into a clinical trial where possible. In the absence of a clinical trial, there is sufficient expert consensus to proceed with combination therapy while the patient's response to treatment is carefully monitored.

Balloon atrial septostomy (IIa C)

Atrial septostomy is a palliative or bridging procedure for patients with severe PAH who are failing on medical therapy.

Transplantation (I C)

Transplantation should be considered in all patients presenting in WHO III or IV. All candidates should be treated with disease-targeted therapy before undergoing transplantation, and if treatment is failing then transplantation should be performed if the patient is suitable.

Further reading

Galie N et al. (2004). Guidelines on diagnosis and treatment of pulmonary arterial hypertension. The Task Force on Diagnosis and Treatment of Pulmonary Arterial Hypertension of the European Society of Cardiology. Eur Heart J 25:2243–78.
National Pulmonary Hypertension Centres of the UK and Ireland (2008). Consensus statement on the management of pulmonary hypertension in clinical practice in the UK and Ireland. Heart 94:1–41.

Clinical trials

AIR (Aerolized Iloprost Randomized Study Group)[1]

- Patients in NYHA III or IV with IPAH or APAH (scleroderma, anorexigen induced, inoperable thromboembolic).
- 1° endpoint: combined outcome of 10% increase in 6MWD *and* improvement in NYHA.
- 2° endpoint: change in NYHA, increase in 6MWD, quality of life (QoL).
- Results: 16.8% reached 1° outcome compared with 4.9% in placebo (*P*=0.03).
- 2° outcome improvements in NYHA (*P*=0.03), QoL (*P*=0.026)

A Comparison of Continuous Intravenous Epoprostenol (Prostacyclin) with Conventional Therapy for Primary Pulmonary Hypertension[2]

- First trial to show a treatment which improves survival in severe IPAH. Also showed improvements in exercise capacity and QoL. Potential problem with trial is that it was not double blind so it is not possible to exclude investigator or patient bias, particularly with exercise tolerance.
- NYHA III/IV IPAH. Compared conventional therapy with combined conventional therapy and continuous IV epoprostenol.

References

1 *N Engl J Med* 2002; **347**:322–9.
2 *N Engl J Med* 1996; **334**:296–335.

Aortic and peripheral vascular disease

Peripheral arterial disease

Background

Peripheral arterial disease (PAD)—sometimes termed peripheral vascular disease—refers to atherosclerosis, usually of the lower limbs, with obstruction to blood supply. This usually gives rise to intermittent claudication and may progress to critical limb ischaemia characterized by rest pain, ulceration, and gangrene. Symptoms may become acutely worse due to atherothrombosis or acute embolization. PAD is increasingly recognized as a marker of arterial disease in other vascular beds as atherosclerosis is usually widespread.

Diagnosis

When a history suggests intermittent claudication, assessment of ABPI (ankle–brachial pressure index) is essential in establishing a diagnosis of PAD.

ABPI ≤0.9 is diagnostic of PAD and ABPI ≤0.4 is indicative of severe PAD. Additional tests such as arterial duplex may be necessary to confirm the diagnosis, and more detailed imaging to define the vascular anatomy is required if revascularization is being considered. Diagnosis should prompt a full cardiovascular assessment looking specifically at lower limb pulses, examination for popliteal or abdominal aortic aneurysms, and assessing risk factors for cardiovascular disease. Once PAD is diagnosed, the patient should undergo annual cardiovascular review to assess and monitor risk factors.

Preventative management

Preventative treatment aims to reduce the risk of coronary and cerebrovascular atherothrombosis and reduce the progression of the PAD. This involves risk-factor modification through lifestyle changes and/or pharmacotherapy. The most important considerations are controlling diabetes, hyperlipidaemia, and BP, and supporting smoking cessation through formal stop smoking clinics and encouraging regular exercise. Antithrombotic therapy is also very important for reducing the risk of occlusive vascular events and for symptomatic benefit.

Systemic hypertension

Hypertension should be managed as per national guidelines with clinic sitting BP targets of 140/90mmHg for non-diabetics and 130/80mmHg for diabetics. Whilst traditionally β-blockers have been avoided in patients with PAD, there is no compelling evidence to support them having a detrimental effect due to peripheral vasoconstriction. Newer β-blockers are vasoneutral and some such as nebivolol may be mild peripheral vasodilators, and as such may be preferred in more severe PAD.

In a PAD subgroup of the HOPE study, the ACEI ramipril was shown to be similarly beneficial in hypertensive and non-hypertensive patients in reducing cardiovascular mortality and occlusive events. This may reflect the increased cardiovascular risk in these patients, which is reduced by ACEI therapy (see 📖 p.84).

Lipid lowering

A PAD subgroup analysis of the Heart Protection Study in which patients with cholesterol >3.5mmol/L were randomized to simvastatin 40mg or placebo showed a highly significant reduction in vascular events in the treatment group. Risk reduction was 25% over 5 years. In the LEADER study (see further reading), bezafibrate 400mg od reduced the rate of non-fatal coronary events compared with placebo in men with PAD. There is some evidence supporting improvement in claudication symptoms following statin use.

Antithrombotic treatment

The use of antiplatelet medication for prevention of occlusive vascular events was systematically reviewed by the Antithrombotic Trialists' Collaboration (ATC). For those with PAD:

- antiplatelet treatment conferred a 23% reduction in major cardiovascular events
- similar benefits were seen for patients with claudication (22%), peripheral arterial grafts (22%), and peripheral angioplasty (29%)
- in most of these studies aspirin was the agent used but the CAPRIE study (Clopidogrel versus Aspirin in Patients at Risk of Ischaemic Events) which compared aspirin 325mg with clopidogrel 75mg, demonstrated superiority of clopidogrel overall and the benefit was more marked in the group with PAD (6.7% risk of major adverse cardiac events in the clopidogrel group vs. 8.6% for aspirin)
- AHA/ACC and Scottish Intercollegiate Guidelines Network (SIGN) both recommend aspirin as 1st-line antiplatelet treatment for PAD based on cost and evidence base
- in trials comparing different aspirin doses in cardiovascular disease, 75–150mg was as effective as 160–325mg. The SIGN guidelines recommend 75–150mg to avoid GI side effects, whereas the AHA/ACC guidelines support 75–325mg
- the CHARISMA trial suggested that combination therapy with aspirin and clopidogrel may have a slight benefit over individual therapy, albeit with a greater bleeding risk
- anticoagulation with warfarin has been shown to reduce graft occlusion after revascularization but is not superior to antiplatelet treatment and confers a greater risk of major haemorrhage. Appropriate when there is comorbidity such as AF, mechanical heart valve, DVT, etc
- other antiplatelet agents have proven efficacy in PAD but are not widely used: ticlopidine (thienopyridine)—risk of thrombotic thrombocytopenic purpura and bd dosing makes this unfavourable; and picotamide (thromboxane antagonist)—bd dosing and not widely available in the UK
- patients with a history of stroke or TIA may benefit from combination therapy with aspirin and dipyridamole MR as shown by the ESPS2 study, although there is little evidence to suggest any specific benefit of dipyridamole in PAD
- the POPADAD study in 2008 showed no reduction in cardiovascular events with aspirin vs. placebo in patients with type 2 diabetes and asymptomatic PAD.

Symptomatic treatment

Cilostazol (100mg twice daily) is a phosphodiesterase inhibitor and increases cyclic adenosine monophosphate (cAMP), thereby leading to vasodilatation. It also inhibits the response to several prothrombotic factors. Since phosphodiesterase inhibitors have been found to reduce survival in patients with HF, cilostazol is contraindicated in these patients. However, in large RCTs, cilostazol was found to increase claudication distance by 50–76%, with the best results obtained in those with short claudication distances prior to commencing treatment. If no benefit is obtained after 3 months of treatment, or if side effects intervene, the drug should be discontinued and an alternative sought.

Pentoxifylline is a PDE4 inhibitor increasing intracellular cAMP and stimulating protein kinase A activity, and is an inhibitor of tumour necrosis factor (TNF)-α. It may be considered at a dose of 400mg tds as 2nd-line alternative therapy to *cilostazol* to improve walking distance in patients with intermittent claudication. The likely benefit is marginal.

Naftidrofuryl (initial dose is 100mg tds but can be increased to 200mg) is a vasodilator that improves tissue oxygenation, increases adenosine triphosphate (ATP) levels, and reduces lactic acid. It is approved in Europe but not in the USA. In clinical trials, it has been found to have a positive effect on quality of life.

Other drugs used in intermittent claudication include inositol nicotinate, and cinnarizine, but there is little evidence to support their benefit.

In critical limb ischaemia, vasodilator prostaglandins such as prostaglandin E_1 and iloprost administered IV may improve ischaemic pain and help with ulcer healing but only a small percentage are likely to benefit.

Drugs for the future treatment of PAD may include angiogenic factors and vitamin-derived compounds such as carnitine. Revascularization using percutaneous transluminal angioplasty and stenting or surgical bypass procedures are indicated in patients with disabling symptoms who are not responding to optimum medical therapy.

Further reading

Belch J et al. (2008). The prevention of progression of arterial disease and diabetes (POPADAD) trial: factorial randomised placebo controlled trial of aspirin and antioxidants in patients with diabetes and asymptomatic peripheral arterial disease. *BMJ* **337**:a1840.

Bhatt DL et al. (2006). Clopidogrel and aspirin versus aspirin alone for the prevention of atherothrombotic events. *N Engl J Med* **354**:1706–17. (CHARISMA)

CAPRIE Steering Committee (1996). A randomised controlled trial of clopidogrel versus aspirin in patients at risk of ischaemic events (CAPRIE). *Lancet* **348**:1329–39.

Diener HC et al. (1996). European Stroke Prevention Study 2. *J Neurol Sci* **143**:1–13.

Meade T et al. (2002). Benzafibrate in men with lower extremity arterial disease: randomised controlled trial. *BMJ* **325**:1139.

Scottish Intercollegiate Guidelines Network (2006). *Diagnosis and management of peripheral arterial disease. A national clinical guideline.* Edinburgh: SIGN. www.sign.ac.uk/pdf/sign89.pdf (accessed 19 May 2010).

Aortic aneurysms

Risk-factor modification is the key intervention for reducing the formation and enlargement of both thoracic and abdominal aortic aneurysms (AAAs). It is also important, as atherosclerotic disease is almost inevitably present in other vascular beds.

Antihypertensive agents

- β-blockers, particularly *propranolol*, are the most extensively studied agents with respect to AAA growth. While their use has shown a significant growth rate reduction in cohort studies, RCTs have not supported this finding. Trials involving *propranolol* generally reported a large number of patients suffering side effects and discontinuing treatment.
- CCBs hold promise for reducing the expansion rate but the use of diuretics has not been shown to delay the progression of AAA size.
- Progression of atherosclerosis and AAA formation has been linked to the effects of angiotensin II; *captopril* and *losartan* have been shown to prevent aneurysm expansion in rodent models. A retrospective Canadian database showed ACEI use in the preceding 3–12 months was less frequent among those admitted with a ruptured aneurysm, suggesting a protective effect from ACEIs.

Anti-inflammatory agents

- Tetracycline and macrolide antibiotic agents have been shown to reduce the activity of matrix metalloproteinase (MMP), an enzyme implicated in the formation and expansion of AAAs. Furthermore, macrolides are used in the treatment of *Chlamydia pneumoniae,* a bacterium associated with AAA and atherosclerosis formation.
- Statin therapy has been shown in cohort studies to reduce the rate of progression of AAAs. They may reduce collagen degradation via suppression of MMP. This effect is more evident in those with smaller aneurysms (<4cm). RCTs are unlikely to ever take place, because of the widespread use of statins in 2° prevention of cardiovascular disease.

Regular follow-up is warranted especially for larger aneurysms. The aim is to identify growth of the aneurysm—either an absolute size of >5.5cm, or rate of expansion >0.5cm per year.

Perioperative pharmacotherapy

Medical therapy to reduce cardiovascular risk is particularly critical around the time of operative intervention to repair AAA, when the mortality from endoluminal and open surgery is approximately 2% and 5% respectively. The main cause of mortality is perioperative cardiac events.

- β-blockade has been indicated for patients prior to AAA repair, although clinical trials have produced conflicting evidence. The ACC/AHA guidelines support the use of β-blockers in those undergoing vascular surgery who are high risk because of a finding of ischaemia on preoperative testing, pre-existing coronary heart disease, or those with >1 risk factor, but the guidelines state that the usefulness of β-blockers is uncertain in those with only one cardiovascular risk factor.

- Use of statins is deemed beneficial in those undergoing vascular surgery. The ACC/AHA guidelines support the use of preoperative statin therapy in those undergoing vascular surgery with or without clinical risk factors.[1]
- In a meta-analysis, preoperative statin therapy was associated with a 59% reduction in risk of mortality after vascular surgery. Furthermore, a RCT published in 2004 has shown a statistically significant reduction in cardiac death in those treated preoperatively with atorvastatin for an average of 30 days prior to vascular surgery.[2]

References

1 Hirsch AT et al. (2006). ACC/AHA 2005 guidelines for the management of patients with peripheral arterial disease (lower extremity, renal, mesenteric, and abdominal aortic): executive summary. A collaborative report from the American Association for Vascular Surgery/Society for Vascular Surgery, Society for Cardiovascular Angiography and Interventions, Society for Vascular Medicine and Biology, Society of Interventional Radiology, and the ACC/AHA Task Force on Practice Guidelines (Writing Committee to Develop Guidelines for the Management of Patients With Peripheral Arterial Disease) endorsed by the American Association of Cardiovascular and Pulmonary Rehabilitation; National Heart, Lung, and Blood Institute; Society for Vascular Nursing; TransAtlantic Inter-Society Consensus; and Vascular Disease Foundation. *J Am Coll Cardiol* **47**:1239–1312.

2 Durazzo AE et al. (2004). Reduction in cardiovascular events after vascular surgery with atorvastatin: a randomized trial. *J Vasc Surg* **39**:967–75.

Aortic dissection

Acute aortic dissection classically involves the rapid development of an intimal flap, creating a false lumen for aortic blood flow thus compromising the systemic circulation. Intramural haemorrhage may be associated with dissection or can exist as a separate entity due to spontaneous bleeding into the aortic wall. Aetiological factors are varied but the most important are hypertension and connective tissue disorders (e.g. Marfan syndrome, Ehlers–Danlos syndrome).

For type A dissection (ascending aortic origin), definitive surgical management with aortic/aortic root repair/replacement is usually necessary to prevent aortic rupture and haemopericardium, and to maintain perfusion to vital organs.

In type B dissection (descending aortic origin), although surgical and endovascular repair may be possible, the focus is more on medical management to prevent aortic rupture.

Medical management

Acute care

- 2 large-bore IV lines, oxygen, respiratory monitoring, and monitoring of cardiac rhythm, BP, and urine output.
- Administer IV morphine to relieve pain and associated hypertension and tachycardia
- SBP should be controlled at a level of 100–120mmHg.
- β-blockers should be given regardless of whether hypertension is present or not. The dose should be incrementally increased until the heart rate is 60–80bpm. There is no real preference as to which β-blocker is used.
- If the patient is hypotensive, then rapid volume expansion is needed.
- Vasopressors such as noradrenaline or phenylephrine may be indicated in refractory hypotension. Dopamine is avoided except if renal perfusion needs to be improved. If needed, it is used at very low doses as it can increase LV outflow.
- If the patient becomes cardiovascularly unstable, this is indicative of cardiac tamponade or aortic rupture, and urgent surgical intervention should be sought.

Definitive medical management is preferred to surgery in stable patients with acute distal dissection, arch dissection, or those with chronic dissection. Endovascular repair is considered by many to be the gold standard in acute complicated type B dissection, as the duration of surgery and recovery time are significantly shorter than with open repair.

Surgery is used when medical management fails or when distal dissection is complicated by rupture, organ compromise, or extension into the ascending aorta. Surgery is also the treatment of choice for acute proximal dissection and dissection in Marfan syndrome.

Ongoing management
- Long-term BP control with a SBP of <130mmHg is indicated for all patients. The agent used for long-term control can be the same as that used in the acute setting and depends on the clinical situation.
- Long-term follow-up is needed to detect any progression or recurrence of the dissection, aneurysm formation, or aortic regurgitation.
- Follow-up should be 3-monthly for the first year, 6-monthly for the next year, and then annually thereafter. Patients are at highest risk immediately after hospitalization and during the first 2 years.
- The 5-year survival rate is about 75% whether the patient is treated medically or surgically.

Treatment options (Table 12.1)

Table 12.1 Treatment options in aortic dissection

Agent	Uses/notes	Dosing
Esmolol	Short $t_{1/2}$—useful in cases where abrupt withdrawal may be necessary, e.g. labile BP, risk of bronchospasm. In practice it is rarely used	Loading dose of 0.5mg/kg over 2–5min followed by an infusion of 0.10–0.20mg/kg/min
Labetalol	Lowers both the BP and LV outflow	2mg/min IV infusion or 50mg IV over >1min repeated every 5min until satisfactory response. Max total dose 200mg
Sodium nitroprusside	β-blocker needs to be simultaneously instituted otherwise the dissection may propagate if sodium nitroprusside is used alone as it increases stroke volume	Initial dose is 0.25mcg/kg/min
CCBs (if β-blocker contraindicated)	Diltiazem and verapamil have both vasodilator and negative inotropic effects. Nifedipine can be given sublingually and therefore can be utilized while other drugs are being prepared. However, it has little effect in slowing the heart rate or reducing contractility	Verapamil 5–10mg IV over 2–3min, repeated again after 5min if necessary
ACEIs	ACEIs may be used to treat hypertension caused by excess renin secretion. This usually occurs when the dissection flap reduces flow through the renal arteries	

Large-vessel vasculitis

Takayasu arteritis

Clinical features

This disease classically affects young women. It progresses through three stages.

- Stage 1 is manifested by constitutional symptoms such as malaise and fever.
- Stage 2 is characterized by features of vascular inflammation: arterial stenoses, aneurysms, symptoms of vascular insufficiency such as paraesthesia, claudication (more frequent in upper than lower limbs), and visual disturbances. Aneurysms most commonly affect the aortic root, and may lead to AR. Vasculitis can affect the renal vessels and may lead to hypertension. Neurological manifestations include amaurosis fugax, stroke, TIAs, hemiplegia, seizures, and paraplegia.
- Stage 3 is manifested by fibrosis and remission; however, patients may relapse. In terms of cardiac manifestations, morbidity and mortality are 2° to poorly controlled hypertension and AR, as well as vasculitis affecting the coronary vessels. If coronary vessels do become involved, the coronary ostia are usually affected.

Management

Early intensive treatment with high-dose corticosteroids has been shown to induce remission and should be started in active disease.

- Initial dose of prednisolone is 1mg/kg (max 60mg) per day. This dose should be maintained for at least 1 month and gradually tapered. NB tapering should *not* be alternate-day dosing as this may lead to relapse.
- If symptomatic relapse occurs whilst the patient is still on glucocorticoid treatment, a step up of dose by 5–10mg is usually sufficient.
- Ensure adequate bone protection therapy is in place as per local policy.

Takayasu arteritis can remain active subclinically and often requires a steroid-sparing immunosuppressive regimen:

- azathioprine (2mg/kg/day) or methotrexate (20–25mg weekly) may help maintain control of disease and reduce the requirement for steroid
- cyclophosphamide has been used in steroid-resistant cases.

Reconstructive surgery should be performed in the quiescent phase and only in specialist centres.

Giant cell arteritis

Also known as temporal arteritis, giant cell arteritis (GCA) principally affects the elderly. As in Takayasu arteritis, women are more frequently affected than men, although the ratio is not as great. It can lead to a variety of systemic, neurological, and ophthalmological complications with visual loss being one of the most significant causes of morbidity.

Management

As with Takayasu arteritis, the initial treatment aims to induce remission with high-dose corticosteroids. IV methylprednisolone may be helpful if visual symptoms manifest early.

- Prednisolone (1mg/kg, max 60mg per day) should be initiated if high suspicion exists. Arrangements for temporal artery biopsy should not delay treatment.
- Inflammatory markers (C-reactive protein (CRP)/ESR) should be monitored to detect relapses. If already on reducing-dose steroids, the daily dose of prednisolone should be increased by 5–10mg or otherwise restarted as described earlier.
- GCA usually requires long-term corticosteroid treatment, and steroid-sparing agents such as methotrexate (10–15mg/week) have some effect at preventing relapse and reducing the cumulative dose of steroid.
- The combination of anti-TNF-α agent infliximab with corticosteroids has not proven to be any more effective than steroids alone.
- Antiplatelet treatment with low-dose aspirin should be prescribed allowing for contraindications as patients with GCA have a higher risk of coronary and cerebrovascular events.
- There is little evidence to suggest that statins are beneficial in GCA.
- Suitable bone protection should be given.

Further reading

Mukhtyar C et al. (2009). EULAR recommendations for the management of large vessel vasculitis. *Ann Rheum Dis* **68**:318–23.

A–Z of cardiac drugs

Abciximab

A hybrid murine–human monoclonal antibody Fab fragment directed against the glycoprotein IIb/IIIa receptor.

CV indications

1. Patients undergoing PCI
2. Patients with UA not responding to conventional medical therapy when PCI is planned within 24h

Mechanism of action

Abciximab inhibits platelet aggregation by preventing the binding of fibrinogen, von Willebrand factor, and other adhesive molecules to GP IIb/IIIa receptor sites on activated platelets. Abciximab also inhibits the vitronectin receptors that take part in coagulation and as a result abciximab is more efficient than other GP IIb/IIIa receptor antagonists.

Pharmacodynamics

Abciximab has been studied in phase 3 RCTs in patients undergoing PCI: at high risk for abrupt closure of the treated coronary vessel (EPIC), in a broader group of patients (EPILOG), in unstable angina patients not responding to conventional medical therapy (CAPTURE), and in patients suitable for either conventional angioplasty/atherectomy or 1° stent implantation (EPILOG Stent; EPISTENT).

The EPIC trial evaluated abciximab in patients undergoing percutaneous transluminal coronary angioplasty or atherectomy and the 1° endpoint was death, MI, the need for urgent intervention for recurrent ischaemia within 30 days compared to placebo. There was a 4.5% lower incidence in the bolus plus infusion abciximab group including all high-risk subgroups.[1]

In the EPILOG trial, the 1° composite endpoint of death or MI occurring within 30 days of PCI was lower in the abciximab group; this benefit was sustained after 6 months[2] and 12 months.[3] Major bleeding was not significantly different in the abciximab and in the placebo arm.

The CAPTURE trial evaluated abciximab in UA patients not responding to conventional medical therapy for whom PCI was planned, but not immediately performed. The combined 1° endpoint was death, MI, or urgent intervention within 30 days of PCI.[4] The results are consistent with EPIC results.

The ISAR-REACT 2 trial evaluated whether abciximab provides incremental benefit in high-risk patients with NSTEACS undergoing urgent PCI after pretreatment with 600mg clopidogrel at least 2h before the procedure. Abciximab reduced the composite 30-day endpoint of death, MI, target vessel revascularization by 25%.[5] This benefit was maintained after 1 year (RRR 30% in the combined incidence of death, MI, or target vessel revascularization and RRR 26% in the combined incidence of death or MI).[6]

Abciximab was tested in comparison with tirofiban in the TARGET trial in patients with recent NSTEACS. Abciximab was superior to tirofiban in reducing the risk of death, non-fatal MI, or urgent revascularization at 30 days, primarily by reducing non-fatal MI.[7] Follow-up at 6 months revealed no significant difference in 1° outcomes between abciximab and tirofiban (14.3% vs. 14.8%).[8]

EPISTENT evaluated 3 different treatment strategies in patients undergoing PCI: conventional PTCA with abciximab plus low-dose heparin, 1° intracoronary stent implantation with abciximab plus low-dose heparin, and 1° intracoronary stent implantation with placebo plus standard-dose heparin.[9] The results demonstrated benefit in both abciximab arms (i.e. with and without stents) compared with stenting alone on the composite of death, MI, or urgent intervention within 30 days of PCI.

Pharmacokinetics

Initial $t_{1/2}$ <10min and a 2nd phase $t_{1/2}$ of about 30min although abciximab remains in the circulation for 15 days or more. Platelet function generally recovers over the course of 48h after discontinuation. However, the antibody remains platelet bound in circulation up to 15 days. Its action can be reversed by platelet transfusion. Elimination is unknown but is suggested to be by catabolism or proteolytic degradation.

Practical points

⚗ Doses

IV bolus: 0.25mg/kg administered 10–60min before PCI
Continuous IV infusion: 0.125mcg/kg/min (to a maximum of 10mcg/min) for 12h

☺ Common side effects

- Bleeding: major (3.8%), minor (4.8%)
- Thrombocytopenia (0.5–2.4%)
- Other: hypotension (14.4%), bradycardia (4.5%), abdominal pain (6.1%), nausea or vomiting (20.9%), back pain (17.6%), chest pain (11.4%), headache (6.4%), puncture site pain (3.6%), peripheral oedema (1.6%)

Interactions

Increased risk of bleeding when co-administered with heparins, other anticoagulants, thrombolytics, antiplatelet agents, dextran solutions, prostacyclin, and NSAIDs.

Cautions/notes

Administration of abciximab may result in human antichimeric antibody (HACA) formation that could potentially cause allergic or hypersensitivity reactions, thrombocytopenia, or diminished benefit in approximately 6%. Patients with HACA titres may have allergic or hypersensitivity reactions when treated with other diagnostic or therapeutic monoclonal antibodies.

It is not recommended for use in children and adolescents <18 years of age, due to a lack of data on safety and efficacy.

Pregnancy and lactation

Safety of abciximab in pregnancy and breastfeeding has not been established. It should not be used during pregnancy unless clearly necessary (*pregnancy category C*). Interruption of breastfeeding during the treatment period is recommended.

Contraindications

- Active internal bleeding
- Recent (within 6 weeks) GI or GU bleeding of clinical significance
- History of cerebrovascular accident (CVA) within 2 years, or CVA with a significant residual neurological deficit
- Bleeding diathesis
- Administration of oral anticoagulants within 7 days unless prothrombin time is 1.2× control
- Thrombocytopenia (<100,000/µL)
- Recent (within 6 weeks) major surgery or trauma
- Intracranial neoplasm, arteriovenous malformation, or aneurysm
- Severe uncontrolled hypertension
- Presumed or documented history of vasculitis
- Acute pericarditis
- Cirrhosis or other clinically significant liver disease
- Use of IV dextran before PCI, or intent to use it during an intervention.
- Patients with known hypersensitivity to any component of this product or to murine proteins (abciximab)

References

1 Topol EJ *et al.* for the EPIC Investigators (1997). Long-term protection from myocardial ischemic events in a randomized trial of brief integrin blockade with percutaneous coronary intervention. *JAMA* 278:479–84.

2 The EPILOG Investigators (1997). Platelet glycoprotein IIb/IIIa receptor blockade and low-dose heparin during percutaneous coronary revascularization. *N Engl J Med* 336:1689–96.

3 Lincoff AM *et al.* for the EPILOG Investigators (1999). Sustained suppression of ischemic complications of coronary intervention by platelet GP IIb/IIIa blockade with abciximab. *Circulation* 99:1951–8.

4 The CAPTURE Investigators (1997). Randomised placebo-controlled trial of abciximab before and during coronary intervention in refractory unstable angina. *Lancet* 349:1429–35.

5 Kastrati A *et al.*; Intracoronary Stenting and Antithrombotic: Regimen Rapid Early Action for Coronary Treatment 2 (ISARREACT 2) Trial Investigators (2006). Abciximab in patients with acute coronary syndromes undergoing percutaneous coronary intervention after clopidogrel pretreatment: the ISAR-REACT 2 randomized trial. *JAMA* 295:1531–8.

6 Ndrepepa G *et al.* (2008). One-year clinical outcomes with abciximab vs. placebo in patients with non-ST-segment elevation acute coronary syndromes undergoing percutaneous coronary intervention after clopidogrel pre-treatment. *Eur Heart J* 29:455–61.

7 Topol E *et al.* (2001). Comparison of two platelet glycoprotein IIb/IIIa inhibitors, tirofiban and abciximab, for the prevention of ischemic events with percutaneous coronary revascularization. *N Engl J Med* 244:1888–94.

8 Moliterno DJ *et al.* for the TARGET Investigators (2002). Outcomes at 6 months for the direct comparison of tirofiban and abciximab during percutaneous coronary revascularisation with stent placement: The TARGET follow-up study. *Lancet* 360:355–60.

9 EPISTENT Investigators (1998). Randomised placebo-controlled and balloon angioplasty-controlled trial to assess safety of coronary stenting with use of platelet glycoprotein-IIb/IIIa blockade. *Lancet* 352:87–92.

Adenosine

(See also 📖 Antiarrhythmic drugs: classification, p.362)

IV purine nucleoside.

CV indications

Rapid conversion of paroxysmal SVT to sinus rhythm.

Mechanism of action

Adenosine is a purine nucleoside, which is present in all cells of the body. It acts via 4 known adenosine G-coupled receptor subtypes. Cardiac effects are mediated via the Gi-coupled A_1 receptor subtype located in the SA and AV nodes. Adenosine produces cell hyperpolarization through the activation of the adenosine-sensitive inward rectifier K^+ channel and inhibits adenyl cyclase, decreasing cAMP-mediated Ca^{2+} influx through L-type calcium channels. Hence, IV administration of adenosine has a negative chronotropic effect on the SA node and a negative dromotropic effect on the AV node (prolongs the PR interval), causing transient heart block and interrupting the re-entry pathways through the AV node. Stimulation of A_2 receptors in vascular smooth muscle causes vasodilatation and may contribute to BP effects.

Pharmacodynamics

The IV bolus dose of 6 or 12mg adenosine usually has no systemic haemodynamic effects. When larger doses are given by infusion, adenosine decreases BP by decreasing peripheral vascular resistance.

In patients with paroxysmal SVT, cumulative response rates of conversion to sinus rhythm with IV adenosine of 3, 6, 9, and 12mg given in sequence were 35.2%, 62.3%, 80.2%, and 91.4% in patients who received maximum doses of 3, 6, 9, and 12mg respectively compared with placebo (8.9%, 10.7%, 14.3%, and 16.1%). Compared with verapamil, cumulative rates of conversion with adenosine 6 and 12mg in sequence were 57% (cf 81% with verapamil 5mg) and 93% (cf 91% with verapamil 7.5mg).[1]

Adenosine does not modify cardiac contractility or conduction via accessory pathways.

Pharmacokinetics

IV-administered adenosine is rapidly cleared from the circulation via cellular uptake, primarily by erythrocytes and vascular endothelial cells. As adenosine is present throughout the body, it is difficult to study its pharmacokinetics. The $t_{1/2}$, as measured in whole blood, is <10s. Adenosine does not require hepatic or renal function for its activation or inactivation, so hepatic and renal failure would not be expected to alter its effectiveness or tolerability.

Practical points

⚖ Doses

1st dose: 6mg (0.05–0.25mg/kg) as rapid IV bolus over 2s
2nd dose: 12mg rapid IV bolus is given 1–2min after the 1st injection
3rd dose: 12mg rapid IV bolus may be repeated in 1–2min

The 2nd and 3rd doses can be given if SVT has not been eliminated by previous dose. Additional or higher doses thereafter are not recommended.

☺ Common side effects
(>10%): facial flushing, shortness of breath/dyspnoea, bradycardia, asystole, sinus pause, AV block, atrial extrasystoles, skipped beats, ventricular excitability disorders, degeneration of atrial flutter or paroxysmal SVT to AF.

(1–10%): headache, lightheadedness, apprehension, nausea, chest pressure, and/or burning sensation.

Interactions
Dipyridamole inhibits the uptake of adenosine and so may potentiate the effects of adenosine (hypotension); thus, the dose of adenosine should be reduced. Digoxin and verapamil when associated with adenosine may produce synergistic depressing effects on the SA and AV nodes.

The effects of adenosine are antagonized by methylxanthines (caffeine and theophylline). Thus larger doses may be required where these have been concomitantly taken.

Cautions/notes
- Due to the possibility of transient cardiac arrhythmias arising during conversion of the SVT to normal sinus rhythm, adenosine should only be used in hospital and with cardiac monitoring. Also, patients who develop high-level AV block at a particular dose should not be given further dosage increments.
- Due to interactions, reduced doses of adenosine may be required in the presence of dipyridamole.
- Adenosine does not convert atrial flutter, AF, or VT to normal sinus rhythm. In the presence of atrial flutter or AF, a transient modest slowing of ventricular response may occur immediately following adenosine administration; when an accessory bypass tract is present, adenosine may develop increased conduction down the anomalous pathway.
- Due to the possible risk of torsades de pointes, adenosine should be used with caution in patients with a prolonged QT interval, whether this is congenital or acquired.
- In patients with asthma or COPD, adenosine may precipitate bronchospasm lasting >30min.

In the absence of evidence regarding its effects during pregnancy and lactation, adenosine should be used only when absolutely necessary (pregnancy category C).

Contraindications
- 2nd- or 3rd-degree AV block (except from patients with a functioning artificial pacemaker)
- Sick sinus syndrome (except in patients with a functional artificial pacemaker)
- Long QT syndrome
- Bronchospasm, asthma
- Known hypersensitivity to adenosine

Reference
1 DiMarco JP et al. (1990). Adenosine for paroxysmal supraventricular tachycardia: dose ranging and comparison with verapamil. Assessment in placebo-controlled, multicenter trials. The Adenosine for PSVT Study Group. Ann Intern Med **113**:104–10.

Agalsidase alfa

Agalsidase alfa is the recombinant human protein α-galactosidase A.

CV indications

Fabry disease, an X-linked deficiency of the enzyme α-galactosidase A.

Mechanism of action

Fabry disease is a glycosphingolipid storage disorder that is caused by α-galactosidase A deficiency. This results in accumulation of globo-triaosylceramide (GL-3). Clinical manifestations of Fabry disease include renal failure, cardiomyopathy, and CVAs. Agalsidase alfa catalyses the hydrolysis of GL-3 and other α-galactyl-terminated neutral glycosphin-golipids to ceramide dihexoside and galactose. Agalsidase alfa provides an exogenous source of α-galactosidase A to limit the accumulation of these glycolipids in the tissues.

Pharmacodynamics

Agalsidase alfa reduces accumulation of GL-3 in many cell types, including endothelial cells (of the kidney, heart, and skin) and parenchymal cells. It reduces pain scores and improves renal function and myocardial contractility. Its effect may be limited in those with advanced renal disease. Plasma GL-3 levels were reduced to normal levels and remained at normal levels after up to 60 months of treatment.

Pharmacokinetics

Following a single IV dose of 0.2mg/kg, agalsidase alfa had a biphasic distribution and elimination profile from the circulation. In the single-dose pharmacokinetic studies there was early distribution throughout the blood volume, followed by uptake into liver, spleen, lungs, heart, kidney, and bone marrow within a few hours, and it is retained in these viscera for >24–48h. Elimination $t_{1/2}$ was 89–110min and V_d was approximately 17% body weight. Agalsidase alfa is cleared from the circulation faster in children than adults. Agalsidase alfa is a protein, its metabolism occurs by peptide hydrolysis, and the kidneys are considered to be a minor clearance pathway. The pharmacokinetic properties are essentially unaffected by the dose of the enzyme, and unmodified by impaired liver or renal function.

With prolonged treatment (6 months and greater), altered pharmacokinetics may be observed with an apparent increase in clearance and a lower systemic exposure. This is due to the development of IgG antibodies against agalsidase alfa, which could serve as an additional clearance. However, the apparent change in clearance does not result in a change in the elimination half-life.

Practical points

♣ Doses
0.2mg/kg by IV infusion over 40min every alternate week

☻ Side effects
The most serious are anaphylactic and allergic reactions.

(≥5%): headache, chills, pyrexia, feeling hot or cold, increased sweating, dyspnoea, nausea, vomiting, diarrhoea, paraesthesia, fatigue, pruritus, pain in extremity, myalgia, back pain, peripheral oedema, urticaria, rash, and somnolence.

Others: malaise, cough, sore or tight throat, hoarseness, ataxia, vertigo, acne, pruritus, altered taste perception, rhinorrhoea, tinnitus.

Cardiovascular: tachycardia, bradycardia, palpitations, facial flushing, hypotension, chest pain.

Infusion reactions occur in some patients after receiving pretreatment with antipyretics, antihistamines, and oral steroids. Because of the potential for severe infusion reactions, appropriate medical support measures should be readily available when agalsidase alfa is administered.

An important number of patients developed IgG antibodies to agalsidase alfa within the first 3 months of exposure.

Serious/life-threatening reactions
See 'Cautions/notes' section.

Interactions
As agalsidase alfa is a protein, drug–drug interactions are not expected. However, it should not be co-administered with drugs (chloroquine, amiodarone, monobenzone, and gentamicin) that potentially inhibit intracellular α-galactosidase activity.

Cautions/notes
Serious infusion reactions are reported uncommonly, including tachycardia, urticaria, nausea/vomiting, angioneurotic oedema with stridor, and tongue swelling. These gradually reduce over time. These reactions ameliorate with slowing the infusion rate, temporarily stopping the infusion, and/or when antipyretics, antihistamines, or corticosteroids are given prior to commencing the infusion.

Patients with advanced Fabry disease have a compromised cardiac function; they should be monitored closely because they may have a higher risk of severe complications from infusion reactions.

Pregnancy and lactation
Animal studies do not indicate direct or indirect harmful effects with respect to pregnancy or development of the fetus and no adverse effects on the mother and baby have been demonstrated (pregnancy category B). It is not known whether it penetrates to the fetus nor if it passes into milk. Therefore, caution should be taken when prescribing to pregnant or breastfeeding women.

Contraindications
Hypersensitivity reactions to agalsidase alfa.

Further reading
Schaefer RM et al. (2009). Enzyme replacement therapy for Fabry disease: a systematic review of available evidence. *Drugs* **69**:2179–205.

Agalsidase beta

Agalsidase beta is the recombinant human protein α-galactosidase A.

CV indications

Fabry disease, an X-linked deficiency of the enzyme α-galactosidase A.

Mechanism of action

(See 📖 Agalsidase alfa, p.335)

Pharmacodynamics

After IV infusion, agalsidase beta is rapidly removed from the circulation and taken up by vascular endothelial and parenchymal cells into lysosomes. Agalsidase beta reduces GL-3 deposition in a dose-dependent manner in capillary endothelium of kidney, heart, and skin and in the plasma (plasma levels are normalized within 20 weeks of treatment). As with agalsidase alfa, the effect of agalsidase beta treatment on the kidney function is limited in some patients with advanced renal disease.

Pharmacokinetics

Agalsidase beta follows non-linear pharmacokinetics and seems to be affected by the formation of IgG antibodies against it. Repeated infusions results in a progressive increase in the uptake of agalsidase beta into leucocytes, but it is unclear as to whether or not these changes will affect long-term drug efficacy. As pharmacokinetic parameters are not altered by impaired renal function, elimination of agalsidase beta by the kidneys is *considered* to be a minor clearance pathway. $t_{1/2}$ is ~90min. Agalsidase beta is a protein and metabolism is expected to occur by peptide hydrolysis. Therefore, impaired liver function is not expected to affect the pharmacokinetics of agalsidase beta in a clinically significant manner.

Practical points

🔧 Doses

The initial infusion rate should be 0.25mg/min to minimize the potential infusion-associated reactions. Once patient tolerance is established, the infusion rate may be increased with subsequent infusions up to 1mg/kg (15mg/h) every 2 weeks.

Patients who have had a positive skin test to agalsidase beta or who have tested positive for anti-agalsidase beta IgE may be successfully rechallenged with agalsidase beta at a lower infusion rate.

😊 Side effects

(See 📖 Agalsidase alfa, p.335)

Interactions

None

Cautions/notes

The majority of patients develop IgG antibodies to agalsidase beta, although some develop IgE. However, over time many patients develop tolerance. Patients with antibodies to agalsidase beta have a greater potential to experience infusion-associated reactions and hypersensitivity reactions.

If infusion reactions occur, patients should be managed in the same way as with agalsidase alfa.

Pregnancy and lactation

No adverse effects on the mother and baby have been demonstrated (pregnancy category B). However, as data are limited, agalsidase beta should only be used when necessary. Animal studies do not indicate direct or indirect harmful effects with respect to pregnancy or development of the fetus. It is not known whether agalsidase beta is excreted in human milk, so caution should be taken when prescribing to pregnant or breast-feeding women.

Contraindications

Hypersensitivity reactions to agalsidase beta.

Reference

1 Schaefer RM *et al.* (2009). Enzyme replacement therapy for Fabry disease: a systematic review of available evidence. *Drugs* **69**:2179–205.

Aldosterone antagonists

(See also 📖 Spironolactone, p.588 and 📖 Eplerenone, p.449)

Aldosterone is a mineralocorticoid hormone released in response to angiotensin II, adrenocorticotropic hormone, and increased potassium. It plays an important role in the regulation of Na^+ and K^+ homeostasis, extracellular fluid volume, and BP. Aldosterone binds to mineralocorticoid receptors in both epithelial (e.g. kidney) and nonepithelial (e.g. heart, blood vessels, and brain) tissues. In the kidney it binds to the mineralocorticoid receptor in cells of the collecting duct. It exerts its effects via the mineralocorticoid receptor and the resultant activation-opening of specific amiloride-sensitive sodium channels (ENaC) and increase in the number and activity of Na^+/K^+-ATPase pumps. Reabsorbed sodium is pumped out of the cell by the Na^+–K^+–ATPase pump in the basolateral (peritubular) membrane. Thus, aldosterone is responsible for the reabsorption of about 2% of filtered sodium in the kidneys and the excretion of K^+, contributing to the genesis of oedema. In addition, aldosterone can cause endothelial dysfunction (increases NADPH and decreases NOS activity), increases both sympathetic tone and the vasoconstrictor response to angiotensin II, produces cardiovascular fibrosis and hypertrophy, and may lead to cardiac arrhythmias.

Plasma aldosterone levels increase in HF patients due to an increased synthesis in response to angiotensin II and decreased hepatic clearance, contributing to deleterious cardiac remodelling. In this setting, increased aldosterone levels decrease initially, in response to ACEIs and ARBs, but levels have been shown to return to control values during chronic therapy with these agents. Spironolactone and eplerenone are aldosterone antagonists and will be discussed in this book under specific sections.

Aliskiren

A direct renin inhibitor.

CV indications

Treatment of essential hypertension.

Mechanism of action

Renin catalyses the first rate-limiting step of the RAAS, and cleaves angiotensinogen to angiotensin I, the only route to angiotensin II formation. Renin and prorenin bind to the (pro)renin receptor and stimulate signalling pathways independently from angiotensin II synthesis. Aliskiren binds to the active site of renin (subpocket S3^{SP}), inhibiting the conversion of angiotensinogen to angiotensin I by renin and thereby the synthesis of angiotensin II by ACE and ACE-independent pathways, without affecting kinin metabolism. ACEIs and ARBs increase, while aliskiren inhibits plasma renin activity.

Pharmacodynamics

Hypertension: a meta-analysis[1] has shown that BP reductions with aliskiren are: ≈15.8–14.1/12.3–10.3mmHg with 300mg od and ≈13.0–8.7/10.3–7.8mmHg 150mg od. Antihypertensive effects appear to last for days–weeks after its withdrawal and are increased when combined with a diuretic. Aliskiren suppressed the increase in plasma renin activity induced by ACEIs, ARBs, diuretics, and dihydropyridines.

DBP lowering from baseline with aliskiren 300mg in combination with valsartan 320mg od (12.2mmHg) was significantly greater than with either aliskiren (9.0mmHg) or valsartan (9.7mmHg) monotherapy.[2]

Diabetic nephropathy: RRR 20% in the mean urinary albumin-to-creatinine ratio by 20%, with a reduction of 50% or more in 24.7% of the patients treated with losartan 100mg od who received aliskiren (150–300mg od) for 6 months) as compared to 12.5% in the placebo group.[3] This benefit was independent of the small difference in BP observed between the treatment groups at the end of the study.

Heart failure: in hypertensive patients with congestive HF, aliskiren, when added on top of the current medication (β-blockers, ACEIs/ARBs, and aldosterone antagonist), reduced LV filling pressures, plasma renin activity, levels of NT-proBNP, BNP, and urinary aldosterone concentrations.[4]

Pharmacokinetics

Aliskiren is rapidly absorbed following oral administration, but presents a low oral bioavailability (2.5%), reaching peak plasma levels within 1–3h. High-fat meals decreases AUC and C_{max} 71% and 85%, respectively. It is approximately 50% protein-bound and has a mean V_d of 1.9L/kg. It is metabolized in the liver via CYP3A4 and excreted almost completely via the faecal route (99% corresponding to non-absorbed drug) and 0.6% is recovered in the urine. $t_{1/2}$ of ≈24–40h. Steady state levels are reached in 5–7 days.

⁙ Dose 150–300mg od.

☺ Common side effects

(1–10%): diarrhoea; hyperkalaemia (particularly when used with ACEIs in patients with diabetes), hypotension (particularly in volume-depleted patients), rash, elevated uric acid, and renal stones. Cases of angio-oedema have been reported.

Interactions

Plasma levels of aliskiren are elevated when it is administered with potent (e.g. ciclosporin) and moderate P-gp inhibitors (e.g. ketoconazole, clarithromycin, erythromycin, amiodarone, atorvastatin).

Aliskiren shows no clinically relevant pharmacokinetic interactions with warfarin, lovastatin, atenolol, celecoxib, digoxin, or cimetidine. Aliskiren reduces furosemide serum concentrations.

Effects may be attenuated when used with NSAIDs. Concomitant use with agents that can raise serum K^+ levels is likely to lead to rises in K^+ levels. Use with NSAIDs may reduce the effect of aliskiren and also increase the risk of renal impairment.

Cautions/notes

- Routine monitoring of U&Es is recommended in patients with diabetes, kidney disease, or HF.
- Due to its mechanism of action, aliskiren needs to be used with caution with other RAAS blockers or in patients who are volume- or salt-depleted, and stopped with persistent diarrhoea or dehydration due to risks of hyperkalaemia.
- Aliskiren has not been used in hypertensive patients with renal impairment and GFR <30mL/min, a history of dialysis, nephrotic syndrome, or renovascular disease. Thus, it should be used with caution in these patient groups. It should also be used with caution in patients with NYHA class III–IV HF.

Pregnancy and lactation

There are no data on aliskiren in pregnancy. Other inhibitors of RAAS are associated with serious fetal malformations and neonatal death (pregnancy category D). Aliskiren is not recommended in breastfeeding and is contraindicated in pregnancy.

Contraindications

1. Pregnancy
2. History of angio-oedema with aliskiren
3. Hyperkalaemia
4. Bilateral renal stenosis, severely impaired renal function

References

1 Weir MR et al. (2007). Antihypertensive efficacy, safety, and tolerability of the oral direct renin inhibitor aliskiren in patients with hypertension: a pooled analysis. J Am Soc Hypertens 21:264–77.
2 Oparil S et al. (2007). Efficacy and safety of combined use of aliskiren and valsartan in patients with hypertension: a randomised, double-blind trial. Lancet 370:221–9.
3 Parving HH et al.; AVOID Study Investigators (2008). Aliskiren combined with losartan in type 2 diabetes and nephropathy. N Engl J Med 358:2433–2446.
4 McMurray JJ et al. for the Aliskiren Obsrevation of Heart Failure Treatment (ALOFT) Investigators (2008). Effects of the oral direct renin inhibitor aliskiren in patients with symptomatic heart failure. Circ Heart Fail 1:17–24.

Alpha₁-adrenoreceptor blockers

(See also 📖 Doxazosin, p.438, 📖 Phenoxybenzamine, p.546, 📖 Prazosin, p.551)

CV indications

1. Hypertension
2. Pheochromocytoma

Other indications

Benign prostatic hyperthrophy

Mechanism of action

α_1-adrenoreceptor blockers act as antagonists to the binding of noradrenaline released by sympathetic nerves synapsing on vascular smooth muscle. Consequently, they antagonize the vasoconstrictor effect of sympathetic stimulation of α_1-adrenoceptors located on the vascular smooth muscle, producing arteriolar and venous vasodilatation. Although α_1-adrenoreceptor blockers antagonize the underlying basal vasoconstrictor tone to reduce BP, they are relatively more effective under conditions of elevated sympathetic activity (e.g. stress; phaeochromocytoma).

Pharmacodynamics

Hypertension: α_1-blockers are considered particularly helpful in hypertensive patients with benign prostatic hypertrophy and metabolic syndrome.

α_1-blockers effectively reduce BP (mean BP fall ≈11.7/6.9mmHg in patients with mean baseline BP of 159/89mmHg).[1] α_1-blockers do not appear to cause adverse metabolic effects.

In addition, α_1-blockers inhibit platelet aggregation induced by adrenaline, collagen, or ADP.

Pharmacokinetics

(See 📖 individual drug)

Practical points

💊 Doses

(See 📖 individual drug)
Initiation at lowest possible doses at bedtime; gradual uptitration may help limit incidence of unwanted side effects.

☺ Side effects

Dizziness (>10% of patients); orthostatic hypotension (due to loss of reflex vasoconstriction upon standing); 1st-dose hypotension (orthostatic hypotension and fainting, especially in the elderly); drowsiness, headache, syncope, vertigo; tachycardia and palpitations.

Others: oedema, fatigue, general malaise; nausea, diarrhoea; rhinitis, nasal congestion (due to dilation of nasal mucosal arterioles). Urinary incontinence, especially in females, often resulting in drug discontinuation.

Interactions

Alpha-blockers should be used cautiously with antihypertensives and PDE-5 inhibitors due to potential of hypotension. Avoid intake of alcohol or other sedating medications to prevent excessive drowsiness and dizziness.

Cautions/notes

- Syncope is the most severe orthostatic effect but other symptoms of lowered BP, such as dizziness, lightheadedness, or vertigo can occur, especially at initiation of therapy or at the time of dose increases. Avoid getting up too fast from a sitting or lying position; get up slowly and steady yourself to prevent a fall. Tolerance due to Na^+ and water retention may develop during chronic therapy, requiring increased doses or added diuretic therapy. If tachycardia is excessive, it may be necessary to use a β-blocking agent concomitantly.
- Intraoperative floppy iris syndrome (a variant of small pupil syndrome) has been observed in patients on α-blockers (predominantly tamsulosin) undergoing cataract surgery.
- Should be administered with caution in patients with impaired hepatic function or to patients receiving drugs known to influence hepatic metabolism.

Pregnancy and lactation (see individual drugs)

Contraindications

(See also individual drugs)
- Known hypersensitvity to quinazolines (e.g. doxazosin, prazosin)
- HF (doxazosin)

Reference

1 Chapman N *et al.*; ASCOT Investigators (2008). Effect of doxazosin gastrointestinal therapeutic system as third-line antihypertensive therapy on blood pressure and lipids in the Anglo-Scandinavian Cardiac Outcomes Trial. *Circulation* **118**:424–8.

Alteplase

(See also 📖 Thrombolytic agents, p.608)

A single-chain tissue plasminogen activator produced by recombinant DNA technology (rTPA, 70 kDa).

CV indications

Treatment of:
1. STEMI: in the absence of contraindications if 1° PCI can not be performed within 2h
2. acute ischaemic stroke: within 3h after the onset of stroke symptoms and after exclusion of intracranial haemorrhage by a cranial CT scan or other diagnostic imaging method sensitive for the presence of haemorrhage
3. acute pulmonary embolism: when the pulmonary embolism is accompanied by unstable haemodynamics
4. central venous access devices (CVADs) blocked.

Mechanism of action

When introduced into the systemic circulation alteplase is more active on fibrin-bound plasminogen than on the plasma plasminogen (i.e. clot-selective). Thus, it binds to fibrin in a thrombus and converts the entrapped plasminogen to plasmin. This initiates local fibrinolysis with limits systemic proteolysis.

Recombinant tPA is not antigenic and is indicated in patients who are allergic to streptokinase or likely to have antibodies to streptokinase.

Pharmacodynamics

The *ASSET study* compared activase to placebo in patients with AMI. Patients infused with alteplase within 5h of the onset of symptoms experienced improved 30-day survival (45% vs. 72%) compared with those treated with placebo.[1]

The *GUSTO study* evaluated 4 thrombolytic regimens in patients with AMI. The regimens included accelerated infusion of alteplase plus IV heparin, streptokinase plus IV heparin, streptokinase plus SC heparin, and alteplase plus streptokinase. The incidence of 30-day mortality in the accelerated infusion of alteplase group was 14% lower than in the other groups.[2]

Pharmacokinetics

Alteplase is rapidly cleared from the plasma with an initial $t_{1/2}$ of 4–8min, so it should given as an IV bolus followed by an infusion. There is no difference in the dominant initial plasma $t_{1/2}$ between the 3h and accelerated regimens in the AMI. The initial V_d is 0.1L/kg. The plasma clearance (380–570mL/min) is mediated primarily by the liver and <2% is excreted by urine.

Practical points

♪ Doses

In MI: 2 regimens of alteplase are used:
- *accelerated infusion*: 15mg IV bolus followed by 0.75mg/kg infused over the next 30min (not to exceed 50mg) and then 0.5mg/kg over

the next 60min (not to exceed 35mg). Total dosage not to exceed 100mg
- *3-h infusion*: 100mg administered as 60mg in the 1st hour (of which 6–10mg is administered as a bolus), 20mg over the 2nd hour, and 20mg over the 3rd hour.

In acute ischaemic stroke: 0.9mg/kg infused over 60min with 10% of the total dose administered as an initial IV bolus over 1min. Total dosage not to exceed 90mg.

In acute pulmonary embolism: 100mg administered by IV infusion over 2h.

In lysis of venous thrombus: a catheter-directed infusion of 1–1.5mg/h for 12–24h has been used.

In CVADs

tPA is available in a 2mg/2mL vial, a volume sufficient to fill most catheter lumens. For patients ≥30kg, 2mg in 2mL saline is used. Patients ≤30kg, fill 100% of the internal lumen volume of the catheter. It should dwell for 0.5–2h and then be withdrawn. The dose may be repeated. If this is unsuccessful, an infusion of tPA 2mg/50mL over 4h may be used.

Peripheral arterial disease: 0.05–0.1mg/kg/h intra-arterially.

☺ Common side effects
- Bleeding: GI 5%, GU 4%, ecchymosis 1%, retroperitoneal, epistaxis, and gingival <1%; haemorrhagic stroke 0.7%. If serious, haemorrhage can be treated with tranexamic acid, fresh plasma or coagulation factors.
- Allergic reactions (anaphylactoid reaction, laryngeal or orolingual oedema, rash, and urticaria): <1%.
- Other adverse reactions reported in the AMI: arrhythmias, AV block, cardiogenic shock, HF, cardiac arrest, recurrent ischaemia, myocardial reinfarction, myocardial rupture, electromechanical dissociation, pericardial effusion, pericarditis, MR, cardiac tamponade, thromboembolism, pulmonary oedema, nausea, vomiting, and hypotension.

Interactions
- The risk of bleeding increases when combined with anticoagulants, platelet antiaggregants, NSAIDs, dextran solutions.
- Nitroglycerin appears to impair thrombolytic effects of tPA.

Cautions/notes
IM injections and non-essential handling of the patient should be avoided during treatment with alteplase.

In the following conditions, the risk of alteplase therapy may be increased and should be weighed against the anticipated benefits:
- recent major surgery (CABG, obstetric delivery, organ biopsy, previous puncture of non-compressible vessels)
- CVD

- recent GI or GU bleeding
- recent trauma
- hypertension: SBP/DBP >180/110mmHg
- high likelihood of left heart thrombus (ex. mitral stenosis with AF)
- acute pericarditis
- subacute bacterial endocarditis
- suspected aortic dissection
- haemostatic defects, including those 2° to severe hepatic or renal disease
- severe hepatic dysfunction
- severe anaemia
- diabetic proliferative retinopathy
- acute pancreatitis
- pregnancy
- diabetic haemorrhagic retinopathy or other haemorrhagic ophthalmic conditions
- septic thrombophlebitis
- occluded AV cannula at seriously infected site
- advanced age (>75 years) with suspicion of cerebral arteriosclerotic vascular degeneration, agitation, or confusion
- patients currently receiving oral anticoagulants
- recent administration of GP IIb/IIIa inhibitors
- any other condition in which bleeding constitutes a significant hazard or would be particularly difficult to manage because of its location

Coronary thrombolysis may result in arrhythmias associated with reperfusion. These arrhythmias are not different from those often seen in the ordinary course of AMI and may be managed with standard antiarrhythmic measures.

There have been post-marketing reports of orolingual angio-oedema associated with the use of alteplase, particularly in patients with acute ischaemic stroke receiving concomitant ACEIs.

Pregnancy and lactation

Alteplase has an embryocidal effect in rabbits. There are no adequate and well-controlled studies in pregnant women. Alteplase should be used during pregnancy only if the potential benefit justifies the potential risk to the fetus (pregnancy category C). It is not known whether alteplase is excreted in human milk; caution should be exercised when it is administered to a nursing woman.

Contraindications

Hypersensitivity to alteplase or any component of the formulation

In MI or pulmonary embolism:
- active internal bleeding
- history of CVA
- intracranial or intraspinal surgery or trauma within 2 months
- intracranial neoplasm, arteriovenous malformation, or aneurysm
- known bleeding diathesis
- severe uncontrolled hypertension

- hypersensitivity to the active substance alteplase and to any of the excipients.

In acute ischaemic stroke:
- evidence of intracranial haemorrhage on pre-treatment evaluation
- suspicion of subarachnoid haemorrhage on pre-treatment evaluation
- recent (within 3 months) intracranial or intraspinal surgery, serious head trauma, or previous stroke
- history of intracranial haemorrhage
- uncontrolled hypertension at time of treatment (SBP >185mmHg or DBP >110mmHg)
- seizure at the onset of stroke
- active internal bleeding
- intracranial neoplasm, arteriovenous malformation, or aneurysm.

References

1 Vaage-Nilsen M *et al.* (1993). The prevalence of myocardial ischemia six months after thrombolytic treatment of acute coronary episodes. A subset of a placebo controlled, randomised trial, the ASSET Study. *Int J Cardiol* **39**:187–93.
2 The GUSTO Investigators (1993). An international randomized trial comparing four thrombolytic strategies for acute myocardial infarction. *N Engl J Med* **1329**:673–82.

Ambrisentan

Relatively selective antagonist of the ET_A receptor.

CV indications

PAH to improve exercise capacity and symptoms in patients with WHO class II or III symptoms.

Mechanism of action

Pharmacodynamics

Ambrisentan improves haemodynamics (increases cardiac index and reduces pulmonary artery pressure, pulmonary vascular resistance, and mean right atrial pressure) and exercise capacity and decreases progression of clinical symptoms.

Ambrisentan (5 or 10mg) once daily for 12 weeks improves exercise capacity (+22.8m and +49.4m for the 5- and 10-mg doses, respectively), and −7.8m in the placebo group (ARIES-1 trial); in ARIES-2 changes were +22.2 and +49.4m for the 2.5- and 5-mg doses and −10.1m for the placebo.[1] The 2° endpoint of time to clinical worsening was improved with active therapy in ARIES-2.

Pharmacokinetics

Absorption is rapid, reaching peak plasma levels in ≈2h. Protein-binding is 99%, and it is metabolized by CYP3A4, CYP2C19, and uridine 5'-diphosphate glucuronosyltransferases (UGTs) and is excreted as active and inactive metabolites predominantly in faeces. Terminal $t_{1/2}$ is 15h.

Practical points

⁑ Doses

5mg PO qd initially; increase to 10mg PO qd if 5mg/day tolerated; do not chew, crush, or split the tablet.

☺ Side effects

Aminotransferase elevations >3 × ULN at 1 year 2.8%.[1] Lower-extremity oedema is more frequent (29%) and severe in patients >65 years of age, and nasal congestion.

Cautions/notes

Similar to bosentan
Adverse events are generally unrelated to dose, including the elevated serum aminotransferase concentrations.

Contraindications

Similar to bosentan
Ambrisentan may produce serious birth defects if used by pregnant women, as this effect has been seen consistently in animals.

Reference

1 Galie N *et al.* (2008). Ambrisentan for the treatment of pulmonary arterial hypertension: results of the Ambrisentan in Pulmonary Arterial Hypertension, Randomized, Double-Blind, Placebo-Controlled, Multicenter, Efficacy (ARIES) study 1 and 2 (abstr). *Circulation* **117**:3010–19.

Amiodarone

(See also 📖 Antiarrhythmic drugs: classification, p.362)

Antiarrhythmic with predominantly Vaughan Williams class III effects.

Oral amiodarone is indicated only for severe cardiac arrhythmias not reponding to other treatments or when other treatments cannot be used including:

- Tachyarrhythmias associated with WPW
- Atrial flutter and fibrillation when other drugs cannot be used
- All paroxysmal tachyarrhythmias including: supraventricular, nodal and ventricular tachycardias, ventricular fibrillation (when other treatment cannot be used).

It should be initiated and usually monitored under hospital/specialist supervision.

Mechanism of action

Amiodarone exhibits class III antiarrhythmic effects, lengthening the cardiac APD and refractory periods in all cardiac tissue without slowing intracardiac conduction. In addition, it blocks several K^+ channels and the L-type Ca^{2+} channel, and exhibits non-competitive α- and β-adrenergic inhibition at the SA and AV nodes. It also inhibits inactivated Na^+ channels at high stimulation rates, reducing cardiac excitability and conduction velocity. Thus, amiodarone presents class I, II, III, and IV activity.

Pharmacodynamics

Amiodarone prolongs the APD (QT interval) and refractoriness in all cardiac tissues with minimal frequency dependence, so that it can suppress arrhythmias with a short excitable gap. Amiodarone makes the APD more uniform, reducing the heterogeneity of repolarization and possible reentry. The blockade of Ca^{2+} channels explains the slowing in SA driving rate (10–15%) and AV nodal conduction (prolongation of the PR), the suppression of early/delayed afterdepolarizations and the systemic and coronary vasodilatory effect, as well as the low incidence of torsades de pointes. In chronic treatments and at fast driving rates amiodarone decreases cardiac excitability and conduction velocity and increases VF threshold.

Amiodarone reduces the slope of phase 4 diastolic depolarization in automatic cells, decreasing sinus rate (10–20%) and suppressing ectopic pacemaker activity.

Haemodynamically, IV amiodarone causes vascular smooth muscle relaxation, reduces afterload, and slightly increases cardiac index. After oral dosing, it does not appear to cause reduction in LVEF, even in patients with reduced LVEF; after acute IV dosing, amiodarone may have a mild negative inotropic effect.

Pharmacokinetics

Following oral administration, amiodarone is slowly and variably absorbed. Bioavailability is variable (22–86%). Food increases the rate of absorption and the area under the plasma concentration–time curve (AUC) and the peak plasma concentration (C_{max}) of amiodarone increases by 2.3 and 3.8×, respectively. Peak plasma levels are reached after 6–8h. However, the onset of action may occur in 2–3 days, but more commonly takes 1–3 weeks, even with loading doses. It is almost completely bound to proteins (99%) and widely distributed throughout the body (V_d 70L/kg), mainly in the adipose tissue, liver, heart, and lungs; the concentration in the myocardium is 10–15× that in plasma. It is metabolized in the liver by CYP450 3A4 and 2C8, leading to various active metabolites (desethylamiodarone), and excreted primarily by hepatic and biliary routes with almost no elimination via the renal route; amiodarone is not dialysable. Mean $t_{\frac{1}{2}}$ is 58 days (range 15–142 days). Therapeutic plasma levels: 1–2.5mcg/mL.

Practical points

♣ Doses

PO: loading dose 200–400mg tds for 1–3 weeks (occasionally longer) until initial therapeutic response occurs. Maintenance: 200mg od.

Minimum effective maintenance dose should be used. Neurological (tremor, ataxia, and peripheral neuropathy) and GI (nausea and vomiting) side effects are common during loading with high daily doses and usually improve once maintenance doses are begun.

IV: 150mg over 10min (15mg/min), then 360mg over 6h (1mg/min), then 540mg over the remaining 18h (0.5mg/min). Higher doses may induce hypotension.

☻ Common side effects

Side effects are very common with amiodarone. They occur in up to 75%, causing discontinuation in 7–18%; and some may be potentially fatal.

(>10%): reversible corneal microdeposits usually only discernible under slit-lamp examination (with overall ≈1.5% requiring discontinuation due to halos or blurred vision); photosensitivity (may persist for many months after discontinuation). Optic neuropathy/neuritis (1–2%). Thus, periodic eye examinations are recommended.

(1–10%): sinus bradycardia (elderly) and conduction disturbances, congestive HF (≈3%). Torsades de pointes may occur in patients with hypokalaemia, bradycardia, or receiving QT-prolonging drugs.

Due to the iodine content, amiodarone produces hypothyroidism (6%, TSH >10mU/L) or hyperthyroidism (0.9%, TSH <0.35mU/L).

Skin: blue/grey skin discoloration (slowly reverses but may not disappear); rashes, especially photosensitivity.

GI symptoms: nausea, vomiting, constipation, and anorexia (10–25%); reversible increase in transaminase levels.

Neurological: malaise, fatigue, peripheral neuropathy, ataxia, tremors, nightmares, and sleep disturbances.

Pulmonary toxicity: mainly bronchiolitis obliterans organizing pneumonia, and chronic interstitial pneumonitis occurs in patients receiving chronic doses ≥400mg/day. Risk factors include pre-existing lung disease; may cause cough and progressive dyspnoea associated with functional or radiological changes, diagnosis of which may be delayed by cardiac failure.

Interactions
- Additive proarrhythmic effects with QT-prolonging drugs (class I and III drugs, thiazides, tricyclic antidepressants, phenothiazines).
- Amiodarone inhibits the action of the cytochrome P450 isozyme family, increasing the plasma levels of: atorvastatin, ciclosporin, digoxin, flecainide, procainamide, sildenafil, simvastatin, tacrolimus, theophylline, and trazodone. Amiodarone inhibits p-glycoprotein and other CYP450 isoenzymes (CYP1A2, CYP2C9, CYP2D6), which can result in unexpectedly high plasma levels of other drugs which are metabolized by those CYP450 enzymes or are substrates of p-glycoprotein.
- Amiodarone potentiates the effects of oral anticoagulants (i.e. decrease the dose of warfarin 30–50%). The effect of amiodarone on the warfarin concentration can be as early as a few days after initiation of treatment, or can be delayed a few weeks. Amiodarone may decrease the antiplatelet activity of clopidogrel.
- Amiodarone increases plasma levels of phenytoin; colestyramine and colestipol decrease, while cimetidine increases the plasma levels of amiodarone.
- Combination with atorvastatin or simvastatin may increase the risk of myopathy and rhabdomyolysis.
- Antihypertensives: possible risk of hypotension, particularly with IV amiodarone.
- Combination with digoxin, verapamil, or diltiazem increases the risk of bradycardia and AV block; with β-blockers, verapamil or diltiazem increases the risk of HF.
- Higher IV doses of dopamine and dobutamine are needed in patients receiving amiodarone.

Cautions/notes
Amiodarone can cause serious adverse reactions affecting the eyes, heart, lung, liver, thyroid gland, skin, and peripheral nervous system. Because these reactions may be delayed, patients on long-term treatment should be carefully supervised. As undesirable effects are usually dose related, the minimum effective maintenance dose should be given.

Monitoring
In 1° care, patients on amiodarone should undergo blood monitoring of liver and thyroid function at least every 6 months.

Pregnancy and lactation
Amiodarone is embryotoxic in animals. Amiodarone and its metabolite, desethylamiodarone, cross the placenta to the fetus. Hypothryoidism and hyperthyroidism, growth retardation, VSDs, bradycardia, and prolonged QT interval can be observed in some amiodarone-newborns (pregnancy category D). Amiodarone is excreted in significant quantities in breast milk, so its use is contraindicated in breastfeeding.

Contraindications
- Sinus bradycardia and SA heart block
- Cardiogenic shock
- Lactation; pregnancy (except in exceptional circumstances)
- Evidence or history of thyroid dysfunction
- In combination with other drugs that may cause torsades de pointes
- Known hypersensitivity to amiodarone or to iodine

Amlodipine

(See also 📖 Calcium-channel blockers, p.390)

Oral dihydropyridine derivative L-type CCB.

CV indications

1. Treatment of hypertension
2. Symptomatic treatment of chronic stable angina
3. Treatment of vasospastic angina (Prinzmetal's variant angina)
4. Patients with recently documented CAD and without HF or a LVEF <40% to reduce the risk of hospitalization due to angina and of a coronary revascularization procedure

Mechanism of action

(See 📖 Calcium-channel blockers, p.390)

Amlodipine presents a slow rate of association and dissociation from its receptor site in the L-type Ca^{2+} channel, resulting in a gradual onset of its effect. Amlodipine also exhibits antioxidant and antiproliferative effects.

Pharmacodynamics

Hypertension and CVD: amlodipine (5–10mg od) reduces BP by ~13/11mmHg in patients with hypertension (baseline DBP: 90–109mmHg) and CHD.[1] The antihypertensive effect is maintained for at least 24h.

The ALLHAT study showed that the combined 1° endpoint (fatal CHD and non-fatal MI) was similar (11.3%) in hypertensive patients with ≥1 risk factor for CHD treated with amlodipine 2.5–10mg od (as 1st step with additional antihypertensives as required) compared to lisinopril (11.4%) or chlortalidone (1.4%) and followed up for a mean of 4.9 years.[2] Similar benefit was observed in diabetic and non-diabetic patients, and in diabetic patients amlodipine produces similar benefits to ACEIs.[3]

The ASCOT study found an 11% RR in the 2° endpoint of all-cause mortality (HR=0.89; 95% CI 0.81–0.99, P=0.02) but not in the 1° endpoint (fatal CHD and non-fatal MI) in hypertensive patients with ≥3 other risk factors for CHD treated for 5.5 years with amlodipine (5–10mg od) in combination with perindopril (4–8mg od) as compared to atenolol combined with bendroflumethiazide.[4] Individuals on amlodipine had fewer fatal and non-fatal strokes (27%), total CV events and procedures (16%), and all-cause mortality (11%) and less incidence of developing diabetes (30%).

In hypertensive patients at high CV risk, amlodipine reduced cardiac morbidity and mortality and all-cause mortality in the same way as valsartan.[5] The amlodipine group had a significantly lower incidence of MI and higher rate of new-onset diabetes than in the valsartan group. The most consistent difference between the groups was that amlodipine-based therapy was significantly more efficacious in reducing BP, especially during the early phases of treatment.

CHD: amlodipine (uptitrated to 10mg od) improved exercise tolerance testing (symptom-limited ETT time, time to moderate angina, and time to 1mm ST depression) compared to placebo.[6]

Amlodipine had no demonstrable effect on the progression of coronary atherosclerosis or the risk of major CV events in patients with angiographically documented CHD but was associated with fewer hospitalizations for UA (35%) and revascularizations (33%). However, amlodipine significantly slowed the 36-month progression of carotid artery atherosclerosis.[7]

Heart failure: no changes in all-cause mortality and cardiac morbidity (defined by life-threatening arrhythmia, AMI, or hospitalization for worsened HF), NYHA classification, or symptoms of HF between amlodipine and placebo were observed in patients with HF (NYHA class III–IV) treated with standard therapy.[8] No differences between amlodipine and placebo in all-cause mortality were observed in patients with NYHA class III or IV HF of non-ischaemic origin followed for a mean of 33 months.[9] Thus, amlodipine can be used in patients with HF on standard therapy with uncontrolled BP or angina.

Pharmacokinetics

After oral administration its bioavailability (60–90%) is unaffected by food, reaching peak plasma levels within 6–12h. It is approximately 95% protein bound, presents a V_d of 16L/kg and is metabolized slowly but extensively in the liver into inactive metabolites; 10% of the drug and 60% of the metabolites are excreted via urine. $t_{1/2}$ is ≈35–50h, and time to steady state is ≈7–8 days. The AUC increases 40–60% in elderly patients and patients with hepatic insufficiency or HF.

Practical points

⌁ Doses

5–10mg od. Elderly individuals, or patients with hepatic insufficiency may be started on 2.5mg od.

☺ Side effects

(See 📖 Calcium-channel blockers, p.390)

Interactions

(See 📖 Calcium-channel blockers, p.390)
In clinical trials, amlodipine has been safely used with thiazide diuretics, β-blockers, ACEIs, long-acting nitrates, sublingual glyceryl trinitrate, digoxin, warfarin, cimetidine, NSAIDs, antibiotics, phenytoin, sildenafil, and oral hypoglycaemic drugs.

Cautions/notes

Caution should be exercised in patients with impaired hepatic function and the elderly.

Pregnancy and lactation

(See 📖 Calcium-channel blockers, p.390)

Contraindications

(See 📖 Calcium-channel blockers, p.390)

References

1 Pepine CJ et al. (2003). Comparison of effects of nisoldipine-extended release and amlodipine in patients with systemic hypertension and chronic stable angina pectoris. *Am J Cardiol* **91**:274–9.

2 ALLHAT Officers and Coordinators for the ALLHAT Collaborative Research Group (2002). The Antihypertensive and Lipid-Lowering Treatment to Prevent Heart Attack Trial. Major outcomes in high-risk hypertensive patients randomized to angiotensin-converting enzyme inhibitor or calcium channel blocker vs diuretic: The Antihypertensive and Lipid-Lowering Treatment to Prevent Heart Attack Trial (ALLHAT). *JAMA* **288**:2981–97.

3 Whelton PK et al.; ALLHAT Collaborative Research Group (2005). Clinical outcomes in antihypertensive treatment of type 2 diabetes, impaired fasting glucose concentration, and normoglycemia: Antihypertensive and Lipid-Lowering Treatment to Prevent Heart Attack Trial (ALLHAT). *Arch Intern Med* **165**:1401–9.

4 Dahlöf B et al.; ASCOT Investigators (2005). Prevention of cardiovascular events with an antihypertensive regimen of amlodipine adding perindopril as required versus atenolol adding bendroflumethiazide as required, in the Anglo-Scandinavian Cardiac Outcomes Trial-Blood Pressure Lowering Arm (ASCOT-BPLA): a multicentre randomised controlled trial. *Lancet* **366**:895–906.

5 Julius S et al.; VALUE trial group (2004). Outcomes in hypertensive patients at high cardiovascular risk treated with regimens based on valsartan or amlodipine: the VALUE randomised trial. *Lancet* **363**:2022–31.

6 Frishman WH et al. (1999). Comparison of controlled-onset, extended-release verapamil with amlodipine and amlodipine plus atenolol on exercise performance and ambulatory ischemia in patients with chronic stable angina pectoris. *Am J Cardiol* **83**:507–14.

7 Pitt B et al. (2003). Effect of amlodipine on the progression of atherosclerosis and the occurrence of clinical events. PREVENT Investigators. *Circulation* **102**:1503–10.

8 Packer M et al. (1996). for The Prospective Randomized Amlodipine Survival Evaluation Study Group (1996). Effect of amlodipine on morbidity and mortality in severe chronic heart failure. *N Engl J Med* **335**:1107–14.

9 de Vries RJ et al. (2000). Efficacy and safety of calcium channel blockers in heart failure: focus on recent trials with second-generation dihydropyridines. *Am Heart J* **139**:185–94.

Angiotensin-converting enzyme inhibitors

e.g.: captopril, (📖 p. 397) enalapril (📖 p. 444), lisinopril (📖 p. 505) ramipril (📖 p. 562), perindopril (📖 p. 543), trandolapril (📖 p. 617)

Others: benazepril, cilazapril, fosinopril, imidapril, moexipril, quinapril

Indications

1. Management of hypertension
2. Management of HF to reduce CV death and HF hospitalizations
3. Treatment of haemodynamically stable patients with acute MI within 24h
4. Nephropathy, diabetic or non-diabetic
5. Slow progression of renal disease in patients with type 1 diabetes with microalbuminuria
6. Cardiovascular protection (HOPE, EUROPA, PEACE trials)

Mechanism of action

(See 📖 RAAS inhibitors, p.568)

ACEIs prevent the conversion of angiotensin I to angiotensin II and so inhibit the RAAS. In addition, ACE is identical to kininase II, so that ACEIs inhibit the breakdown of bradykinin. Bradykinin stimulates its endothelail receptors and promotes the release of nitric oxide (NO) and vasodilatory prostaglandins (I_2 and E_2), which exert vasodilatory, antiaggregant and antiproliferative effects.

Pharmacodynamics

(See 📖 RAAS inhibitors, p.568 and individual ACEIs)

Hypertension: ACEIs produce an arterial and venous vasodilatation due to: (a) inhibition of angiotensin II synthesis; (b) inhibition of the sympathetic tone and of the release of aldosterone, endothelin-1, and vasopressin; (c) an increase in the release of kinins, NO, and prostaglandins I_2 and E_2.

ACEIs improve endothelial dysfunction and peripheral (skeletal muscle, coronary and cerebral) blood flow, reduce LVH, and increase arterial distensibility. They are indicated in hypertensives with HF or LV dysfunction, post-MI, type 1 diabetes, renal disease or microalbuminuria, metabolic syndrome, and asymptomatic atherosclerosis.[1] More effective in white patients; less in black patients, especially in the elderly, which can be overcome by adding low-dose diuretics.

HF: ACEIs reduce pre/afterload, decrease signs and symptoms, improve haemodynamics (increase cardiac output, reduce pulmonary capillary wedge and LV end-diastolic pressures), exercise tolerance, and diuresis and decrease hospitalizations, progression of the disease, and mortality. They are indicated: (a) in all patients with symptomatic HF and a LVEF <40%; (b) as initial therapy in the absence of fluid retention; in patients with fluid retention together with diuretics; (c) in patients with signs or symptoms of HF after the acute phase of MI, even if the symptoms are transient, to improve survival and to reduce reinfarctions and hospitalizations for HF; and (d) in asymptomatic patients with a documented LV systolic dysfunction.[2]

In type 1 diabetic nephropathy, ACEIs reduce proteinuria and protect against progressive glomerular sclerosis and loss of renal function.[3]

They also reduce the risk of stroke and reduce proteinuria and slow the progression of glomerular sclerosis and loss of renal function in type 2 diabetic nephropathy.[4]

RRR 18% (10.7% vs. 12.8%) for the combined outcomes of CV death, non-fatal MI, or stroke in stable patients with atherosclerosis without known evidence of HF or LV systolic dysfunction.[5] ACEIs also significantly reduced all-cause mortality, cardiovascular mortality, non-fatal MI, all stroke, HF and coronary-artery bypass surgery.

Other effects: ACEIs: (a) decrease myocardial O_2 demands and improve coronary O_2 supply; (b) produce a vasodilatation of the efferent glomerular arteriole, normalize intraglomerular pressure, decrease proteinuria and delay the progression of glomerulosclerosis; (c) inhibit platelet aggregation and increase fibrinolysis.

Practical points

⁙ Doses
(See 📖 individual ACEI)
ACEIs should be initiated under specialist supervision and with careful monitoring in those with severe HF; those receiving multiple or high-dose diuretics or in those with hypovolaemia, hyponatraemia (Na <130mmol/L), pre-existing hypotension (SBP <90mmHg), unstable HF, concomitant high-dose vasodilator therapy, and known renovascular disease.

☺ Side effects
(1–15%): dry, non-productive, cough (thought to be due to increased bradykinin), blurred vision, dizziness, headache, pruritic rash, loss of taste and GI disturbances including diarrhoea and vomiting.

Hypotension is not uncommon, particularly in high renin states (chronic HF, renal artery stenosis, hyponatraemia (<130mmol/L) related to diuretic use or increased serum creatinine 1.5–3mg/dL or 135–265µmol/L). To avoid hypotension discontinue or halve the dose of diuretics 1–2 days before the initial dose.

Hyperkalaemia (especially in renal failure and diabetes).

Angio-oedema (0.3%), which is more common in blacks (1.6%), can be occasionally fatal.[6] Warning signs are facial swelling, unilateral facial oedema, or periorbital oedema.

Deterioration of renal function. The preferential vasodilatation of glomerular efferent arterioles reduces the intraglomerular pressure and may cause an increase of serum creatine initially.

By reducing angiotensin II levels, ACEIs may produce a vasodilatation of efferent arterioles of the glomeruli and reduce GFR. Specifically, ACEIs can induce or exacerbate renal impairment in patients with renal artery stenosis, particularly if the patient is taking an NSAID and a diuretic.

Others: proteinuria (captopril); impotence. Neutropenia, anaemia (0.3g/dL with enalapril), and agranulocytosis are rare.

Interactions
- Risk of hyperkalaemia is increased with renal impairment, diabetes, and especially with concomitant use of K^+-sparing diuretics, ARBs, eplerenone, β-blockers, heparin, or K^+ supplements.
- NSAIDs inhibit the antihypertensive effect and increase the risk of hyperkalaemia. Reduced renal flow induced by NSAIDs can also rarely contribute to renal failure particularly in elderly or dehydrated patients.
- ACEIs decrease the GFR and decrease the renal clearance of other cardiac drugs eliminated by the kidney (atenolol, nadolol, sotalol, flecainide, disopyramide, procainamide).
- Concomitant use of ACEIs with lithium may enhance the effects and risk of toxicity of lithium and so it should be avoided.
- Antihypertensive effects of ACEIs are enhanced when used with other antihypertensives and vasodilators (e.g. nitrates), alcohol, and certain anaesthetic agents, tricyclic antidepressants, and antipsychotics. ACEIs compensate the hypokalaemia produced by thiazides and loop diuretics. The antihypertensive effects of ACEIs are reduced by chronic administration of NSAIDs, ciclosporin, and sympathomimetics.
- It is possible that concomitant use of ACEIs with oral antidiabetic agents may cause an increased glucose-lowering effect, with risk of hypoglycaemia.
- Higher doses of erythropoietin are needed in dialysed patients treated with ACEIs.

Cautions
- Symptomatic hypotension may be seen in patients who are volume depleted or on diuretics. Such patients should be followed closely, particularly those with severe HF where treatment should be started under medical supervision. Use with caution in malignant hypertension, aortic or mitral valve stenosis, LVOT obstruction, and constrictive pericarditis.
- Check baseline renal function and monitor after administration to check for renal impairment. Monitor for hyperkalaemia especially in patients with diabetes, renal insufficiency, on K^+-sparing diuretic or K^+ supplements. Increased risk of hypotension and renal failure in those with renovascular disease, e.g. bilateral renal artery stenosis or artery stenosis of a single functioning kidney. This is usually reversible on stopping therapy.
- Avoid in AMI in those with haemodynamic compromise, particularly if SBP <100mmHg or creatinine is >177umol/L, and discontinue if renal failure (creatinine >203μmol/L or 2.3mg/dL) or if creatinine doubles after initiation. During first 3 days reduce dose if SBP <120mmHg.
- Use of oral hypoglycaemic agents and insulin in patients with diabetes should be monitored during the first few months due to the possibility of increased glucose-lowering effects with ACEIs. In patients undergoing major surgery, hypotension may result, as compensatory renin

release is unable to cause angiotensin-II generation. If required, volume expansion may be used.

- Less commonly, hypersensitivity (resolves with discontinuation) or angio-oedema may occur (discontinue and treat angio-oedema). Angio-oedema is more common in black patients and can rarely be fatal. Anaphylactoid reactions have also been reported in patients dialysed with high-flux membranes (e.g. AN69), LDL apheresis with dextran sulphate and during desensitization.
- Very rarely, ACEIs have been associated with a syndrome of progressive cholestatic jaundice that has led to fulminant necrosis and (sometimes) death.

Pregnancy and lactation

ACEIs are contraindicated in 2nd and 3rd trimester of pregnancy due to increased risk of fetotoxicity (decreased renal function, oligohydramnios, skull ossification retardation) and neonatal toxicity (hyperkalaemia, hypotension, and renal failure). Ultrasound check of renal function and skull should be arranged in the event of exposure to ACEIs in the 2nd trimester. Use of ACEIs in the 1st trimester of pregnancy may be associated with teratogenicity and so is not recommended (pregnancy category D). Alternative antihypertensive agents should be considered in patients planning pregnancy. Not recommended during breastfeeding.

Contraindications

- History of hereditary or idiopathic angiooedema; previous ACEI-related angio-oedema
- Hypotension: SBP <95mmHg
- Pregnancy and breastfeeding
- Hyperkalaemia
- Severe renal failure (serum creatinine >2.5–3mg/dL, or >225–265µmol/L)
- Renal artery stenosis (bilateral, or unilateral with a solitary functioning kidney)

References

1 Mancia G et al. (2007). Guidelines for the management of arterial hypertension: The Task Force for the Management of Arterial Hypertension of the European Society of Hypertension (ESH) and of the European Society of Cardiology (ESC). *Eur Heart J* **28**:1462–536.
2 Dickstein K et al. (2008). ESC Guidelines for the diagnosis and treatment of acute and chronic heart failure 2008: the Task Force for the Diagnosis and Treatment of Acute and Chronic Heart Failure 2008 of the European Society of Cardiology. *Eur Heart J* **29**:2388–442.
3 Schmieder RE et al. (2007). Renin-angiotensin system and cardiovascular risk. *Lancet* **369**:1208–19.
4 Lewis EJ et al. for the Collaborative Study Group (1993).The effect of angiotensin-converting enzyme inhibition on diabetic nephropathy. *New Engl J Med* **229**:1456–62.
5 Dagenais GR et al. (2006). Angiotensin-converting-enzyme inhibitors in stable vascular disease without left ventricular systolic dysfunction or heart failure: a combined analysis of three trials. *Lancet* **368**:581–8.
6 Kostis JB et al. (2004). Omapatrilat and enalapril in patients with hypertension: the Omapatrilat Cardiovascular Treatment vs. Enalapril (OCTAVE) trial. *Am J Hypertens* **17**:103–11.

Angiotensin II (AT$_1$) receptor blockers

Candesartan (📖 p.394), irbesartan (📖 p.492), losartan (📖 p.511), telmisartan (📖 p.599), valsartan (📖 p.625).

Others: eprosartan, olmisartan.

Indications

1. Management of hypertension
2. Management of HF to reduce CV death and HF hospitalizations
3. Slow the progression of nephropathy caused by type 2 diabetes

Mechanism of action

(See 📖 RAAS inhibitors, p.568)

ARBs inhibit the RAAS by antagonizing the effects of angiotensin II at the AT$_1$-receptor site, including vasoconstriction, endothelial dysfunction, cell growth and proliferation, fibrosis, and antinatriuresis. Moreover, in the presence of an ARB, angiotensin II can stimulate AT$_2$ receptors that are not blocked, producing vasodilator, antiproliferative, and natriuretic effects. Thus, the effects of ARBs are due to the blockade of AT$_1$ receptors and the stimulation of AT$_2$ receptors. ARBs avoid bradykinin-related side effects (cough, angio-oedema) of ACEIs.

Pharmacodynamics

(See 📖 RAAS inhibitors, p.568 and individual ARBs, p.359)

Hypertension: a meta-analysis of 50 CTs found that ARBs produced a BP reduction similar to ACEIs, but with better tolerability.[1] Black patients are less likely to respond to ACEIs or ARBs.

ARBs are indicated in hypertensives with ACEI-related cough or intolerance, HF or LV dysfunction, LV hypertrophy, microalbuminuria, type 2 diabetes, chronic renal disease, and metabolic syndrome.[2]

HF and post-MI patients:[3] ACEIs and ARBs have similar efficacy in chronic HF as well as in patients after acute MI with signs of HF or LV dysfunction; ARBs are indicated in symptomatic patients intolerant to ACEIs to improve morbidity and mortality. ARBs can be considered in combination with ACEIs in patients who remain symptomatic, to reduce mortality and hospital admissions for HF.

Renal protection: ARBs reduce proteinuria and slow the progression of glomerular sclerosis and loss of renal function in chronic renal disease, with or without type 2 diabetes.[4–6]

Practical points

↓ Doses

(See individual ARBs, p.359)

Hypertension: the full effect is potentiated by thiazides and loop diuretics or a low-salt diet more than by dose increase.

☺ Side effects
Adverse effects are comparable to placebo.

(1–10%): dizziness, vertigo; fatigue; hypotension; hyperkalaemia, rise in urea and creatinine.

Others: nausea, vomiting; chest infection; headache; angio-oedema has been reported with some ARBs.

Interactions
Antihypertensive effects of ARBs are enhanced when used with other antihypertensives and vasodilators (e.g. nitrates), tricyclic antidepressants, antipsychotics, and baclofen; they are reduced by chronic administration of NSAIDs and sympathomimetics. Antihypertensive effects of diuretics are additive with ARBs.

Risk of hyperkalaemia is increased with renal impairment, and especially with concomitant use of ACEIs, K^+-sparing diuretics, eplerenone, β-blockers, NSAIDs, heparin, or K^+ supplements. Use with NSAIDs can also rarely contribute to renal failure particularly in the elderly, dehydrated, or pre-existing renal impairment.

Concomitant use of ARBs with lithium may enhance effects and risk of toxicity of lithium; and so should be used with monitoring and caution.

The antihypertensive effects of ARBs are additive to those of thiazides and loop diuretics; ARBs compensate the hypokalaemia produced by the diuretics.

Cautions
ARBs should be used in caution in those with a history of angio-oedema, particularly if induced by ACEIs.

Symptomatic hypotension, especially after the 1st dose, may be seen in patients who are volume depleted or on diuretics. Such patients should be followed closely, particularly those with severe HF, where treatment should be started under medical supervision. Use with caution in malignant hypertension, aortic or mitral valve stenosis, LVOT obstruction, or constrictive pericarditis.

Check baseline renal function and monitor after administration to check for renal impairment. Monitor for hyperkalaemia especially in patients with diabetes, renal insufficiency, on K^+-sparing diuretic or K^+ supplements. There is an increased risk of hypotension and renal failure in those with renovascular disease, e.g. bilateral renal artery stenosis or artery stenosis of a single functioning kidney. This is usually reversible on stopping therapy.

Pregnancy and lactation
(See 📖 ACEIs, p.355)
Pregnancy category D.

Contraindications
• History of hereditary or idiopathic angio-oedema; previous ACEI-related angio-oedema
• Hyperaldosteronism

- Hyperkalaemia
- Hypotension
- Pregnancy and breastfeeding
- Severe renal failure (serum creatinine >2.5–3mg/dL, or >225–265µmol/L
- Renal artery stenosis in a solitary kidney or significant bilateral renal artery stenosis

References

1 Matchar DB et al. (2008). Systematic review: comparative effectiveness of angiotensin-converting enzyme inhibitors and angiotensin II receptor blockers for treating essential hypertension. *Ann Intern Med* **148**:16–29.

2. Mancia G et al. (2007). Guidelines for the management of arterial hypertension: The Task force for the Management of Arterial Hypertension of the European Society of Hypertension (ESH) and of the European Society of Cardiology (ESC). *Eur Heart J* **28**:1462–536.

3 Dickstein K et al. (2008). ESC Guidelines for the diagnosis and treatment of acute and chronic heart failure 2008: the Task Force for the Diagnosis and Treatment of Acute and Chronic Heart Failure 2008 of the European Society of Cardiology. *Eur Heart J* **29**:2388–442.

4 Lewis EJ et al.; Collaborative Study Group (2001). Renoprotective effect of the angiotensin-receptor antagonist irbesartan in patients with nephropathy due to type 2 diabetes. *N Engl J Med* **345**:851–60.

5 Parving HH et al. (2001). Irbesartan in Patients with Type 2 Diabetes and Microalbuminuria Study Group (2001). The effect of irbesartan on the development of diabetic nephropathy in patients with type 2 diabetes. *N Engl J Med* **345**:870–8.

6 Brenner BM et al.; RENAAL Study Investigators (2001). Effects of losartan on renal and cardio-vascular outcomes in patients with type 2 diabetes and nephropathy. *N Engl J Med* **345**:861–9.

Antiarrhythmic drugs: classification

The Vaughan Williams classification of antiarrhythmic drugs, proposed in 1970, is still widely used. This system classifies a drug based on the 1° mechanism of its antiarrhythmic action. Four classes were initially proposed (I–IV) according to defined electrophysiological effects on the myocardium. Its dependence on 1° mechanisms is, however, a recognized limitation of the Vaughan Williams classification, as many antiarrhythmic drugs have >1 mechanism of action. A 5th class (V) has been more recently proposed to include drugs such as adenosine, digoxin, and others which do not have a place among classes I to IV.

Class I: Na^+-channel blockade	Reduce phase 0 slope and peak of action potential
Class II: β-adrenergic-blockade	Block sympathetic activity; reduce rate and conduction
Class III: K^+-channel blockade.	Prolong the duration of the cardiac action potential (APD) and refractoriness without affecting intracardiac conduction
Class IV: block L-type calcium channels	Most effective at SA and AV nodes; reduce rate and conduction

See also:
Class Ia antiarrhythmic drugs:
Class Ib antiarrhythmic drugs:
Class Ic antiarrhythmic drugs:
Class III antiarrhythmic drugs:
Class IV antiarrhythmic drugs (see 📖 Calcium-channel blockers, p.390)
Other antiarrhythmic agents:

Aspirin (acetylsalicylic acid)

Cyclo-oxygenase (COX) inhibitor.

CV indications

1. Reduce the combined risk of death and non-fatal stroke in patients who have had ischaemic stroke or transient ischaemia of the brain due to fibrin platelet emboli.
2. Reduce the risk of vascular mortality in patients with suspected AMI.
3. Reduce the combined risk of death and non-fatal MI in patients with a previous MI or UA.
4. Reduce the combined risk of MI and sudden death in patients with chronic stable angina pectoris.
5. Anti-inflammatory agent used in pericarditis, rheumatic fever, and Kawasaki's disease.

Mechanism of action

Aspirin irreversibly inactivates the cyclo-oxygenase (COX) enzyme, preventing the conversion of arachidonic acid to thromboxane (TXA_2) and various prostaglandins. TXA_2 is produced in platelets in response to a variety of stimuli, activates TP receptors and induces platelet aggregation by mediating expression of the glycoprotein complex GP IIb/IIIa in the cell membrane of platelets. Aspirin acetylates the serine residue at position 529 of the COX, leading to an irreversible inhibition of the enzyme, preventing the formation of TXA_2 from arachidonic acid. Endothelial cells regenerate active COX, while mature platelets are unable to synthesize COX, so that the antiplatelet effect of aspirin lasts for the duration of platelet life (~10 days). Thus, by irreversibly inactivating COX, aspirin causes prolonged platelet dysfunction, and prolongs bleeding times. Aspirin also has analgesic, antipyretic, and anti-inflammatory actions due to its inhibitory effect on prostaglandin synthesis. Inhibition of the production of other prostaglandins, including those that are vasoactive or that mediate inflammatory responses, may also contribute to the prevention of CVD.

Pharmacodynamics

34% RR in MI and sudden death and 22–32% RR in vascular events, vascular death, all-cause mortality, and stroke in patients with stable angina (all receiving sotalol) treated with aspirin (75mg od) for 50 months as compared to placebo.[1–3]

11.8% RR in 5-week vascular mortality when given after a suspected AMI.[2] The combination with streptokinase produced an additive effect (42% RR). Aspirin significantly reduced non-fatal MI and non-fatal stroke and was not associated with any significant increase in major bleedings.

Meta-analyses of 287 RCTs,[2] comprising predominantly studies with aspirin, indicate that antiplatelet therapy reduces serious cardiovascular events (non-fatal MI, non-fatal stroke, or vascular deaths) by ~22% in high-risk patients. Absolute risk reductions (/1000) of serious CV events are shown in Table 1.[2] Thus, lifelong aspirin therapy is appropriate for all patients with STEMI in whom it is not contraindicated.[3]

Table 1 Effects of aspirin (75–375mg od) on major cardiovascular events in various risk groups

Patient risk group	Mean duration of treatment (months)	Adjusted % of CV events in antiplatelet group	Adjusted % of CV events in control group	Benefit (/1000 patients)
Previous MI	27	13.5	17.0	~36
AMI	1	10.4	14.2	~38
Previous CVA/TIA	29	17.8	21.4	~36
Acute stroke	0.7	8.2	9.1	~9

Pharmacokinetics

Aspirin is rapidly absorbed from the upper GI tract with oral bioavailability of 45%. It is rapidly hydrolysed in the plasma and tissues to salicylic acid, being indetectable 1–2h after dosing ($t_{1/2}$ ~20min). Salicylic acid binds to plasma proteins (50%), presents a V_d of 0.15L/kg and is glucoconjugated in the liver to several metabolites that are excreted in urine. Salicylic acid has a $t_{1/2}$ of ~6h, but its metabolism is saturable, so that at high doses the $t_{1/2}$ is much longer (15–30h). Urinary excretion is affected by pH; there is a 10–20-fold increase in renal clearance when urine pH is increased from 5 to 8. Plasma salicylate levels increase disproportionately with each dose due to zero-order kinetics.[4,5]

Practical points

♣ Doses

ACS: 75mg–150mg od (for 2° prevention of CVD, following a 300mg initial dose in ACS)

☺ Common side effects

GI: dyspepsia, nausea and vomiting, gastric irritation, ulceration, and haemorrhage.

Use of low-dose asprin increases the risk of upper GI events by 2- to 4-fold, which is not reduced with buffered or enteric-coated preparations. The absolute increase in GI side effects is 0.12% per year.[6]

Others: bruising; water and salt retention; deterioration in renal function; urticaria, angio-oedema, bronchospasm, asthma.

Interactions

Due to pharmacodynamics: (a) increased risk of bleeding with warfarin, heparins, clopidogrel and other NSAIDs; (b) increased risk of GI bleeding with alcohol, corticosteroids, and other NSAIDs.

Due to pharmacokinetics: (a) decreased efficacy when combined with liver enzyme inducers such as phenytoin, phenobarbital, and rifampicin; (b) increased risk of aspirin toxicity with acetazolamide; (c) aspirin displaces a number of drugs from protein-binding sites in the blood, including antidiabetic drugs (increase the risk of hypoglycaemia), phenytoin, valproic acid, and other NSAIDs. Aspirin increases the risk of GI bleeding and ulceration when given with corticosteroids. The pharmacological activity of spironolactone may be reduced by taking aspirin.

Aspirin reduces excretion of methotrexate and uric acid (and hence can precipitate gout) especially in combination with thiazide diuretics. There is also an increased risk of bleeding with antidepressants, such as SSRIs and venlafaxine.

Aspirin can decrease the antihypertensive effects of ACEIs, ARBs, thiazides, and β-blockers.

Cautions/notes

In patients who develop GI side effects while taking aspirin, and in those with an an increased risk of GI bleeding, a PPI should be used. Aspirin may precipitate bronchospasm in patients with asthma. Aspirin has been associated with Reye's syndrome in children. The use of aspirin is avoided in patients with a CrCl of <10mL/min, and with severe hepatic impairment. Aspirin may increase the risk of haemorrhagic stroke.

Patients with haemophilia or other bleeding tendencies should not take aspirin. Aspirin is known to cause haemolytic anaemia in people who have glucose-6-phosphate dehydrogenase deficiency (G6PD).

People with kidney disease, hyperuricaemia, or gout should not take aspirin because aspirin inhibits the kidneys' ability to excrete uric acid.

In up to 25% of patients, aspirin does not have as strong an effect on platelets as for others (aspirin resistance or insensitivity).

The cardioprotective effects of aspirin are potentially blunted by co-administration with non-selective NSAIDs (e.g. ibuprofen).

Pregnancy and lactation

Aspirin should be avoided in pregnancy and lactation (pregnancy category D). Aspirin produces alterations in maternal and neonatal haemostasis, decreases birth weight and increases perinatal mortality, and because of the risk of premature closure of the ductus arteriosus in utero it should be avoided in the 3rd trimester of pregnancy. It should be avoided 1 week before labour and delivery because it may increase the risk of haemorrhage; additionally, it may delay the onset and prolong labour. Aspirin is excreted into breast milk.

Contraindications

- History of GI bleeding, peptic ulcer, haemophilia, or other clotting disorders
- Severe renal and hepatic impairment
- Children under the age of 16
- Relative contraindications include: dyspepsia, iron deficient anaemia, and gout
- Hypersensitivity to aspirin or NSAIDs

References

1 Juul-Moller S et al. (1992). For the Swedish Angina Pectoris Aspirin Trial (SAPAT) Group. Double blind trial of aspirin in primary prevention of myocardial infarction in patients with stable chronic angina pectoris. *Lancet* **340**:1421–5.

2 ISIS-2 Study (1988). Randomised trial of intravenous streptokinase, oral aspirin, both, or neither among 17,187 cases of suspected acute myocardial infarction: ISIS-2. *Lancet* **2**:349–60

3 Antithrombotic Trialists' Collaboration (2002). Collaborative meta-analysis of randomised trials of anti-platelet therapy for prevention of death, myocardial infarction and stroke in high risk patients. *BMJ* **324**:71–86.

4 Bassand JP et al. (2007). Guidelines for the diagnosis and treatment of non-ST-segment elevation acute coronary syndromes. *Eur Heart J* **28**:2–63.

5 Needs CJ, Brooks PM (1985). Clinical pharmacokinetics of the salicylates. *Clin Pharmacokinet* **10**:164–77.

6 American College of Cardiology Foundation Task Force on Clinical Expert Consensus Documents, Bhatt DL et al. (2008). ACCF/ACG/AHA 2008 Expert Consensus Document on Reducing the Gastrointestinal Risks of Antiplatelet Therapy and NSAID Use. *J Am Coll Cardiol* **52**:1502–17.

Atenolol

(See also 📖 β-blockers, p.376)

Cardioselective β_1-adrenergic receptor antagonist.

CV indications
(See 📖 β-blockers, p.376)

Mechanism of action
(See 📖 β-blockers, p.376)

Pharmacodynamics
(See 📖 β-blockers, p.376)

Hypertension and diabetes: 35% RRR in stroke and 27% RRR for the 2° endpoint of clinical non-fatal MI and 32% RRR in major CV events following aggressive treatment for 4.5 years with antihypertensive agents including β-blockers in hypertensive patients.[1] Treatment with β-blockers and diuretics for 65 months reduced the frequency of fatal and non-fatal stroke and MI and other cardiovascular death as well as total mortality in hypertensive patients aged 70–84.[2]

A meta-analysis of clinical trials of antihypertensive drugs found that β-blockers (mainly atenolol) increase the likelihood of new-onset type 2 diabetes.[3]

RRR ≈24% in diabetic endpoints (fatal and non-fatal), 32% in deaths related to diabetes, ≈44% in stroke, ≈37% in microvascular endpoints in hypertensive patients with type 2 diabetes treated aggressively to achieve a BP of <150/80mmHg (using antihypertensives including atenolol) compared to less aggressive BP lowering of <180/105mmHg.[4] There was a significant reduction in progression of diabetic retinopathy, and deterioration in visual acuity.

In contrast, in direct comparisons with other antihypertensives atenolol did not appear to be as effective as a 1st-line antihypertensive agent in reducing major CV events (particularly stroke) when compared to amlodipine;[5] in reducing cardiovascular events in older hypertensive patients;[6] or in reducing LVH when compared to losartan.[7]

Post-MI: RRR ≈15% (absolute rates: 3.9% vs. 4.6%) in 1-week vascular deaths in patients with AMI treated with atenolol (initial 5–10mg IV bolus followed 100mg of PO maintenance for 7 days).[8] The overall vascular mortality was also lower in the atenolol group at 1 year (10.7% vs. 12.0%).

Pharmacokinetics
Rapidly but incompletely absorbed from the GI tract, with oral bioavailability ≈50–60%; peak plasma concentrations are reached in 2–4h. It binds ≈5% to plasma proteins, presents a V_d of 0.7–1.2L/kg and is almost exclusively excreted unchanged in the urine. $t_{1/2}$ ≈6h, but the duration of action is longer (≈24h). The dose may need to be decreased in patients with renal and hepatic impairment.

Practical points

:3 Doses

PO: 50–100mg od or 50mg bd (for angina, dose adjusted to achieve resting heart rate 50–60bpm)

IV: 5–10mg over 10min under careful monitoring; repeat 5min later

☺ **Side-effects**   (see 📖 β-blockers, p.376)

Interactions   (see 📖 β-blockers, p.376)

Cautions/notes   (see 📖 β-blockers, p.376)

Pregnancy and lactation

(See 📖 β-blockers, p.376)

Atenolol crosses the placenta and safety in early pregnancy is not established. Therefore, atenolol should be avoided in early pregnancy (pregnancy category D), but due to the adverse effects of severe maternal hypertension during pregnancy, atenolol may sometimes be used with close monitoring in the 3rd trimester.

Atenolol is excreted in breast milk and if used while breastfeeding, the infant should be monitored for bradycardia, respiratory depression, hypotension, and hypoglycaemia.

Contraindications (see 📖 β-blockers, p.376)

References

1 SHEP Cooperative Research Group (1991). Prevention of stroke by antihypertensive drug treatment in older persons with isolated systolic hypertension. Final results of the Systolic Hypertension in the Elderly Program (SHEP). *JAMA* **265**:3255–64.
2 Dahlöf B et al. (1991). Morbidity and mortality in the Swedish Trial in Old Patients with Hypertension (STOP-Hypertension). *Lancet* **338**:1281–5.
3 Elliott WJ, Meyer PM (2007). Incident diabetes in clinical trials of antihypertensive drugs: a network meta-analysis. *Lancet* **369**:201–7.
4 UKPDS 38 (1998). Tight blood pressure control and risk of macrovascular and microvascular complications in type 2 diabetes: UK Prospective Diabetes Study Group. *BMJ* **317**:703–13.
5 Dahlöf B et al.; ASCOT Investigators (2005). Prevention of cardiovascular events with an antihypertensive regimen of amlodipine adding perindopril as required versus atenolol adding bendroflumethiazide as required, in the Anglo-Scandinavian Cardiac Outcomes Trial-Blood Pressure Lowering Arm (ASCOT-BPLA): a multicentre randomised controlled trial. *Lancet* **366**:895–906.
6 MRC Working Party (1992). Medical Research Council trial of treatment of hypertension in older adults: principal results. *BMJ* **304**:405–12.
7 Lindholm LH et al.; LIFE Study Group (2002). Cardiovascular morbidity and mortality in patients with diabetes in the Losartan Intervention For Endpoint reduction in hypertension study (LIFE): a randomised trial against atenolol. *Lancet* **359**:1004–10.
8 First International Study of Infarct Survival Collaborative Group (1986). Randomised trial of intravenous atenolol among 16 027 cases of suspected acute myocardial infarction: ISIS-1. *Lancet* **2**:57–66.

Atorvastatin

(See also 📖 Statins, p.591)

Oral HMG-CoA reductase inhibitor.

Indications

1. Hypercholesterolaemia: adjunct to diet in 1° hypercholesterolaemia, mixed hyperlipidaemia, homozygous and heterozygous familial hypercholesterolaemia, when response to diet and other non-pharmacological measures is inadequate.
2. Hypertriglyceridaemia and 1° dysbetalipoproteinaemia.
3. 1° prevention in patients without clinically evident CHD, but with multiple risk factors to reduce the risk of MI, stroke, UA or revascularization, as an adjunct to diet.
4. Patients with type 2 diabetes without clinically evident CHD, but with multiple risk factors to reduce the risk of MI and stroke.
5. 2° prevention of cardiovascular events: in patients with clinically evident CHD to reduce the risk of non-fatal MI, fatal and non-fatal stroke, revascularization procedures, hospitalization for CHF or angina.

Mechanism of action

(See 📖 Statins, p.591)

Pharmacodynamics

1° hypercholesterolaemia

Reduces total-C, LDL-C, apolipoprotein B, and triglycerides (Table 2) while producing variable increases in HDL-C.[1]

Table 2 Effects of atorvastatin on lipid profile (adjusted mean % change from baseline)

Dose (mg)	Percentage change					
	Total-C	LDL-C	ApoB	TG	HDL-C	Lp(a)
Placebo	5	8	6	−1	−2	7
10	−30	−41	−34	−14	4	4
20	−35	−44	−36	−33	12	−8
40	−38	−50	−41	−25	−3	3
80	−46	−61	−50	−27	3	−14

1° prevention

36% RRR (1.9% vs. 3.0% absolute rate) in non-fatal and fatal MI with atorvastatin 10mg compared with placebo after 3.3 years in hypertensive patients with total cholesterol levels ≤6.5mmol/L and ≥3 additional predefined CV risk factors.[2] 27% RRR (89 vs. 121) in fatal and non-fatal stroke, 21% RRR (389 vs. 486) in total CV events, and 29% RRR (178 vs. 247) in total coronary events. There was no effect on the total mortality rate or in the incidence of adverse effects.

37% RRR (5.8 vs. 9.0% absolute rate) in major cardiovascular events (MI, acute CHD death, unstable angina, coronary revascularization, or stroke) with atorvastatin 10mg compared with placebo after 3.9 years in patients with diabetes, total cholesterol levels ≤4.14mmol/L and ≥1 additional predefined CV risk factors.[3]

2° prevention and intensive lipid lowering

16% RRR (9.4% vs. 26.3% absolute rates) for a composite endpoint (mortality, MI, ACS rehospitalization, coronary revascularization at 30 days, and stroke) with atorvastatin 80mg daily compared with pravastatin 40–80mg daily for 2 years who had been hospitalized for an ACS within the preceding 10 days.[4] This was the 1st clinical trial to demonstrate an added clinical benefit of a more intensive lipid-lowering strategy.

Reduction of 22% in HR (2.2% absolute reduction) has been shown for major CV events with atorvastatin 80mg daily compared with 10mg daily in patients with stable CHD and LDL-cholesterol <3.4 mmol/l.[5] RRR 13% in major CV events (any major coronary event plus stroke), RRR 16% in CHD events (any major coronary event, any coronary revascularization procedure, or UA) and RRR 26% in any CV events (any of the former plus heart failure, PAD, and stroke) in patients with a prior MI treated for 4.8 years with atorvastatin 80 mg/day when compared with simvastatin 20 mg/day.[6] However, there were no differences in the 1° endpoint (time to a major coronary event, defined as coronary death, nonfatal MI, or cardiac arrest with resuscitation).

Acute treatment of ACS

RRR 16% (absolute value 17.4% vs. 14.8%) in the 1° endpoint (death, non-fatal AMI, resuscitated cardiac arrest with resuscitation, or recurrent symptomatic myocardial ischaemia with objective evidence and requiring emergency rehospitalization) in patients with ACS or non-Q-wave AMI treated 24–96h after hospital admission with atorvastatin (80mg) vs. placebo for 4 months.[6] There were no significant differences in risk of death, non-fatal MI, or cardiac arrest between groups, although the atorvastatin group had a lower risk of symptomatic ischaemia requiring emergency rehospitalization.

Coronary atherosclerosis progression

In patients with CAD, coronary angiography with >20% stenosis, intensive lipid-lowering treatment with atorvastatin 80mg reduced progression of coronary atherosclerosis (−0.4%; CI −2.4–1.5% of baseline) compared with moderate lipid-lowering with pravastatin 40mg (2.7%; 95% CI 0.2–4.7% vs. baseline) over a period of 18 months.[8]

Stroke

16% RRR (absolute value 11.2% vs. 13.1%) in fatal or non-fatal stroke, 35% RRR in major coronary vascular events and 45% in any revascularization procedures in patients with recent TIA or stroke, no known CHD, and hypercholesterolaemia treated for 4.9 years with high-dose atorvastatin (80mg) as compared to placebo.[9]

The SPARCL trial randomized patients with TIA or stroke within 1 to 6 months without CAD and LDL-C 100 to 190 mg/dL to atorvastatin 80 mg od or placebo. 33% RRR in any stroke, 43% RRR in major coronary events and 56% RRR in revascularizations in patients with carotid artery stenosis treated with atorvastatin od cf placebo.[10] These results indicate that intense lipid lowering with atorvastatin reduced the risk of cerebro- and cardiovascular events in patients with and without carotid stenosis.

Homozygous familial hypercholesterolaemia
Effective in reducing LDL-C, in a population that has not usually responded to lipid-lowering medication. Mean reductions from baseline with 6 weeks of atorvastatin 80mg were 18.0% for LDL-C, 17.9% total cholesterol and 11.7% ApoB (part of a crossover trial with 80mg rosuvastatin, resulting in 19.1%, 17.6%, and 11.4% reduction respectively).[11]

Pharmacokinetics
Atorvastatin is rapidly absorbed, but presents a low bioavailability ($\approx$12%) due to pre-systemic clearance in GI mucosa and/or hepatic 1^{st}-pass metabolism; reaches peak plasma concentrations within 1–2h. Antacids can decrease drug absorption. It is metabolized by CYP450 3A4 into active metabolites, binds to plasma proteins ($\geq$98%), and present a large V_d ($\approx$5.3L/kg). Atorvastatin is also a substrate of the intestinal P-glycoprotein efflux transporter, which pumps the drug back into the intestinal lumen during drug absorption. Elimination is primarily via hepatic biliary excretion with <2% of atorvastatin recovered in the urine. Plasma elimination $t_{\frac{1}{2}}$ is $\approx$14h and $t_{\frac{1}{2}}$ of inhibitory activity $\approx$20–30h due to active metabolites. Plasma concentrations are markedly increased in chronic alcoholic liver disease and in patients with Child–Pugh B disease. In patients >65 years old the mean AUC and C_{max} values are higher (40% and 30%, respectively) and show a greater pharmacodynamic response to atorvastatin.

Practical points

♣ Doses
10mg daily (maximum: 80mg daily).
- Doses may be individualized according to baseline LDL-C levels, the goal of therapy, and patient response.
- Adjustment of dosage should be made at intervals of 4 weeks or more. No dose adjustment is needed in patients with renal dysfunction.

☺Side effects
(See 📖 Statins, p.591)
Elevated serum ALT levels reported in 0.4–1.3%. Clinically important (>3× upper limit) elevations in serum ALT occurred in 0.7%, were dose-related and reversible.

Elevated serum CPK levels (>3× upper limit in 2.5%; >10× upper limit in 0.4%). Only 0.1% had concurrent muscle pain, tenderness, or weakness.

Interactions
(See 📖 Statins, p.591)
- When patients are receiving drugs that increase the plasma concentration of atorvastatin, the starting dose of atorvastatin should be 10mg od.
- In the case of ciclosporin, clarithromycin, and itraconazole, caution should be used when the dose exceeds 20mg.
- Atorvastatin increases the plasma levels of digoxin. Patients taking digoxin should be monitored appropriately.
- Atorvastatin increases AUC values for some oral contraceptives (norethisterone and ethinylestradiol).

Cautions/notes (see 📖 Statins, p.591)

Pregnancy and lactation (see 📖 Statins, p.591)

Contraindications (see 📖 Statins, p.591)

References

1 Nawrocki JW et al. (1995). Reduction of LDL cholesterol by 25% to 60% in patients with primary hypercholesterolemia by atorvastatin, a new HMG-CoA reductase inhibitor. *Arterioscler Thromb Vasc Biol* **155**:678–82.
2 Sever PS et al. (2003). Prevention of coronary and stroke events with atorvastatin in hypertensive patients who have average or lower-than-average cholesterol concentrations, in the Anglo-Scandinavian Cardiac Outcomes Trial–Lipid Lowering Arm ASCOT-LLA): a multicentre randomised controlled trial. *Lancet* **361**:1149–58.
3 Colhoun HM et al. (2004). Primary prevention of cardiovascular disease with atorvastatin in type 2 diabetes in the Collaborative Atorvastatin Diabetes Study (CARDS): multicentre randomised placebo-controlled trial. *Lancet* **364**:685–96.
4 Cannon CP et al. (2004). Comparison of Intensive and Moderate Lipid Lowering with Statins after Acute Coronary Syndromes (PROVE IT-TIMI 22). *N Engl J Med* **350**:1495–504.
5 LaRosa JC et al.; Treating to New Targets (TNT) Investigators (2005). Intensive lipid lowering with atorvastatin in patients with stable coronary disease. *N Engl J Med* **352**:1425–35.
6 Pedersen TR et al.; Incremental Decrease in End Points Through Aggressive Lipid Lowering (IDEAL) Study Group (2005). High-dose atorvastatin vs usual-dose simvastatin for secondary prevention after myocardial infarction: the IDEAL study: a randomized controlled trial. *JAMA* **294**:2437–45.
7 Schwartz GG et al. (2001). Effects of atorvastatin on early recurrent ischemic events in acute coronary syndromes. The MIRACL study: a randomized controlled trial. *JAMA* **285**:1711–18.
8 Nissen SE et al.; REVERSAL Investigators (2004). Effect of intensive compared with moderate lipid-lowering therapy on progression of coronary atherosclerosis: a randomized controlled trial. *JAMA* **291**:1071–100.
9 Amarenco P et al.; Stroke Prevention by Aggressive Reduction in Cholesterol Levels (SPARCL) Investigators (2006). High-dose atorvastatin after stroke or transient ischemic attack. *N Engl J Med* **355**:549–59.
10 Sillesen H et al.; Stroke Prevention by Aggressive Reduction in Cholesterol Levels Investigators (2008). Atorvastatin reduces the risk of cardiovascular events in patients with carotid atherosclerosis: a secondary analysis of the Stroke Prevention by Aggressive Reduction in Cholesterol Levels (SPARCL) trial. *Stroke* **39**:3297–302.
11 Marais AD et al. (2008). A dose-titration and comparative study of rosuvastatin and atorvastatin in patients with homozygous familial hypercholesterolaemia. *Atherosclerosis* **197**:400–6.

Atropine

(See also 📖 Antiarrhythmic drugs: classification, p.362)

Muscarinic receptor antagonist.

CV indications

1. Treatment of asystole or sinus bradycardia during CPR
2. Treatment of sinus bradycardia induced by toxin
3. Management of bradycardia of AMI
4. Prevention of cholinergic effects on the heart (e.g. arrhythmias, bradycardia) during surgery

Other indications

As preoperative medication for the reduction of salivary and bronchial secretion; in combination with neostigmine during reversal of effect of non-depolarizing muscle relaxants.

Mechanism of action

Inhibits the effects of vagal stimulation on SA and AV nodes.

Pharmacodynamics

Enhances the rate of discharge of the SA node and improves AV conduction. However, it does not modify cardiac contractility and BP.

Pharmacokinetics

Atropine disappears rapidly from the blood following IV injection and is distributed throughout the body. Atropine binds poorly (20%) to plasma proteins, is hydrolysed particularly in the liver, and 50% of the dose is excreted unchanged in the urine. The elimination half-life (2h) is more than doubled in children under 2 years and the elderly (>65 years old) compared to other age groups.

Practical points

♪ Doses

- *Cardiac arrest*: 1mg IV, repeated in 2–5min if necessary (max dose 3mg, 0.04mg/kg).
- *Severe bradycardia*: 0.5mg every 5min (max dose 2mg).

☺ Common side effects

Common: dryness of the mouth, blurred vision, photophobia, tachycardia, constipation and difficulty in micturition. Confusion, dissociative hallucinations, and excitation are common in the elderly. VF, SVT, or VT.

Interactions

Amantadine, tricyclic antidepressants (anticholinergic effects), phenothiazine antipsychotics, diphenhydramine, and disopyramide exert anticholinergic effects and potentiate those of atropine.

Pregnancy and lactation

It is not known whether atropine can cause fetal harm when given to a pregnant woman or can affect reproduction capacity (pregnancy category C).

Contraindications

- Glaucoma
- Pyloric stenosis
- Prostatic hypertrophy

Bendroflumethiazide

(See also 📖 Thiazide and related diuretics, p.604)

Oral thiazide diuretic.

CV and other indications

(See 📖 Thiazide and related diuretics, p.604)

Mechanism of action

(See 📖 Thiazide and related diuretics, p.604)

Pharmacodynamics (Tables 3 and 4)
Doses above 2.5mg od do not appear to be associated with increased antihypertensive effects but are associated with other effects.

Table 3 BP lowering (mmHg) with different doses of bendroflumethiazide after 4 and 10–12 weeks' treatment[1]

	1.25mg od	2.5mg od	5mg od	10mg od
4 wks	−6.4/7.5	−11.3/8.7	−11.5/8.1	−11.7/9.0
10–12 wks	−12.7/9.8	−14.3/10.8	−13.4/10.1	−17.0/10.8

Table 4 Change in biochemical parameters after 10 weeks' treatment with bendroflumethiazide at different doses[1]

	1.25mg od	2.5mg od	5mg od	10mg od
K⁺ (mmol/L) (baseline ≈4.3)	−0.16	−0.20	−0.33	−0.45
Urate (µmol/L) (baseline ≈320)	19.0	29.0	63.0	68.0
Creatinine (µmol/L) (baseline ≈80)	2.4	2.5	NS	2.8
Glucose (mmol/L) (baseline ≈4.3)	NS	NS	NS	0.27
Cholesterol (mmol/L)l (baseline ≈6)	NS	NS	NS	0.25

The MRC Trial of treatment of mild hypertension[2] showed that compared to placebo, bendroflumethiazide 10mg od over a mean of 5.5 years reduced stroke rate (1.4 cf 2.6/1000 patients years) and rate of all CV events (6.7 cf 8.2/1000 patient years) in patients with mild hypertension (DBP: 90–109mmHg). All-cause mortality was shown in a post hoc analysis to be reduced with bendroflumethiazide in men (7.1 cf 8.2/1000 patient years) but not women. Bendroflumethiazide was associated with significant increase in glucose intolerance, impotence, gout, headache, constipation, dizziness, and nausea.

Pharmacokinetics

It is completely absorbed from the GI tract (bioavailability 100%). It is bound to plasma proteins (96%), presents a V_d of 1–1.5kg/L, is extensively metabolized and $\approx$30% is excreted unchanged in the urine. The onset of diuretic action of the thiazides following oral administration occurs within 2h and the peak effect between 3–6h after administration. The duration of the diuretic action is between 18–24h.

Practical points

♪ Doses

For hypertension: 1.25–10mg od.
For oedema: initially 5–10mg od or alternate days to 5–10mg 1–3 times weekly.

☻ Side effects (see 📖 Thiazide and related diuretics, p.604)

Interactions

(See 📖 Thiazide and related diuretics, p.604)
Prolongation of clotting times has been reported when administered concomitantly with warfarin.

Cautions/notes

(See 📖 Thiazide and related diuretics, p.604)
Fluid and electrolyte balance should be monitored regularly and carefully, especially when administered with loop diuretics.

Pregnancy and lactation (see 📖 Thiazide and related diuretics, p.604)

Contraindications (see 📖 Thiazide and related diuretics, p.604)

References

1 Carlsen JE et al. (1990). Relation between dose of bendrofluazide, antihypertensive effect, and adverse biochemical effects. BMJ 300:1465–56.
2 Medical Research Council Working Party (1985). MRC trial of treatment of mild hypertension: principal results. BMJ 291:97–104.

β-blockers

See also 📖 Atenolol, p.367
        📖 Bisoprolol, p.384
        📖 Carvedilol, p.399
        📖 Labetalol, p.499
        📖 Metoprolol, p.522
        📖 Sotalol, p.586

Cardioselective β_1-adrenergic receptor antagonists: acebutolol, atenolol, bisoprolol, celiprolol, metoprolol, nebivolol.

Non-selective β-blockers: nadolol, pindolol, propranolol, sotalol, timolol.

α- and β-adrenergic receptor blockers: carvedilol, labetalol.

CV indications

1. Long-term management of chronic stable angina
2. Treatment of hypertension
3. Cardiac arrhythmias
4. HF
5. Reduction of early mortality and improvement of long-term prognosis following AMI

Other indications

Anxiety; thyrotoxicosis; migraine prophylaxis; glaucoma; essential tremor; phaeochromocytoma (in conjunction with α-blocker).

Mechanism of action

β_1-adrenergic receptor antagonists bind and block the effects of noradrenaline and adrenaline at β_1-adrenoceptors sites. The latter are Gs-coupled receptors and, within the heart, mediate positive chronotopic, inotropic, and dromotropic effects in response to stimulation by noradrenaline and adrenaline. By antagonizing these effects, cardioselective β_1-adrenoceptor blockers reduce heart rate, cardiac output, and conduction velocity. Stimulation of β_1-adrenoceptors also increases renin release from juxtaglomerular cells, lipolysis in adipose tissue, aqueous humour production, and cardiac apoptosis

Angina and CHD: β-blockers reduce myocardial oxygen demands by reducing heart rate, contractility and cardiac afterload. The decrease in heart rate also increases diastolic filling time and improves subendocardial coronary perfusion. β-adrenergic blockers also decrease mortality in patients with previous MI, not only through improving the oxygen supply/demand mismatch but also through their antiarrhythmic properties and their ability to inhibit subsequent cardiac remodelling.

Hypertension: the mechanism of the antihypertensive effects of β_1-blockers is unknown, but several possible mechanisms have been proposed:

- blockade of prejunctional β_2-adrenoceptors, leading to a decrease in noradrenaline release
- a central effect leading to reduced sympathetic peripheral outflow
- inhibition of renin release from the kidney (and of the RAAS), which causes hyponatraemia and hyperkalaemia
- reduction of cardiac output (due to decrease in heart rate and contractility).

They are 1st-choice drugs in hypertensive patients with CHD, HF, AF, tachyarrhythmias, pregnancy, and phaeochromocytoma (in conjunction with α-blockers).

Arrhythmia: β_1-adrenoceptor antagonists inhibit sympathetic influences on cardiac electrical activity (class II effects) and so reduce sinus rate and decrease conduction velocity and increase the effective refractory period in the AV node. In the ischaemic myocardium they decrease the dispersion of ventricular repolarization and increase VF threshold. These effects contribute to their antiarrhythmic actions. Sotalol has additional class III antiarrhythmic properties and prolongs cardiac action potential duration and refractoriness through K^+-channel blockade.

Heart failure: the mechanism of action by which β_1-adrenoceptors confer benefit in HF is uncertain but may include a decrease in heart rate that increases the ejection fraction despite its initial reduction, their antiarrhythmic and anti-anginal actions and the inhibition of neurohumoral activation (RAAS and sympathetic tone). In addition, high plasma catecholamine levels have been documented in severe HF and it is possible that the benefits of β-blockers may derive from attentuation of catecholamine toxicity and cardiac remodelling.

Pharmacodynamics (Table 5)

Effects of different β-blockers vary depending on their cardioselectivity. 1st-generation β-blockers developed were relatively non-selective and so blocked both β_1- and β_2-adrenoceptors. 2nd-generation β-blockers are more selective for β_1- whilst 3rd-generation agents possess vasodilator actions through blockade of α-adrenoceptors. In addition, β-blockers also differ in their intrinsic sympathomimetic activity (ISA), α-antagonism, lipid solubility, and antioxidant properties. However, β_1-cardioselectivity diminishes with increased doses.

Table 5

β-blocker	β_1-selectivity	ISA	α-antagonism	Lipid solubility
Acebutolol	+/−	+	−	+
Atenolol	+	−	−	−
Bisoprolol	+++	−	−	+
Carvedilol	β_1 and β_2	−	+	++
Celiprolol	+	+	−	+
Labetalol	β_1 and β_2	−	+	++
Metoprolol	+	−	−	++
Nebivolol	++	−	−	+
Propranolol	β_1 and β_2	−	−	+++
Sotalol	β_1 and β_2	−	−	−

Angina and post-MI: β-blockers reduce the frequency of chronic stable angina symptoms and raise the angina threshold through reduction in heart rate and contractility, by lowering peak heart rate and BP during exercise and improving diastolic flow to ischaemic areas (due to a decrease in heart rate). In patients with chronic stable angina, β-blockers reduce the risk of CV death and AMI by 30%.[1] β-blockers used in the treatment of angina are long-acting, cardioselective drugs without intrinsic sympathomimetic activity. However, there do not appear to be differences in efficacy in the treatment of angina between the various β-blockers.

β-blockers are not indicated in vasospastic angina due to a predominance of α-vasoconstriction.

Hypertension: reductions in BP are significantly greater with β-blockers compared to placebo or no treatment; and associated with reductions in stroke (RR=0.80; 95% CI: 0.66–0.96; NNT=200 for 5 years) and all CVD (RR=0.88; 95% CI: 0.79–0.97; adjusted RR 0.7%; NNT=140 for 5 years) but not in all-cause mortality, CV mortality or CHD.[2] However, all-cause mortality (RR=1.07; 95% CI: 1.00–1.14; NNH=200 for 5 years) and risk of CVD (RR=1.18; 95% CI: 1.08–1.29; NNH=80 for 5 years) was significantly greater with β-blockers than CCBs, but not different from diuretics or RAAS inhibitors. In addition, patients on β-blockers were more likely to discontinue treatment due to side effects than those on diuretics (RR=1.86; 95% CI: 1.39–2.50; NNH=16) and RAAS inhibitors (RR=1.41; 95% CI: 1.29–1.54; NNH=18), but not CCBs.

Compared to placebo, 1st-line β-blockers plus supplementary antihypertensives reduced BP by ≈11/6mmHg. However, compared to diuretics, CCBs, or RAAS inhibitors, the mean BPs at the end of the trials were 0–2mmHg higher with β-blockers.[3]

β-blockers have been relegated to third- or fourth-line initial choice of treatment in the management of hypertension as they are not as effective as other antihypertensive drugs at preventing cardiovascular events (particularly stroke) and as they increase the incidence of diabetes.[4,5] Although β-blockers reduce brachial blood pressure effectively, they do not lower central systolic blood pressure as much as ACEIs, diuretics, or calcium-channel blockers, and regression of LVH is more closely correlated with central blood pressure than with brachial blood pressure.

Heart failure: bisoprolol, carvedilol, and metoprolol reduce all-cause mortality (RRR ≈34%) and hospital admision for worsening HF (RRR 28–36%) in patients with HF within 1 year of treatment. ARR in mortality is ≈3.8–7.1% with NNT ≈14–23.[6–9] In addition, nebivolol has been shown to reduce mortality and hospital admission for CV disease (RRR 14%) in patients with HF >70 years.[10]

Arrhythmia: β-blockers are safe and effective for control of heart rate in patients with AF and superior to placebo.[11] Rate control in AF is achieved with β-blockers in 70% compared to 54% with CCBs.[12] They are generally not considered as 1st-line treatment for the maintenance of sinus rhythm. However, several studies have suggested moderate efficacy in preventing AF recurrence or reducing frequency of paroxsymal AF, comparable to conventional antiarrhythmic agents. Although unlikely to be efficacious in converting AF or to enhance success of cardioversion or to suppress immediate or late recurrence of AF, β-blockers may reduce subacute recurrences of AF. Treatment with β-blockers improves rate control, ventricular function, and survival in patients with persistent AF and LVF.

β-blockers are very effective against arrhythmias associated with an increase in sympathetic tone: stress, anxiety, HF, CHD (post-MI), hyperthyroidism, surgery and LQTS.

Pharmacokinetics

(See 📖 individual drugs)

Practical points

♪ Doses

(See 📖 individual drugs)

☺ Side effects

Cardiovascular: bradycardia, heart block, deterioration of HF, hypotension, fatigue, dizziness, syncope, cold extremities.

Respiratory: bronchospasm, asthma.

Neurological: confusion, headache, depression, insomnia, paraesthesia, nightmares.

Gastrointestinal: nausea, vomiting, constipation, abdominal cramps, dry mouth.

Endocrine: hypo- and hyperglycaemia, risk of new-onset type 2 diabetes (particularly when co-administered with diuretics).

Dermatological: rash.

Others: dry eyes, blurred vision, impotence, hypokalaemia.

Cardioselective β_1-blockers are thought to cause fewer central nervous system side effects (e.g. depression, nightmares) and have less risk of bronchospasm than non-selective β-blockers. β-blockers with α-antagonist activity (carvedilol) or NO release (nebivolol) may be more prone to cause postural hypotension, but have a better metabolic profile than other β-blockers.

Interactions

Risk of additive hypotension is increased when β-blockers are administered concomitantly with ACEIs, ARBs, nitrates, diuretics, α-blockers (in addition to increased risk of 1st-dose hypotension), tricyclic antidepressants, MAO inhibitors; anaesthetics (e.g. halothane, enflurane); alcohol; vasodilators and benzodiazepines.

Use of β-blockers with diltiazem and verapamil may cause enhanced hypotensive effect, bradycardia, AV block and HF.

There may be an increased risk of myocardial depression when β-blockers are given with antiarrhythmic agents. Specific examples include: bradycardia, AV and myocardial depression when given with amiodarone; and myocardial depression and bradycardia with class I antiarrhythmics. Risk of hypotension and ventricular arrhythmias may be increased when used with antidepressants or antipsychotics (e.g. phenothiazines and tricyclics).

β-blockers can produce hyperkalaemia and increase that produced by ACEIs, ARBs, and K⁺-sparing diuretics.

Other potential interactions include:
- *digoxin*: increased risk of AV block and bradycardia, antagonize the inotropic effect
- *NSAIDs (e.g. indometacin)*: antagonism of antihypertensive effects
- *antidiabetics*: risk of hypoglycaemia may be increased and clinical signs masked
- *OCP*: antihypertensive effects of β-blockers may be antagonized
- *clonidine*: increased risk of hypertension on withdrawal
- *sympathomimetics*: risk of severe hypertension and bradycardia (response to adrenaline may also be reduced)
- *mefloquine*: increased risk of bradycardia
- postural hypotension when combined with alpha-blockers.

Cautions/notes
Use with caution in patients with poor cardiac reserve, as β-blockers decrease myocardial contractility and cardiac output. Abrupt withdrawal of β-blockers (especially in patients with established CAD) may increase risk of exacerbation of angina, rebound hypertension, MI, ventricular arrhythmias, and sudden cardiac death. This may be explained by a return to high myocardial demands while underlying atherosclerosis has worsened, or by a rebound in adrenergic receptor sensitivity. Consequently, β-blockers should be withdrawn gradually over 1–2 weeks.

All β-blockers should be avoided in patients with asthma and other obstructive airway disease due to the risk of bronchospasm, unless a compelling indication is present and close surveillance followed. β-blockers should also not be initiated in patients with a phaeochromocytoma without prior α-blockade.

β-blockers are not indicated in vasospastic angina due to a predominance of α-vasoconstriction.

β-blockers may increase sensitivity towards allergens, leading to more severe anaphylactic reactions that are less responsive to treatment with adrenaline. They may exacerbate psoriatic rashes, and unmask or potentiate a myasthenic condition.

β-blockers are diabetogenic, and can mask symptoms of hypoglycaemia (tachycardia, agitation, tremor) and hyperthyroidism.

Pregnancy and lactation
(See 📖 individual blockers)

β-blockers may cause harmful effects in pregnancy and/or the fetus/newborn. In general, β-blockers reduce placental perfusion, which has been associated with growth retardation, intrauterine death, abortion, or early labour. Adverse effects (e.g. hypoglycaemia and bradycardia) may also occur in the fetus and newborn infant. If treatment with β-adrenoceptor blockers is necessary, β₁-selective blockers are preferable. However, in general, β-blockers should be avoided in pregnancy unless clearly necessary (pregnancy category C).

Contraindications

- Severe bradycardia (<45bpm), 2nd- or 3rd-degree heart block; sick sinus syndrome
- Hypotension (<100/60mmHg); cardiogenic shock; unstable HF
- Vasospastic (Prinzmetal type) angina
- Severe peripheral vascular disease
- Untreated phaeochromocytoma
- Severe depression
- Metabolic acidosis
- Asthma and other reversible obstructive airways diseases

Relative contraindications include:

- vasospastic angina
- cold extremities, Raynaud´s phenomenon, absent pulses (avoid non-selective agents; consider carvedilol, nebivolol)
- prediabetes or metabolic syndrome: β-blockers increase glycaemia and new-onset diabetes and impair insulin sensitivity (particularly when co-administered with thiazides). Consider carvedilol, nebivolol
- insulin-requiring diabetes (non-selective agents decrease reactions to hypoglycaemia: tachycardia, tremor)
- renal failure (avoid/reduce dose of agents eliminated by kidney: atenolol, sotalol)
- liver disease (avoid drugs with a high hepatic clearance (acebutolol, carvedilol, metoprolol, propranolol, timolol).

References

1 López-Sendón J et al.; Task Force On Beta-Blockers of the European Society of Cardiology (2004). Expert consensus document on beta-adrenergic receptor blockers. *Eur Heart J* **25**: 1341–62.

2 Mancia et al. (2007). 2007 Guidelines for the Management of Arterial Hypertension: The Task Force for the Management of Arterial Hypertension of the European Society of Hypertension (ESH) and of the European Society of Cardiology (ESC). *Eur Heart J* **28**:1462–53.

3 Wiysonge CS et al. (2007). Beta-blockers for hypertension. *Cochrane Database Syst Rev* (**1**):CD002003.

4 Lindholm LH et al. (2005). Should beta blockers remain first choice in the treatment of primary hypertension? A meta-analysis. *Lancet* Oct 29–Nov 4; **366**(9496):1545–53.

5 Elliott WJ, Meyer PM (2007). Incident diabetes in clinical trials of antihypertensive drugs: a network meta-analysis. *Lancet* **369**:201–7.

6 Packer M et al. for the US Carvedilol Heart Failure Study Group (1996). The effect of carvedilol on morbidity and mortality in patients with chronic heart failure. *N Engl J Med* **334**: 1349–55.

7 MERIT-HF Study Group (1999). Effect of metoprolol CR/XL in chronic heart failure: Metoprolol CR/XL Randomized Intervention Trial in Congestive Heart Failure (MERIT-HF). *Lancet* **353**:2001–7.

8 CIBIS II Investigators and Committee (1999). The Cardiac Insufficiency Bisoprolol Study II: a randomized trial. *Lancet* **353**:9–13.

9 Packer M et al. for the Carvedilol Prospective Randomized Cumulative Survival Study Group (2001). Effect of carvedilol on survival in severe chronic heart failure. *N Engl J Med* **344**: 1651–8.

10 Flather M et al. (2005). Randomized trial to determine the effect of nebivolol on mortality and cardiovascular hospital admission in elderly patients with heart failure (SENIORS). *Eur Heart J* **26**:215–25.

11 Fuster V et al. (2006). ACC/AHA/ESC 2006 Guidelines for the Management of Patients with Atrial Fibrillation. *Circulation* **114**:e257–354.

12 Olshansky B et al. (2004). The Atrial Fibrillation Follow-up Investigation of Rhythm Management (AFFIRM) study: approaches to control rate in atrial fibrillation. *J Am Coll Cardiol* **43**:1201–8.

Bezafibrate

(See also 📖 Fibrates, p.462)

Oral PPAR-alpha receptor agonist.

CV indications

Hyperlipidaemias of type IIa, IIb, III, IV, and V.

Mechanism of action

(See 📖 Fibrates, p.462)

Bezafibrate is also a PPAR-γ agonist that stimulates enzymes regulating glucose metabolism. It reduces fasting blood glucose, which may be useful in diabetic patients, and serum fibrinogen level in hyperfibrinogenaemic patients.

Pharmacodynamics

At the daily dose of 600mg, it lowered total (17%) and LDL-C (19.6%), VLDL (44.3%), triglyceride (13.7%), and ApoB (24.0%) and increased HDL-C (15.3%) plasma levels.[1]

In young male survivors of MI treated for 5 years, bezafibrate (300mg tds) significantly retarded the progression of coronary atheroma and coronary events, as assessed by changes in minimum lumen diameter.[2] This positive outcome is most likely due to the beneficial effects on the levels of serum triglycerides (−31%), plasma fibrinogen (−12%), and HDL-C (+9%).

In patients with normal triglyceride and elevated LDL-C levels it produces a non-significant (7.3%) RRR in the rate of major cardiac events after a mean follow-up period of 6.2 years, possibly owing to increasing use of non-study lipid-lowering drugs (LLDs) during the trial.[3] However, in a post hoc analysis, a significant reduction was shown in patients with elevated triglyceride and low HDL-C levels. Moreover, in an extended follow-up study, bezafibrate (400mg/day) produced an 18% RR in cardiac death or non-fatal MI among study subjects who were not treated with concurrent LLDs during follow-up or before non-randomized treatment with these medications was initiated.[4]

In patients with impaired glucose tolerance, bezafibrate may delay progress to diabetes[5] and in patients with CHD and type 2 diabetes, bezafibrate attenuated the development of insulin resistance and the progressive failure of pancreatic β-cell function.[6]

Pharmacokinetics

Standard preparations: rapid and complete oral absorption (bioavailability 100%), reaching peak concentrations 2h after ingestion. The relative bioavailability of bezafibrate retard compared to the standard form is about 70%. Protein binding in serum is ~95% (Vd 0.24L/kg). Excretion is almost exclusively (95%) renal and the elimination $t_{1/2}$ is ~1–2h (longer in renal dysfunction). The drug is non-dialysable.

Practical points

Doses
Standard preparation: 200mg bd or tds, after meals.
Modified release: 400mg once daily.

Side effects (see 📖 Fibrates, p.462)

Interactions

(See 📖 Fibrates, p.462)
Should not be administered together with MAO-inhibitors due to hepato-toxic potential.

Cautions/notes

Dose should be adjusted according to renal function:
- GFR 40–60mL/min: 400mg daily; GFR 15–40mL/min: 200mg daily or alternate days. GFR <15mL/min: contraindicated
- modified release is not appropriate in patients with renal dysfunction or on dialysis.

Pregnancy and lactation

(See 📖 Fibrates, p.462)

Contraindications

(See 📖 Fibrates, p.462)
Nephrotic syndrome.

References

1 Schulzeck P et al. (1988). Comparison between simvastatin and bezafibrate in effect on plasma lipoproteins and apolipoproteins in primary hypercholesterolaemia. *Lancet* **331**: 611–13.

2 de Faire U et al. (1996). Secondary preventive potential of lipid-lowering drugs. The Bezafibrate Coronary Atherosclerosis Intervention Trial (BECAIT). *Eur Heart J* 17(Suppl F):37–42.

3 BIP Study Group (2000). Secondary prevention by raising HDL cholesterol and reducing triglyc-erides in patients with coronary artery disease. *Circulation* **102**:21–7.

4 Goldenberg I et al. for the BIP Study Group (2008). Secondary prevention with bezafibrate therapy for the treatment of dyslipidemia: an extended follow-up of the BIP Trial. *J Am Coll Cardiol* **51**:459–65.

5 Tenenbaum A et al. (2004). Peroxisome proliferator-activated receptor ligand bezafibrate for prevention of type 2 diabetes mellitus in patients with coronary artery disease. *Circulation* **109**:2197–202.

6 Tenenbaum H et al. (2007). Long-term effect of bezafibrate on pancreatic beta-cell function and insulin resistance in patients with diabetes. *Atherosclerosis* **194**:265–71.

Bisoprolol

(See also 📖 β-blockers, p.376)
Cardioselective β_1-adrenergic receptor antagonist with high lipid solubility.

CV indications

(See 📖 β-blockers, p.376)

Mechanism of action

(See 📖 β-blockers, p.376)

Bisoprolol exhibits greater cardioselectivity than other 'cardioselective' β-blockers, including atenolol and metoprolol.

Pharmacodynamics

(See 📖 β-blockers, p.376)

Heart failure: HR ≈0.66 (absolute rates: 11.8% vs. 17.3%) in all-cause mortality in patients with NYHA HF III–IV and LVEF <35% established on diuretic and ACEI therapy treated with bisoprolol and followed up for a mean of 1.3 years.[1]

Pharmacokinetics

Well absorbed following PO administration with minimal 1st-pass metabolism (bioavailability ≈90%), reaching peak plasma concentration after 2–4h. Bisoprolol is ≈30% bound to serum proteins, presents a V_d of 3L/kg and is metabolized in the liver; ≈50% of the dose is excreted unchanged in urine. Has a $t_{\frac{1}{2}}$ ≈9–12h.

Practical points

⚕ Doses

5–10mg od (for angina, max dose 20mg/day).
Heart failure: initially 1.25mg od (uptitrated by doubling at intervals of 2 weeks to a maximum of 10mg od)

☻ Side effects (see 📖 β-blockers, p.376)

Interactions (see 📖 β-blockers, p.376)

Cautions/notes (see 📖 β-blockers, p.376)

Pregnancy and lactation

(See 📖 β-blockers, p.376)

Studies of bisoprolol in rats have demonstrated fetotoxicity and maternotoxicity (pregnancy category C) and the presence of bisoprolol in breast milk. Consequently, bisoprolol use is not recommended in breastfeeding.

Contraindications (see 📖 β-blockers, p.376)

Reference

1 (1999). The Cardiac Insufficiency Bisoprolol Study II (CIBIS-II): a randomised trial. *Lancet* **353**(9146):9–13.

Bosentan

Specific, competitive dual endothelin ET_A and ET_B receptor antagonist.

CV indications

Treatment of PAH to improve exercise capacity and symptoms in patients with grade II–IV functional status.

Other indications

To reduce the number of new digital ulcers in systemic sclerosis with ongoing digital ulcer disease.

Mechanism of action

ET-1, a peptide hormone produced by the endothelium, is a powerful vasoconstrictor and also a mediator of vascular smooth muscle cell growth. Its effects are mediated via endothelin ET_A and ET_B receptors. Levels of ET-1 appear to be raised in patients with PAH and correlated with disease severity and prognosis and may contribute to the pulmonary artery hypertension and vascular hypertrophy seen in PAH. Consequently, use of ET-1 antagonist may help limit the detrimental effects of ET-1 in PAH.

Bosentan inhibits vessel constriction and elevation of BP by competitively binding to endothelin-1 receptors ET_A and ET_B in endothelium and vascular smooth muscle.

Pharmacodynamics

In patients with PAH, bosentan improves haemodynamics (increases cardiac index, reduces pulmonary arterial and RA pressures and pulmonary vascular resistances), functional class, exercise capacity (44m in the 6MWT) and symptoms compared to placebo at 12–16 weeks.[1,2] It also decreases the rate of clinical deterioration, a composite morbidity and mortality endpoint.

1st-line therapy with bosentan results in Kaplan–Meir survival estimated of 90–96% and 70–89% at 1 or 2 years, respectively.[3,4]

Pharmacokinetics

Bioavailability after oral administration is 50% and unaffected by food. Highly protein-bound (98%) with a large V_d (18L/kg) and is eliminated by biliary excretion following metabolism in the liver by the CYP450 2C9 and CYP3A4. About <3% of an administered oral dose is recovered in urine. Elimination $t_{1/2}$ is 5.4h.

Practical points

♣ Doses

62.5mg PO bd for 4 weeks (initiation), followed by 125mg PO bd indefinitely

Doses above 125mg bd do not appear to confer sufficient benefit to offset risk of hepatic injury

☺ *Common side effects*

(>10%): headache

(1–10%): flushing, abnormal LFTs, anaemia, leg oedema (all appear dose related); upper respiratory tract infections/nasopharyngitis; weakness; dizziness; hypotension; palpitations

Interactions

Co-administration with CYP3A4 (e.g. atazanavir, ciclosporin, clarithromycin, indinavir, itraconazole, ketoconazole, nefazodone, nelfinavir, ritonavir, saquinavir, telithromycin) or CYP2C19 inhibitors (e.g. omeprazole) increase serum levels and is not recommended. CYP3A and 2C19 inducers (e.g. rifampicin) may increase metabolism and therefore decrease serum levels.

Bosentan may also reduce the efficacy of OCP or statins when given concomitantly. Clinically significant changes in INR do not appear to occur when co-administrated with warfarin.

Hepatotoxicity (liver transaminases) increases with concomitant administration of glybenclamide (glyburide). Ciclosporin A increases the plasma concentrations of bosentan approximately 20-fold.

Cautions/notes

As a class, endothelin receptor antagonists have the potential for liver injury and teratogenicity.

Bosentan should be generally avoided in patients with moderate to severe hepatic impairment. However, many patients with PAH have mild hepatic impairment and it may still be appropriate to try bosentan with caution under specialist supervision.

Dose-dependent elevation of LFTs (alanine aminotransferase and/or aspartate aminotransferase) occurs both early and late during administration, usually progresses slowly, and mostly occurs asymptomatically. There have been rare reports of unexplained liver cirrhosis and liver failure. Therefore, LFTs should be checked prior to administration and monitored monthly. Bosentan should be discontinued with increases in bilirubin levels ≥2× the upper limit.

Dose-related decrease in haemoglobin, predominantly within the 1st few weeks; so Hb levels should be checked 1 and 3 months after commencement and every 3 months thereafter.

Endothelin antagonists as a class may cause testicular atrophy and male infertility. Hormonal methods of birth control may be less effective with concurrent administration of bosentan.

Pregnancy and lactation

Bosentan is expected to cause fetal harm and not recommended in pregnancy and breastfeeding (pregnancy category X). Pregnancy should be excluded before treatment with bosentan and advice regarding contraception sought. A monthly pregnancy test should be performed in women with child-bearing potential.

Contraindications
- Documented hypersensitivity
- Moderate to severe hepatic impairment
- Elevated baseline levels of hepatic aminotransferases (>3× upper limit)
- Concomitant use of ciclosporin or glibenclamide
- Pregnancy; child-bearing age not using reliable contraception

References

1 Channick RN et al. (2001). Effects of the dual endothelin-receptor antagonist bosentan in patients with pulmonary hypertension: a randomised placebo-controlled study. Lancet 358:1119–23.
2 Rubin LJ et al. (2002). Trial bosentan therapy for pulmonary arterial hypertension. (BREATHE-1 Study). N Engl J Med 346:896–903.
3 McLaughlin VV et al. (2005). Survival with first-line bosentan in patients with primary pulmonary hypertension. Eur Respir J 25:244–9.
4 Provencher S et al. (2006). Long-term outcome with first-line bosentan therapy in idiopathic pulmonary arterial hypertension. Eur Heart J 27:589–95.

Bumetanide

(See also 📖 Loop diuretics, p.507)
Potent loop diuretic (PO, IV, IM).

CV indications

(See 📖 Loop diuretics, p.507)
(Not licensed for BP control)

Others: see 📖 Loop diuretics, p.507

Mechanism of action

(See 📖 Loop diuretics, p.507)

Pharmacodynamics

In comparison to furosemide, bumetanide has been shown to be equipotent at $1/40^{th}$ molar dose with a similar pattern of water and electrolyte excretion.[1] The onset of diuresis following PO administration is 30–60min, with peak effect occurring within the 1–2h. The duration of diuretic effect is 4–8h.

Pharmacokinetics

Well absorbed with an oral bioavailability of ≈80–90%. It is ≈95% protein bound, undergoes urinary and hepatic metabolism (by P450 pathways), and is excreted predominantly in urine 45% unchanged. Elimination $t_{\frac{1}{2}}$ is 2–3.5h.

Practical points

🔹 Doses

PO: 0.5–2mg od or bd. 5mg od in severe cases and increased by 5mg every 12–24h according to response.
IV: 1–2mg repeated after 20min (or as infusion: 2–5mg over 30–60min) to a maximum of 10mg daily.
IM: 1mg initially and adjusted according to response.

Dosing may be sufficient at lower levels in the elderly and should be adjusted according to response.

🙂 Common side effects

(See 📖 Loop diuretics, p.507)
Severe, generalized musculoskeletal pain sometimes associated with muscle spasm, occurring 1–2h after administration and lasting up to 12h can occur with high doses in severe chronic renal failure. The lowest reported dose causing this type reaction was 5mg by IV. All patients recovered fully and there was no deterioration in their renal function.

Interactions (see 📖 Loop diuretics, p.507)

Cautions/notes

(See 📖 Loop diuretics, p.507)
Excessively rapid mobilization of oedema, particularly in elderly patients, may give rise to sudden changes in CV pressure–flow relationships with

circulatory collapse. This should be borne in mind when bumetanide is given in high doses intravenously or orally.

Pregnancy and lactation

No teratogenic effects have been seen in animal species but precaution of avoidance in 1st trimester should be observed (pregnancy category C). It is not known whether bumetanide is excreted in breast milk so should either be avoided or used with caution when absolutely necessary.

Contraindications

(See 📖 Loop diuretics, p.507)
• Breastfeeding

Reference

1 Sagar S *et al.* (1984). A comparative randomized double-blind clinical trial of bumetanide and furosemide in congestive cardiac failure and other edema states. *Int J Clin Pharmacol, Ther, Toxicol* **22**(9):473–8.

Calcium-channel blockers

See also 📖 Amlodipine, p.352
📖 Felodipine, p.458
📖 Lercanidipine, p.501
📖 Nifedipine, p.535
📖 Diltiazem, p.425
📖 Verapamil, p.628

There are 3 main classes of CCBs:

1. dihydropyridines, e.g. amlodipine, felodipine, lercanidipine, nifedipine
2. benzothiazepines, e.g. diltiazem
3. phenylalkylamines, e.g. verapamil.

CV indications

(See 📖 individual drugs for specific indications)
1. Essential hypertension
2. Symptomatic treatment of chronic stable angina pectoris and vasospastic angina (Prinzmetal's variant angina)
3. Cardiac arrhythmias (diltiazem and verapamil)

Mechanism of action

CCBs selectively inhibit the entry of Ca^{2+} into the cell through the voltage-gated L-type Ca^{2+} channels located in the cell membrane of vascular smooth muscle, cardiac SA and AV nodes, and cardiomyocytes. These channels are closed at resting membrane potentials but after membrane depolarization they activate-open and allow the influx of Ca^{2+} ions into the cell. By blocking L-type Ca^{2+} channels in vascular smooth muscle cells, CCBs produce arteriolar vasodilatation and decrease peripheral vascular resistance and BP. In addition, CCBs decrease vascular tone and suppress arterial vasospasms. Ca^{2+} influx through L-type calcium channels contributes to phase 0 depolarization in SA and AV nodal cells, and determines the conduction velocity and refractoriness in the AV node; Ca^{2+} entry during the plateau phase of the cardiac action potential is responsible for the excitation–contraction coupling of the cardiomyocytes via the release of Ca^{2+} ions from the sarcoplasmic reticulum. CCBs can also have negative chronotropic, dromotropic (especially at the AV node), and inotropic effects. However, the decrease in BP caused by these agents produces a sympathetic-mediated reflex response characterized by an increase in heart rate (4–6bpm) and contractility. Different CCBs have different effects on the conduction system and BP responses. Thus, the net effect on the CV system depends on the type of CCB used. CCBs do not alter excitability and conduction velocity in atrial or ventricular muscle or Purkinje fibres that generate Na^+-dependent action potentials.

Dihydropyridines exert a greater inhibitory effect on vascular smooth muscle than on cardiac muscle (vascular selectivity). Thus, they do not cause significant changes in heart rate and contractility or AV conduction (PR, PQ, and HV intervals). However, they produce cardiodepressant effects in patients treated with β-adrenergic blockers and those with myocardial diseases.

Diltiazem and verapamil decrease the sinus rate, reduce cardiac contractility, prolong the effective refractory period, and slow conduction through the AV node in a rate-related manner. Thus, they prolong the PR interval of the ECG. This rate-dependent effect on the AV node is the basis for their use to stop nodal reentry tachycardias and to control the ventricular rate in patients with AF/atrial flutter. Therefore, verapamil and diltiazem, but not the dihydropyridines, are classified as Vaughan Williams class IV antiarrhythmic agents (see Table 4.1, p.115). However, verapamil and diltiazem may shorten the antegrade effective refractory period of the accessory bypass tract accelerating the ventricular frequency in patients with AF/atrial flutter and a coexisting WPW syndrome.

Angina: CCBs reduce peripheral resistance (afterload) and myocardial O_2 demand (MVO_2) and cause coronary vasodilatation increasing coronary O_2 supply. In addition, verapamil and diltiazem decrease heart rate and cardiac contractility, which further reduces MVO_2. CCBs also reduce the vascular coronary tone and inhibit coronary vasospasms. These effects are the basis for the use of CCBs in patients with chronic stable angina and those with vasospastic angina pectoris. There is evidence that some CCBs appear beneficial in slowing the progression of carotid hypertrophy and atherosclerosis.[1]

Pharmacodynamics
(See 📖 individual drugs)
CCBs differ in their relative specificity for cardiac and vascular L-type calcium channels. For instance, dihydropyridines have high selectivity for vascular channels, with amlodipine and nifedipine having ~10-fold; felodipine and nicardipine ~100-fold; and lercanidipine ~1000-fold greater vascular selectivity compared to verapamil. By comparison, verapamil is relatively selective for cardiac tissue whilst diltiazem has intermediate selectivity (~7-fold) for vascular calcium channels.

Hypertension: the reduction in BP is correlated with the height of pretreatment elevation (no change is observed in normotensive individuals), but independent from Na^+ intake. CCBs provide a slightly better protection against stroke, but they show a reduced ability, as compared with conventional therapy, to protect against the incidence of HF. Dihydropyridines are recommended in isolated systolic hypertension (elderly) and in patients with LVH, angina pectoris, carotid/coronary atherosclerosis, and pregnancy, and in black hypertensives; verapamil and diltiazem are recommended also in patients with SVTs.[1] In diabetic patients, CCBs can improve the outcome.[2]

Antianginal effects: CCBs reduce the frequency of angina attacks and improve ETT (symptom-limited ETT time, time to moderate angina, and time to 1mm ST depression).

Renal effects: CCBs decrease afferent arteriolar resistance and increase renal blood flow, while GFR remains unchanged. Mild diuresis, natriuresis, and kaliuresis are observed during the 1st week of therapy.

Pharmacokinetics
(See 📖 individual drugs)

CCBs are extensively metabolized in the liver via the CYP3A4 and the metabolites are eliminated in the urine. The AUC of CCBs increases with age and in patients with hepatic disease (the clearance is reduced); however, renal insufficiency does not alter the pharmacokinetics.

Practical points

◦♪ Doses
(See 📖 individual drugs)
Due to the marked differences among the different preparations of each drug, patients may require different doses.

☺ Side effects
(1–10%): somnolence, dizziness, headache, fatigue; palpitations, flushing (especially on initiation of treatment); abdominal pain, nausea, dyspepsia; peripheral oedema (due to precapillary vasodilatation).

Cardiovascular: bradycardia, hypotension, tachycardia, postural hypotension, nasal congestion.

Others: lightheadedness, giddiness, weakness, gingivitis, and gum hyperplasia.

Interactions

CCBs administered concomitantly with other antihypertensive agents, vasodilators (nitrates), phenothiazines, or alcohol, have an additive effect on lowering BP.

Due to its metabolism by CYP3A4, efficacy of dihydropyridine CCBs may be reduced by CYP3A4 inducers (e.g. carbamazepine, phenytoin, rifampicin), and increased by inhibitors (ketoconazole, itraconazole, ritonavir, erythromycin, fluoxetine, valproic acid, cimetidine, other CCBs, HIV protease inhibitors, grapefruit juice). Therefore, caution is advised when administered concomitantly with such drugs.

Conversely, concomitant administration of CCBs with other drugs metabolized by CYP3A4 leads to an increase of their plasma levels (ciclosporin, tacrolimus, ketoconazole, carbamazepine, sildenafil); thus, the doses of these drugs may need to be reduced when given with a CCB. Ciclosporin plasma levels should be closely monitored.

Co-administration of β-blockers with dihydropyridine CCBs is usually well tolerated in patients with hypertension or angina, even when the combination may increase the likelihood of congestive HF, severe hypotension, bradycardia, or AV block. The risk of cardiodepressant effects markedly increases with the combination of β-blockers with verapamil or diltiazem.

CCBs potentiate the depression of cardiac contractility, conduction and automaticity and the vasodilatation produced by general anaesthetics.

Cautions/notes

CCBs are eliminated via hepatic metabolism. Therefore, in patients with impaired renal or hepatic function, and elderly patients, dosage should commence at the lower level and be increased slowly.

Pregnancy and lactation
(See 📖 individual drugs)
Some CCBs produce teratogenic findings in animals. There are no well-controlled studies in pregnant women and thus they should be used during pregnancy only if the potential benefit justifies the potential risk to the fetus (pregnancy category C). In general, CCBs are not recommended during pregnancy and breastfeeding.

Contraindications
(See 📖 individual drugs)
● Cardiogenic shock, UA, severe AS, obstructive cardiomyopathy, severe hypotension, HF, AMI
● Pregnancy and lactation; women of childbearing potential unless effective contraception is used

References

1 Mancia G *et al.* (2007). 2007 Guidelines for the management of arterial hypertension: The Task Force for the Management of Arterial Hypertension of the European Society of Hypertension (ESH) and of the European Society of Cardiology (ESC). *Eur Heart J* **28**:1462–536.
2 Hansson L *et al.* (1998). Effects of intensive blood-pressure lowering and low-dose aspirin in patients with hypertension: principal results of the Hypertension Optimal Treatment (HOT) randomised trial. HOT Study Group. *Lancet* **351**:1755–62.

Candesartan cilexetil

(See also 📖 Angiotensin II (AT$_1$) receptor blockers, p.359)

Angiotensin receptor blocker (prodrug).

Indications

(See 📖 Angiotensin II (AT$_1$) receptor blockers, p.359)
1. Treatment of essential hypertension
2. Treatment of HF (NYHA class II–IV) in patients with LV systolic dysfunction (ejection fraction ≤ 40%) as add-on therapy or when ACEIs are not tolerated

Mechanism of action

(See also 📖 Renin–angiotensin–aldosterone system inhibitors, p.568 and 📖 Angiotensin II (AT$_1$) receptor blockers, p.359)

Pharmacodynamics

(See also 📖 Renin–angiotensin–aldosterone system inhibitors, p.568 and 📖 Angiotensin II (AT$_1$) receptor blockers, p.359)

Hypertension and prehypertension

RR ≈15.6% in 1° endpoint development of clinical hypertension at 4 years in patients with pre-hypertension (BP 130–139/<89mmHg or ≤139/85–89mmHg) treated with candesartan 16mg od for 2 years compared with placebo.[1] Clinical hypertension was defined in this study as an average clinic SBP ≥140 and/or DBP ≥90mmHg at 3 visits during the 4 years of the study, an average clinic BP ≥160/100mmHg at any visit, finding of target organ damage or need for pharmacological treatment; or mean clinic BP >140/90mmHg at 48 months. Consequently, prevention of hypertension may have been overestimated and reflected greater masking.

RRR 27.8% in the risk of non-fatal strokes (7.4 vs. 10.3 events per 1000 patient-years), but not of all stroke, and RRR 10.9% in combined 1° outcome (CV death, non-fatal CVA and non-fatal MI) in hypertensive patients (70–79 years) treated with candesartan (titrated to 32mg od with additional open-labelled antihypertenisves as required) for 3.7 years as compared to placebo.[2] However, there were no differences in MI, CV mortality, or in the cognitive function measured by the Mini Mental State Examination (MMSE) scores. BP reductions in the study were greater in the candesartan compared to placebo group (mean difference in adjusted BP 3.2/1.6mmHg).

RRR 42% (7.2 vs. 12.5/1000 patient-years) in fatal/non-fatal strokes in patients with isolated systolic hypertension treated with candesartan as compared to placebo, despite little difference in BP reduction (2/1mmHg).[3] There were no differences between groups in other CV endpoints or all-cause mortality.

Diabetic nephropathy: reduction of DBP (9.5mmHg) and urinary creatinine:albumin ratio (UCAR, 30%) in hypertensive patients with micro-albuminuria and type 2 diabetes treated with candesartan 16mg od at 12 weeks and comparable to lisinopril 20mg od.[4] Reductions in DBP and

UCAR were greater in this study with combination of candesartan and lisinopril compared with monotherapy.

Heart failure: adjusted HR ≈0.90 (absolute rate 23% vs. 25%) of death in patients with HF (class II–IV) with LVEF <40% treated with candesartan (target dose of 32mg od) and followed up for 37.7 months compared with placebo.[5] RRR 22% in new-onset diabetes and RRR 23.4% in non-fatal MI. Fewer CV deaths (unadjusted HR 0.87) and hospital admissions (20% vs. 24%) in the candesartan group. There was no significant heterogeneity for candesartan results across the component trials.

HR ≈0.85 (absolute rate 38% vs. 42%) of combined endpoint of CV death or HF hospitalization in patients with NYHA II–IV and LVEF <40% taking ACEIs treated with candesartan (target dose of 32mg od) for 41 months compared with placebo.[6] Candesartan reduced each of the components of the 1° outcome significantly, as well as the total number of hospital admissions for chronic HF.

Adjusted HR 0.70 (absolute rate 33% vs. 40%) in CV death or hospitalizations for chronic HF in patients with symptomatic chronic HF and intolerance to ACEIs treated with candesartan (target dose of 32mg od) for 33.6 months compared with placebo.[7] Each component of the 1° outcome was reduced, as was the total number of hospital admissions for chronic HF.

Adjusted HR 0.86 RRR 11% (absolute rate 22% vs. 24.3%) in cardiovascular death or admission to hospital for chronic HF in patients with preserved systolic function and class II–IV HF and LVEF >40% treated with candesartan (target dose of 32mg od) for 36.6 months.[8] CV death did not differ between groups, but fewer patients were hospitalized for chronic HF in the candesartan group.

Diabetes: in hypertensive patients, candesartan (alone or in combination with felodipine) was associated after 1 year with less new-onset diabetes (0.5% vs. 4.1%) and lower fasting levels of both serum insulin and plasma glucose than hydrochlorothiazide (HCTZ, alone or in combination with atenolol).[9] The ratio LDL-C/HDL-C was reduced in the candesartan group and increased in the HCTZ group; a minor increase in plasma triglycerides levels was observed with candesartan and a larger increase with HCTZ.

Pharmacokinetics

Following oral administration, candesartan cilexetil is converted to the active metabolite candesartan. The absolute bioavailability of candesartan is ≈14% and is not significantly affected by food. Serum concentrations peak at 3–4h and increase linearly with increasing doses in the therapeutic dose range. Candesartan is highly bound to plasma protein (>99%) with an apparent V_d of 0.1L/kg. Candesartan is mainly eliminated unchanged via urine (33%), bile (77%), and to a minor extent by hepatic metabolism. Renal elimination of candesartan is both by glomerular filtration and active tubular secretion. The terminal $t_{1/2}$ is ≈9h. Candesartan is not removed by dialysis.

Practical points

.5 *Doses*

Initial dose: 4mg od (for HF)–8mg od (for hypertension) (increased to maximum of 32mg od).

A reduced initial dose of 2mg od should be used in hepatic impairment and 4–6mg od in renal impairment.

☻ *Side effects*

(See 📖 Angiotensin II (AT$_1$) receptor blockers, p.359)
(1–10%): chest infections; vertigo; headache.

Interactions (see 📖 Angiotensin II (AT$_1$) receptor blockers, p.359)

Cautions (see 📖 Angiotensin II (AT$_1$) receptor blockers, p.359)

Pregnancy and lactation (see 📖 Angiotensin II (AT$_1$) receptor blockers, p.359)

Contraindications (see 📖 Angiotensin II (AT$_1$) receptor blockers, p.359)

References

1 Julius S et al.; Trial of Preventing Hypertension (TROPHY) Study Investigators. Feasibility of treating prehypertension with an angiotensin-receptor blocker. *N Engl J Med* **354**:1685–97.
2 Lithell H et al.; SCOPE Study Group (2003). The Study on Cognition and Prognosis in the Elderly (SCOPE): principal results of a randomized double-blind intervention trial. *J Hypertens* **21**: 875–86.
3 Papademetriou V et al.; Study on Cognition and Prognosis in the Elderly study group (2004). Stroke prevention with the angiotensin II type 1-receptor blocker candesartan in elderly patients with isolated systolic hypertension: the Study on Cognition and Prognosis in the Elderly (SCOPE). *J Am Coll Cardiol* **44**:1175–80.
4 Mogensen CE et al. (2000). Randomised controlled trial of dual blockade of renin-angiotensin system in patients with hypertension, microalbuminuria, and non-insulin dependent diabetes: the candesartan and lisinopril microalbuminuria (CALM) study. *BMJ* **321**:1440–4.
5 Pfeffer MA et al.; CHARM Investigators and Committees on mortality and morbidity in patients with chronic heart failure: the CHARM-Overall programme. *Lancet* **362**:759–66.
6 McMurray JJ et al.; CHARM Investigators and Committees (2003). Effects of candesartan in patients with chronic heart failure and reduced left-ventricular systolic function taking angiotensin-converting-enzyme inhibitors: the CHARM-Added trial. *Lancet* **362**:767–71.
7 Granger CB et al; CHARM Investigators and Committees (2003). Effects of candesartan in patients with chronic heart failure and reduced left-ventricular systolic function intolerant to angiotensin-converting-enzyme inhibitors: the CHARM-Alternative trial. *Lancet* **362**:772–6.
8 Yusuf S et al.; CHARM Investigators and Committees (2003). Effects of candesartan in patients with chronic heart failure and preserved left-ventricular ejection fraction: the CHARM-Preserved Trial. *Lancet* **362**:777–81.
9 Lindholm LH et al. (2003). Metabolic outcome during 1 year in newly detected hypertensives: results of the Antihypertensive Treatment and Lipid Profile in a North of Sweden Efficacy Evaluation (ALPINE study). *J Hypertens* **21**:1563–74.

Captopril

(See also 📖 Angiotensin-converting enzyme inhibitors, p.355)

Orally active ACEI.

Indications

(See 📖 Angiotensin-converting enzyme inhibitors, p.355)

Mechanism of action

(See also 📖 Angiotensin-converting enzyme inhibitors, p.355)

Pharmacodynamics

(See also 📖 Renin–angiotensin–aldosterone system inhibitors, p.568 and 📖 Angiotensin-converting enzyme inhibitors, p.355)

AMI and HF: RRR ≈7% (absolute rate 7.2% vs 7.7%) in death in patients given captopril (6.25mg titrated to 50mg bd) for 1 month within 24h of AMI compared with placebo.[1]

RRR ≈19% (absolute rate 20% vs 25%) in all-cause mortality, RRR ≈37% of development of severe HF and RRR ≈25% of recurrent MI in patients with 3–14 days post-MI with LVEF <40% without overt HF given captopril (titrated to 12.5–25mg tds as inpatient to 50mg tds as long term) for ≈42 months compared with placebo.[2]

Hypertension: no difference in 1° composite endpoint of fatal and non-fatal MI, stroke, and other CV deaths in hypertensive patients treated with captopril 50mg (in 1 or 2 doses daily) compared conventional antihypertensive agents (diuretics, β-blockers, or both).[3] Interpretation of data from this trial including the finding of increased risk of stroke with captopril is complicated by differences in baseline and treated BPs in the 2 groups; and by dosing regimen for captopril.

Diabetes: BP lowering to <150/85mmHg with captopril has been shown to be similar to atenolol and associated with similar reductions in macro- (44% reductions in stroke) and microvascular (37% reduction, predominantly in photocoagulation) endpoints compared with placebo.[4]

Pharmacokinetics

Rapidly absorbed by oral route, reaching peak plasma levels within 1–1.5h. **Food reduces absorption (33%), so it should be administered orally 1h before meals**. Approximately 25–30% protein bound. Elimination $t_{1/2}$ is ≈2–3h with 95% excreted in urine (40–50% unchanged and remainder as inactive metabolites). Effects on BP appear within 30min, with a peak effect in 1–2h and duration of 8–12h.

Practical points

💊 Doses

(See 📖 Angiotensin-converting enzyme inhibitors for initiation under supervision, p.562)

Hypertension: 12.5–50mg bd on an empty stomach

Heart failure: 6.25–12.5mg bd or tds (titrated up to daily maximum of 150mg based on responses) under close medical supervision

Post-MI: 6.25mg test dose (followed by 12.5mg tds for 2 days and then 25mg tds) from 3 days in stable post-MI and titrated over several weeks to a daily dose of 75–150mg

Diabetic nephropathy: 75–100mg daily in divided doses.

Due to potential accumulation in renal impairment, dose should be reduced accordingly (Table 6)

Table 6 Recommended doses of captopril according to creatinine clearance

Creatinine clearance	Starting dose	Maximum daily dose
>40mL/min/1.73m^2	25–50mg	150mg
21–40mL/min/1.73m^2	25mg	100mg
10–20mL/min/1.73m^2	12.5mg	75mg
10mL/min/1.73m^2	6.25mg	37.5mg

☺ **Side effects**
(See 📖 Angiotensin-converting enzyme inhibitors, p.355)
Neutropenia especially in collagen vascular renal disease; proteinuria, skin reactions (4–10%)

Interactions (see 📖 Angiotensin-converting enzyme inhibitors, p.355)

Cautions
(See 📖 Angiotensin-converting enzyme inhibitors, p.355)
Monitor neutrophil counts in patients with pre-existing collagen vascular disease.

Co-administration with allopurinol may increase the risk of hypersensitivity reactions (Stevens–Johnson syndrome, skin eruptions, anaphylaxis, fever and arthralgias).

Pregnancy and lactation (See 📖 Angiotensin-converting enzyme inhibitors, p.355)

Contraindications
(See 📖 Angiotensin-converting enzyme inhibitors, p.355)
• Immune-based vascular renal disease
• Pre-existent neutropenia

References

1 ISIS-4 (Fourth International Study of Infarct Survival) Collaborative Group (1995). ISIS-4: a randomised factorial trial assessing early oral captopril, oral mononitrate, and intravenous magnesium sulphate in 58,050 patients with suspected acute myocardial infarction. *Lancet* **345**:669–85.
2 Pfeffer MA *et al.* (1992). Effect of captopril on mortality and morbidity in patients with left ventricular dysfunction after myocardial infarction. Results of the survival and ventricular enlargement trial. The SAVE Investigators. *N Engl J Med* **327**:669–77.
3 Hansson L *et al.* (1999). Effect of angiotensin-converting-enzyme inhibition compared with conventional therapy on cardiovascular morbidity and mortality in hypertension: the Captopril Prevention Project (CAPPP) randomised trial. *Lancet* **353**:611–16.
4 UKPDS 38 (1998). Tight blood pressure control and risk of macrovascular and microvascular complications in type 2 diabetes: UKPDS 38. UK Prospective Diabetes Study Group. *BMJ* **317**:703–13.

Carvedilol

(See also 📖 β-blockers, p.376)

Non-selective, lipid-soluble β-adrenergic receptor antagonist with α-antagonism and antioxidant properties.

CV indications

(See 📖 β-blockers, p.376)

Mechanism of action

(See 📖 β-blockers, p.376)

Pharmacodynamics

(See 📖 β-blockers, p.376)

Heart failure: RRR ≈35% (absolute rate: 12.8% vs. 19.7%) in all-cause mortality in patients with severe, stable CHF (mean LVEF <25%) treated with carvedilol (target dose: 25mg bd) compared with placebo and followed up for a mean of 10.4 months.[1] Rates of hospitalization and worsening heart failure were also reduced with carvedilol compared with placebo (absolute values 425 vs. 507).

RRR ≈17% (absolute rate: 34% vs. 40%) in all-cause mortality in patients with HF (NYHA class II–IV, LVEF 26%) treated with carvedilol (target dose 25mg bd) compared to metoprolol tartrate-IR, target dose 50mg bd).[2] The reduction of all-cause mortality was consistent across predefined subgroups.

Pharmacokinetics

Bioavailability of carvedilol is ≈25% following PO administration, with peak plasma levels occurring at ≈1–3h. Carvedilol is 98–99% plasma protein bound and has V_d ≈2L/kg. Elimination is mainly biliary with excretion in faeces (16% in urine). Its $t_{1/2}$ is ≈6–10h. Due to significant 1st-pass hepatic metabolism (CYP2D6, CYP2C9), bioavailability may be up to 4× higher in hepatic impairment. Plasma levels appear ≈50% higher in the elderly.

Practical points

💊 Doses

Heart failure: 3.125mg bd (uptitrated by doubling at intervals of 2 weeks to the highest tolerated dose and a maximum of 25mg bd). Monitor for hypotension (systolic <100mmHg), worsening renal function, or HF before dose increase. If transient worsening of HF, treat by adjusting diuretic, ACEIs (ARBs), or temporarily stop carvedilol.

Hypertension and angina: 12.5mg od (increase after 2 days to 25mg od up to a maximum of 50mg od or in divided doses).

In general there is no dose adjustment in the elderly or those with renal impairment.

☺ *Side effects* (see 📖 β-blockers, p.376)

Interactions

(See 📖 β-blockers, p.376)

Carvedilol may prolong AV conduction time when given with digoxin and increase trough levels of digoxin by 16% in hypertensive patients. Thus, monitoring of digoxin levels is recommended when initiating or adjusting carvedilol doses.

Care may be required in those concomitantly receiving inducers (e.g. rifampicin, which may decrease serum levels of carvedilol) or inhibitors (e.g. cimetidine, which may increase carvedilol levels) of mixed function oxidases.

Modest increases in trough ciclosporin levels have been seen in renal transplant patients with approximately 20% requiring ≈30% reduction in dosage.

Cautions/notes

(See 📖 β-blockers, p.376)

Monitor renal function in HF patients with hypotension, CHD, diffuse vascular disease, or underlying renal insufficiency as renal function may deteriorate and is reversible with stopping or dose reduction.

Pregnancy and lactation

Inadequate data in pregnant women. However, carvedilol has been shown to cross the placental barrier and so should not be used in pregnancy unless clearly necessary (pregnancy category C). Although it is not known if it is excreted in human milk, carvedilol has been demonstrated in animal breast milk and so is not recommended during breastfeeding.

Contraindications (see 📖 β-blockers, p.376)

References

1 Packer M *et al.*; Carvedilol Prospective Randomized Cumulative Survival Study Group (2001). Effect of carvedilol on survival in severe chronic heart failure. *N Engl J Med* **344**:1651–8.
2 Poole-Wilson PA *et al.*; Carvedilol Or Metoprolol European Trial Investigators (2003). Comparison of carvedilol and metoprolol on clinical outcomes in patients with chronic heart failure in the Carvedilol Or Metoprolol European Trial (COMET): randomised controlled trial. *Lancet* **362**:7–13.

Chlortalidone

(See also 📖 Thiazide and related diuretics, p.604)

Oral thiazide diuretic.

CV and other indications

(See 📖 Thiazide and related diuretics, p.604)
1. HF
2. Oedema due to nephrotic syndrome
3. Ascites due to cirrhosis

Mechanism of action

(See 📖 Thiazide and related diuretics, p.604)

Pharmacodynamics

Office SBP is reduced by ≈17mmHg and mean ambulatory 24h SBP by ≈12mmHg with chlortalidone 25mg od after 8 weeks in hypertensive patients (mean baseline BP=145/96mmHg).[1] In a number of large clinical trials, BP reduction with chlortalidone (12.5–25mg od) has been shown to reduce stroke, CV endpoints, as well as all-cause mortality, but at the cost of increased diabetes and hypokalaemia.[2–5] It is also possible that the reduction of risk of HF may be greater with chlortalidone compared with the ACEI lisinopril or the CCB amlodipine.[6]

RRR 36% of stroke compared to placebo, RRR 13% of all-cause mortality and RRR 27% for the 2° endpoint (non-fatal MI plus coronary death) in elderly patients (mean age=72 years; mean baseline BP=170/77mmHg) with chlortalidone 25mg od after a mean of 4.5 years.[2] The 6-year rate of composite endpoint of fatal CHD and non-fatal MI is ≈11.6% in hypertensive patients with one additional CV risk factor treated with chlortalidone 12.5–25mg (not significantly different from amlodipine 2.5–10mg od or lisinopril 10–40mg od).[3]

Causes a greater loss of K^+ than equivalent doses of HCTZ.

Pharmacokinetics

Oral bioavailability is ≈65%. Following absorption, chlortalidone is ≈98% bound to erythrocytes, where it binds carbonic anhydrase, and plasma proteins and its V_d is 0.14L/kg. It has a long $t_{1/2}$ of ≈40–60h and is excreted unchanged in the urine. The diuretic effect begins within 2.5h, concentration peaks in 3–6h, and duration of action is up to 72h.

Practical points

♣ Doses

• For hypertension: 12.5–50mg od
• For HF: 25–50mg od increased up to 100–200mg/day

☺ Side effects (see 📖 Thiazide and related diuretics, p.604)
Interactions (see 📖 Thiazide and related diuretics, p.604)
Cautions/notes (see 📖 Thiazide and related diuretics, p.604)

Pregnancy and lactation (see 📖 Thiazide and related diuretics, p.604)
Contraindications (see 📖 Thiazide and related diuretics, p.604)

References

1 Ernst ME et al. (2006). Comparative antihypertensive effects of hydrochlorothiazide and chlortha-lidone on ambulatory and office blood pressure. *Hypertension* **47**(3):352–8.

2 SHEP Cooperative Research Group (1991). Prevention of stroke by antihypertensive drug treatment in older persons with isolated systolic hypertension. Final results of the Systolic Hypertension in the Elderly Program (SHEP). *JAMA* **265**:3255–64.

3 ALLHAT Officers and Coordinators for the ALLHAT Collaborative Research Group (2002). The Antihypertensive and Lipid-Lowering Treatment to Prevent Heart Attack Trial. Major outcomes in high-risk hypertensive patients randomized to angiotensin-converting enzyme inhibitor or calcium channel blocker vs diuretic: The Antihypertensive and Lipid-Lowering Treatment to Prevent Heart Attack Trial (ALLHAT). *JAMA* **288**:2981–97.

4 The Multiple Risk Factor Intervention Trial Research Group (MRFIT) (1990). Mortality rates after 10.5 years for hypertensive participants in the Multiple Risk Factor Intervention Trial. *Circulation* **82**:1616–28.

5 Neaton JD et al. (1993). Treatment of Mild Hypertension Study. Final results. Treatment of Mild Hypertension Study Research Group. *JAMA* **270**:713–24.

6 Wright JT Jr et al. for the ALLHAT Collaborative Research Group (2009). ALLHAT Findings Revisited in the Context of Subsequent Analyses, Other Trials, and Meta-analyses. *Arch Intern Med* **169**:832–42.

Class Ia antiarrhythmic drugs

(See also 📖 Disopyramide, p.430, 📖 Procainamide, p.553, and 📖 Quinidine, p.559)

Class I antiarrhythmic agents: mechanism of action

Functional cardiac Na^+ channels result from the coassembly of the pore-forming α-subunit Nav 1.5 (encoded by the *SCN5A* gene) and accessory β-subunits. In atrial and ventricular muscle and in Purkinje fibres, the rapid upstroke (phase 0) of the action potential is due to the activation (opening) of the sodium channels generating the fast inward Na^+ current, which determines cellular excitability, conduction velocity of the cardiac action potential, and the QRS complex of the ECG. Na^+ channels open transiently, for 1–3ms, upon membrane depolarization but then rapidly inactivate and remain closed during the plateau phase of the action potential. At the end of repolarization, Na^+ channels change from the inactivated to the resting state, a process called reactivation. Once in the resting state, the channel can re-open.

Class I antiarrhythmic drugs inhibit Na^+ entry, decreasing the slope of phase 0 and amplitude of the fast cardiac action potentials generated in non-nodal cardiomyocytes (widening the QRS complex). This results in a reduction in excitability and conduction block suppressing re-entrant rhythms that depend on unidirectional or conduction pathways operating at a low margin of safety. Class I agents have a high affinity for both activated and inactivated channels (the latter predominates in ischaemic-depolarized cardiac tissue) and prolong the reactivation of the channel thus affecting cardiac refractoriness independently of changes in APD. The effect of class I drugs increases at fast driving rates (increase the time the channel spends in the active/inactive state) and in depolarized (ischaemic) cardiac tissues because the depolarization of the resting membrane potential inactivates the Na^+ channels. According to the prolongation of channel reactivation, class I antiarrhythmics can be subclassified into 3 subgroups: Ia (reactivation time prolonged 1–4s), Ib (300–500ms), and Ic (>5s).

In Purkinje fibres, class I drugs reduce the slope of phase-4 depolarization and shift the threshold voltage to less negative values; these effects reduce the automaticity of cardiac ectopic pacemakers (mainly in the His–Purkinje system). They also raise the fibrillation thresholds of the atria and ventricles. Class Ia drugs prolong the APD (and QT interval) due to the blockade of several K^+ currents; they can also block the L-type Ca^{2+} current and thus decrease cardiac contractility. In contrast, class Ic drugs shorten the APD due to the blockade of the late Na^+ currents.

However, class I antiarrhythmic agents can paradoxically facilitate the appearance of severe (and sometimes lethal) reentrant arrhythmias by two main mechanisms: slowing intracardiac conduction; and by producing an inhomogeneous prolongation of the APD. The risk of proarrhythmia increases in patients with structural heart disease (CAD, LVH, CCF).

Clopidogrel

A selective ADP receptor antagonist of the thienopyridine family.

CV indications

Prevention of atherothrombotic events in patients with:
1. recent MI, recent ischaemic stroke, or established PAD
2. acute coronary syndromes (UA, NSTEMI, or STEMI)

Mechanism of action

Platelets release adenosine diphosphate (ADP), a pro-aggregatory agonist. The binding of ADP to its G_i-coupled $P2Y_{12}$ receptor leads to the inhibition of adenylyl cyclase and lowers the platelet cAMP levels. This inhibits the cAMP-mediated phosphorylation of vasodilator-stimulated phosphoprotein (VASP), which is closely related to the inhibition of glyprotein IIb/IIIa receptor activation.

Clopidogrel competitively and irreversibly inhibits the platelet $P2Y_{12}$ receptor and the subsequent ADP-mediated activation of the glycoprotein GP IIb/IIIa complex, thereby inhibiting platelet aggregation. Because the inhibition is irreversible, platelets exposed to clopidogrel are affected for their lifespan (7–10 days). Clopidogrel also inhibits the platelet aggregation induced by agonists other than ADP by blocking the amplification of platelet activation by released ADP.

Pharmacodynamics

- Clopidogrel inhibits platelet aggregation (≈40–60% of ADP-induced aggregation maximally after 5–7 days) and increases bleeding times. The delayed onset of effect can be reduced by using a loading dose of 300–600mg.
- ≈20% RRR (9.3% vs 11.4%) in 1° composite (CV death, non-fatal MI, or stroke) at the end of 12 months in CV death, MI, stroke, or refractory ischaemia in patients with NSTEMI treated with clopidogrel (300mg followed by 75mg/day for 3–12 months) vs. placebo.[1] Major bleeding increase in the clopidogrel group (3.7% vs. 2.7%), but no differences were found in the rates of fatal bleeding or haemorrhagic stroke.
- 20% RR (9.3% vs 11.4%) in a composite of death from CV causes, non-fatal MI, or stroke, and 14% RR in first 1° outcome or refractory ischaemia, in patients with NSTEMI treated with clopidogrel (300mg, followed by 75mg od) or placebo in addition to aspirin for 3–12 months.[2] The percentages of patients with in-hospital refractory or severe ischaemia, HF, or revascularization procedures were also significantly lower with clopidogrel.
- 30% RR (4.5% vs. 6.4%) in CV death, MI, or urgent revascularization and 25% RR in CV death or MI 30 days and 8 months after PCI in patients with NSTEMI pretreated with clopidogrel or placebo in addition to aspirin.[3] Patients were treated for a median of 6 days before PCI and for a median of 10 days overall. After PCI, most patients in both groups received open-label thienopyridine for about 4 weeks, after which the study drug was restarted for a mean of 8 months. At follow-up, there was no significant difference in major bleeding between the groups.

- 8.7% RR (5.3% vs. 5.8% per year) in incidence of new ischaemic stroke, new MI, or vascular death in patients with recent history of MI (within 35 days), ischaemic stroke (within 6 months) with at least a week of residual neurological signs, or established PAD treated for 3 years with clopidogrel (75mg daily) as compared with aspirin (325mg daily).[4] The benefit was strongest in patients with PVD and weaker in stroke patients.
- Greater benefit can be obtained from combining clopidogrel with aspirin in patients admitted to hospitals within 24h of suspected AMI onset of symptoms. 7% RR in death from any cause and 9% RR in the risk of reinfarction, stroke, or death in patients with STEMI treated with clopidogrel (75mg/day) or placebo, in addition to aspirin (162mg/day), for 28 days or until hospital discharge, whichever came first.[5]
- 36% RR in hospital infarct-related arterial occlusion, death, or recurrent MI before angiography in patients who presented within 12h after the onset of an STEMI treated with clopidogrel (300mg loading dose, followed by 75mg daily) or placebo and a thrombolytic, aspirin, and, when appropriate, weight-adjusted heparin.[6] 20% RR of 30-day CV death, recurrent MI, or urgent revascularization. The rates of major bleeding were similar in the 2 groups.
- 46% RR in the occurrence of CV death, recurrent MI or stroke after 30 days in patients with STEMI who received fibrinolysis and then underwent PCI treated with clopidogrel (300mg, followed by 75mg/day until coronary angiography) compared with placebo.[7]
- 26.9% RR in death, MI or stroke in patients treated with clopidogrel (300mg followed by 75mg/daily for 28 days) 3–24h before PCI as compared with placebo; all patients received aspirin.[8]
- Clopidogrel therapy for 6–12 months in addition to long-term aspirin is the standard therapy in patients receiving a drug-eluting stent.[9]

Pharmacokinetics

Clopidogrel is an inactive prodrug that is rapidly absorbed after oral administration (bioavailability 30–50%), a process that is not influenced by food, reaching peak plasma levels after 45min. Clopidogrel binds to plasma proteins (97%), has a V_d of 5.3–8.5L/kg and is metabolized by CYP450 enzymes (CYP 3A4, 2C9, 1A2, and 2B6), firstly to 2-oxo-clopidogrel and then to a thiol derivative (SR 26334) that binds rapidly and irreversibly to the platelet $P2Y_{11}$ receptor, thus inhibiting platelet aggregation. Clopidogrel and its active metabolite are reversibly protein bound (98% and 94% respectively) and excreted in urine (50%) and faeces (50%). Plasma $t_{1/2} \approx$20–50h.

Clopidogrel pharmacokinetics and antiplatelet effects differ according to polymorphisms of gene coding for $P2Y_{11}$ receptor or for cytochrome CYP2C19 or CYP3A4. Patients with an impaired metabolizer status (intermediate and poor combined) have lower levels of the active metabolite of clopidogrel, less inhibition of platelets, and a higher rate of CV events (death, MI, and stroke) or stent thrombosis compared to extensive metabolizers.[10]

In CYP2 C19 poor metabolizers, a high-dose regimen (600mg loading dose followed by 150mg od) increases antiplatelet response.

Practical points

♪ Doses

ACS: loading dose 300mg, maintenance 75mg/day
Patients with STEMI: a loading dose of 300mg at least 6h before PCI or, if this is not possible, a dose of 600mg at least 2h before

After implantation of a bare-metal stent clopidogrel should be continued at 75mg/daily for 4–6 weeks; after a drug-eluting stent for 12 months.[9,11]

No dose adjustment is needed in elderly patients or patients with renal disease.

☺ Common side effects

(1–10%): bleeding; diarrhoea, abdominal pain, dyspepsia.
The absolute risk of major bleeding associated with clopidogrel is ≈1.4% (cf 1.6% with aspirin), with ≈2.0% (cf ≈2.7% with aspirin) GI bleeds and 0.7% (cf ≈1.1% with aspirin) GI bleeds requiring hospitalization.[4]

Others: fever, myalgia, arthralgia, urticaria, hypotension, agranulocytosis.

The absolute risk of major bleeding with clopidogrel from major trials[1] (in which patients at high risk of bleeding were excluded) is ≈3.7% (an increase of ≈1%) when added to aspirin (NNH ≈100 over 9 months).

Interactions

Main interactions include those relating to increased risk of bleeding with other agents. In particular, use with warfarin is not recommended due to the risk of increased intensity of bleeding. As with other antiplatelet agents, clopidogrel should be used with caution in those at risk of bleeding and in those receiving aspirin, NSAIDs, heparins, antiplatelet agents, or thrombolytics.

Drugs that inhibit CYP2 C19 (omeprazole) reduce plasma levels of the active metabolite of clopidogrel and its clinical efficacy and should be avoided.

Clopidogrel should not be given with PPIs as these agents can reduce its antiaggregant efficiency.

Cautions/notes

Due to its long $t_{1/2}$, discontinuation 5–7 days before CABG may be recommended. Co-administration with naproxen in healthy individuals has been shown to increase faecal occult blood. Hence, co-administration with NSAIDs should also be with caution.

In the elderly, plasma concentrations and $t_{1/2}$ have been shown to be prolonged but do not appear to be associated with additional differences in bleeding times or platelet aggregation; so dose adjustment is not required. Experience is limited in patients with renal and hepatic impairment.

Pregnancy and lactation

Animal studies indicate excretion of clopidogrel and its metabolites into breast milk but there is no evidence of harm in pregnancy. However, there are no clinical data and use in pregnancy is not preferable (pregnancy category B).

Contraindications

- Active pathological bleeding (e.g. intracranial haemorrhage or GI bleed)
- Severe liver impairment
- Breastfeeding

References

1 The Clopidogrel in Unstable Angina to Prevent Recurrent Events Trial Investigators (2001). Effects of clopidogrel in addition to aspirin in patients with acute coronary syndromes without ST-segment elevation. *N Engl J Med* **345**: 494–502.

2 Yusuf S *et al.*; Clopidogrel in Unstable Angina to Prevent Recurrent Events Trial Investigators (2001). Effects of clopidogrel in addition to aspirin in patients with acute coronary syndromes without ST-segment elevation. *N Engl J Med* **345**:494–502.

3 Mehta SR *et al.* for the Clopidogrel in Unstable angina to prevent Recurrent Events Trial (CURE) Investigators (2001). Effects of pretreatment with clopidogrel and aspirin followed by long-term therapy in patients undergoing percutaneous coronary intervention: the PCI-CURE study. *Lancet* **358**:527–33.

4 CAPRIE Steering Committee (1996). A randomised, blinded, trial of clopidogrel versus aspirin in patients at risk of ischaemic events (CAPRIE). *Lancet* **348**:1329–39.

5 Chen ZM *et al.*; COMMIT (ClOpidogrel and Metoprolol in Myocardial Infarction Trial) collaborative group (2005). Addition of clopidogrel to aspirin in 45,852 patients with acute myocardial infarction: randomised placebo-controlled trial. *Lancet* **366**:1607–21.

6 Sabatine MS *et al.*; CLARITY-TIMI 28 Investigators (2005). Addition of clopidogrel to aspirin and fibrinolytic therapy for myocardial infarction with ST-segment elevation. *N Engl J Med* **352**:1179–89.

7 Sabatine MS *et al.* for the Clopidogrel as Adjunctive Reperfusion Therapy (CLARITY)-Thrombolysis in Myocardial Infarction (TIMI) 28 Investigators (2005). Effect of clopidogrel pretreatment before percutaneous coronary intervention in patients with ST-elevation myocardial infarction treated with fibrinolytics: the PCI-CLARITY study. *JAMA* **294**:1224–32.

8 Steinhubl SR *et al.* for the CREDO Investigators (2006). Optimal timing for the initiation of pretreatment with 300mg clopidogrel before percutaneous coronary intervention. *J Am Coll Cardiol* **47**:939–43.

9 Silber S *et al.* (2005). Guidelines for percutaneous coronary interventions. The Task Force for Percutaneous Coronary Interventions of the European Society of Cardiology. *Eur Heart J* **26**:804–47.

10 Mega JL *et al.* (2009). Cytochrome P-450 polymorphisms and response to clopidogrel. *N Engl J Med* **360**:354–62.

11 Bassand JP *et al.* (2007). Guidelines for the diagnosis and treatment of non-ST-segment elevation acute coronary syndromes. *Eur Heart J* **28**:2–63.

Colesevelam

Oral (tablet) bile acid sequestrant.

CV indications

It is indicated as an adjunct to diet and exercise to:
1. reduce elevated LDL-C in patients with 1° hyperlipidemia (Fredrickson type IIa) as monotherapy or in combination with an HMG-CoA reductase inhibitor
2. to improve glycaemic control in adults with type 2 diabetes mellitus.

Mechanism of action

(See 📖 Colestyramine, p.410)
In type 2 diabetes, colesevelam improves glycaemic control, as reflected by a reduction in haemoglobin A_{1c}; this effect reached maximal or near-maximal effect after 12–18 weeks of treatment.

Pharmacodynamics

1° hypercholesterolaemia: 2.3–4.5g daily for 24 weeks decreases LDL-C (9–18%), total cholesterol (4–10%), and ApoB (6–12%) levels, while it increases HDL-C (3–4%) and triglycerides (up to 10%) levels.[1]

Co-administration of colesevelam and an HMG-CoA reductase inhibitor produces an additive reduction of LDL-C levels (8–16%) above that produced with the HMG-CoA reductase inhibitor alone.

Mixed hyperlipidaemia: in patients already treated with fenofibrate (160mg daily), combination therapy with colesevelam (3.75g daily) for 6 weeks reduces LDL-C (10.4%), non-HDL-C (7.5%), total cholesterol (5.9%), and ApoB (7.3% ApoB) compared to addition of placebo to fenofibrate (2.3%, 2.2%, 1.6% and 0.8% respectively).[2]

So far, no studies conducted have directly demonstrated whether monotherapy or combination therapy has any effect on morbidity or mortality.

Type 2 diabetes: colesevelam in combination with metformin, sulfonylureas, and insulin reduces haemoglobin A_{1c} (0.5%) and lipid parameters.[3]

Pharmacokinetics

Not absorbed from the GI tract

Practical points

⚡ Doses

Hyperlipidaemia: combination therapy (with statin): 4–6 tablets (2.5–3.75g) per day, either once or twice a day. Monotherapy: 6–7 tablets (3.75–4.375g) per day

Type 2 diabetes mellitus: 6 tablets od or 3 tablets tds

Colesevelam should be taken with a meal and liquid

☹ Side effects

Common: constipation, dyspepsia, nausea, asthenia, pharyngitis, raised tri-glyceride levels
Uncommon: isolated transaminase elevations, myalgia
Combination with statins did not result in any frequent unexpected adverse reactions compared to statins alone.

Interactions

(See 📖 Colestyramine, p.410)
Colesevelam has no significant effect on the bioavailability of digoxin, fenofi-brate, lovastatin, metoprolol, quinidine, valproic acid, warfarin, verapamil, and pioglitazone.

Cautions/notes

Should be taken orally with a meal and liquid. Prior to therapy, patients should be on a cholesterol-lowering diet, lipid profile performed, and 2° causes of hypercholesterolaemia excluded.

Safety and efficacy are not established for patients with triglyceride levels >3.4mmol/L, since such patients were excluded from the clinical studies.

Safety and efficacy have not been established in children/adolescents; therefore it is not recommended.

Pregnancy and lactation

There are no well-controlled studies of colesevelam in pregnant women (pregnancy category B). Colesevelam is not expected to be excreted in human milk.

Contraindications

• Hypersensitivity to the active substance or the excipients
• History of bowel or biliary obstruction
• A history of hypertriglyceridemia-induced pancreatitis
• Patients with type 1 diabetes

References

1 Insull W Jr *et al.* (2001). Effectiveness of colesevelam hydrochloride in decreasing LDL cho-lesterol in patients with primary hypercholesterolemia: a 24-week randomized controlled trial. *Mayo Clin Proc* **76**:971–82.
2 Bays HE *et al.* (2008). Colesevelam hydrochloride therapy in patients with type 2 diabetes mel-litus treated with metformin: glucose and lipid effects. *Arch Intern Med* **168**:1975–83.
3 McKenney J *et al.* (2005). Safety and efficacy of colesevelam hydrochloride in combination with fenofibrate for the treatment of mixed hyperlipidemia. *Curr Med Res Opin* **21**:1403–12.

Colestyramine

Oral bile acid sequestrant.

CV indications

1. As adjunctive therapy to dietary changes for the reduction of elevated serum cholesterol in patients with 1° hypercholesterolaemia (elevated LDL-C) who do not respond adequately to diet alone

Non-CV indications

1. Relief of pruritus associated with partial biliary obstruction and 1° biliary cirrhosis
2. Relief of diarrhoea in diabetic vagal neuropathy, ileal resection or Crohn's disease
3. Management of radiation-induced diarrhoea

Mechanism of action

Colestyramine resin adsorbs and combines with the bile acids in the intestine to form an insoluble complex that is excreted in the faeces. This results in the partial removal of bile acids from the enterohepatic circulation by preventing their reabsorption. The increased faecal loss of bile acids leads to an increased oxidation of cholesterol to form bile acids. As a result there is an overall hepatic depletion of cholesterol. This increases the expression of LDL receptors and increases activity of the HMG-CoA reductase in the hepatocytes. Both effects increase the clearance of LDL-C from the blood and decrease cholesterol and LDL-C serum levels. Serum TG levels, however, may remain unchanged or increase (if so, it may be necessary to add nicotinic acid or a fibrate to control this increase).

In partial biliary obstruction, a reduction in serum bile acid levels reduces the amount of bile acids deposited in the dermal tissue and results in a decrease in pruritus.

Pharmacodynamics

1° hypercholesterolaemia: colestyramine produces reductions in plasma total- and LDL-C levels of 8.5% and 12.6% greater than placebo, and a 19% RRR (absolute rates 7% vs. 8.6%) in definite CHD death and/or non-fatal MI, over an average of 7.4 years in middle-aged men with 1° hypercholesterolaemia as compared to placebo.[1]

In another study, after 5 years of treatment with colestyramine arteriography showed a reduction in the progression of CAD as compared with placebo (32% vs. 49%).[2]

Pharmacokinetics

Not absorbed from the digestive tract.

Practical points

🥄 Doses

Colestyramine should be taken in its dry form; mix the powder with water or other fluids before ingesting.

1° hypercholesterolaemia: initial introduction over a 3–4-week period, 2–4 sachets (8–16g) per day, either as a single daily dose or in divided doses up to 4 times daily. The maximum recommended daily dose is 24g.

To relieve pruritus: 4g or 8g daily.

To relieve diarrhoea: dose as for reduction of cholesterol, but if a response is not seen within 3 days, alternative therapy should be initiated.

☺ Side effects
Constipation (frequently disappears on continued use); large doses can cause diarrhoea. Abdominal discomfort and/or pain, flatulence, nausea, vomiting, eructation, anorexia, and steatorrhoea can all occur.

Increased bleeding tendency due to hypoprothrombinaemia associated with vitamin K deficiency (usually responds to parenteral vitamin K).

Others: skin irritation, taste disturbance.

Interactions
When administered simultaneously with colestyramine can affect the bio-availability of other drugs (warfarin, digoxin, thiazide diuretics, propranolol, tetracycline, oral contraceptives containing ethinylestradiol and norethis-terone, levothyroxine and glibenclamide). Thus, it is recommended that concurrent drugs should be taken either at least 1h before or 4–6h after colestyramine.

Bile acid sequestrants both reduce absorption of vitamin K and interfere with the effect of warfarin. Anticoagulant therapy, and the INR should be monitored.

Cautions/notes
Colestyramine may interfere with the absorption of fat-soluble vitamins. Therefore, supplementation with vitamins A, D and K during prolonged high-dose administration should be considered.

Pregnancy and lactation
Safety has not been established in pregnant women (pregnancy category C). Possibility of interference of absorption of fat-soluble vitamins should be considered. Thus, it is not recommended in pregnant and breastfeeding women.

Contraindications
- Hypersensitivity to any of its product ingredients
- Complete biliary obstruction (as colestyramine cannot be effective)

References
1 (1984). The Lipid Research Clinics Coronary Primary Prevention Trial results. I. Reduction in incidence of coronary heart disease. *JAMA* **251**:351–64.

2 Brensike JF et al. Effects of therapy with cholestyramine on progression of coronary arteriosclerosis: results of the NHLBI type II coronary intervention study. *Circulation* 1984; **69**:313–24.

Dabigatran

Dabigatran etexilate is an oral prodrug that is rapidly converted to dabigatran, a potent, direct, competitive inhibitor of thrombin.

CV indications

1. Prophylaxis of venous thromboembolic events (VTEs) in adults who have undergone elective total hip- or total knee-replacement surgery
2. Currently under investigation for stroke prophylaxis in patients with AF and in ACSs

Mechanism of action

Dabigatran is an oral reversible direct thrombin inhibitor. It binds directly to exosite 1 on thrombin, a site specific for fibrin, preventing cleavage of fibrinogen to fibrin by thrombin to block the final step of the coagulation cascade and thrombus development. Unlike heparin, dabigatran reversibly inhibits both fibrin-bound thrombin and free circulating fibrin, providing more effective thrombin inhibition than heparins (which block mainly free thrombin).

It also inhibits platelet activation induced by thrombin (the most potent stimulus for platelet activation), and activation of clotting factors V, VIII, and XI by thrombin (even small amounts of thrombin can initiate the up-regulation of these clotting factors).

Pharmacodynamics

Dabigatran has a predictable anticoagulant effect, without the need for coagulation monitoring. Ecarin clotting time (ECT) and thrombin time (TT) are very sensitive to dabigatran and show a linear correlation with its plasma concentration.

3 CTs analysed the efficacy and safety in the prevention and treatment of VTE (2 following total knee replacement, 1 following total hip replacement). Patients were randomized to dabigatran (75 or 110mg orally within 1–4h of surgery followed by 150 or 220mg daily thereafter) or enoxaparin (40mg as a SC injection 12h prior to surgery and daily thereafter).[1] Dabigatran was as effective as enoxaparin for preventing the composite of total VTE (including pulmonary embolism, proximal and distal DVT) and all-cause mortality. There were no differences in major bleeding rates or in the frequency of increase in liver enzymes between both drugs.

Dabigatran (50, 150, or 300mg tds) with or without aspirin (81 or 325mg daily) was compared with warfarin (INR 2–3) for stroke prevention in patients with AF and additional risk factors for thromboembolism (hypertension, diabetes mellitus, congestive HF or LV dysfunction, previous ischaemic stroke or TIA, or age >75 years).[2] After 12 weeks, major haemorrhages were limited to patients treated with dabigatran 300mg plus aspirin and the incidence was significant versus 300mg dabigatran alone.[2] Patients receiving dabigatran 50mg tds had a higher stroke rate than other active groups, while at 150mg tds there were no thrombotic events or changes in D-dimer.

RR 9% (*P*<0.001 for non-inferiority) and 34% (*P*<0.001 for superiority) in the annualized rates of stroke or systemic embolism (1.69% vs. 1.53% and 1.11%) in patients with AF and at least 1 non-AF stroke risk factor treated for 2 years in a blinded fashion with fixed doses of dabigatran, 110mg or 150mg bd, or, in an unblinded fashion, adjusted-dose warfarin.[3] The annualized rates of major bleeding were 3.36% on warfarin and 2.71% (*P*=0.003) and 3.36% on dabigatran 110mg and 150mg, and the rates of haemorrhagic stroke 0.38%, 0.12% (69% RR), and 0.10% (74% RR), respectively. The annualized mortality rates were 4.13% on warfarin and 3.74% and 3.64% on dabigatran 100mg and 150mg. However, the annualized MI rates were higher in the dabigatran groups than in the warfarin group (0.72% and 0.74% vs. 0.53%). Thus, in patients with AF, dabigatran 110mg is associated with similar rates of stroke and systemic embolism to warfarin, and lower rates of major haemorrhage. Dabigatran 150mg is associated with lower rates of stroke and systemic embolism than warfarin, and similar rates of major haemorrhage.

Pharmacokinetics
Dabigatran etexilate is a prodrug that is rapidly absorbed, and rapidly hydrolysed by unspecific plasma and hepatic esterases to the active form (bioavailability 6.5%), dabigatran, which reaches peak plasma concentrations within 2–3h. Absorption is unrelated to food but may be decreased with co-administration of proton pump inhibitors. Dabigatran binds to plasma proteins (25–30%) and is rapidly distributed (V_d 1L/kg). The cytochrome P450 system does not play a major role in the metabolism of dabigatran, which is a substrate of P-glycoprotein (P-gp). About 85% of the dose is excreted unchanged in urine; the remainder undergoes conjugation with glucuronic acid to active acylglucuronides which are excreted via the bile in the faeces. Its serum $t_{1/2}$ is 12–17h, and it does not require regular monitoring. Subjects with CrCl <50mL/min present prolonged excretion rates and elevated plasma concentrations of dabigatran. Dabigatran is dialysable.

Practical points
♣ Doses
Preventing VTE after orthopaedic surgery: 150mg od
Maximum dose: 300mg bd; experience in elderly is limited

😊 Common side effects
Common (in at least 3% of patients): dyspepsia, nausea, vomiting, constipation, pyrexia, wound secretion, hypotension, insomnia, peripheral oedema, anaemia, dizziness, diarrhoea, and headache. Moderate increases in ALT of more than 3× the upper limit of normal have a 2% frequency after 12 months.

Haemorrhage occurs rarely. There is less minor bleeding than with warfarin; but similar rates of major bleeding as enoxaparin.

Interactions
Concomitant use of aspirin, other platelet inhibitors, and NSAIDs significantly increases the risk of bleeding. Co-administration with pantoprazole

decreases the AUC of dabigatran by 30%. Dabigatran does not alter the metabolism of drugs that are substrates of CYP2C9 and 3A4, but concomitant use with potent P-gp inhibitors, e.g. quinidine, clarithromycin, verapamil, is contraindicated. Amiodarone (CYP 2C9, 2D6 and 3A4, and P-gp inhibitor) increases plasma concentration of dabigatran.

Cautions/notes

Caution should be exerted in elderly, patients with body weight <50kg, recent surgery, history of acute intracranial disease, haemorrhagic stroke; major surgery, trauma, uncontrolled hypertension, or MI in the past 3 months, bleeding disorders, active GI ulceration, concomitant use of drugs that increase risk of bleeding, GI or urogenital bleeding, or ulcer disease in past 6 months, bacterial endocarditis, renal impairment (avoid if CrCl is <30mL/min), severe liver disease, anaesthesia with postoperative indwelling epidural catheter (give initial dose at least 2h after catheter removal and monitor neurological signs).

Caution in patients with liver transaminases concentrations >2× the upper limit of normal or treated with NSAIDs.

Pregnancy and lactation

Animal reproductive studies have shown toxicity. Since there are no adequate and well-controlled studies in pregnant women, dabigatran should not be given to a pregnant woman.

Contraindications

- Active bleeding, history of acute intracranial disease, haemorrhagic stroke; major surgery or major trauma in past 3 months, uncontrolled hypertension, or MI in the past 3 months; GI or urogenital bleeding, or ulcer disease in past 6 months; severe liver disease
- Impaired haemostasis
- Severe renal failure (Crcl <30ml/min)
- Hypersensitivity to any component of the product

References

1 Wolowacz SE et al. (2009). Efficacy and safety of dabigatran etexilate for the prevention of venous thromboembolism following total hip or knee arthroplasty. A meta-analysis. *Thromb Haemost* **101**:77–85.

2 Ezekowitz MD et al. (2007). Dabigatran with or without concomitant aspirin compared with warfarin alone in patients with nonvalvular atrial fibrillation (PETRO Study). *Am J Cardiol* **100**:1419–26.

3 Connolly SJ et al.; the RE-LY Steering Committee and Investigators (2009). Dabigatran versus warfarin in patients with atrial fibrillation. *N Engl J Med* **361**:1139–51.

Dalteparin

(See also 📖 Heparin, p.479 and 📖 Low-molecular-weight heparins, p.516)

CV indications

(See 📖 Heparin, p.479)
1. Prophylaxis of ischaemic complications in UA and NSTEMI
2. Prophylaxis of DVT, which may lead to PE
3. Treatment of symptomatic VTE (proximal DVT and/or PE), to reduce the recurrence of VTE in patients with cancer

Mechanism of action

(See 📖 Heparin, p.479)

Pharmacodynamics

2 trials confirmed that dalteparin may be an alternative to UFH in the acute treatment of UA or NSTEMI. In 1 study, patients with UA or NSTEMI were treated with dalteparin (120 IU SC every 12h) plus aspirin (75mg/day) within 72h of the event and continued for 5–8 days; then 7500 IU for the next 35–45 days.[1] 63% RR in death and new MI at 6 days in patients treated with dalteparin and aspirin (1.8%) in comparison to aspirin alone (4.8%); however, 4–5 months after the end of treatment, the benefit was no longer apparent.

In another study, patients with UA or NSTEMI were assigned from days 1 to 6 to dalteparin (120 IU/kg SC) or dose-adjusted IV infusion of UFH; from days 6 to 45, patients received SC either dalteparin (7,500 IU od) or placebo. The rate of death, MI, recurrence of angina or revascularization procedures was similar in both groups.[2]

In patients with cancer and acute DVT and/or PE, SC dalteparin (200 IU/kg od) was more effective than an oral anticoagulant in reducing the risk of recurrent embolic events (HR 0.48; P=0.002) without increasing the risk of bleeding.[3]

Pharmacokinetics

(See 📖 Heparin, p.479)
After a single SC injection absolute bioavailability, measured as the anti-factor Xa activity, is 87%, reaching peak levels after 4h. The V_d for dalteparin anti-factor Xa activity is 0.13L/kg and the terminal $t_{1/2}$ is 3–5h.

Practical points

💊 Doses

Treatment in UA and NSTEMI: 120 IU/kg SC every 12h for 5–8 days.

Prophylaxis of VTE following hip replacement surgery: 2500 IU 2h before surgery, 2500 IU 4–8h after surgery, and then 5000 IU daily for 5–10 days.

Prophylaxis in patients undergoing abdominal surgery: 2500 IU od, starting 1–2h prior to surgery and repeated od postoperatively for 5–10 days.

Extended treatment of symptomatic VTE in patients with cancer: the first 30 days administer 200IU/kg SC od (maximum daily dose 18,000 IU); 150IU/kg od during months 2 through 6.

Prophylaxis of VTE in medical patients: 5000 IU sc every 24h.

Treatment for DVT or PE: 7500 IU sc daily for body weight <46 kg, 10000 IU sc daily for body weight 46–56 kg, 12500 IU sc daily for body weight 57–68 kg, 15000 IU sc daily for body weight 69–82 kg, 18000 IU sc daily for body weight >83 kg.

☻ *Common side effects* (see 📖 Heparin, p.479)

Interactions (see 📖 Heparin, p.479)

Cautions/notes (see 📖 Heparin, p.479)

Pregnancy and lactation (see 📖 Heparin, p.479)

Contraindications (see 📖 Heparin, p.479)

Patients undergoing regional anaesthesia should not receive dalteparin for UA/NSTEMI or cancer for extended treatment of symptomatic VTE.

References

1 The FRISC Study Group (1996). Low molecular weight heparin during instability in coronary artery disease. *Lancet* **347**:561–8.
2 Klein W et al. (1997). Comparison of low-molecular-weight heparin with unfractionated heparin acutely and with placebo for 6 weeks in the management of unstable coronary artery disease. Fragmin in unstable coronary artery disease study (FRIC). *Circulation* **96**:61–8.
3 Lee AY et al. (2003). Randomized Comparison of Low-Molecular-Weight Heparin versus Oral Anticoagulant Therapy for the Prevention of Recurrent Venous Thromboembolism in Patients with Cancer (CLOT) Investigators. Low-molecular-weight heparin versus a coumarin for the prevention of recurrent venous thromboembolism in patients with cancer. *N Engl J Med* **349**:146–53.

Diazoxide

Potassium channel activator—intravenous direct vasodilator and oral management of intractable hypoglycaemia

CV indications

Hypertensive emergencies (IV preparation).

Other indications

(PO formulation): intractable hypoglycaemia due to hyperinsulinism (idiopathic hypoglycaemia in infancy; functional islet cell tumours, extrapancreatic neoplasms producing hypoglycaemia; glycogen storage disease; hypoglycaemia of unknown origin).

Mechanism of action

Diazoxide activates K^+ channels sensitive to ATP in vascular smooth muscle cells; this results in a hyperpolarization of the resting membrane potential, decreases the open probability of L-type Ca^{2+} channels, and produces arteriolar vasodilatation that decreases peripheral vascular resistance and BP. It also increases blood glucose levels primarily by inhibition of insulin release from the pancreas but also through peripheral mechanisms: including stimulating catecholamine release or increasing hepatic release of glucose.

Pharmacodynamics

By IV route, diazoxide lowers BP very rapidly achieving maximum effect in 2–5min and the effect persists for 2–12h. Diazoxide produces a dose-related increase in blood glucose. It also increases heart rate and serum uric acid levels and decreases sodium and water excretion.

In a small uncontrolled study, diazoxide reduced an average DBP from 139 to 98mmHg within 10min; and was judged to be successful in 38 of 41 patients.[1] In another small study, BP was effectively lowered with a 15mg mini-bolus of diazoxide in patients with hypertensive crises in labour in 19min compared to 34min with hydralazine.[2] However, experience with diazoxide remains limited and meta-analyses do not support its use in hypertensive crises in pregnancy.[3]

Pharmacokinetics

Following IV administration, diazoxide is extensively bound to plasma proteins (>90%), metabolized in the liver, and excreted via the kidneys (50% unchanged). Plasma $t_{1/2}$ after IV administration is ~28h (longer in patients with impaired renal function). The plasma $t_{1/2}$ is much longer than the hypotensive effect, and accumulation occurs with repeated doses.

Practical points

Doses

IV: 1mg/kg every 8h; maintenance: 3–8mg/kg daily in 2–3 doses, given every 8–12h

☺ *Side effects*

Common (>1%): transient hyperglycaemia (due to an inhibition of insulin release from the pancreas); hypotension, nausea, vomiting, headache, dizziness and weakness; sodium and fluid retention that may precipitate congestive HF.

Others: hyperuricaemia, hyperlipidemia, diabetic ketoacidosis, hyperosmolar non-ketotic coma, neutropenia, thrombocytopenia, hirsutism that subsides on discontinuation of the drug. Anorexia, diarrhoea, transient loss of taste, palpitations, tachycardia.

Interactions

Should not be administered within 6h of hydralazine, reserpine, alphaprodine, methyldopa, β-blockers, prazosin, minoxidil, nitrites and other papaverine-like compounds.

It can potentiate the effects of other antihypertensives.

Diazoxide may displace oral anticoagulants from plasma proteins, increasing their plasma levels; the INR should be periodically determined.

Concomitant administration of diazoxide and phenytoin may result in a loss of seizure control. Co-administration with thiazides potentiates the hyperglycaemic and hyperuricaemic effects of diazoxide.

Cautions/notes

As diazoxide causes a transient hyperglycaemia, blood glucose levels should be carefully monitored until the patient's condition has stabilized. It should be used with caution in patients with diabetes mellitus, although hyperglycaemia is usually responsive to usual management. As diazoxide causes sodium retention, repeated injection may precipitate congestive cardiac failure, which is usually responsive to diuretic therapy in the presence of adequate renal function.

Diazoxide increases heart rate and cardiac output and should be used with care in patients with coronary or cerebrovascular insufficiency, HF, or aortic aneurysm. It is not recommended for >10 days and is ineffective against hypertension due to phaeochromocytoma.

When used for the management of hypertensive crises in pregnancy, diazoxide can cause delay in 2nd stage of labour. Diazoxide should only be used when other agents such as hydralazine or labetalol have been shown to be ineffective.

Due to high alkalinity, care should be taken to ensure administration directly into a vein and not surrounding tissue.

Pregnancy and lactation

Diazoxide crosses the placenta and produces fetal alterations in animals. Because the safety in pregnant women has not been established, it should only be used when hypertension is considered life threatening (pregnancy category C). Diazoxide causes cessation of labor in eclamptic patients, although oxytocin will reverse this effect. Information is not available regarding presence in breast milk. Thus, it is not recommended in nursing mothers.

Contraindications
- Compensatory hypertension (e.g. coarctation of aorta), acute aortic dissection
- Patient's hypersensitivity to diazoxide, other thiazides, or other sulphonamide-derived drugs

References

1 MacDonald WJ *et al.* (1977). Intravenous diazoxide therapy in hypertensive crisis. *Am J Cardiol* **40**:409–15.
2 Hennessy A *et al.* (2007). A randomised comparison of hydralazine and mini-bolus diazoxide for hypertensive emergencies in pregnancy: the PIVOT trial. *Aust N Z J Obstet Gynaecol* **47**(4):279–85.
3 Duley L *et al.* (2006). Drugs for treatment of very high blood pressure during pregnancy. *Cochrane Database Syst Rev* **3**:CD001449.

Digoxin

Cardiac glycoside

CV indications

1. Congestive HF, especially with systolic dysfunction and ventricular dilatation
2. AF with uncontrolled ventricular response

Mechanism of action

Digoxin is a potent inhibitor of cellular Na^+-K^+ ATPase. Inhibition of this pump leads to an increase in intracellular Na^+ and $2°$ accumulation of intracellular Ca^{2+} via the Ca^{2+}/Na^+ exchange system. Within cardiac tissue, accumulation of intracellular Ca^{2+} allows more Ca^{2+} to be released from sarcoplasmic reticulum, thereby increasing availability for binding of troponin-C and contractility. Within vascular smooth muscle this mechanism and depolarization resulting from Na^+-K^+ ATPase inhibition may contribute to vascular smooth muscle contraction and vasoconstriction.

Digoxin decreases neurohumoral activation. It inhibits sympathetic outflow, the release of renin from the kidney, and the plasma levels of renin and angiotensin II; moreover, it also increases cardiac output, which counteracts neurohumoral activation, resulting in vasodilatation and afterload reduction.

Digoxin slows the sino-atrial node and in the AV node slows conduction (prolongs the PR interval) and increases refractory period, thus reducing ventricular rate. These effects are due to an increase in cardiac vagal tone, a decrease in sympathetic activity and a direct depressant effect. Digoxin shortens atrial and ventricular action potentials decreasing the QT interval in the ECG.

Pharmacodynamics

Heart failure

Digoxin reduces signs and symptoms, improves haemodynamics (increases stroke volume and cardiac output, reduces PCWP and LV end-diastolic pressure), inhibits neurohumoral activation, and reduces HF hospitalizations. Digoxin is indicated in patients with congestive HF, and also in patients with hypotension (SBP <100mmHg) where vasodilators are contraindicated.

A poor response is expected in low- (valvular stenosis, chronic pericarditis) and high-output states (cor pulmonale, thryrotoxicosis), and conditions increasing digoxin sensitivity (hypokalaemia, post-MI, chronic pulmonary disease, acute hypoxaemia, myocarditis).

Digoxin appears to improve morbidity in terms of reducing risk of hospitalization (RR=0.79 cf placebo over a mean follow-up of 37 months)[1] and the combined outcome of death related to HF, or hospitalization related to HF (RR=0.80, 1041 vs. 1291 patients), but not mortality in HF.[1,2] NNT for the prevention of hospitalization over 3 years is ≈10–12. Digoxin reduced death or hospitalization caused by worsening HF in patients with class II–IV HF with LVEF <25% or with cardiothoracic ratio >0.5. Post hoc subgroup analysis has suggested that mortality in HF may be positively related to levels of digoxin, with those with levels ≥ 1.2ng/mL and ≤ 0.8 had an 11.8% increase and 6.3% decrease in absolute mortality.[3]

Electrophysiological effects

Digoxin decreases the slope of phase 4 depolarization in the SA node and increases automaticity of ectopic pacemakers. The increase in $[Ca^{2+}]_i$ increases the appearance of delayed afterdepolarizations.

It shortens atrial and ventricular APD and depolarizes the resting membrane potential, decreasing intracardiac conduction velocity; both effects facilitate the appearance of re-entrant arrhythmias.

Digoxin reduces ventricular rate in patients with AF, particularly in elderly sedentary people. It should be used in combination with β-blockers, verapamil, or diltiazem for rate control during exercise. Not indicated when AF occurs without HF or when AF is due to thyrotoxicosis.

Pharmacokinetics

Rapid oral absorption (bioavailability 60–75%); effects occur within 0.5–2h and reach the maximum effect at 2–6h. Food delays the absorption, although the total amount absorbed is unchanged. In 10% of patients, intestinal flora convert digoxin to an inactive metabolite. Steady-state levels are reached within 5–7 days. IV administration of a loading dose produces a pharmacological effect within 5–30min; with maximal effect within 1–5h. Digoxin has a large V_d (6L/kg), indicating that digoxin is extensively bound to body tissues with highest concentrations in the heart, liver, kidney, and skeletal muscle. Of the small proportion of digoxin circulating in plasma, $\approx 25\%$ is bound to proteins. Digoxin is primarily excreted through the kidneys unchanged and 30% by a non-renal route (faeces, hepatic metabolism). $t_{\frac{1}{2}}$ is 35h (up to 80–140h in renal failure).

Therapeutic plasma levels: 0.5–2ng/mL. Determination of serum digoxin levels should be made no earlier than 6h after the last dose of digoxin.

Practical points

Doses

They should be titrated according to the patient's age, lean body weight, renal function, and concomitant disease states, concurrent medications, or other factors likely to alter the pharmacokinetic or pharmacodynamic profile of digoxin.

Loading dose (PO): 0.125–0.375mg tds for 1 day (a 70kg patient requires 0.75 to 1.25mg).

Maintenance dose (PO): 0.125 (>70 years) or 0.25mg/day (<70 years), preferably at bedtime. In renal impairment, the maintenance dose is lower (0.0625mg in patients with marked renal impairment).

Supraventricular tachyarrhythmias: 0.065–0.250mg loading dose can be achieved either through: (a) rapid: 0.75–1.5mg one-off dose; or (b) slow: 0.25–0.75mg for 7 days.

IV: 0.75–1.25mg as an infusion over 2h or more, depending on age, renal function and body weight.

Doses for PO administration should be reduced by ≈33% compared to IV doses.

☺ *Side effects*

Cardiovascular: arrhythmias, conduction disturbances, bigeminy, trigeminy, PR prolongation, sinus bradycardia, supraventricular tachyarrhythmia, atrial tachycardia, junctional tachycardia, ventricular arrhythmia, ventricular premature contractions, ST segment depression.

Others: anorexia, nausea, vomiting, diarrhoea, xanthopsia, dizziness, headache, gynaecomastia.

Serious/life-threatening reaction: digoxin may lead to death from cardiac manifestations of toxicity (rhythm disturbances).

Treatment of digoxin toxicity: stop digoxin, discontinue diuretics, normalize kalaemia, check the dose used and adjust to weight, age, and creatinine clearance. Digoxin-specific antibodies in patients with life-threatening ventricular tachyarrhythmias or hypokalaemia (>5.5mEq/L).

Tachyarrhythmias: lidocaine.

Bradyarrhythmias: atropine and temporary pacing.

Interactions

- With class Ia and Ic antiarrhythmics: increased risk of bradycardia, conduction block, and arrhythmias. Amiodarone and propafenone reduce clearance of digoxin and increase digoxinaemia (25–75%); decrease the dose of digoxin by 50%.
- β-blockers and calcium-channel antagonists (diltiazem, felodipine, nicardipine, nifedipine, verapamil) increase the risk of bradycardia and AV block; combination with verapamil may result in bradycardia and asystole.
- Calcium and vitamin D if administered rapidly, can precipitate arrhythmias in patients on digoxin.
- ACEIs decrease renal elimination and can increase serum digoxin levels. Spironolactone falsely increases digoxin assay.
- Hydralazine and nitroprusside increase the renal excretion of digoxin.
- Amphotericin B, β₂-adrenegic agonists, carbenoxolone, glucocorticoids, insulin, laxatives, loop diuretics, and thiazides cause hypokalaemia and increase sensitivity to digoxin

See Table 7 for other drugs that affect serum digoxin levels.

Table 7 Drugs that alter serum digoxin levels

Increase digoxin levels	Decrease digoxin levels
AINEs, alprazolam, amiloride, amiodarone, atorvastatin, ciclosporin, diphenoxylate with atropine, flecainide, gentamicin, indometacin, itraconazole, macrolide antibiotics (e.g. clarithromycin, erythromycin), prazosin, propafenone, propantheline, quinidine, quinine, spironolactone, tetracycline, triamterene, trimethoprim, verapamil	Acarbose, adrenaline, antacids, bulk laxatives, colestyramine, cimetidine, colestipol, kaolin-pectin, metoclopramide, neomycin, PAS, penicillamine, phenytoin, rifampicin, salbutamol, St John's wort, sulfasalazine

Cautions/notes
- Lower doses should be administered in the elderly due to decreased renal function; this together with low lean body mass leads to an increased risk of digoxin toxicity. Hypokalaemia sensitizes the myocardium to the actions of cardiac glycosides and must be avoided, and serum digoxin levels should be checked regularly to determine if digoxin is in the therapeutic or toxic range.
- In addition to hypokalaemia, hypoxia, hypomagnesaemia, myocarditis, and AMI increase myocardial sensitivity to cardiac glycosides. Hyperkalaemia increases the risk of AV block.
- In hypothyroidism, digoxin doses may need to be reduced while hyperthyroidism decreases digoxin sensitivity, necessitating an increase in dose. During the course of treatment of thyrotoxicosis, dosage should be gradually reduced.
- Patients with malabsorption syndrome or GI reconstructions may require larger doses of digoxin as it is absorbed in the stomach and proximal part of the small intestine.
- Digoxin should be withheld for 24h before cardioversion. In emergencies, such as cardiac arrest, the lowest effective energy should be applied when attempting cardioversion. DCCV is inappropriate in the treatment of arrhythmias caused by cardiac glycosides.
- The use of inotropic drugs in some patients post MI may result in increased myocardial O_2 demand that may lead to ischaemia.
- Digoxin should not be used in HOCM or constrictive pericarditis unless it is used to control ventricular rate in AF.

Pregnancy and lactation
Animal studies failed to reveal evidence of teratogenicity, but there are no controlled data in human pregnancy (pregnancy category C). Breast-feeding is not contraindicated, although small amounts of digoxin can be detected in breast milk.

Contraindications
- Digitalis toxicity
- Advanced AV block (except with a functioning pacemaker)
- Bradycardia or sick sinus syndrome (except in patients with a functioning pacemaker)
- WPS syndrome with AF. Digoxin accelerates anterograde conduction over the accessory pathway and may precipitate VT/VF
- Ventricular premature beats, VT/VF
- Marked hypokalaemia

References

1 Ahmed A et al. (2006). Digoxin and reduction in mortality and hospitalization in heart failure: a comprehensive post hoc analysis of the DIG trial. *Eur Heart J* **27**:178–86.
2 The Digitalis Investigation Group (1997). The effect of digoxin on mortality and morbidity in patients with heart failure. *N Engl J Med* **336**:525–33.

Diltiazem

(See also 📖 Calcium-channel blockers, p.390)

An oral benzothiazepine (non-dihydropyridine) L-type selective calcium-channel blocker with direct cardiac effect and class IV antiarrhythmic activity.

CV indications

1. Treatment of hypertension
2. Treatment of chronic stable and vasospastic angina pectoris
3. Treatment and prophylaxis of paroxysmal SVT and control of ventricular rate in atrial flutter/AF

Mechanism of action

(See 📖 Calcium-channel blockers, p.390)

Pharmacodynamics

Reduction in BP of ~13/8mmHg (vs 5/1mmHg) from baseline (mean BP ~165/101mmHg) with diltiazem (240–360mg/day) compared to placebo.[1]

Angina: diltiazem (180–420mg od) increases total duration of exercise, time to onset of angina and also time to ≥1mm ST segment depression in patients with stable chronic angina.[2]

Hypertension: RR ~1.00 (16.6 vs. 16.2/1000 patient-years) of combined 1° endpoint (fatal and non-fatal stroke, MI, and other CV death) in hypertensive patients with DBP ≥100mmHg treated with diltiazem (180–360mg daily) as 1st-line compared to β-blocker and diuretic, with additional stepped antihypertensive agents as required to achieve DBP <90mmHg and followed up for ~5 years.[3]

Atrial fibrillation: HR ~1.15 (95% CI: 0.99–1.34, *P*=0.08; absolute rate = 23.8 vs. 21.3% at 5 years) in total mortality in patients with AF and high risk of death or stroke treated by rate control with drugs including diltiazem compared to rhythm control using antiarrhythmic agents.[4]

Pharmacokinetics

Oral diltiazem is almost completely absorbed, but has a low bioavailability (bioavailability 40%) due to hepatic 1st-pass metabolism. The pharmacokinetics vary widely between preparations and brands. Diltiazem is available in a range of formulations, including standard (onset of action 15min, peak plasma concentrations after 1–4h, and plasma $t_{1/2}$ of 4–8h) and longer-acting (peak plasma concentrations approximately 8–11h after dosing, and average plasma $t_{1/2}$ of 6–8h). Diltiazem binds to plasma proteins (~80%) and has a high V_d of 3.3L/kg. It is metabolized extensively (to desacetyl-diltiazem) and is excreted in urine (35%, only 1–3% unchanged) and faeces (65%).

Practical points

.💊 Doses

Diltiazem is available in a variety of preparations from different manufacturers, and due to different pharmacokinetics, the doses may vary and the following is a general guide. To ensure consistency of response, once established on a particular modified-release formulation, it is not advisable to substitute different brands for another, hence they should be prescribed by brand names.

Hypertension: short-acting formulations: 120–360mg bd or tds; modified-release formulations: initial daily dose of 180mg od or tds up to a daily dose of 180–540mg depending on formulation and manufacturer.

Chronic angina: standard formulation: starting at 60mg tds, increasing to a daily dose of 360–480mg/day. Modified-release formulations: initial daily dose of 180mg od or tds up to a daily dose of 240–480mg depending on manufacturer.

Rate control in patients with AF/atrial flutter: 0.25mg/kg over 2min monitoring BP and ECG; maintenance dose: 5–15mg/h IV. Maintenance dose: 120–360mg daily in divided doses.

🙁 Side effects
(See 📖 Calcium-channel blockers, p.390)

Others: sinus bradycardia; 1st-degree AV block; fatigue, rash.

Rare: gingival hyperplasia (disappearing on cessation of treatment); exfoliative dermatitis, angioneurotic oedema, erythema multiforme, vasculitis, transient increased liver transaminases and isolated cases of clinical hepatitis resolving after withdrawing treatment.

Interactions
(See 📖 Calcium-channel blockers, p.390)
Diltiazem also increases the plasma levels of quinidine (50%) and lovastatin (3- to 4-fold), and dose adjustment is required. Unlike verapamil, diltiazem does not interact with digoxin.

Co-administration with drugs such as β-blockers, antiarrhythmics, or cardiac glycosides may increase the risk of bradycardia, AV block, and hypotension. Patients with pre-existing conduction defects should not receive the combination of diltiazem and β-blockers. IV β-blockers should be discontinued during therapy with diltiazem.

Diltiazem can be combined with dihydropyridines in patients with resistant coronary artery vasospasm.

Risk of lithium-induced neurotoxicity is also increased. High doses of vitamin D and/or high intake of calcium salts leading to elevated serum calcium levels may reduce the response to diltiazem.

Diltiazem increases the AUC and the elimination time of buspirone, midazolam, and triazolam, so dose adjustments are needed.

Cautions/notes
(See 📖 Calcium-channel blockers, p.390)
Diltiazem should be used with caution in patients with reduced LV function, mild bradycardia, 1st-degree AV block, or prolonged PR interval; and under close supervision, and doses should not be increased if bradycardia (heart rate <50/min) occurs.

Pregnancy and lactation (see 📖 Calcium-channel blockers, p.390)

Contraindications

(See 📖 Calcium-channel blockers, p.390)

- Bradycardia, sick sinus syndrome, 2nd- or 3rd-degree AV block and sick sinus syndrome except in the presence of a functioning ventricular pacemaker
- Hypotension (SBP <90 mmHg)
- Decompensated HF, LV dysfunction (LVEF <40%) or severe hypotension following MI
- AF/atrial flutter and simultaneous presence of a WPW syndrome
- Patients with AMI and pulmonary congestion documented by X-ray on admission
- Hypersensitivity to the drug

References

1 Nikkila MT *et al.* (1989). Antihypertensive effect of diltiazem in a slow-release formulation for mild to moderate essential hypertension. *Am J Cardiol* **63**:1227–30.

2 Glasser SP *et al.* (2005). Efficacy and safety of a once-daily graded-release diltiazem formulation dosed at bedtime compared to placebo and to morning dosing in chronic stable angina pectoris. *Am Heart J* **149**:E1–E9.

3 Hansson L *et al.* (2000). Randomised trial of effects of calcium antagonists compared with diuretics and β-blockers on cardiovascular morbidity and mortality in hypertension: the Nordic Diltiazem (NORDIL) study. *Lancet* **356**:359–65.

4 Wyse DG *et al.*; Atrial Fibrillation Follow-up Investigation of Rhythm Management (AFFIRM) Investigator (2002). A comparison of rate control and rhythm control in patients with atrial fibrillation. *N Engl J Med* **347**:1825–33.

Dipyridamole

Platelet aggregation inhibitor.

CV indications

1. Dipyridamole is indicated as an adjunct to coumarin anticoagulants in the prevention of postoperative thromboembolic complications of cardiac valve replacement.
2. Combination of low-dose aspirin and dipyridamole is considered an acceptable option for 2° prevention of stroke and TIA.
3. Dipyridamole-echocardiography test for diagnosis and prognosis of coronary artery disease.

Mechanism of action

Dipyridamole inhibits the uptake of adenosine into platelets, endothelial cells, and erythrocytes in a dose-dependent manner. This inhibition results in an increase in local concentrations of adenosine which acts on the platelet A_2-receptor thereby stimulating platelet adenylate cyclase and increasing platelet cAMP levels. Via this mechanism, platelet aggregation is inhibited in response to various stimuli such as platelet-activating factor, ADP, and collagen.

Dipyridamole also inhibits cyclic-3',5'-guanosine monophosphate-PDE (cGMP-PDE), thereby augmenting the increase in cGMP produced by nitric oxide.

Dipyridamole produces a marked vasodilatation in healthy coronary arteries, whereas stenosed arteries remain narrowed. This creates a 'steal' phenomenon, so that coronary blood flow will increase to the dilated healthy vessels compared to the stenosed arteries, which can be detected by clinical symptoms of chest pain, ECG, and echocardiography when it causes ischaemia.

Pharmacodynamics

In a meta-analysis of 6 RCTs in patients with prosthetic heart, the combination of dipyridamole (225 to 400mg per day) with anticoagulants reduced the risk of thromboembolic events (fatal or nonfatal) by 56% when compared with the use of anticoagulants alone. 64% RR in fatal and in nonfatal thromboembolic events and 40% RR in overall mortality rate.[1] In another meta-analysis, aspirin and dipyridamole reduced mortality similarly (RRR of 49% (95% CI: 29% to 63%) and an NNT of 27).[2]

Dipyridamole (SR 200mg bd) combined with aspirin (30–325mg od) for 6 months results in a significant reduction in the occurrence of stroke (37% RRR for the combination, 15% for dipyridamole, and 18% for aspirin) and death.[3]

Pharmacokinetics

Oral bioavailability 60%, reaching peak plasma levels in 1.5 hr. It is highly bound to plasma proteins (99%) and is metabolized in the liver where it is conjugated as a glucuronide and excreted with the bile. The decline in plasma concentration fits a two-compartment model. The alpha half-life is approximately 40 minutes and the beta half-life approximately 10 hr.

Practical points

♪ Doses

Oral: 75–100mg 4 times daily (maximum dosage 600mg/day).
Dipyridamole stress echocardiography protocol: IV infusion of 0.84mg/kg over 10 min in 2 separate infusions (0.56mg/kg over 4 min followed by 4min of no dose; if still negative, an additional dose of 0.28mg/kg over 2 min).

☺ Common side effects

- Dizziness (13.6%), abdominal distress (6.1%), headache (2.3%), rash (2.3%), hypotension, palpitations
- It may increase ischaemia and angina due to coronary steal
- *Uncommon*: diarrhoea, vomiting, flushing, pruritus and angina

Interactions

- Adenosine: dipyridamole increases the plasma levels and CV effects of adenosine; thus, the dose of adenosine should be halved.
- Cholinesterase inhibitors: dipyridamole may counteract the anticholinesterase effect of cholinesterase inhibitors, thereby potentially aggravating myasthenia gravis.

Cautions/notes

- Dipyridamole has a vasodilatory effect and should be used with caution in patients with severe coronary artery disease.
- Elevations of hepatic enzymes and hepatic failure have been reported in association with dipyridamole administration.
- Dipyridamole should be used with caution in patients with hypotension since it can produce peripheral vasodilatation.
- Safety and effectiveness in the pediatric population below the age of 12 years have not been established.

Pregnancy and lactation

Dipyridamole should be used during pregnancy only if clearly needed (pregnancy category B). Dipyridamole is excreted in human milk.

Contraindications

- Hypersensitivity to dipyridamole and any of the other components
- UA and immediately after MI

References

1 Pouleur J, Buyse M (1995). Effects of dipyridamole in combination with anticoagulant therapy on survival and thromboembolic events in patients with prosthetic heart valves: a meta-analysis of the randomized trials. *J Thorac Cardiovasc Surg* **110**:463–72.

2 Massel D, Little SH (2001). Risks and benefits of adding anti-platelet therapy to warfarin among patients with prosthetic heart valves: a meta-analysis. *J Am Coll Cardiol* **37**:569–78.

3 ESPRIT Study Group, Halkes PH *et al.* (2006). Aspirin plus dipyridamole versus aspirin alone after cerebral ischaemia of arterial origin (ESPRIT): randomised controlled trial. *Lancet* **367**: 1665–73.

Disopyramide

(See also 📖 Class Ia antiarrhythmic drugs, p.403)
Oral sodium-channel blocker with class Ia antiarrhythmic properties.

Mechanism of action

(See 📖 Class Ia antiarrhythmic drugs, p.403)

Pharmacodynamics

Compared with other class I antiarrhythmics, disopyramide is a moderate sodium-channel blocker. As with other class Ia drugs, it slows heart rate, prolongs the QRS, PR, and QT and exerts an anticholinergic effect, most prominent in the SA and AV nodes due to extensive vagal innervation, such that SA rate and AV conduction may be increased.

Pharmacokinetics

Disopyramide is rapidly and completely absorbed (bioavailability 60–83%) reaching peak plasma levels in 1–2h. It binds to plasma proteins (50–65%) and presents a V_d of 0.6L/kg and a $t_{1/2}$ of 6–8h (longer in renal insufficiency or MI). About 50% of a given dose is excreted unchanged in urine but 50% is metabolized in the liver to a mono-N-dealkylated derivate by the liver (CYP3A4) and 10% to other metabolites. Therapeutic plasma levels: 2–6mcg/mL.

Practical points

💊 Doses

Oral: 100–200mg q 4h. A dose reduction is recommended in the elderly and may be required in renal and hepatic impairment.
IV: 20mg/kg in 15min followed by 0.4–4mg/kg/h.

☺ Common side effects

(>10%): urinary retention (anticholinergic effect).

(1–10%): other anticholinergic effects (blurred vision, xerostomia (dry mouth), abdominal pain, constipation), erectile dysfunction, anorexia, diarrhoea, dizziness, headache, bradycardia, and hypotension.

There appears to be a risk of hypoglycaemia with disopyramide, particularly in the elderly, malnourished and those treated for diabetes, or with cardiac or renal failure. Rapid infusion may cause profuse sweating.

Although disopyramide is generally accepted as having weak arrhythmogenic potential, it may worsen or provoke arrhythmia (particularly with hypokalaemia and in patients with structural heart disease). ECG changes include: intracardiac conduction abnormalities, QT interval prolongation, widening of the QRS complex, AV block, and bundle–branch block. Because of its negative inotropic effect, episodes of severe HF or even cardiogenic shock have also been described particularly in patients with severe structural heart disease.

Interactions

Combinations with other antiarrhythmics are not well studied and should be avoided. As disopyramide prolongs the QT interval, it should be used with caution with other drugs that prolong the QT interval or predispose to torsades de pointes. There is no interaction with digoxin.

Combination with other drugs metabolized by CYP3A should be avoided as the effect is unpredictable. Drugs that induce hypokalaemia may reduce its effect or potentiate proarrhythmia. Atropine and other anticholinergic drugs potentiate the atropine-like effect of disopyramide; pyridostigmine (90–180mg tds) reduces these anticholinergic affects.

Disopyramide increases the negative inotropic effects and the depressant effects of diltiazem, verapamil, digoxin, and β-blockers on SA and AV nodes. Risk of hypotension if associated with β-blockers, diltiazem, or verapamil.

Cautions/notes

Special caution must be paid when using this drug in patients with structural heart disease. Due to effects of class Ic agents in post-MI patients,[1] disopyramide is generally not recommended in patients with structural heart disease.

There have been reports of VT, VF, and torsades de pointes with disopyramide, usually in association with widening of the QRS or prolongation of the QT interval. Consequently these ECG features should be monitored and disopyramide discontinued if either become present. It should be used with caution in atrial flutter or atrial tachycardia with block.

Owing to its negative inotropic effects, disopyramide should be used with caution in patients with HF.

Blood glucose and potassium levels should be monitored due to risk of hypoglycaemia and exacerbation of arrhythmias respectively. Also, given its atropine-like effects, disopyramide may increase the risk of: ocular hypertension in narrow-angle glaucoma, urinary retention in prostatic hypertrophy, and aggravation of myasthenia gravis.

Pregnancy and lactation

Although there is no evidence of teratogenicity in animal models, safety of disopyramide in pregnancy has not been established (pregnancy category C). The drug crosses the placenta and may induce labour. It is also secreted in breast milk. Thus, in either pregnancy or breastfeeding it should be used with caution.

Contraindications

- Conduction abnormalities: un-paced 2nd- or 3rd-degree AV block or trifascicular block, bifascicular block, pre-existing long QT; severe sinus dysfunction
- Glaucoma, myasthenia gravis, hypotension, and prostatic hypertrophy causing urinary retention
- Severe HF (unless due to arrhythmia)
- In combination with other antiarrhythmics or drugs likely to provoke ventricular arrhythmia
- The sustained release form is contraindicated in liver or renal impairment

Reference

1 The Cardiac Arrhythmia Suppression Trial (CAST) Investigators (1989). Preliminary report: effect of encainide and flecainide on mortality in a randomized trial of arrhythmia suppression after myocardial infarction. *N Engl J Med* **321**:406–12.

Dobutamine

Synthetic analogue of dopamine used as a positive inotropic agent.

CV indications

1. To provide inotropic support in the short-term treatment of adults with cardiac decompensation due to depressed contractility resulting either from organic heart disease or from cardiac surgical procedures
2. To increase or maintain cardiac output during positive end expiratory pressure (PEEP) ventilation
3. Echocardiographic stress testing (as an alternative to exercise in patients in whom routine exercise cannot be satisfactorily performed)

Mechanism of action

Dobutamine directly stimulates β_1-adrenergic receptors; it also has mild β_2- and α_1-adrenergic receptor agonist effects ($\beta_1 > \beta_2 > \alpha$). Unlike dopamine, dobutamine does not cause renal or mesenteric vasodilatation or a release of endogenous catecholamines.

Pharmacodynamics

Acute HF: dobutamine increase cardiac contractility and cardiac output, but produces less increase in heart rate than dopamine. It reduces systemic vascular resistances but SBP is usually stable. However, stimulation of β_2-receptors may lead to a fall in DBP and reflex tachycardia. Experience with IV dobutamine in controlled trials does not extend beyond 48h of repeated boluses and/or continuous infusions.

Dopamine and dobutamine improve signs, symptoms, and haemodynamics in patients with acute HF but do not reduce the risk of hospitalization and death.[1]

Coronary blood flow and myocardial oxygen consumption are usually increased due to enhanced myocardial contractility. The improved diuresis observed with dobutamine is the result of increased renal blood flow in response to improved cardiac output.

Pharmacokinetics

Dobutamine is given by IV infusion; the onset of action occurs within 2min, and peak plasma concentration and effects are reached within 10min. Due to its short $t_{1/2}$ (2min), the effects of dobutamine cease shortly after discontinuation of the infusion. Dobutamine is mainly metabolized in the liver and other tissues by catechol-*O*-methyltransferase (COMT) to an inactive compound, 3-0-methyldobutamine and by conjugation with glucuronic acid. These metabolites are excreted in urine and, to a minor extent, in faeces.

Practical points

Due to its short $t_{1/2}$, dobutamine should be given as a continuous IV infusion. Dobutamine must be diluted to at least 50mL (in glucose or saline solution) prior to IV administration. Patients should gradually have their dose reduced as opposed to sudden cessation of infusion. In prolonged infusion (>48–72h), partial tolerance develops requiring higher doses to maintain the same effects.

♨ Doses

For inotropic support: starting dose 0.5–1mcg/kg/min, titrated at intervals of a few minutes up to 40mcg/kg/min, guided by the patient's response.

Cardiac stress testing: 5mcg/kg/min, with incremental increases of 5mcg/kg/min up to 20mcg/kg/min. Each incremental dose should be infused for 8min.

Continuous cardiac monitoring is essential and the infusion should be terminated if the following occur: 3mm ST segment depression, development of ventricular tachyarrhythmias, maximum heart rate is achieved, or SBP >220mmHg.

☺ Side effects

Cardiovascular: palpitations, tachyarrhythmias, hypertension, hypotension, anginal pain, myocardial ischaemia, coronary artery spasm

Other: nausea, headache, hypokalaemia, dyspnoea, rash, fever, asthma, bronchospasm, phlebitis and cutaneous necrosis

Serious/life-threatening side effects: cardiac rupture, LV outflow obstruction, VT/VF, MI

Interactions

- Cyclopropane and halogenated anaesthetics: increased risk of ventricular arrhythmias
- Entacapone: may enhance effect of dobutamine because of COMT inhibition.
- β-blockers: antagonize the inotropic effect of dobutamine. Co-administration of a non-selective β-blocker can result in elevated BP (due to α-mediated vasoconstriction) and reflex bradycardia. Carvedilol, which possesses α- and β-receptor antagonist activity, may cause hypotension during concomitant use of dobutamine due to vasodilatation caused via stimulation of β_2 receptors.

Cautions/notes

- During the administration of dobutamine ECG, BP, PCWP, and cardiac output should be continuously monitored.
- In patients with atrial flutter or AF, dobutamine facilitates AV conduction, which may lead to rapid ventricular responses.
- Dobutamine may be ineffective in patients treated with β-blocking drugs; in these patients the peripheral vascular resistances may increase.
- Care is required with dobutamine use in patients with AMI, as increases in heart rate or arterial pressure may intensify ischaemia.
- Dobutamine does not improve haemodynamics in patients with impaired ventricular filling or outflow caused by mechanical obstruction or those with reduced ventricular compliance (includes cardiac tamponade, valvular AS, and idiopathic hypertrophic subaortic stenosis).
- Care is needed when considering cardiac stress testing in patients with a recent MI, as cardiac rupture is a potential complication, especially in those with a dyskinetic or thinned ventricle.

- Hypovolaemia should be corrected when necessary before administering dobutamine. If arterial BP remains low or decreases progressively during administration of dobutamine despite adequate ventricular filling pressure and cardiac output, the concomitant use of a peripheral vasoconstrictor agent (DA or noradrenaline) may be needed.
- Dobutamine should not be diluted in alkaline solutions, with other drugs in the same solution or with other agents or diluents containing both sodium bisulphite and ethanol.

Pregnancy and lactation

There are no well-controlled studies in pregnant women (pregnancy category B). It is not known whether dobutamine crosses the placenta or is distributed into breast milk. Thus, dobutamine should not be used during pregnancy unless the potential benefits outweigh the potential risks to the fetus.

Contraindications

Phaeochromocytoma, idiopathic hypertrophic subaortic stenosis and hypersensitivity to dobutamine (sulphites in dobutamine may cause allergic-type reactions, including anaphylactic symptoms and asthmatic episodes in certain susceptible people).

Dobutamine is not recommended for exercise testing in patients with any cardiac condition that could make them unsuitable for exercise stress testing.

Reference

1 Dickstein K et al. (2008). ESC Guidelines for the diagnosis and treatment of acute and chronic heart failure 2008: the Task Force for the Diagnosis and Treatment of Acute and Chronic Heart Failure 2008 of the European Society of Cardiology. Developed in collaboration with the Heart Failure Association of the ESC (HFA) and endorsed by the European Society of Intensive Care Medicine (ESICM). *Eur Heart J* **29**:2388–442.

Dopamine

Inotropic catecholamine.

CV indications

1. To correct haemodynamic instability present in the shock syndrome due to MI, trauma, endotoxic septicaemia, cardiac surgery, renal failure, and acute HF
2. To treat hypotension due to inadequate cardiac output
3. To improve renal blood flow and diuresis in decompensated HF with hypotension and low urine output

Mechanism of action

Pharmacodynamics

Dopamine (DA) is a natural catecholamine formed by the decarboxylation of 3,4-dihydroxyphenylalanine (DOPA); it is also a precursor of noradrenaline in noradrenergic nerves and a neurotransmitter in certain areas of the CNS (i.e. nigrostriatal tract), and in a few peripheral sympathetic nerves.

At doses of 0.5–2mcg/kg/min, DA stimulates predominantly dopaminergic receptors. Stimulation of DA_1 receptors in renal, mesenteric, coronary, and intracerebral vascular beds causes vasodilatation; stimulation of presynaptic DA_2 receptors decreases the release of noradrenaline and renin. In patients with renal hypoperfusion and failure, these doses of DA increase renal blood flow, GFR, sodium excretion, and urine flow, and increase the response to diuretic agents.

At doses of 2–5mcg/kg/min, DA activates β_1-adrenergic receptors and also increases the release of noradrenaline from storage sites in sympathetic nerve terminals which counteracts the effects on DA_2 receptors; both effects increase heart rate and contractility, cardiac output, and SBP, with either no effect or a slight increase in DBP.

At higher doses, dopamine activates α_1-adrenoceptors producing a combined inotropic and vasoconstrictor effect that increases BP. These doses can reduce the circulation of the limbs and counteract the renal effects of dopamine, reversing renal dilation and natriuresis.

It is believed that α-adrenergic effects result from inhibition of adenylyl cyclase and reduction of the cellular levels of cAMP, whereas β-adrenergic effects result from stimulation of adenyl cyclase activity and an increase in cAMP levels. In cardiac myocytes, the increase in cAMP increases intracellular Ca^{2+} levels, leading to an increase in heart rate and contractility; in vascular smooth muscle cells, cAMP decreases intracellular Ca^{2+} levels leading to vasodilator response.

Pharmacokinetics

DA is inactive orally and following an IV bolus it has a $t_{1/2}$ of ≈2min (1h if MAO inhibitors are present); so it is given by continuous IV infusion.

Via this route its effects reach steady state within 5–10min, but on termination of the infusion they persist for <10min. It is widely distributed, but does not cross the blood–brain barrier substantially, and is metabolized in the liver, kidney, and plasma by MAO and COMT to the inactive compounds homovanillic acid (HVA) and 3,4-dihydroxyphenyl acetic acid (DOPAC), that are excreted in the urine. About 25% of a dose of DA is stored in adrenergic nerve terminals, where it is hydroxylated to form noradrenaline.

Practical points

- DA should not be diluted in alkaline solutions.
- At the infusion site DA can cause local vasoconstriction; hence, it should be infused into a large vein to prevent the possibility of extravasation.
- During the treatment, BP, urine flow, myocardial function, and ECG should be monitored with periodic measurements of cardiac output and PCWP.

Doses

Starting dose infusion: 2.5mcg/kg/min (5mcg/kg/min may be utilized in more severe cases), increased gradually in 5–10mcg/kg/min increments up to 20–50mcg/kg/min according to the patient's response. In patients who do not respond to these doses, additional increments of DA may be given in an effort to achieve adequate BP, urine flow, and perfusion generally.

In the presence of a decline of urine flow rate, increasing tachycardia, or development of new arrhythmias, one should consider decreasing or temporarily suspending the dosage.

Side effects

Cardiovascular: ectopic heart beats, tachycardia, angina, palpitations, hypotension, vasoconstriction, aberrant conduction, bradycardia, widened QRS complex, hypertension. Fatal ventricular arrhythmias have been reported on rare occasions.

Other: nausea, vomiting, headache, dyspnoea, azotaemia, mydriasis, piloerection.

Gangrene of the feet has occurred when high doses were administered for prolonged periods or in patients with pre-existing vascular disease.

DA extravasation may cause necrosis and sloughing of surrounding tissue; thus, the infusion site should be continuously monitored for free flow.

Interactions

- *Anaesthetics*: cyclopropane or halogenated hydrocarbon anaesthetics sensitize the myocardium to catecholamine-induced arrhythmias. Even when ventricular arrhythmias can be reversed by propranolol, this combination should therefore be avoided.
- *α- and β-blockers*: β-adrenergic-blocking agents antagonize the cardiac effects of DA. The peripheral vasoconstriction caused by high doses

of DA is antagonized by α-adrenergic-blocking agents. DA-induced renal and mesenteric vasodilatation is not antagonized by either α- or β-adrenergic blocking agents, but, in animals, is antagonized by butyrophenones (e.g. haloperidol), phenothiazines, and opiates.

- *MAO inhibitors*: potentiate the effect of DA and its duration of action. Patients treated with MAO inhibitors within 2–3 weeks prior to the administration of DA should receive one-tenth of the usual dose of DA.
- *Phenytoin*: in combination with DA, may result in hypotension and bradycardia; avoid, if possible, this combination.
- Co-administration of low-dose DA and diuretic agents may produce an additive effect on urine flow.
- Tricyclic antidepressants may potentiate the cardiovascular effects of DA.
- The use of vasoconstricting agents (ergot alkaloids) and some oxytocic drugs may result in severe hypertension.

Cautions/notes

β_2-adrenergic stimulation causes hypokalaemia with enhanced risk of arrhythmias; serum potassium should be checked to minimize arrhythmias.

Precautions

Circulating blood volume should be restored with a suitable plasma expander or whole blood prior to DA infusion.

The dose of DA should be adjusted according to the patient's response (urine flow rate, heart rate). When discontinuing the infusion, it may be necessary to gradually decrease the dose of DA while expanding blood volume with IV fluids, to avoid unnecessary hypotension.

Patients with a history of peripheral vascular disease should be closely monitored for any changes in colour or temperature of the skin of the extremities; these changes may be reversed by decreasing the rate or discontinuing the infusion. IV administration of phentolamine mesylate 5–10mg reverses the ischaemia. DA should be used with care in AS.

Glucose solutions should be used with caution in patients with known subclinical or overt diabetes mellitus.

Safety and effectiveness of DA in children have not been established.

Pregnancy and lactation

Animal studies have shown no evidence of teratogenic effects with dopamine, but its effect on the human fetus is unknown, so it should be used during pregnancy only if the potential benefit justifies the potential risk to the fetus (pregnancy category C). It is not known if DA is excreted in breast milk.

Contraindications

- Patients with phaeochromocytoma or hyperthyroidism
- Presence of atrial or ventricular tachyarrhythmias or VF

Doxazosin

(See also 📖 Alpha$_1$-adrenoreceptor blockers, p.342)
Selective post-synaptic competitive α_1-adrenoreceptor blocker.

CV indications
(See 📖 Alpha$_1$-adrenoreceptor blockers, p.342)

Mechanism of action
(See 📖 Alpha$_1$-adrenoreceptor blockers, p.342)

Pharmacodynamics
(See 📖 Alpha$_1$-adrenoreceptor blockers, p.342)

Hypertension: the addition of doxazosin (mean dose ≈7mg) as 3rd-line treatment effectively reduces BP (mean BP fall ≈11.7/6.9mmHg in patients with mean baseline of 159/89mmHg).[1] Doxazosin does not appear to cause adverse metabolic effects. It lowers total plasma cholesterol, LDL-C, and triglycerides and increases HDL-C levels. In diabetic patients, it reduces insulin resistance.

RR ≈1.26 of 2° endpoint of stroke (absolute 4-year rates: 5.5/100 vs. 4.1/100) and RR ≈1.20 (absolute 4-year rates: 28.6/100 vs. 25.1/100) of 2° endpoint of combined CVD (particularly risk of HF) in hypertensive patients with an additional CHD risk factor treated with 1st-line doxazosin compared with chlortalidone and followed for mean of 3.2 years.[2]

Heart failure: the doxazosin arm in the ALLHAT trial was terminated because of an excess in combined CV 2° endpoint.[3] However, interpretation of such interim data is not straightforward. The excess comprised mainly of treatment of, or admission for, HF. However, despite inferior BP lowering with doxazosin, there was no increase in 1° endpoint or increased mortality from HF with doxazosin. Furthermore, doxazosin itself can be associated with ankle oedema, a symptom of HF.[5]

Pharmacokinetics
Doxazosin (mesylate) is rapidly absorbed after oral administration (bioavailability ≈66%). It is protein bound (≈98%), extensively metabolized in the liver, and excreted predominantly in faeces. $t_{1/2}$ is ≈22h. Exposure is increased with hepatic impairment. Doxazosin is also available in a modified-release (XL) formulation. With this preparation, plasma levels peak at 8–9h after administration and are about 1/3 those of immediate-release preparations.

Practical points

♣ Doses
Doxazosin: 1mg od (maximum: 16mg od)
Doxazosin XL: 4mg (maximum: 8mg od)

No specific dose changes are specified for hepatic impairment but given extensive hepatic metabolism, doxazosin should be used with caution in such cases.

☺ *Common side effects*
(See ☐ Alpha$_1$-adrenoreceptor blockers, p.342)
(In the THOMS study, the incidence of impotence was lowest in the doxa-zosin group.[4])
Interactions (see ☐ Alpha$_1$-adrenoreceptor blockers, p.342)
Cautions/notes (see ☐ Alpha$_1$-adrenoreceptor blockers, p.342)

Pregnancy and lactation

No data on human pregnancy are available. However, as reduced fetal survival has been observed in animal studies, it should be used with cau-tion in pregnancy (pregnancy category B). Due to accumulation in breast milk, doxazosin is contraindicated in breastfeeding.

Contraindications

(See ☐ Alpha$_1$-adrenoreceptor blockers, p.342)
Lactation

References

1 Chapman N *et al.*; ASCOT Investigators (2008). Effect of doxazosin gastrointestinal therapeu-tic system as third-line antihypertensive therapy on blood pressure and lipids in the Anglo-Scandinavian Cardiac Outcomes Trial. *Circulation* **118**:42–8.

2 Antihypertensive and Lipid-Lowering Treatment to Prevent Heart Attack Trial Collaborative Research Group (2003). Diuretic versus alpha-blocker as first-step antihypertensive therapy: final results from the Antihypertensive and Lipid-Lowering Treatment to Prevent Heart Attack Trial (ALLHAT). *Hypertension* **42**:239–46.

3 Einhorn PT *et al.* (2007). The Antihypertensive and Lipid-Lowering Treatment to Prevent Heart Attack Trial (ALLHAT) Heart failure validation Study: diagnosis and prognosis. *Am Heart J* **153**: 42–53.

4 Grimm RH *et al.* (1997). Long-term effects on sexual function of five antihypertensive drugs and nutritional hygienic treatment in hypertensive men and women. Treatment of Mild Hypertension study (THOMS). *Hypertension* **29**:8–14.

5 Poulter N, Williams B (2001). Doxazosin for the management of hypertension: implications of the findings of the ALLHAT trial. *Am J Hypertens* **14**(11 Pt 1):1170–2.

Dronedarone

(See also 📖 Antiarrhythmic drugs: classification, p.362)

Non-iodinated benzofurane antiarrhythmic drug structurally related to amiodarone, which presents with class I, II, III, and IV actions.

The lack of the iodine moiety minimizes the risk of thyroid toxicity and the addition of a methylsulphonamide group reduces lipophilicity and, thus, the risk of organ toxicity.

CV indications

Adult clinically stable patients with history of, or current, non-permanent AF to prevent recurrence of AF or to lower ventricular rate.

Mechanism of action

Dronedarone exhibits a multiple mechanism of action. It blocks Na^+, L-type Ca^{2+} and several K^+ currents [transient (I_{to}), ultrarapid (I_{Kur}), rapid (I_{Kr}), and slow (I_{Ks}) components of the delayed rectifier, inward rectifier (I_{K1}) and acetylcholine-activated (I_{KAch})]. Like amiodarone, dronedarone produces a non-competitive inhibition of α- and β-adrenergic receptors. Dronedarone produces a vasodilator effect mediated via the L-type Ca^{2+} current blockade.

Dronedarone increases serum creatinine levels due to a partial inhibition of the tubular organic cationic transporter system, rather than a decline in renal function. In fact, the drug does not affect the GFR, renal blood flow, and Na^+ or K^+ excretion.

Pharmacodynamics

Chronic administration of dronedarone prolongs the action potential duration and refractoriness in cardiac tissues independent of the rate of stimulation (e.g. dronedarone does not present reverse use dependence) and reduces transmural dispersion of repolarization.

Dronedarone slows SA nodal automaticity, inhibits the early afterdepolarizations induced by I_{Kr} blockers (e.g. sotalol), and exerts a protective effect against experimental ventricular arrhythmias induced after coronary artery occlusion

ECG: dronedarone prolongs the RR, PR, and QTc intervals as well as the refractory periods of cardiac tissues.

Rhythm control: in patients with persistent AF, dronedarone (800, 1200, or 1600mg daily for 6 months) produced a dose-dependent conversion to sinus rhythm in 5.8%, 8.2%, and 14.8% of patients as compared with 3.1% in the placebo group.[1] Dronedarone delayed the time to first AF recurrence, but only at the dose of 800mg (60 days vs. 5.3 days in the placebo group). At 6 months, 35% of patients treated with 800mg of dronedarone were in sinus rhythm (10% in the placebo group).

Dronedarone (400mg bd) delayed the time to 1st recurrence of AF/AFL, lowering the risk of 1st AF/AFL recurrence during the 12-month study period by about 25%, with an absolute difference in recurrence rate of about 11% at 12 months in patients in sinus rhythm with at least 1 ECG-documented AF/AFL episode during the 3 months prior to study entry as compared to placebo.[2] Dronedarone also reduced the ventricular rate during AF recurrence. A post hoc analysis revealed a 27% RR in all-cause hospitalization.

Rate control: the addition of dronedarone (400mg bd) to standard rate-control therapy reduced the ventricular rate (11.7 bpm) on day 14, and the effect was maintained after 6 months. The decrease of heart rate was more pronounced during exercise (26bpm), without any reduction in tolerance.[3]

Mortality and morbidity: 24% RR of hospitalization due to CV events or death in patients with a recent history of paroxysmal or persistent AF or atrial flutter who were in sinus rhythm or to be converted to sinus rhythm and treated for a mean of 21 months with dronedarone (400mg bd) as compared to placebo.[4] This difference was entirely attributable to a 26% RR for 1st hospitalization due to CV events. 16% RR for death from any cause, and 29% RR for death from CV causes, mainly due to a 45% RR in death from cardiac arrhythmias. There was also a 26% RR in first hospitalization due to CV events, driven mainly by a 37% RR in hospitalizations due to AF. The reduction in CV hospitalization or death from any cause was consistent in all subgroups based on baseline characteristics (age, sex, HF, LV dysfunction) or medications (ACEIs or ARBs; β-blockers, digoxin, statins, CCBs, diuretics). In a post hoc analysis, dronedarone reduced the risk of stroke from 1.8% per year to 1.2% per year (HR 0.66); this was similar whether or not patients were receiving oral anticoagulant therapy, and there was a significantly greater effect of dronedarone in patients with higher CHADS2 scores.[5]

Dronedarone increased the mortality rate (8.1%) as compared with placebo (3.8%), in patients with NYHA class III or IV congestive HF and LV ejection fraction <35% (or referred to a specialty HF clinic, for worsening symptoms of HF, notably shortness of breath) primarily due to worsening congestive HF leading to death.[6] The risk of death and hospitalization was higher in patients with the most severe LV systolic dysfunction.

Pharmacokinetics

Dronedarone is well absorbed after oral administration, but it undergoes an extensive 1st-pass metabolism, so that oral bioavailability is ~5%, increasing to 15% when it is administered with a high-fat meal. Peak plasma concentrations of dronedarone and the main circulating active metabolite (*N*-debutyl metabolite) are reached within 3–6h and steady-state plasma concentrations after 5–8 days. Dronedarone and its active metabolite bind to plasma proteins (>98 %) and are widely distributed (V_d 20L/kg), crossing the blood–brain and placental barriers. It is excreted into breast milk in animals. Dronedarone is extensively metabolized, mainly by CYP3A, to active (*N*-debutyl metabolite) and inactive metabolites. Dronedarone is excreted in urine (6%) and faeces (84%), mainly as metabolites. Its elimination $t_{1/2}$ is 13–19h.

No pharmacokinetic difference was observed in patients with mild to severe renal impairment or moderate hepatic impairment.

Practical points

⚚ Doses
400mg bd

☺ Side effects
Frequent: GI disorders (diarrhoea, nausea, abdominal pain, vomiting, dyspepsia), asthenia, bradycardia, and QT prolongation

Other (<1%): skin reactions (rashes, pruritus, eczema, dermatitis, allergic dermatitis, photosensitivity), and dysgeusia

Dronedarone is not associated with thyroid, neurological, ocular, or pulmonary toxicity.

Interactions
Dronedarone is a moderate inhibitor of CYP3A4. Thus, it would be expected that potent CYP3A4 inhibitors [antifungals (ketoconazole, itraconazole, voriconazole), ciclosporin, macrolides (telithromycin, clarithromycin), protease inhibitors (nefazodone, and ritonavir)] increase the plasma levels of dronedarone. In fact, ketoconazole may increase dronedarone exposure by 17-fold. When co-administered with moderate CYP3A4 inhibitors (e.g. verapamil, diltiazem, sirolimus, tacrolimus, grapefruit), lower doses of concomitant drugs should be used. On the contrary, CYP3A inducers (rifampin, carbamazepine, phenytoin, and St John's wort) markedly decreased dronedarone exposure.

Dronedarone produces a 2- to 4-fold increase in simvastatin levels, with a potential risk of statin-induced myopathy.

Treatment with class I or III antiarrhythmics (e.g. amiodarone, flecainide, propafenone, quinidine, disopyramide, dofetilide, sotalol) should be avoided.

Dronedarone increases (1.7–2.5-fold) the digoxin plasma levels, possibly due to a P-glycoprotein-mediated interaction in the kidney. Thus, the dose of digoxin should be halved and the digoxin concentration should be monitored.

AV nodal blocking agents (β-blockers, diltiazem, verapamil) may increase the depressant effects of dronedarone on SA and AV nodes.

Dronedarone inhibits CYP2D6 and slightly increases the exposure of CYP2D6 substrates (propranolol, metoprolol, tricyclic antidepressants, and SSRIs).

Drugs that prolong the QTc interval (phenothiazines, tricyclic antidepressants) may induce torsades de pointes and, therefore, are contraindicated.

Cautions/notes
Hypokalaemia induced by K^+-depleting diuretics increases dronedarone-induced QT prolongation.

Pregnancy and lactation

Dronedarone may cause fetal harm when administered to a pregnant woman, and is contraindicated in women who are or may become pregnant (pregnancy category X). It should also be avoided in nursing mothers.

Contraindications

• Patients with NYHA class IV or NYHA class II–III HF with a recent decompensation
• 2nd- or 3rd-degree AV block (PR >280ms) or sick sinus syndrome except when used in conjunction with a functioning pacemaker
• Bradycardia <50bpm
• Concomitant use of a strong CYP3A inhibitor
• QT-prolonging drugs (phenothiazines, tricyclic antidepressants, some macrolide antibiotics, and class I and III antiarrhythmics) and QTc Bazett interval ≥500ms
• Severe hepatic impairment
• Pregnancy and nursing mothers

References

1 Touboul P *et al.* (2003). Dronedarone for prevention of atrial fibrillation: a dose-ranging study. *Eur Heart J* **24**:1481–7.
2 Singh BN *et al.* (2007). Dronedarone for maintenance of sinus rhythm in atrial fibrillation or flutter. *N Engl J Med* **357**:987–99.
3 Davy JM *et al.* (2008). Dronedarone for the control of ventricular rate in permanent atrial fibrillation: the Efficacy and safety of dRonedArone for the cOntrol of ventricular rate during atrial fibrillation (ERATO) study. *Am Heart J* **156**:527–9.
4 Hohnloser SH *et al.* (2009). Effect of dronedarone on cardiovascular events in atrial fibrillation. *N Engl J Med* **360**:668–78.
5 Connolly SJ *et al.*; for the ATHENA Investigators (2009). Analysis of Stroke in ATHENA: A Placebo-Controlled, Double-Blind, Parallel-Arm Trial to Assess the Efficacy of Dronedarone 400mg BID for the Prevention of Cardiovascular Hospitalization or Death From Any Cause in Patients With Atrial Fibrillation/Atrial Flutter. *Circulation* **120**:1174–80.
6 Kober L *et al.* (2008). Increased mortality after dronedarone therapy for severe heart failure. *N Engl J Med* **358**:2678–87.

Enalapril

(See also 📖 Angiotensin-converting enzyme inhibitors, p.355)
Orally active ACEI (prodrug).

Indications

(See 📖 Angiotensin-converting enzyme inhibitors, p.355)
(Enalapril does not have a specific indication for AMI or diabetic nephropathy.)

Mechanism of action

(See 📖 Renin–angiotensin–aldosterone system inhibitors, p.568 and 📖 Angiotensin-converting enzyme inhibitors, p.355)

Pharmacodynamics

(See 📖 Renin–angiotensin–aldosterone system inhibitors, p.568 and 📖 Angiotensin-converting enzyme inhibitors, p.355)

Heart failure: RRR ≈29% of death or development of HF in patients with asymptomatic HF and LVEF <35% given enalapril (titrated to 2.5–20mg/day) for ≈37 months compared with placebo.[1] A 12-year follow-up revealed that treatment with enalapril for 3–4 years extended median survival by 9.4 months.[2]

RRR ≈16% (absolute rate 35.2% vs. 39.7%) of death (mainly from progressive HF) in patients with HF (NYHA class II–III) and LVEF <35% given enalapril (titrated to 2.5–20mg/day) for ≈41 months compared with placebo.[3] RRR 26% in death or hospitalization for worsening HF.

RRR ≈31% in severe CHF (NYHA class IV) patients after 1 year treatment with enalapril cf placebo.[4] The reduction in total mortality was found to be among patients with progressive HF (a reduction of 50%), whereas no difference was seen in the incidence of sudden cardiac death.

Hypertension: RRR ≈30% (absolute rate 5.15 vs. 7.3%) of death of major non-fatal CV with enalapril 5mg/day (BP lowering of ≈14.7/11.5mmHg from baseline) compared with placebo (BP lowering 9.1/8.6mmHg from baseline) after a median 4.4 years in patients with mild hypertension with DBP <100mmHg receiving lifestyle advice.[5]

AMI: Mortality at 6 months was not significantly reduced in patients given IV infusion of enalapril within 24h of AMI and BP above 100/60mmHg compared with placebo (10.2% vs. 11.0%).[6]

Pharmacokinetics

Rapidly absorbed, reaching peak plasma levels within ≈1h; oral bioavailability ≈60% without influence of meals. Following absorption, enalapril is rapidly and extensively de-esterified to enalaprilat, a potent and active ACEI, whose levels peak within 4h of enalapril administration. Enalapril binds to protein (88%) and is excreted mainly by the kidney (40% enalaprilat, 20% enalapril). Exposure is increased in renal impairment and especially when CrCl is <30mL/min. It can be removed by dialysis. Terminal $t_{1/2}$ of ≈11h.

Practical points

♪ Doses
(See 📖 Angiotensin-converting enzyme inhibitors for initiation under supervision, p.355)

Hypertension: 5–20mg initially to maximum of 40mg/day

Heart failure: 2.5mg od initially to maximum of 40mg/day

Due to potential accumulation in renal impairment, dose should be reduced accordingly:

Creatinine clearance	Starting dose
30–80mL/min	5–10mg
10–30mL/min	2.5mg
<10mL/min	2.5mg on dialysis days

😊 **Side effects** (see 📖 Angiotensin-converting enzyme inhibitors, p.355)
Interactions (see 📖 Angiotensin-converting enzyme inhibitors, p.355)
Cautions (see 📖 Angiotensin-converting enzyme inhibitors, p.355)

Pregnancy and lactation
(See 📖 Angiotensin-converting enzyme inhibitors, p.355)
Limited pharmacokinetic data demonstrate very low concentrations of enalapril in breast milk. Although likely to be clinically irrelevant, its use in breastfeeding is not recommended for preterm infants or for the 1st few weeks after delivery. In the case of older infants, its use in breast-feeding may be considered, if this treatment is necessary for the mother and the child is observed for any adverse effect.

Contraindications (see 📖 Angiotensin-converting enzyme inhibitors, p.355)

References

1 The SOLVD Investigators (1992). Effect of enalapril on mortality and the development of heart failure in asymptomatic patients with reduced left ventricular ejection fractions. *N Engl J Med* **327**:685–91.
2 Jong P *et al.* (2003). Effect of enalapril on 12-year survival and life expectancy in patients with left ventricular systolic dysfunction: a follow-up study. *Lancet* **361**:1843–88.
3 The SOLVD Investigators (1991). Effect of enalapril on survival in patients with reduced left ventricular ejection fractions and congestive heart failure. *N Engl J Med* **325**:293–302.
4 Consensus Trial Study Group (1987). Effects of enalapril on mortality in severe congestive heart failure: Results of the Cooperative North Scandinavian Enalapril Survival Study (CONSENSUS). *N Engl J Med* **316**:1429–35.
5 Neaton JD *et al.* (1993). Treatment of Mild Hypertension Study. Final results. Treatment of Mild Hypertension Study Research Group. *JAMA* **270**:713–24.
6 Swedberg K *et al.* (1992). Effects of the early administration of enalapril on mortality in patients with acute myocardial infarction. Results of the Cooperative New Scandinavian Enalapril Survival Study II (CONSENSUS II). *N Engl J Med* **327**:678–84.

Enoxaparin

(See also 📖 Heparin, p.479 and 📖 Low-molecular-weight heparins, p.516)
LMWH.

CV indications

(See 📖 Heparin, p.479)
1. Prophylaxis of DVT
2. Treatment of DVT
3. Treatment following UA and NSTEMI
4. Treatment of acute STEMI receiving thrombolysis and being managed medically or with PCI

Mechanism of action

(See 📖 Heparin, p.479)

Pharmacodynamics

In aspirin-treated patients with NSTEMI, enoxaparin (1mg/kg SC bd administered for a minimum of 48h to a maximum of 8 days) reduced at 14 days the risk of death, MI, and urgent revascularization as compared to UFH (16.6% vs. 19.8%, $P=0.019$).[1] At 30 days, the risk of this composite endpoint and the need for revascularization procedures remained significantly lower in the enoxaparin group. The 30-day incidences of major bleeding complications were similar in both groups, but the incidence of bleeding overall was significantly higher in the enoxaparin group.

OR 0.82 in death, MI, or urgent revascularization occurred by 8 days (OR 0.85 by 45 days) in patients with UA/NSTEMI treated with enoxaparin during both the acute phase (30mg IV bolus followed by 1.0mg/kg SC every 12h) and the outpatient phase (injections every 12h) as compared to UFH.[2] There was no difference in the rate of major haemorrhage in the treatment groups during hospitalization, but there was an increase in the rate of major haemorrhage during the outpatient phase.

12% RR in death, MI, or refractory ischaemia at 7 days in patients with non-ST-elevation ACS treated with enoxaparin (1mg/kg every 12h) as compared with UFH who received tirofiban and aspirin.[3]

In elective PCI, enoxaparin (0.5 and 0.75mg/kg IV) reduced the rate of bleeding in the first 48h, as compared with UFH (5.9% vs 8.5%).[4] Target anticoagulation levels were reached in significantly more patients who received enoxaparin (79% and 92%) than in those who received UFH (20%).

Pharmacokinetics

Mean absolute bioavailability 100% after mg/kg given SC, reaching maximum anti-factor Xa activity after 3–5hr and steady state on the second day of treatment. The V_d of anti-factor Xa activity is about 0.12L/kg. Enoxaparin is metabolized in the liver to lower-molecular-weight species with much reduced biological potency that are eliminated in urine. Elimination $t_{1/2}$ based on anti-factor Xa activity is 4h after a single SC dose (7h after repeated dosing). In patients with severe renal impairment (CrCl <30 mL/min), the AUC of enoxaparin increases by 65%.

Practical points

◆ Doses
UA and NSTEMI: 1mg/kg SC every 12h (with 75–325mg daily of aspirin unless contraindicated) for 2–8 days. 1mg/kg od in patients with moderate renal impairment. Elderly: 0.75mg bd.

STEMI: single IV bolus of 30mg plus a 1mg/kg SC dose followed by 1mg/kg administered SC every 12h (all patients on aspirin unless contraindicated). When administered in conjunction with a thrombolytic, enoxaparin should be given between 15min before and 30min after the start of fibrinolytic drug. The duration of treatment may be longer than 8 days or until hospital discharge, whichever came first.

☺ Common side effects
(See 📖 Heparin, p.479)
Serious adverse reactions: spinal/epidural haematoma, increased risk of haemorrhage and thrombocytopenia

Fever, nausea, anaemia, oedema, reversible elevations of AST and ALT levels >3× the upper limit (6%)

Local reactions: irritation, pain, hematoma, ecchymosis, and erythema

Interactions
(See 📖 Heparin, p.479)

Cautions/notes
(See 📖 Heparin, p.479)
• Monitoring anticoagulant activity (anti-Xa levels) is not necessary except in patients with renal failure and in pregnant women.
• Bleeding is only partly reversed with protamine.
• Regular platelet counts are required and LMWH should be stopped if platelets <100,000/mm^3.

Pregnancy and lactation
(See 📖 Heparin, p.479)
Pregnancy category B

Contraindications
(See 📖 Heparin, p.479)
Severe renal impairment

References

1 Cohen M et al. (1997). A comparison of low-molecular-weight heparin with unfractionated heparin for unstable coronary artery disease. Efficacy and Safety of Subcutaneous Enoxaparin in Non-Q-Wave Coronary Events Study Group. *N Engl J Med* **337**:447–52.

2 Antman EM et al. (1999). Enoxaparin prevents death and cardiac ischemic events in unstable angina/non-Q-wave myocardial infarction. Results of the thrombolysis in myocardial infarction (TIMI) 11B trial. *Circulation* **100**:1593–601.

3 Blazing MA et al. for A to Z Investigators (2004). Safety and efficacy of enoxaparin vs unfractioned heparin in patients with non-ST-segment elevation acute coronary syndromes who receive tirofiban and aspirin: a randomized controlled trial. *JAMA* **292**:55–64.

4 Montalescot G et al.; STEEPLE Investigators (2006). Enoxaparin versus unfractionated heparin in elective percutaneous coronary intervention. *N Engl J Med* **355**:1006–17.

Eplerenone

(See also 📖 Aldosterone antagonists, p.339)

Selective aldosterone receptor antagonist (K⁺-sparing diuretic).

CV indications

1. Adjunctive therapy in stable LV systolic dysfunction and clinical evidence of congestive HF after an AMI
2. Treatment of hypertension

Mechanism of action

(See 📖 Spironolactone, p.588)
Compared to spironolactone, the presence of an epoxy group within the lactone ring in eplerenone results in minimal binding to glucocorticoid, androgen, and progesterone receptors, minimizing anti-androgenic (gynaecomastia, impotence) and antiprogesterone side effects of spironolactone, while maintaining mineralocorticoid receptor blockade.

Pharmacodynamics

It reduces BP in a dose-dependent manner (≈15/9mmHg with 40mg od).[1]
It is equally effective in white and black patients.[2]

In patients with AMI complicated by LV dysfunction and HF (NYHA class III–IV, LVEF ≤40%) eplerenone (mean dose of 42.6mg od), in combination with standard therapies, over 16 months of follow-up, produces 15% RRR in total mortality, 17% RRR in cardiovascular mortality (17%), and 13% RRR in CV death or hospitalization or hospitalization for cardiovascular events cf placebo.[3] There was also a 21% RRR in sudden death from cardiac causes. RRR all-cause mortality in post-MI groups with hypertension and/or diabetes and LVEF ≤30% by 43% and SCD by 58% at 30 days.

Pharmacokinetics

Oral bioavailability of eplerenone is ≈69% and absorption is not affected by food. Maximum concentrations are reached after ≈2hrs and steady state reached within 2 days. It binds to plasma proteins (50%), has a V_d ≈0.7L/kg, is metabolized by cytochrome P450 CYP3A4 and excreted mainly in the urine (67%) and partly (32%) in faeces. Elimination $t_{1/2}$ is ≈3–6h. Steady-state C_{max} and AUC are increased with renal impairment, liver insufficiency, HF, and in the elderly, and reduced in blacks.

Practical points

🎜 Doses

25–50mg od (maximum 50mg od). 25mg od when plasma K⁺ level >5.5mmol/L or creatinine plasma levels >2.5mg/dL; at higher levels, eplerenone is contraindicated

☺ Common side effects

(>1%): hyperkalaemia; hypotension, dizziness, headache; nausea, diarrhoea; rash, altered renal function, flu-like symptoms (e.g. fever, chills, unusual tiredness) and increased creatinine concentration

Interactions

Concomitant use with ACEIs, ARBs, other K⁺-sparing diuretics (e.g. amiloride, spironolactone, triamterene), K⁺ supplements, trimethoprim can precipitate serious hyperkalaemia, particularly in renal impairment. Concomitant use with α-blockers, tricyclic antidepressants, neuroleptics, amifostine, and baclofen may lead to potentiation of antihypertensive effects and postural hypotension. Ciclosporin and tacrolimus may impair renal function and increase risk of hyperkalaemia.

Levels of lithium should be monitored when used with eplerenone, due to potential risk of toxicity. Risk of acute renal failure may be increased when used with NSAIDs. Glucocorticoids reduce the antihypertensive effect of eplerenone.

Use of eplerenone with strong CYP3A4 inhibitors such as clarithromycin, ketoconazole, itraconazole, ritonavir, nelfinavir, erythromycin, telithromycin, and nefazodone is contraindicated due to potential enhanced effects. With mild to moderate CYP3A4 inhibitors (e.g. erythromycin, troleandomycin, amiodarone, diltiazem, verapamil, and fluconazole), eplerenone should not be used at doses above 25mg.

CYP3A4 inducers (e.g. rifampicin, carbamazepine, phenytoin, phenobarbital, St John's wort) decrease eplerenone efficacy, and their concomitant use is not recommended.

There are no pharmacokinetic interactions when eplerenone is administered with digoxin, warfarin, midazolam, cisapride, ciclosporin, simvastatin, glibenclamide, or oral contraceptives (norethisterone/ethinylestradiol).

Cautions/notes
K⁺ levels should be monitored at initiation and on change of dosage. Electrolyte levels should be monitored regularly, particularly in the elderly, and in those with renal and hepatic impairment. Eplerenone should not be used concomitantly with CYP3A4 inducers or lithium, ciclosporin, or tacrolimus. Tablets contain lactose and should not be administered in patients with rare hereditary problems of galactose intolerance, the Lapp lactase deficiency, or glucose-galactose malabsorption.

Pregnancy and lactation
Due to inadequate data, caution is required in pregnancy (pregnancy category B). Balance of risk/benefits should be made in breastfeeding due to detection of eplerenone in rat breast milk.

Contraindications
- Moderate and severe renal impairment (CrCl <30mL/min)
- Hyperkalaemia (>5mEq/L) at initiation
- Severe (Child–Pugh score C) hepatic impairment
- Concomitant treatment with drugs that produce hyperkalaemia and strong inhibitors of CYP3A4

References
1 Weinberger MH et al. (2002). Eplerenone, a selective aldosterone blocker, in mild-to-moderate hypertension. Am J Hypertens **15**:709–16.
2 Flack JM et al. (2003). Efficacy and tolerability of eplerenone and losartan in hypertensive black and white patients. J Am Coll Cardiol **41**:1148–55.
3 Pitt B et al. (2003). Eplerenone, a selective aldosterone blocker, in patients with left ventricular dysfunction after myocardial infarction. N Engl J Med **348**:1309–21.

Epoprostenol

(See also 📖 Prostanoids, p.558). Also known as prostacyclin (PGI_2), (member of the family of eicosanoids).

CV indications

Pulmonary arterial hypertension in WHO class III and IV patients.

Non-CV indications

Can be given to inhibit platelet aggregation during renal dialysis either alone or with heparin.

Mechanism of action

Pharmacodynamics

IV epoprostenol has been evaluated in controlled clinical trials in idiopathic PAH and PAH associated with scleroderma. It improves functional class, symptoms, exercise capacity, and haemodynamics; it is the only treatment to be shown in RCTs to improve survival in idiopathic PAH.[1,2]

Inhibits platelet aggregation.

Pharmacokinetics

Epoprostenol has an immediate onset of action. It is rapidly hydrolysed in the stomach and in plasma, which explains its poor tissue distribution (V_d 357mL/kg) and its short $t_{1/2}$ (4–6min). Thus, it must be administered by IV infusion via a central venous catheter coupled to a perfusion pump. Through this route it reached steady-state levels within 15min. Epoprostenol is metabolized to active metabolites that are eliminated in urine (93%). The dose should be halved in patients with hepatic insufficiency. Epoprostenol is only stable for 8h at room temperature and as such must be kept cool by using cold packs.

Practical points

⚬ Doses

Starting dose: 2–4ng/kg/min IV under close monitoring; the dose is further adjusted based on symptoms of PAH and side effects of the drug. Dose titration should be carried out in hospital due to the risk of pulmonary oedema. Optimal dose range for chronic therapy is 25–40ng/kg/min; doses >40ng/kg/min after 1 year of therapy are not uncommon.

☻ Side effects

Common side effects include: headache, flushing, hypotension, nausea, diarrhoea, skin rash, jaw pain, and musculoskeletal pain.

Infections and infusion interruptions can be life threatening.

Chronic overdose sometimes results in high cardiac output failure.

Interactions

Since PGI_2 is a *vasodilator*, additive hypotensive effects are expected when co-administered with antihypertensive agents or vasodilating agents.

Epoprostenol inhibits platelet aggregation, thereby increasing the risk of bleeding when co-administered with other antiplatelet drugs (e.g. aspirin) or anticoagulants (e.g. warfarin, heparin).

Contraindications
Patients with known hypersensitivity to the drug or to structurally related compounds.

Cautions/notes
Epoprostenol must be delivered by continuous IV infusion through a central venous catheter using an ambulatory infusion pump. Patients must learn the techniques of sterile preparation of the medication, operation of the ambulatory infusion pump, and care of the central venous catheter. Given the complexity, epoprostenol use should be limited to centres experienced with its administration and with systematic follow-up of patients.

Sudden discontinuation or reduction in therapy may result in rebound pulmonary hypertension.

Co-administration with anticoagulants reduces the risk of thromboembolism but this combination may increase the risk of bleeding.

Caution is advised when administering to patients with impaired kidney or liver function.

Pregnancy and lactation
Fetal risk in animal studies (FDA category class B). It is not known whether epoprostenol is excreted in breast milk. Thus, caution is advised when administering this medication to nursing women.

References

1 Sitbon O et al. (2002). Long-term intravenous epoprostenol infusion in primary pulmonary hypertension: prognostic factors and survival. *J Am Coll Cardiol* **40**:780–8.
2 McLaughlin VV et al. (2002). Survival in primary pulmonary hypertension: the impact of epoprostenol therapy. *Circulation* **106**:1477–82.

Eptifibatide

Cyclic heptapeptide glycoprotein IIb/IIIa receptor antagonist.

CV indications

1. In patients undergoing PCI
2. Prevention of early MI in patients with UA or NSTEMI with the last episode of chest pain occurring within 24h, ECG changes, and/or elevated
   cardiac enzymes

Mechanism of action

Eptifibatide reversibly inhibits platelet aggregation by preventing the binding of fibrinogen, von Willebrand factor, and other adhesive ligands to the
glycoprotein (GP)IIb/IIIa receptors.

Pharmacodynamics

The pivotal clinical trial for use of the eptifibatide in UA/non-Q wave
MI was the *PURSUIT trial*. In this trial, eptifibatide significantly reduced
the incidence of death from any cause or new MI within 30 days and this
reduction was maintained through 3 months. Bleeding was more common
in the eptifibatide group, although there was no increase in the incidence
of haemorrhagic stroke.[1]

The *ESPRIT trial* evaluated eptifibatide in patients undergoing non-urgent
PCI with intracoronary stenting. Eptifibatide significantly reduced the
incidence of 1° endpoints (composite of death, MI, urgent target vessel
revascularization).[2]

Pharmacokinetics

The effect of eptifibatide is observed immediately after administration of
IV bolus. It binds to plasma proteins (25%) and its V_d is 0.25L/kg. Platelet
inhibition was readily reversed (>50% platelet aggregation) 4h after stopping the continuous infusion. Plasma elimination $t_{1/2}$ is 3h. Renal excretion
≈50%.

Practical points

Doses

IV bolus: 90–180mcg/kg

IV infusion: 0.5–2mcg/kg/min for up to 72h. Reduce the dose to 0.5mcg/kg/
min at time of PCI, then for 20–24h after PCI

Common side effects

- Bleeding: minor bleeding (13%), major bleeding (10%)
- Thrombocytopenia 0.2%
- Other adverse events: AF, hypotension, congestive HF, cardiac arrest
  and allergic (anaphylactic) reactions

Interactions

(See 📖 Abciximab, p.330)

Cautions/notes
- Decrease doses in patients with moderate renal impairment (CrCl ≥30 to <50mL/min): an IV bolus of 180mcg/kg followed by a continuous infusion dose of 1.0mcg/kg/min.
- Experience in patients with hepatic impairment is very limited. It should be administered with caution to patients in whom coagulation could be affected.
- It is not recommended for use in children and adolescents, due to a lack of data on safety and efficacy.

Pregnancy and lactation
(See 📖 Abciximab, p.330)

Contraindications
- Hypersensitivity to the active substance or to any of the excipients
- Evidence of GI bleeding, gross GU bleeding, or other active abnormal bleeding within the previous 30 days of treatment
- History of stroke within 30 days or any history of haemorrhagic stroke
- Known history of intracranial disease (neoplasm, arteriovenous malformation, aneurysm)
- Major surgery or severe trauma within past 6 weeks
- History of bleeding diathesis
- Thrombocytopenia (<100,000 cells/mm^3)
- Prothrombin time >1.2× control or INR ≥2.0
- Severe hypertension (SBP >200mmHg or DBP >110mmHg on antihypertensive therapy)
- Severe renal impairment (CrCl <30mL/min) or dependency on renal dialysis
- Clinically significant hepatic impairment
- Concomitant or planned administration of another parenteral GP IIb/IIIa inhibitor

References

1 The PURSUIT Trial Investigators (1998). Inhibition of platelet glycoprotein IIb/IIIa with eptifibatide in patients with acute coronary syndromes. *N Engl J Med* **339**:436–43.
2 ESPRIT (2000). Novel dosing regimen of eptifibatide in planned coronary stent implantation: a randomized placebo controlled trial. *Lancet* **256**:2037.

Ezetimibe

Oral cholesterol-absorption inhibitor.

CV indications

As adjuvant therapy to diet in the management of:
1. 1° (heterozygous familial and non-familial) hyperlipidaemia (in combination with a statin) or mixed hyperlipidaemia (in combination with fenofibrate)
2. homozygous familial hypercholesterolaemia (heterozygous LDL receptor defect): co-administered with a statin
3. homozygous sitosterolaemia (phytosterolaemia).

Mechanism of action

Of the cholesterol available for absorption, 50% comes from hepatic secretions, 31% from dietary sources, and 19% from sloughing of epithelial cells. Of the total cholesterol available, 50% is absorbed and 50% is excreted in the faeces. Thus, a low-cholesterol diet reduces dietary intake of cholesterol from 31% to 15%, but this has little impact on overall plasma cholesterol levels, given the large contribution from the other sources.

Ezetimibe binds to the Niemann–Pick C1-Like 1 (NPC1L1) protein, which is responsible for the intestinal uptake of cholesterol and phytosterols, and inhibits the transport of cholesterol at the brush border membrane of the intestinal wall. The decreased cholesterol absorption leads to a decrease in the delivery of intestinal cholesterol to the liver, an upregulation of LDL receptors on the surface of cells, and an increased LDL-C uptake into cells, thus decreasing its plasma levels.

Pharmacodynamics

1° hypercholesterolaemia: 10mg ezetimibe daily (vs. placebo) reduced LDL-C by 18.5%, and increased HDL-C by 3.5% over 12 weeks.[1]

In a meta-analysis of 5 RCTs (5039 patients), combination ezetimibe/statin was superior to placebo/statin at reducing total cholesterol (16.1%) and LDL-C (23.6%) and increasing HDL-C (1.7%).[2]

Homozygous familial hypercholesterolaemia: ezetimibe co-administered with atorvastatin (40 or 80mg) or simvastatin (40 or 80mg) significantly reduced LDL-C by 20.7% compared with increasing the dose of simvastatin or atorvastatin monotherapy from 40 to 80mg (6.7% reduction) over 12 weeks in patients with or without concomitant LDL apheresis.[3]

Homozygous sitosterolaemia: ezetimibe 10mg/day (in addition to any current therapy) over 2 years led to significant reductions in sitosterol (43.9%), campesterol (50.8%), LDL-sterols (13.1%), total sterols (10.3%), and ApoB (−10.1%) plasma levels. The effects on morbidity and mortality in this population are not known.[4]

No incremental benefit of ezetimibe (10mg) plus simvastatin (80mg) on CV morbidity and mortality over that demonstrated for simvastatin. There was also no significant difference in carotid artery intima–media thickness between patients with familial hypercholesterolaemia taking ezetimibe and simvastatin for 2 years as compared with simvastatin alone, despite decreases in levels of LDL-C and C-reactive protein.[5] However, in this study many patients had already received lipid-lowering therapy and were starting with lower baseline intima–media thickness levels than in patients naïve to LDL-lowering therapy, which would result in smaller decreases in intima–media thickness over the course of the trial.[6]

The combination of simvastatin and ezetimibe reduced LDL-C levels by 50%, but did not reduce the composite outcome of combined aortic-valve events and ischaemic events in patients with AS.[7]

Pharmacokinetics

Ezetimibe is rapidly absorbed, reaching peak plasma levels after 1–2h; food has no effect on drug absorption. It is extensively conjugated in the liver and small intestine to a phenolic glucuronide (active metabolite); both parent drug and metabolite inhibit cholesterol absorption. Ezetimibe and its metabolite undergo repeated enterohepatic circulation, which returns it to the intestine. Ezetimibe binds to plasma proteins (90%), and approximately 78% and 11% of the administered dose is excreted in faeces and urine, respectively. Terminal $t_{1/2}$ is 22h. In patients with a moderate or severe hepatic impairment, the mean AUC values for total ezetimibe are increased approximately 3–4-fold, and 5–6-fold respectively.

Practical points

Doses

10mg PO od. A combination preparation ezetimibe/simvastatin (10mg of ezetimibe with 20, 40, or 80mg of simvastatin) is also available.

There is also a combination of ezetimibe (10mg) with fenofibrate (160mg) for patients with mixed hyperlipidaemia.

Adverse effects

GI, headache, mylagia, arthralgia, upper respiratory tract infection, diarrhoea. *Rare*: hypersensitivity reactions (rash, urticaria, angio-oedema, and anaphylaxis), hepatitis; very rarely pancreatitis, cholelithiasis, thrombocytopenia, myopathy, and rhabdomyolysis. A slightly higher percentage of patients have elevated levels (≥3× the upper limit of normal) of liver enzymes with ezetimibe and a statin combined than with a statin alone.

In combination with a statin: headache, fatigue, abdominal pain, constipation, diarrhoea, flatulence and nausea.

In combination with fenofibrate: abdominal pain.

Interactions

Ezetimibe does not affect the absorption of vitamin A, D, and C and does not interact with statins, fibrates, nicotinic acid, digoxin, warfarin, oral contraceptives, or cimetidine.

Colestyramine decreases the mean AUC of ezetimibe (55%) and the expected additional reduction in LDL-C; therefore dosing should occur either ≥2h before or ≥4h after colestyramine.

Co-administration with fenofibrate: possible risk of cholelithiasis and gall-bladder disease.

In combination with ciclosporin, it increases the plasma levels of both drugs. Thus, ciclosporin concentrations should be monitored.

Cautions/notes

Ezetimibe is not recommended in patients with moderate (Child–Pugh score 7–9) or severe (score >9) liver dysfunction. During co-administration with a statin, transaminases elevations (≥3× the upper limit) have been observed. Therefore LFTs should be assessed at initiation of therapy and at regular intervals during treatment.

Rhabdomyolysis has been reported very rarely in monotherapy or with the addition of other agents known to be associated with increased risk of rhabdomyolysis.

- If myopathy is suspected or confirmed by a creatine phosphokinase level >10× upper limit of normal, ezetimibe and any statin should be immediately discontinued.
- All patients starting therapy with ezetimibe should be advised of the risk of myopathy and asked to report any unexplained muscle pain, tenderness, or weakness.

Patients with rare hereditary problems, such as galactose intolerance, the Lapp lactase deficiency, or glucose-galactose malabsorption, should not take this drug.

Pregnancy and lactation

No clinical data available regarding use during pregnancy, and thus it should be given in pregnancy only if clearly necessary (pregnancy category C). Combination with statins is contraindicated in pregnancy (see 📖 Statins, p.591). It is unknown if ezetimibe is excreted into human breast milk and so it should not be used during lactation.

Contraindications

- Hypersensitivity to the active substance or the excipients
- Active liver disease or unexplained persistent elevations in hepatic transaminase levels
- Women who are pregnant or may become pregnant

References

1 Bays HE *et al.* (2001). Effectiveness and tolerability of ezetimibe in patients with primary hypercholesterolemia: pooled analysis of two phase II studies. *Clin Ther* **23**:1209–30.
2 Mikhailidis DP *et al.* (2007). Meta-analysis of the cholesterol-lowering effect of ezetimibe added to ongoing statin therapy. *Curr Med Res Opin* **23**:2009–26.
3 Gagné C *et al.* (2002). Efficacy and safety of ezetimibe co-administered with atorvastatin or simvastatin in patients with homozygous familial hypercholesterolemia. *Circulation* **105**:2469–75.
4 Lütjohann D *et al.* (2008). Long-term efficacy and safety of ezetimibe 10mg in patients with homozygous sitosterolemia: a 2-year, open-label extension study. *Int J Clin Pract* **62**:1499–510.
5 Kastelein JJP *et al.*; ENHANCE investigators (2008). Simvastatin with or without ezetimibe in familial hypercholesterolemia. *N Eng J Med* **358**:1431–43.
6 Brown BG, Taylor AJ (2008). Does ENHANCE diminish confidence in lowering LDL or in ezetimibe? *New Eng J Med* **358**:1504–47.
7 Rossebø AB *et al.* for the SEAS Investigators (2008). Intensive lipid lowering with simvastatin and ezetimibe in aortic stenosis. *N Eng J Med* **359**:1343–56.

Felodipine

(See also 📖 Calcium-channel blockers, p.390)
Oral dihydropyridine derivative L-type CCB.

CV indication

Treatment of hypertension.

Mechanism of action

Felodipine is vascular selective, and has no effect on cardiac conduction or contractility at therapeutic concentrations.

Pharmacodynamics

(See 📖 Calcium-channel blockers, p.390)
Felodipine appears to have a mild natriuretic/diuretic effect, reducing the reabsorption of filtered sodium.

Hypertension: it provides clinically significant, dose-dependent reductions in BP lasting at least 24h (trough DBP reduction is 11.3, 9.5, and 7.8mmHg with 10, 5, and 2.5mg of felodipine, respectively, compared with 5.3mmHg with placebo).[1]

Aggressive BP lowering to DBP ≤80 mmgHg compared to ≤90mmHg with baseline felodipine and additional antihypertensive agents as required in hypertensive patients (mean DBP ~105mmHg) and followed up for a mean 3.8 years is associated with a reduction of MI (2.6 vs. 3.6 events/1000 patient years) and of major CV events in diabetic patients (11.9 vs. 24.4 events/1000 patient years).[2]

Angina: compared to placebo, felodipine improves exercise tolerance, increasing the time until 1mm ST-segment depression on ETT as well as workload at time of 1mm ST-depression.[3]

HF: in patients with congestive HF felodipine (5mg bd) added to standard therapy (including enalapril and diuretics) exerts a well-tolerated additional sustained vasodilator effect, but has no effect on mortality or hospitalization rates.[4]

Pharmacokinetics

It is completely absorbed from the GI tract (unaffected by the concomitant intake of food), with a bioavailability of ~15%. Peak plasma concentrations are reached in 2.5–5h. It is ~99% protein bound, its V_d is 10L/kg, and it is extensively metabolized in the liver into inactive metabolites. About 70% is excreted in urine and 10% in the faeces. $t_{1/2}$ is ~14h with no significant accumulation in long-term treatment.

Practical points

🥄 Doses

5–10mg od (to maximum of 20mg od)
😊 **Side effects** (see 📖 Calcium-channel blockers, p.390)
Interactions (see 📖 Calcium-channel blockers, p.390)

Cautions/notes

(See also 📖 Calcium-channel blockers, p.390)

Should be used with caution in severe LV dysfunction.

Pregnancy and lactation

(See 📖 Calcium-channel blockers, p.390)

Contraindications

- Uncompensated HF; within 1 month after an AMI
- Pregnancy and lactation

References

1 Weber MA *et al.* (1994). Extended-release felodipine in patients with mild to moderate hyper-tension. Felodipine ER Dose-Response Study Group. *Clin Pharmacol Ther* **55**:346–52.

2 Hansson L *et al.* (1998). Effects of intensive blood-pressure lowering and low-dose aspirin in patients with hypertension: principal results of the Hypertension Optimal Treatment (HOT) randomised trial. HOT Study Group. *Lancet* **351**:1755–62.

3 Ekelund LG *et al.* (1994). Effects of felodipine versus nifedipine on exercise tolerance in stable angina pectoris. *Am J Cardiol* **73**:658–60.

4 Cohn JN *et al.* (1997). Effect of the calcium antagonist felodipine as supplementary vasodilator therapy in patients with chronic heart failure treated with enalapril: V-HeFT III. Vasodilator-Heart Failure Trial (V-HeFT) Study Group. *Circulation* **96**:856–63.

Fenofibrate

(See also 📖 Fibrates, p.462)

Oral PPAR-alpha receptor agonist.

CV indications

Severe dyslipidaemia (types IIa, IIb, III, IV, and V) where dietary measures alone have failed to produce an adequate response.

Mechanism of action

(See 📖 Fibrates, p.462)

Fenofibrate also has a uricosuric effect, potentially benefiting the ~20% of hyperlipidaemic patients with elevated plasma uric acid levels.

Pharmacodynamics

Fenofibrate 300mg daily reduces total cholesterol (18–20%), LDL-C (20–31%), ApoB (25%), and triglyceride (40–45%), and increases HDL-C (11%) levels compared to placebo over 6 months. The greatest effectiveness in the lowering of atherogenic lipoproteins was recorded in dyslipidaemia type IIa and III, while good effectiveness was experienced in type IV. In the case of type IIb the effectiveness was limited only to VLDL.[1] However, another study indicated similar improvement in lipid profiles in type IIb.[2]

11% RRR (5.2% vs. 5.9% absolute rate) in coronary events and CHD mortality, 24% RRR (3.2% vs. 4.2% absolute rate, P=0.01) in non-fatal MI and 21% RRR (5.9% vs. 7.4% absolute risk) in coronary revascularization, albuminuria progression, and retinopathy needing laser treatment, comparing micronized fenofibrate 200mg daily with placebo over an average of 5 years in patients aged 50–70 with type 2 diabetes mellitus and at increased risk of CV disease.[3]

After 39.6 months of treatment, fenofibrate (200mg/daily) reduced the progression of CHD in type 2 diabetic patients, with non-significant reduction of CV events.[4]

Pharmacokinetics

Fenofibrate is a prodrug that is well absorbed from the GI tract (bioavailability 60%), reaching peak plasma levels after 2–3h. It binds to plasma proteins (99%) and is rapidly hydrolysed by esterases to the active metabolite, fenofibric acid, which reaches peak plasma levels within 4–8h. Fenofibric acid is primarily conjugated with glucuronic acid and then excreted in urine (65%) and faeces (25%). Plasma $t_{1/2}$ of elimination is ~20h.

Practical points

·ℑ Doses

Starting dose 200mg od, up to the maximum dose of 267mg daily, and reduced in renal impairment

With the suprabioavailable formulation 'Supralip®', 160mg is equivalent to 200mg of the previous formulations.

☺ *Side effects* (see 📖 Fibrates, p.462)

Interactions (see 📖 Fibrates, p.462)

Cautions/notes

The use of fenofibrate should be avoided in patients with severe renal impairment; dose reduction is required in patients with mild to moderate renal impairment.

'*Supralip®*' *preparation:* should be stopped in case of an increase in creatinine levels >50% ULN.

Pregnancy and lactation
(See 📖 Fibrates, p.462)

Contraindications
(See 📖 Fibrates, p.462)
Hypersensitivity, known photoallergy or phototoxic reaction during treatment with ketoprofen

Chronic or acute pancreatitis (except acute pancreatitis due to severe hypertriglyceridaemia)

References

1 Canzler H, Bojanovski D (1980). Lowering effect of fenofibrate (procetofene) on lipoproteins in different types of hyperlipoproteinemias. *Artery* **8**:171–8.
2 Brown WV *et al.* (1986). Effects of fenofibrate on plasma lipids. Double-blind, multicenter study in patients with type IIA or IIB hyperlipidemia. *Arteriosclerosis* **6**:670–8.
3 Keech A *et al.* (2005). Effects of long-term fenofibrate therapy on cardiovascular events in 9795 people with type 2 diabetes mellitus (the FIELD study): randomised controlled trial. *Lancet* **366**:1849–61.
4 Vakkilainen J *et al.*; DAIS Group (2003). Relationships between low-density lipoprotein particle size, plasma lipoproteins, and progression of coronary artery disease: the Diabetes Atherosclerosis Intervention Study (DAIS). *Circulation* **107**:1733–7.

Fibrates

(See also 📖 Bezafibrate, p.382, 📖 Fenofibrate, p.460, 📖 Gemfibrozil, p.475.)

Oral PPAR-α receptor agonists.

CV indications

1. Hyperlipidaemias of type IIa, IIb, III, IV, and V, especially in hypertriglyc-eridaemia or low HDL-C when dietary measures alone have failed to produce an adequate response
2. Considered when statins are inappropriate, not tolerated or not suf-ficiently efficacious as monotherapy
3. To reduce the risk of pancreatitis in patients with high triglyceride plasma levels

Mechanism of action

The mechanism of action has not been definitively established, and it is unclear if all fibrates act via the same pathways.

Fibrates are amphiphatic carboxylic acids acting as agonists of the peroxi-some proliferator-activated receptor type-alpha (PPAR-α), a nuclear tran-scription factor, in skeletal muscle, liver, and other tissues. This modulates lipoprotein metabolism, increasing the expression of lipoprotein lipase (LPL) and of ApoA-I and ApoA-II, while reducing the expression of ApoC-III genes.[1]

It is suggested that fibrates potentially alter lipoprotein levels by 5 mechanisms:[1]

- increased lipoprotein lipolysis of triglyceride-rich remnant lipoproteins and VLDL due to an increase in LPL activity or a reduction of ApoC-III (an inhibitor of LPL activity)
- induction of the hepatic β-oxidation pathway with a concomitant decrease in fatty acid (FA) synthesis resulting in a lower availability of FAs for triglyceride production and VLDL synthesis
- increased removal of LDL particles. Fibrates result in the formation of LDLs with a higher affinity for the LDL receptor, which are thus catabolized more rapidly
- reduction in triglyceride exchange between VLDL and HDL-C may result from decreased plasma levels of triglyceride-rich particles
- increased synthesis of ApoA-I and ApoA-II in the liver, which may contribute to the increase of plasma HDL concentrations and a more efficient reverse cholesterol transport

(See 📖 individual drugs for additional proposed mechanisms of action)

Pharmacodynamics

A meta-analysis of 10 RCTs revealed:

- a significant decrease in non-fatal MI in the fibrate group (OR 0.78, 95% CI 0.71–0.86, $P<0.00001$, including clofibrate studies; OR 0.75, 95% CI 0.67–0.85, $P<0.00001$, without clofibrate studies)
- no significant effect on all-cause or CV mortality

- non-CV mortality is increased in the fibrate group including clofibrate studies (OR 1.16, 95%CI 1.05–1.29, $P<0.05$). However, in the analysis of currently available fibrates (excluding clofibrate), there are no statistical differences in non-cardiovascular mortality.[2]

(See 📖 individual drugs for specific trial data)

Pharmacokinetics
(See 📖 individual drugs)

Practical points

📖 Doses (see 📖 individual drugs)

☺ Side effects
Common: nausea, loss of appetite, vomiting, diarrhoea, constipation, dyspepsia, flatulence, abdominal discomfort, cholelithiasis (women, obese, diabetics)

CNS: dizziness, somnolence, paraesthesia, depression, decreased libido, headache, blurred vision

Others: impotence, anaemia, leukopenia, eosinophilia, rash, dermatitis, pruritus

Musculoskeletal: myopathy (muscle pain with CPK elevations), myalgia, painful extremities. Isolated cases of rhabdomyolysis leading to renal failure have been described. Risk may be increased in renal impairment, hypothyroidism, severe infection, trauma, surgery, or electrolyte imbalance and a high alcohol intake.

Clinical laboratory: increases in liver transaminases, bilirubin, alkaline phosphatase and creatine phosphokinase

(See 📖 individual drugs for specific side effects)

Interactions
Combination therapy with statins increases the risk of liver and muscle toxicity. Risks and benefits should be assessed prior to initiation of combination therapy.

Anticoagulants: fibrates may potentiate effects of oral anticoagulants. The dose of anticoagulants should be reduced (e.g. 2/3 to 1/2 normal dose), and frequent INR determinations should be performed until its level is stabilized.

Isolated cases of reversible impairment of renal function have been reported when bezafibrate or fenofibrate (but potentially not gemfibrozil) are co-administered with ciclosporin in organ transplant patients.

Resins potentiate the lipid-lowering effects of fibrates, but may reduce oral bioavailability of fibrates. Fibrates should be taken at least 1h before or 4–6h after resins.

High-dose niacin (>1g/day) can increase the risk of myopathy.

Fibrates displace other drugs (phenytoin, oral hypoglycaemic agents, levothyroxine) from plasma proteins and increase their free plasma levels; doses of these drugs should be reduced as needed.

(See 📖 individual drugs for specific interactions)

Cautions/notes

Monitoring for muscular disorders:

- In most subjects who have had unsatisfactory lipid responses to either statins or fibrates alone, the possible benefits of combined therapy do not outweigh the risks of severe myopathy, rhabdomyolosis, and acute renal failure.
- Creatine phosphokinase (CPK) level should be measured before starting such a combination in patients with predisposing factors for rhabdomyolysis—renal impairment, hypothyroidism, alcohol abuse, age >70 years, personal or family history of hereditary muscular disorders, previous history of muscular toxicity with another fibrate or statin.
- Myopathy should be suspected in patients presenting with diffuse myalgia, myositis, muscular cramps and weakness, and/or marked increases in CPK, e.g. ≥5× normal range.
- CPK should not be measured following strenuous exercise or in the presence of any plausible alternative cause of CPK increase, as this makes value interpretation difficult.

Monitoring of LFTs is recommended prior to therapy, periodically after, and in patients who develop any signs or symptoms suggestive of liver injury:

- Stopping fibrates should be considered in transaminase elevations to ≥3× upper limit of normal or ≥100 IU.
- Patients who develop increased transaminase levels should be monitored until resolution.

Periodic determinations of serum lipids are necessary during treatment with fibrates.

- Sometimes a paradoxical increase of (total and LDL) cholesterol can occur in patients with hypertriglyceridaemia.
- If the response is insufficient after 3 months of therapy at recommended doses, treatment should be discontinued and alternative treatment methods considered.

Fibrates may also activate PPAR-γ, hence improving glucose utilization:

- Careful monitoring is recommended in diabetic patients.
- Hypoglycaemia has been reported with gemfibrozil, but not regularly reported with bezafibrate or fenofibrate.

Dose adjustment may be required in elderly and in patients with renal dysfunction (see 📖 individual drugs for specifics).

Pregnancy and lactation

Animal models suggest deleterious effects in pregnancy. In general, not recommended in pregnant and breastfeeding women (pregnancy category C).

Contraindications

- Hypersensitivity to (any) fibrate or the excipients

- Severe hepatic impairment and patients with 1° biliary cirrhosis and persistent liver function abnormalities
- Severe renal impairment (see 📖 individual drugs)
- Pre-existing gallbladder or biliary tract disease, with or without cholelithiasis

(See 📖 individual drugs for specific contraindications)

References

1 Staels B et al. (1998). Mechanism of action of fibrates on lipid and lipoprotein metabolism. Circulation 98:2088–93.
2 Saha SA et al. (2007). The role of fibrates in the prevention of cardiovascular disease—a pooled meta-analysis of long-term randomized placebo-controlled clinical trials. Am Heart J 154:943–53.

Flecainide

(See also 📖 Antiarrhythmic drugs: classification, p.362)

Na$^+$ channel blocker with class Ic properties.

CV indications

Oral formulation:
1*. Paroxysmal supraventricular tachycardias (PSVT), including AV nodal reentrant tachycardia, AV reentrant tachycardia and other arrhythmias associated with WPW syndrome and similar conditions with accessory pathways associated with disabling symptoms
2*. Paroxysmal or persistent atrial fibrillation (and flutter) in patients without structural heart disease. Flecainide can also be used for maintenance of sinus rhythm after cardioversion by other means
3*. Symptomatic sustained VT
4. Premature VCs and/or non-sustained VT causing disabling symptoms, which are resistant to other therapy or when other treatment has not been tolerated.

*Intravenous formulation: indicated when the rapid control of ventricular rate is required in these situations.

Mechanism of action

Flecainide blocks fast Na$^+$ channels that are responsible for the rapid depolarization (phase 0) of fast-response cardiac action potentials found in non-nodal cardiomyocytes. By inhibiting rapid Na$^+$ entry into cells, flecainide decreases the slope of phase 0, amplitude of the action potential, and conduction velocity, particularly in the His–Purkinje system, and thus results in negative dromotropy. Flecainide also reduces automaticity by decreasing the slope of phase 4, via a mechanism unrelated to its action on fast Na$^+$ channels (general class I effects). Flecainide has no effect on the duration of the ventricular action potential (APD) but extends the effective refractory period by prolonging the reactivation of the Na$^+$ channel and blocking several K$^+$ currents. However, flecainide prolongs atrial APD and refractoriness. The marked depression of conduction velocity, together with a heterogeneous prolongation of the APD, may explain the proarrhythmic effects of flecainide.

Pharmacodynamics

Flecainide does not modify heart rate, although bradycardia and tachycardia have been reported. ECG changes: it prolongs the PR and QRS intervals (particularly at fast heart rates), while the QTc interval remains unaffected. Flecainide decreases intracardiac conduction in all parts of the heart with the greatest effect on the His–Purkinje system.

Flecainide increases endocardial pacing thresholds.

At a median dose of 300mg od, flecainide prevented PAF in 31% (cf 9% with placebo) over a 16-week period and increased median time to 1st episode of PAF to 15 days (cf 3 days with placebo).[1]

In selected, risk-stratified patients with recurrent AF, out-of-hospital self-administration of flecainide (pill-in-the-pocket approach) is feasible and safe, with a high rate of compliance by patients, a low rate of adverse effects and a marked reduction in emergency room visits and hospital admissions.[2]

Pharmacokinetics

Flecainide is readily absorbed after oral administration (bioavailability 95%), reaching peak plasma levels in 2–3h. Food or antacids do not affect absorption. Milk, however, may inhibit absorption in infants. $t_{1/2}$ is approximately 20h (12–27h); elimination $t_{1/2}$ after IV administration appears to be 9–17h). Flecainide excretion depends on renal function (i.e. 35% appears in urine as unchanged drug); the remainder is metabolized by the cytochrome P450 2D6 isoenzyme in the liver. Therapeutic plasma levels: 3–8mcg/ml.

Practical points

♣ Doses

PO: 50mg bd (max: 300mg/day) for SVTs
100–200mg bd (max: 400mg/day) for ventricular arrhythmias

Dose reduction is recommended in renal impairment (GFR <35mL/min/1.73m²). After 3–5 days, dose should be lowered to minimal effective dose. Given long $t_{1/2}$, increases in doses should not be more frequently than approximately once every 4 days.

IV: where required, dilution should be with 5% dextrose; otherwise a volume >500mL of 0.9% NaCl to avoid precipitation
- IV bolus injection: 2mg/kg (max bolus dose: 15mg) (over no less than 10min or in divided doses; or diluted in 5% dextrose and given as mini-infusion). A bolus dose can be administered in an emergency or when rapid response is required. ECG monitoring is recommended for all patients receiving a bolus dose
- IV infusion: (1) 2mg/kg over 0.5h; followed by (2) 1.5mg/kg for 1st hour; then (3) 0.1–0.25mg/kg/h (max recommended dose over 24h: 600mg)

Prolonged parental administration over 24h is generally not recommended. Where necessary, monitor plasma levels in those receiving doses at the upper limit. Doses should be halved in patients with renal impairment (GFR <35ml/min/1.73m²). Transition to oral administration should be achieved as soon as possible.

☺ Common side effects

(>10%): dizziness; visual disturbances; dyspnoea

(1–10%): headache, nausea, fatigue, palpitation, chest pain, abdominal pain, constipation, tremor, oedema

Cardiovascular: bradycardia, tachycardia, hypo/hypertension, AV block, cardiac arrest, proarrhythmia. In AF, flecainide may induce atrial flutter with 1:1 conduction leading to a rapid ventricular response.

Nervous: nightmares, tremor, confusion, numbness, paraesthesias, tinnitus, vertigo.

Interactions

Flecainide interacts with other antiarrhythmic drugs. There are added negative inotropic and AV nodal depressant effects when added to β-blockers, propafenone, verapamil, and diltiazem. Decrease in intracardiac conduction when added to class Ia drugs.

Levels of flecainide, risk of toxicity, or arrhythmia may be increased during concomitant use with amiodarone (inihibits CYP2D6), cimetidine, antivirals (ritonavir, lopinavir, and indinavir), terfenadine, fluoxetine, paroxetine, tricyclic antidepressants, and clozapine. Flecainide increases digoxin levels. Use of flecainide with other sodium-channel blockers is not recommended.

Cautions/notes

- In post-MI patients (up to 2 years after MI) with asymptomatic ventricular non-sustained arrhythmias, flecainide was associated with increased risk of death of 5.1% (cf 2.3% with placebo).[3]
- Flecainide is known to increase endocardial pacing thresholds, and thus should be used with caution in patients with permanent pacemakers or temporary pacing electrodes; it should not be administered to patients with existing poor thresholds or non-programmable pacemakers unless suitable pacing rescue is available.
- It should be used with caution in patients with acute onset of AF following cardiac surgery. Monitoring of levels may be helpful in patients with renal failure, given its slower excretion in such patients.

Pregnancy and lactation

Flecainide has been shown to cross placenta to fetus (pregnancy category C). It is also known to be excreted in human milk, with levels reflecting maternal blood levels.

Contraindications

- Structural heart disease (HF, CAD, cardiogenic shock) or with abnormal LV function
- Post-MI patients with asymptomatic VCs or non-sustained VT
- Severe bradycardia, sinus node dysfunction, atrial conduction defects, 2nd-degree or greater AV block, bundle branch block or distal block—unless pacing rescue is available
- Severe electrolyte balance (hypo/hyperkalaemia)

References

1 Anderson JL et al. (1989). Prevention of symptomatic recurrences of paroxysmal atrial fibrillation in patients initially tolerating antiarrhythmic therapy. A multicenter, double-blind, crossover study of flecainide and placebo with transtelephonic monitoring. Flecainide Supraventricular Tachycardia Study Group. *Circulation* **80**:1557–70.

2 Alboni P et al. (2004). Outpatient treatment of recent-onset atrial fibrillation with the 'pill-in-the-pocket' approach. *Engl J Med* **351**:2384–91.

3 The Cardiac Arrhythmia Suppression Trial (CAST) Investigators (1989). Preliminary report: effect of encainide and flecainide on mortality in a randomized trial of arrhythmia suppression after myocardial infarction. *N Engl J Med* **321**:406–12.

Fluvastatin

(See also 📖 Statins, p.591)

Oral HMG-CoA reductase inhibitor.

CV indications

1. 1° hypercholesterolaemia, heterozygous familial hypercholesterolaemia or mixed dyslipidaemia, as an adjunct to diet, when response to non-pharmacological treatments is inadequate
2. 2° prevention of coronary events

Mechanism of action

(See 📖 Statins, p.591)

Pharmacodynamics

1° hypercholesterolaemia

Reduces LDL-C, total cholesterol, triglycerides and increases HDL-C (Table 8).

Table 8 Effects of fluvastatin on lipid profile (mean adjusted % change from baseline)

Dose (mg)	Percentage change			
	Total chol	LDL chol	HDL chol	TG
Placebo	−2.0	−1.0	−1.0	+9.0
20	−17.0	−22.0	+3.0	−12.0
40	−19.0	−25.0	+4.0	−14.0
80	−25.0	−35.0	+6.0	−19.0

2° prevention

22% RRR of recurrent cardiac events (181 vs. 222 patients) and 32% RRR of late revascularization procedures (CABG or PCI) with fluvastatin 80mg compared with placebo after 3.9 years in patients with CHD who had undergone a PCI.[1]

28% RRR of major adverse cardiac events (MACE) among patients with UA treated for 3.9 years with fluvastatin 80mg/day after a first PCI compared to patients on placebo.[4] 35% RRR in coronary atherosclerotic events (MACE excluding restenosis) in patients with UA (31% RRR in patients with stable angina).

Pharmacokinetics

Fluvastatin is absorbed rapidly and completely (bioavailability 9–50%), with peak concentrations reached in 0.5–1.5h. Administration of a high-fat meal delayed the absorption and increased the bioavailability by 50%. Fluvastatin is ≈98% bound to plasma proteins (V_d is ≈0.35L/kg). Fluvastatin is metabolized in the liver via CYP2C9 (75%), CYP2C8 (~5%), and CYP3A4 (~20%) isoenzymes. Fluvastatin is primarily (about 90%) eliminated in the faeces as metabolites, with <2% present as unchanged drug. Urinary excretion is about 5%. Plasma elimination $t_{1/2}$ is 3h.

Practical points

♣ Doses
20–80mg od (taken at night)
Dose adjustments for mild to moderate renal impairment are not necessary

☺ Side effects
(See 📖 Statins, p.591)
Persistent transaminase elevations (>3× ULN on 2 consecutive weekly measurements) occurred in 0.2%, 1.5%, and 2.7% of patients treated with 20, 40, and 80mg.

Interactions
(See 📖 Statins, p.591)
- CYP2C9 inhibitors increase the plasma levels of fluvastatin; reduce the dose of fluvastatin.
- Fluvastatin increases the plasma levels of S-warfarin (monitor the INR).
- Patients treated with glibenclamide (glyburide) and fluvastatin should be monitored when the fluvastatin dose is increased to 40mg bd.
- Cimetidine/ranitidine/omeprazole reduce (24–33%) fluvastatin plasma clearance and increase fluvastatin C_{max} (43%, 70%, and 50%, respectively).
- Concomitant use of fluvastatin and phenytoin increases the plasma levels of both drugs.

Cautions/notes (see 📖 Statins, p.591)

Pregnancy and lactation (see 📖 Statins, p.591)

Contraindications (see 📖 Statins, p.591)

References
1 Serruys PW et al.; Lescol Intervention Prevention Study (LIPS) Investigators (2002). Fluvastatin for prevention of cardiac events following successful first percutaneous coronary intervention: a randomized controlled trial. *JAMA* **287**:3215–22.
2 Holdaas H et al. (2003). Effect of luvastatin on cardiac outcomes in renal transplant recipients: a multicenter, randomised, placebo-controlled trial. *Lancet* **361**:2024–31.
3 LCAS Investigators (1997). Effects of fluvastatin on coronary atherosclerosis in patients with mild to moderate cholesterol elevations (Lipoprotein and Coronary Atherosclerosis Study [LCAS]). *Am J Cardiol* **80**:278–86.
4 Lee CH et al. (2004). Beneficial effects of fluvastatin following percutaneous coronary intervention in patients with unstable and stable angina: results from the Lescol intervention prevention study (LIPS). *Heart* **90**:1156–61.

Fondaparinux

A synthetic pentasaccharide (1728Da) that acts as a specific inhibitor of activated factor X.

CV indications

1. Prophylaxis of VTE in patients immobilized because of acute illness, and patients undergoing major orthopaedic surgery of the legs or abdominal surgery who are at risk for thromboembolic complications
2. Treatment of acute DVT and pulmonary embolism, administered in conjunction with warfarin
3. Treatment of UA, NSTEMI, or STEMI

Mechanism of action

The antithrombotic activity of fondaparinux is the result of antithrombin III (ATIII)-mediated selective inhibition of factor Xa. By selectively binding to and potentiating the action of ATIII, fondaparinux potentiates (about 300×) the innate neutralization of factor Xa by ATIII. Neutralization of factor Xa interrupts the blood coagulation cascade and thus inhibits thrombin formation and thrombus development.

Fondaparinux does not inactivate thrombin (factor IIa), has no known effect on platelet function, and does not affect fibrinolytic activity or bleeding time.

The effect of fondaparinux is derived from fondaparinux plasma concentrations quantified via anti-factor Xa activity; this activity increases with increasing drug concentration, reaching maximum values in approximately 3h.

Pharmacodynamics

The clinical programme has focused on prophylaxis of vein thrombosis after orthopaedic surgery, acute therapy of vein thrombosis, 2° prevention of recurrent vein thrombosis, and ACSs.

In 4 RCTs, fondaparinux (2.5mg od) initiated 6h after major orthopaedic surgery reduced the incidence of VTE by day 11 compared with enoxaparin (6.8% vs. 13.7%), with an odds reduction of 55.2%.[1] Although major bleeding occurred more frequently in the fondaparinux-treated group, the incidence of clinically relevant bleeding (leading to death or reoperation or occurring in a critical organ) did not differ between groups.

Fondaparinux (7.5mg od) for 5 days was at least as effective as enoxaparin (1mg/kg SC bd) in the initial treatment of symptomatic DVT; major bleeding (1.1% vs. 1.2%) and mortality rates (3.8% vs. 3%) were similar in both groups.[2]

In the OASIS trial, no difference (5.8% vs. 5.7%) in death, MI, or refractory ischaemia at 9 days was observed in patients with UA or NSTEMI treated with SC fondaparinux 2.5mg/day or SC enoxaparin (1mg/kg tds or od in those with renal dysfunction) for a mean of 6 days. The efficacy was maintained for up to 6 months.[3] Fondaparinux was associated with a 50% reduction in major bleeding at 9 days, resulting in a benefit:risk balance favouring fondaparinux.

13% RRR (11% vs. 9.7%) in death or recurrent MI at 30 days in patients with STEMI treated with SC fondaparinux 2.5mg/day given for up to 8 days compared with control patients (receiving placebo or IV UFH).[4] This benefit was marked in patients who received thrombolytics (OR 0.80) or no reperfusion therapy (OR 0.79). There were no differences in the incidence of major bleeding between these groups, resulting in a benefit:risk balance favouring fondaparinux. Thus, overall, fondaparinux was non-inferior to enoxaparin in patients with UA or NSTEMI, and was more effective in those with STEMI.

Fondaparinux (2.5mg daily) is similar to enoxaparin (1mg/kg tds) in reducing the risk of death, MI, or refractory ischaemia, major bleeding, and their combination, at 9 and 180 days in patients with ACS, but it substantially reduces major bleeding and improves long-term mortality and morbidity.[5] The rate of major bleeding at 9 days was markedly lower with fondaparinux than with enoxaparin.

Pharmacokinetics

After SC injection, fondaparinux is rapidly and completely absorbed (bioavailability 100%), reaching peak plasma concentrations within 2–3h. It distributes mainly in blood and only to a minor extent in extravascular fluid (V_d ~0.15L/kg). In vitro, fondaparinux sodium is highly (at least 94%) and specifically bound to ATIII and does not bind significantly to other plasma proteins. Up to 77% of the dose is eliminated unchanged in urine in 72h. The elimination $t_{1/2}$ is 17–21h (longer in elderly patients with renal failure).

The specificity and selectivity of fondaparinux, combined with its long $t_{1/2}$ and 100% bioavailability, allows once-daily anticoagulation without the need for monitoring activated clotting time.

Practical points

₰ Doses

Fondaparinux is provided in a single dose, prefilled syringe with an automatic needle protection system. It should be administered SC (not IM).

Prophylaxis of VTE after surgery: 2.5mg 6h after surgery; then 2.5mg od for 5–9 days (longer after hip surgery)

Prophylaxis of VTE in medical patients: 2.5mg od usually for 6–14 days

ACS: 2.5mg SC for up to 8 days (or until hospital discharge if sooner)

Treatment of DVT and pulmonary embolism: 5mg (body weight <50kg), 7.5mg (body weight 50–100kg) or 10mg (>100kg) SC every 24h; usually for at least 5–9 days (and until adequate oral anticoagulation established)

☻ Common side effects

Bleeding, purpura, anaemia; less commonly GI disturbances (nausea, vomiting, dyspepsia), oedema, hepatic impairment, chest pain, dyspnoea, thrombocytopenia (but no HIT has been reported), thrombocythaemia, rash, pruritus; rarely hypotension, flushing, cough, vertigo, dizziness, anxiety, drowsiness, confusion, headache, hypokalaemia, hyperbilirubinaemia, injection-site reactions; also reported AF, tachycardia, and pyrexia.

Interactions

There are no known drug or food interactions.

The concomitant use of oral anticoagulants (warfarin), platelet inhibitors (acetylsalicylic acid), NSAIDs, and digoxin did not significantly affect the pharmacokinetics/pharmacodynamics of fondaparinux sodium.

Agents that may enhance the risk of haemorrhage should be discontinued prior to initiation of therapy with fondaparinux sodium. If co-administration is essential, close monitoring may be appropriate.

Cautions/notes

- Bleeding disorders, active GI ulcer disease; recent intracranial haemorrhage; brain, spinal, or ophthalmic surgery; spinal or epidural anaesthesia (risk of spinal haematoma); risk of catheter thrombus during PCI; low body weight; elderly patients; concomitant use of drugs that increase risk of bleeding; hepatic impairment; renal impairment. The anticoagulant effect of fondaparinux may be reversed with recombinant factor VII.
- The clearance of fondaparinux decreases in elderly people and with renal impairment; thus, the dose should be adjusted according to creatinine clearance.
- The occurrence of major bleeding is doubled in patients with a body weight <50kg.

Pregnancy and lactation

Animal studies have revealed harm to the fetus. However, there are no adequate and well-controlled studies in pregnant women (pregnancy category B). It is not known whether this drug is excreted in human milk, and caution should be exercised when fondaparinux is administered to a nursing mother.

Contraindications

- Active major bleeding, impaired haemostasis, infective endocarditis
- Severe renal impairment (creatinine clearance <30mL/min)
- Patients with thrombocytopenia associated with a positive in vitro test for antiplatelet antibody in the presence of fondaparinux

References

1 Turpie AG et al. (2002). Fondaparinux vs enoxaparin for the prevention of venous thromboembolism in major orthopedic surgery: a meta-analysis of 4 randomized double-blind studies. *Arch Intern Med* **162**:1833–40.

2 Büller HR et al.; Matisse Investigators (2004). Fondaparinux or enoxaparin for the initial treatment of symptomatic deep venous thrombosis: a randomized trial. *Ann Intern Med* **140**:867–73.

3 Yusuf S et al. (2006). Comparison of fondaparinux and enoxaparin in acute coronary syndromes. *N Engl J Med* **354**:1464–76.

4 Yusuf S et al.; The OASIS-6 Trial Group (2006). Effects of fondaparinux on mortality and reinfarction in patients with acute ST-elevation myocardial infarction. The OASIS-6 randomized trial. *JAMA* **295**:1519–30.

5 Fifth Organization to Assess Strategies in Acute Ischemic Syndromes Investigators et al. (2006). Comparison of fondaparinux and enoxaparin in acute coronary syndromes. *N Engl J Med* **354**: 1464–76.

Furosemide

(See also 📖 Loop diuretics, p.507)

Loop diuretic (PO, IM, IV).

CV indications (see 📖 Loop diuretics, p.507)

Others: (see 📖 Loop diuretics, p.507)

Mechanism of action

(See 📖 Loop diuretics, p.507)

Pharmacodynamics

The onset of diuresis following PO administration is within 1.5h, with peak effect occuring within 1–2h. The duration of diuretic effect is 3–6h. By IV route, diuresis peak effects are observed within 15min.

Pharmacokinetics

(See 📖 Loop diuretics, p.507)

Rapidly absorbed from the GI tract, with low and variable bioavailability (26–65%). Food reduces the absorption of furosemide and it should be taken with an empty stomach. It is 99% bound to plasma proteins and is glucuronidated in the liver, but is largely excreted (60–80%) unchanged in urine. Elimination $t_{1/2}$ is 1.5–3h.

Practical points

⚡ Doses

PO: 10–40mg bd for hypertension; 20–80mg 2–3 times daily for CHF (adjusted according to response); bd doses should be given early in the morning and mid-afternoon to avoid nocturia.

IV: 20–40mg over 20min (increased in 20mg steps if necessary not less than every 2h; to maximum of 1.5g daily).

In patients with refractory HF with severe renal failure, furosemide (160–320mg) plus metolazone may be required to promote diuresis. When GFR <20mL/min high doses (up to 2g daily) may be needed because of reduced luminal excretion.

☺ **Common side effects** (see 📖 Loop diuretics, p.507)

Interactions (see 📖 Loop diuretics, p.507)
Furosemide does not decrease the renal excretion of lithium.

Cautions/notes (see 📖 Loop diuretics, p.507)

Pregnancy and lactation

Crosses the placental barrier. It is also excreted in breast milk, albeit in amounts probably too small to be harmful, and can impair lactation. Hence, should be avoided in pregnancy and breastfeeding (pregnancy category C).

Contraindications (See 📖 Loop diuretics, p.507)

Gemfibrozil

(See also 📖 Fibrates, p.462)

Oral PPAR-α receptor agonist.

CV indications

1. Adult patients with very high triglyceride levels (types IV and V hyper-lipidaemia) who present a risk of pancreatitis and who do not respond adequately to diet
2. To prevent CHD in patients without a history or symptoms of existing CHD who have high LDL-C and triglycerides and low HDL-C levels with an inadequate response to non-pharmacological and pharmacological therapy

Mechanism of action

(See also 📖 Fibrates, p.462)

Gemfibrozil also inhibits synthesis of VLDL in the liver. Gemfibrozil increases the HDL2 and HDL3 subfractions as well as ApoA-I and ApoA-II.

Pharmacodynamics

34% RRR (2.7% vs. 4.1% absolute rate) in cumulative rate of serious coronary events (sudden cardiac deaths plus fatal and non-fatal MI) and 37% RRR (2.2% vs. 3.5% absolute rate) in non-fatal MI in male subjects aged 40–55, with 1° dyslipidaemia, but no previous history of CAD, treated for over 5 years compared with placebo.[1] This benefit was associated with a significant reduction in triglycerides (43%), total cholesterol (11%), and LDL-C (10%), and a significant increase in HDL-C (10%). Diabetic patients and patients with severe lipid fraction deviations showed a 68% and 71% RRR of the above CHD endpoints, respectively.[1] After an 18-year follow-up, there was a 32% RRR in CHD mortality in the patients treated with gemfibrozil, but there were no differences in all-cause or cancer mortality. Subgroup analyses showed that participants with high BMI, high triglyceride level, or low HDL-C level at baseline benefited most from an early start of treatment.[2]

24% RRR (21.7% vs. 17.3%) in death from CHD, non-fatal MI, and stroke in men with CHD, HDL-C levels ≤40mg/dL (1.0mmol/L) and LDL-C levels ≤140mg/dL (3.6mmol/L) treated for 5.1 years with gemfibrozil (1200mg per day) as compared to placebo.[3] At the end of the trial, HDL-C levels were 6% higher and triglyceride levels 31% lower in the gemfibrozil group than in the placebo group, while LDL-C did not change. There were no differences in the rates of coronary revascularization, hospitalization for UA, and total mortality. Thus, reduction of total cholesterol and LDL-C levels was not essential to achieve benefit.

Pharmacokinetics

Gemfibrozil is completely absorbed after oral administration (bioavailability 100%), reaching peak plasma levels after 1–2h. The presence of food decreases drug bioavailability. It binds to plasma proteins (97%) and its V_d at steady state is 0.14L/kg.

Gemfibrozil undergoes oxidation of a ring methyl group to form successively a hydroxymethyl and a carboxyl metabolite (the main metabolite) and ~70% of the dose is excreted in the urine, mainly as conjugates and its metabolites, <6% is excreted unchanged in the urine and 6% is found in faeces. The elimination $t_{1/2}$ is ~1.3–1.5h. Pharmacokinetics are linear with therapeutic doses.

Practical points

♪ Doses
Ranges from 900mg daily (once a day) to 1200mg daily (600mg twice daily, 30min before morning and evening meal).

☺ Side effects
(See 📖 Fibrates, p.462)
Gallstones, hyperaesthesia, paraesthesia, viral and bacterial infections (common cold, cough, urinary tract infections)

Interactions
(See 📖 Fibrates, p.462)
Potently inhibits CYP2C8, CYP2C9, CYP2C19, CYP1A2, UGTA1, and UGTA3, and the interaction profile of gemfibrozil is complex resulting in an increased exposure of many medicinal products

Hypoglycaemic agents: concomitant use (oral and/or insulin) has resulted in reports of hypoglycaemic reactions. Monitoring of glucose levels recommended.
- Combination with repaglinide is contraindicated due to risk of hypogly-caemic reactions.
- Combination with rosiglitazone should be approached with caution, due to increase in rosiglitazone exposure.

Combination with bexarotene is not recommended due to increases in plasma concentrations of bexarotene.

Cautions/notes
Dose adjustment in renal impairment. In patients with GFR ≥30mL/min a starting dose of 900mg daily; assess renal function before increasing dose. Contraindicated when GFR <30mL/min.

Pregnancy and lactation
Potential risk is unknown (pregnancy category C) and there are no data on excretion of gemfibrozil in milk. Should not be used in pregnancy or when breastfeeding.

Contraindications
(See 📖 Fibrates, p.462)
Concomitant use of repaglinide

References
1 Frick MH et al. (1987). Helsinki Heart Study: primary-prevention trial with gemfibrozil in middle-aged men with dyslipidemia. Safety of treatment, changes in risk factors, and incidence of coronary heart disease. *N Engl J Med* **317**:1237–45.
2 Tenkanen L et al. (2006). Gemfibrozil in the treatment of dyslipidemia: an 18–year mortality follow-up of the Helsinki Heart Study. *Arch Intern Med* **166**:743–8.
3 Rubins HB et al.; Veterans Affairs High-Density Lipoprotein Cholesterol Intervention Trial Study Group (1999). Gemfibrozil for the secondary prevention of coronary heart disease in men with low levels of high-density lipoprotein cholesterol. *N Engl J Med* **341**:410–18.

Glyceryl trinitrate

(See also 📖 Nitrates, p.538)

Rapid-acting nitrate.

CV indications

(See also 📖 Nitrates, p.538)
1. Acute relief of attack or prophylaxis of angina pectoris
2. Management of severe hypertension (IV formulation)

Mechanism of action

(See 📖 Nitrates, p.538)

Pharmacodynamics

(See 📖 Nitrates, p.538)

IV GTN is very effective in the treatment of pain in patients with ACS.

In acute pulmonary oedema, GTN relieves dyspnoea, reduces LV filling pressure, and increases cardiac output.[1] In patients hospitalized for decompensated HF, IV nesiritide decreased PCWP at 3h more than either GTN or placebo and improved dyspnoea compared with placebo but not when compared with GTN. At 24h, the reduction in PCWP was greater in the nesiritide group than the GTN group, but patients reported no significant differences in dyspnoea. No differences in 30-day rehospitalization or 6-month mortality were observed among groups.[2] Hypotension was more common and more prolonged with nesiritide (2.2h vs. 0.7h), while headache was more frequent with GTN (8% vs. 20%).

Pharmacokinetics

GTN is available for administration through sublingual, transdermal, PO, and IV routes. GTN is rapidly absorbed from mucous membranes, skin, and GI tract. When given orally, it undergoes extensive 1st-pass metabolism. It is metabolized in the liver by a reductase and by extrahepatic mechanisms (red blood cells and vascular wall), to 1,2- and 1,3-dinitroglycerols. Its V_d is 3L/kg and it has $t_{1/2}$ ~1–3min. After sublingual administration clinical response is usually within 5–10min and its effects persists for 20–30min.

Steady-state plasma concentrations of GTN are reached by about 2h after application of a patch and are maintained for the duration of wearing the system. Upon removal of the patch, the plasma concentration declines with a $t_{1/2}$ of 1h.

Practical points

ꙮ Doses
Transdermal:
• Patches: 0.1–0.8mg/h (patch on for 12h/off for 12h)
• Ointment: 2% 1-3 inches every 3-4 hours if required
The onset of action of transdermal GTN is not sufficiently rapid to be useful in aborting an acute attack.

Sublingual: 0.3–0.6mg (maximum dose 1.5mg). Peak levels at 2min and $t_{\frac{1}{2}}$ of 7–10min. Take tablets in the sitting position (standing promotes light-headedness, especially just after rising from a recumbent or seated position) every 5min until the pain disappears (maximum 4 tablets).

Spray: 0.4mg/metered dose, with 1 or 2 doses under tongue at onset of angina or 2–3min before provoking activity. Doses should be administered 5min apart and no more than 3 doses at once. Special interest in patients with dry mouth.

Buccal: 1–3mg tds (5mg in severe angina). Effects begin within minutes and last 3–5h.

PO: 2.5–6.5mg bd/tds.

IV: 5–200mcg/min. The high doses (>350mcg/min) that may be required in UA to overcome tolerance contain propylene glycol that may reduce the anticoagulant effect of heparin.

☻ *Side effects* (see 📖 Nitrates, p.538)
Interactions (see 📖 Nitrates, p.538)
Cautions/notes (see 📖 Nitrates, p.538)

Acute interruption of IV GTN infusion in patients with UA is often associated with acute myocardial ischaemia.

Pregnancy and lactation (see 📖 Nitrates, p.538)
Contraindications (see 📖 Nitrates, p.538)

References

1 Bussmann WD et al. (1978). Effect of sublingual nitroglycerin in emergency treatment of classic pulmonary edema. *Minerva Cardiol* **26**:623–32.
2 Publication Committee for the VMAC Investigators (2002). Intravenous nesiritide vs nitroglycerin for treatment of decompensated congestive heart failure: a randomized controlled trial. *JAMA* **287**:1531–40.
3 Figueras J et al. (1991). Rebound myocardial ischaemia following abrupt interruption of intravenous nitroglycerin infusion in patients with unstable angina at rest. *Eur Heart J* **12**:405–11.

Heparin

(See also 📖 Unfractionated heparin, p.623, 📖 Low-molecular-weight heparins, p.516)

Heparin is a heterogeneous mucopolysaccharide with extremely complex effects on the coagulation mechanism and on blood vessels.

CV indications

1. Prophylaxis and treatment of venous thrombosis and its extension
2. Treatment of DVT and pulmonary embolism in patients undergoing major abdominothoracic surgery or who, for other reasons, are at risk of developing thromboembolic disease
3. AF with embolization
4. Diagnosis and treatment of acute and chronic consumptive coagulopathies (disseminated intravascular coagulation)
5. Prevention of clotting in arterial and cardiac surgery
6. Prophylaxis and treatment of peripheral arterial embolism
7. As an anticoagulant in blood transfusions, extracorporeal circulation, and dialysis procedures and in blood samples for laboratory purposes

Mechanism of action

UFH is a sulphated mucopolysaccharide with a MW range of 3–30kDa (mean, 15kDa, ~45 monosaccharide chains). Heparin binds through a high-affinity pentasaccharide, which is present on about 1/3 of heparin molecules, to antithrombin III (AT). The heparin–AT complex inactivates a number of coagulation enzymes, including thrombin (factor IIa), factors IXa, Xa, XIa, and XIIa. Thrombin and factor Xa are most responsive to inhibition, but human thrombin is about 10-fold more sensitive to inhibition by the heparin–AT complex than factor Xa. To inhibit thrombin, UFH must bind to both the AT via the pentasaccharide and thrombin by its 13 additional saccharide units, but to inhibit factor Xa it is sufficient that UFH binds to AT. By inactivating thrombin, heparin prevents fibrin formation and inhibits thrombin-induced activation of factor V and factor VIII. UFH also prevents the formation of a stable fibrin clot by inhibiting the activation of the fibrin stabilizing factor.

LMWHs are produced from UFH to yield smaller polysaccharides with average MW of 4–5 kDa. These shorter molecules retain the anti-Xa activity, with some inhibition of thrombin.

UFH and LMWH also induce secretion of tissue factor pathway inhibitor by vascular endothelial cells and reduce the procoagulant activity of tissue factor–factor VIIa complex, an effect that may contribute to their anti-thrombotic action. UFH does not have fibrinolytic activity and does not inactivate factor Xa in the prothrombinase complex or thrombin bound to fibrin or to subendothelial surfaces.

UFH binds to platelets, and can either induce or inhibit platelet aggregation. The interaction of UFH with platelets and endothelial cells may contribute to heparin-induced bleeding by a mechanism that is independent of its anticoagulant effect.

UFH inhibits the proliferation of vascular smooth muscle cells, suppresses osteoblast formation, and activates osteoclasts that promote bone loss.

Pharmacokinetics

Heparin is not absorbed by oral administration and should be given by intermittent IV injection, IV infusion, or deep SC injection. Peak plasma levels are achieved immediately by IV route or after 2–4h following SC administration. UFH binds to a number of plasma proteins, endothelial cells, and macrophages, which reduces its anticoagulant activity at low concentrations; this explains the marked variability of the anticoagulant response to UFH among patients with thromboembolic disorders and the phenomenon of heparin resistance. Heparin clearance involves a rapid saturable, dose-dependent mechanism (due to its binding to receptors on endothelial cells and macrophages where it is depolymerized) and a much slower 1st-order renal mechanism. At therapeutic doses, heparin is cleared predominantly through the rapid mechanism. As a result, the $t_{1/2}$ of heparin increases from approximately 30min following an IV bolus of 25U/kg, to 60min with a bolus of 100U/kg, and to 150min with a bolus of 400U/kg. Thus, to obtain a rapid and persistent effect, UFH is given IV as a bolus followed by a perfusion. The $t_{1/2}$ increases in patients with renal or hepatic insufficiency.

Practical points

♣ Doses
(See 📖 Unfractionated heparin, p.623, 📖 Low-molecular-weight heparins, p.516)

The anticoagulant response to heparin varies among patients with thromboembolic disorders. The dosage of heparin is adequate when the APTT (a test sensitive to the inhibitory effects of heparin on factor IIa, IXa, and Xa) is 1.5–2.5× the control value (50–75s) or the ACT is elevated approximately 2.5–3× the control value (100–190s). APTT should be determined every 4h when heparin is given by continuous IV infusion; when it is administered IV intermittently, tests should be performed before each injection at the beginning of treatment and at appropriate intervals thereafter. Tests are best performed on samples drawn 4–6h after SC or IV injection. Periodic platelet counts, haematocrits, and tests for occult blood in stool are recommended during the treatement, regardless of the route of administration.

UFH overdose is treated by stopping the drug and giving protamine sulphate (1% solution, <50mg in 10min).

☺ Side effects
Haemorrhage is the main complication from heparin therapy. HIT occurs in 3–5% of patents treated with UFH for >5 days (<1% in those receiving LMWH); of these, 20–50% develop HIT and venous and arterial thrombosis (HITT). There are 2 types of HIT: type I is an early-onset, mild and reversible decline in platelet count due to the direct platelet-aggregating

effect of heparin; type II occurs 2–5 days after the initial heparin exposure and is due to formation of antibodies (of the IgG or IgM class) against heparin when it is bound to platelet factor 4 (PF4) leading to irreversible aggregation of platelets. To reduce the risk of HIT, IV UFH should not be given for >48h and all patients receiving UFH should have platelet counts on day 1 and every 2 days during days 2–14 of treatment. Thrombocytopenia can be accompanied by severe thromboembolic complications (skin necrosis, gangrene of the extremities that may lead to amputation, MI, pulmonary embolism, stroke, and possibly death). Patients with HIT should be treated with thrombin inhibitors (argatroban, bivalirudin, lepirudin), fondaparinux, or danaproid and later with warfarin, when the platelet count has recovered.

Injection-site reactions: irritation, erythema, mild pain, haematoma, or ulceration may follow deep SC injection.

Rarely: osteoporosis (lower risk with LMWH), skin necrosis, suppression of aldosterone synthesis, transient alopecia, hyperkalaemia, rebound hyperlipidaemia, priapism, and elevations of SGOT and SGPT.

Heparin hypersensitivity reactions: fever, urticaria, rhinitis, angio-oedema, asthma, and anaphylactoid reactions; itching and burning, especially on the plantar side of the feet, may occur.

Interactions

- Increased risk of bleeding: NSAIDs, dextrans, antiplatelet drugs (aspirin, clopidogrel, dipyridamole, GP IIb/IIIa receptor antagonists), fibrinolytics, oral anticoagulants, alprostadil, and iloprost. These drugs should be co-administered, close clinical and laboratory monitoring is essential.
- Increased risk of hyperkalaemia when combined with ACEIs, angiotensin-II AT_1 receptor blockers, or aliskiren.
- Epoetin, streptokinase, and IV GTN reduce the effects of UF, so the dose of UFH should be adjusted under meticulous laboratory monitoring (APTT).
- Increased risk of hypoglycaemia when UFH is co-administered with sulphonylureas. UFH displaces benzodiazepines from plasma proteins and increases their effects (use lorazepam).
- UFH should not be administered with other drugs, including antibiotics, antihistamines, and corticosteroids or phenothiazines.

Cautions/notes

- The risk of bleeding increases with dose, in the elderly, and in patients receiving other drugs that increase risk of bleeding, with hepatic or renal impairment, or sometimes by surgery, trauma, invasive procedures, or concomitant haemostatic defects.
- The IM route of administration should be avoided because of the frequent occurrence of haematoma at the injection site.
- Heparin may prolong the prothrombin time and when co-administered with an oral anticoagulant, a period of at least 5h after the last IV dose or 24h after the last SC dose should elapse before obtaining a valid blood sample to determine the prothrombin time.
- To reduce the risk of HIT, IV heparin should not be given for >48h.[1] Thrombocytopenia should be monitored closely. If the count falls below 100,000/mm^3 or if recurrent thrombosis develops, heparin

should be promptly discontinued and alternative anticoagulants considered, if needed.

• Some patients present resistance to UFH, possibly related to a deficit of AT, a higher drug clearance, and/or to an increase in fibrinogen, factor VIIa and PF4.

Pregnancy and lactation

Heparins are used for the management of VTE during pregnancy because they do not cross the placenta. However, it is not known whether heparins can cause fetal harm when administered to a pregnant woman (pregnancy category C). Heparins are not excreted in human milk. LMWHs (pregnancy category B) are preferred because they have a lower risk of osteoporosis and of HIT.

Contraindications

• Haemophilia and other haemorrhagic disorders
• Thrombocytopenia (including history of HIT)
• Recent cerebral haemorrhage
• Severe hypertension
• Severe liver disease (including oesophageal varices)
• Peptic ulcer
• After major trauma or recent surgery to eye or nervous system
• Subacute bacterial endocarditis
• Spinal or epidural anaesthesia with treatment doses of heparin
• Hypersensitivity to heparin or to LMWHs
• When blood coagulation tests cannot be performed at appropriate intervals in patients receiving full-dose heparin

Reference

1 Antman EM et al. (2008). 2007 Focused Update of the ACC/AHA 2004 Guidelines for the Management of Patients With ST-Elevation Myocardial Infarction: a report of the American College of Cardiology/American Heart Association Task Force on Practice Guidelines: developed in collaboration With the Canadian Cardiovascular Society endorsed by the American Academy of Family Physicians: 2007 Writing Group to Review New Evidence and Update the ACC/AHA 2004 Guidelines for the Management of Patients With ST-Elevation Myocardial Infarction, Writing on Behalf of the 2004 Writing Committee. *Circulation* **117**:296–329.

Hydralazine

Oral direct peripheral vasodilator.

CV indications

1. Severe hypertension in conjunction with other antihypertensive agents
2. Fixed-dose combination of isosorbide dinitrate and hydralazine is indicated for the treatment of HF as an adjunct to standard therapy in black patients to improve survival, to prolong time to hospitalization for HF, and to improve patient-reported functional status
3. Treatment of hypertensive emergencies and of hypertension with renal complications

Mechanism of action

Hydralazine acts as a direct peripheral vasodilator, primarily of arteries and arterioles. Its precise method of action is not known but observations suggest that it inhibits calcium release from the sarcoplasmic reticulum of the vascular smooth muscle cells induced by inositol trisphosphate (IP3). Hydralazine also opens K^+ channels, which produces a hyperpolarization of the vascular smooth muscle cells and stimulates NO formation, increasing the cellular cGMP level. All these 3 mechanisms reduce intracelluar Ca^{2+} concentration in the arterial wall leading to a vasodilatation and a decrease in peripheral vascular resistances.

Pharmacodynamics

Hydralazine decreases peripheral vascular resistances and BP and induces a reflex sympathetic activation of the heart, increasing heart rate, stroke volume, and cardiac output. It also increases renin release and activates the RAAS, producing sodium and water retention. Hydralazine also maintains or increases renal and cerebral blood flow.

Hydralazine has been traditionally recommended as a treatment of choice in acute and severe hypertension in pregnancy and can be given either through IV or IM administration with falls in mean arterial pressure of ≈33mmHg. However, meta-analyses generally do not support its use in such conditions.[1]

Hypertension: BP reduction ≈25/17mmHg in poorly controlled hypertensive patients (baseline BP ≈174/109mmHg despite treatment with atenolol 100mg od and chlortalidone 25mg od) treated with hydralazine (25–100mg bd); but this reduction is less than that in patients treated with felodipine 5–20mg od (BP reduction ≈39/26mmHg from baseline BP of ≈177/108mmHg).[2]

Heart failure: RR ≈34% (absolute rate: 25.6% vs. 34.3%) in mortality in patients with chronic heart failure (established on digoxin and diuretic therapy) treated for 2.3 years with hydralazine (300mg/day) in combination with isosorbide dinitrate (160mg/day) compared with prazosin (20mg/day) or placebo.[3] 28% RR (18% vs. 25%) in mortality in patients treated for 2 years with enalapril (20mg/day) compared with those in the hydralazine-isosorbide dinitrate arm.[4]

RR ≈44% (absolute rates: 6.2% vs. 10.2%) in mortality and 33% RR in the rate of first hospitalization for HF associated with an improvement in quality of life in African-American patients with NYHA III/IV HF treated with hydralazine in combination with isosorbide dinitrate (target dose of 225mg and 120mg/day, respectively) compared with placebo and followed up for a mean of 10 months.[5]

Pharmacokinetics

Following oral administration, hydralazine is rapidly and completely absorbed (bioavailability of ≈26–55%), reaching peak plasma levels after ≈0.5–1.5h. Binds to plasma proteins (≈90%) and undergoes extensive hepatic metabolism, but is subject to polymorphic acetylation. Hydralazine is excreted mainly in the form of metabolites (90%) in the urine and also in bile. Plasma $t_{1/2}$ ≈2–7h but prolongs up to 16h in severe renal failure and shortens to ≈45min in rapid acetylators. Therefore rapid acetylators often respond inadequately even to doses of 100mg.

Practical points

⚬ Doses

PO:
- Hypertension: 25mg bd, titrated up to dose of 200mg/day.
- Chronic congestive HF: 25mg tds or qds.
- Doses should not be increased beyond 100mg/day without checking the patient's acetylator status.
- In patients with reduced renal or hepatic function, the dose or interval of dosing should be adjusted according to clinical response.

IV: 5–10mg by slow IV injection; or 200–300mcg/min as initial IV infusion initially followed by 50–150mcg/min maintenance.

☻ Side effects

(>10%): tachycardia, palpitations, headache, anorexia, nausea, vomiting, diarrhoea

(1–10%): prolonged treatment (>6 months), especially where daily dose exceeds 100mg and in slow acetylators, may provoke drug-induced lupus erythematosus (accompanied by fever, urticaria, arthralgia, myalgia, pericarditis) that may be associated with an immune-complex glomerulonephritis

Cardiovascular: flushing, hypotension, exacerbation of angina pectoris

Neurological: peripheral neuritis, muscle cramps, difficulty in urination, psychotic reactions

Hypersensitive: rash, urticaria, arthralgia, myalgia, joint swelling, eosinophilia

Interactions

Potentiates the effects of other antihypertensives.

Co-administration with MAO inhibitors may potentiate the decrease in BP.

Cautions/notes

Due to possibility of causing a relatively hyperdynamic circulation, hydralazine should be used with caution in patients with coronary artery disease as it may precipitate/exacerbate angina, with the prior commencement use of β-blockers considered. It should not be used following an AMI. Where possible, withdrawal of hydralazine should be gradual to avoid precipitation or exacerbation of HF. Due to increased cardiac-accelerating effects of adrenaline with hydralazine, the latter should not be used to correct hydralazine-related hypotension in surgery. In patients with valvular disease hydralazine may increase pulmonary arterial pressure.

Prolonged treatment (>6 months) especially in slow acetylators and when given a dose >100g/day may provoke a SLE-type reaction. Clinical assessment including tests such as antinuclear antibodies and urine analysis to monitor for the development of such a reaction should be undertaken at regular intervals with prolonged use.

Pregnancy and lactation
It should be avoided before the 3rd trimester. May be used in later pregnancy if no safer alternative or when disease itself carries serious risks for mother or child (pregnancy category C). There has been no serious adverse event reported with extensive experience in the 3rd trimester. Passes into breast milk but there are no reports so far showing adverse effects on the infant.

Contraindications
- Hypersensitivity to hydralazine or dihydralazine
- Idiopathic SLE
- Severe tachycardia, high-output cardiac failure, isolated right HF 2° to PH, coronary artery disease, and myocardial insufficiency due to mechanical obstruction.

References

1 Magee LA et al. (2003). Hydralazine for treatment of severe hypertension in pregnancy: meta-analysis. *BMJ* **327**:955–60.
2 Cooperative Study Group (1986). Felodipine vs hydralazine: a controlled trial as third line therapy in hypertension. *Br J Clin Pharmacol* **21**(6):621–6.
3 Cohn JN et al. (1986). Effect of vasodilator therapy on mortality in chronic congestive heart failure. Results of a Veterans Administration Cooperative Study. *N Engl J Med* **314**:1547–52.
4 Cohn JN et al. (1991). A comparison of enalapril with hydralazine-isosorbide dinitrate in the treatment of chronic congestive heart failure. *N Engl J Med* **325**:303–10.
5 Taylor AL et al. (2004). Combination of isosorbide dinitrate and hydralazine in blacks with heart failure. *N Engl J Med* **351**:2049–57.

Iloprost

Synthetic analogue of prostacyclin PGI_2. (See also 📖 Prostanoids, p.558)

CV indications

Functional WHO class III and IV PAH.

Other indications

Raynaud's phenomenon or ischaemia of a limb.

Mechanism of action

Iloprost is a prostanoid that can be delivered by an adaptive aerosol device.

Pharmacodynamics

Inhaled iloprost has been evaluated in a 12-week RCT.[1] Inhaled 6–9 times a day, it improves functional class and increases exercise capacity (mean 36m), functional class, and symptoms. Long-term outcomes are conflicting.

Pharmacokinetics

This stable analogue presents a $t_{1/2}$ of 20–25min. It binds to plasma proteins (60%), and is rapidly metabolized in the liver and eliminated in urine (80%). By inhalatory route its effects disappear within 30–90min, so it should be inhaled 6–9 times daily.

Practical points

⚖ Doses

Initial dose: 2.5mcg via nebulizer; if tolerated increase to 5mcg for 2nd dose. Maintenance dose: 5mcg 6–9 times daily; reduce to 2.5mcg 6–9 times daily if higher dose not tolerated.

In Europe, iloprost has been approved for use with 2 compressed air nebulizers with AAD delivery systems (HaloLite® and Prodose®) as well as with 2 ultrasonic nebulizers (Ventaneb® and I-neb®).

☺ Side effects

Headache, flushing, headache, syncope, cough, nausea (13%), vomiting, swelling of the limbs, jaw and limb pain, flu syndrome, hypotension, insomnia and fainting

Other serious adverse effects: congestive HF, chest pain, supraventricular tachycardia, dyspnoea

Interactions (see 📖 Epoprostenol, p.451)

Precautions

Monitor vital signs during initial treatment to decrease syncope risk; avoid eye and skin contact and oral ingestion.

Fetal risk revealed in studies in animals but not established or not studied in humans; may use if benefits outweigh risk to fetus (pregnancy category C).

Contraindications (see 📖 Epoprostenol, p.451)

Reference

1 Olschewski H *et al.* (2002). Inhaled iloprost for severe pulmonary hypertension. *N Engl J Med* **347**: 322–9.

Indapamide

(See also 📖 Thiazide and related diuretics, p.604)

Oral thiazide diuretic with direct vasodilator effects.

CV and other indications:

(See 📖 Thiazide and related diuretics, p.604)
Essential hypertension.

Mechanism of action

(See 📖 Thiazide and related diuretics, p.604)
In addition to its diuretic effects, indapamide exhibits calcium-channel blocking properties, increases the release of prostacyclin, and reduces vascular reactivity to noradrenaline; all these effects reduce peripheral vascular resistances.

Pharmacodynamics

Several large randomized trials have shown that BP reduction with indapamide in combination with an ACEI reduces risk of 2° stroke;[1] risk of 1° stroke and HF in the elderly;[2] and all-cause mortality in type 2 diabetes.[3] Indapamide presents fewer metabolic disturbances than other thiazides.

RRR 28% (absolute rate=10% cf 14%) of stroke treated with indapamide 2.5mg od in combination with perindopril 4mg od for 4 years in patients with a history of stroke or TIA compared with placebo (NNT for 5 years=11).[1]

RRR 30% of stroke (NNT=94), 21% of all-cause mortality (NNT=40), and 64% of rate of HF in hypertensive patients aged >80 years treated with indapamide 2.5mg combined with perindopril 2–4mg od over 2 years.[2]

RRR 14% of all-cause mortality (absolute rate=7.4% cf 8.4%; NNT=79) in patients with type 2 diabetes and additional cardiovascular risk treated with indapamide 1.25mg od in combination with perindopril 4–8mg od compared to placebo.[3]

Regression of LVH with indapamide (1.5mg SR od) better than with enalapril (20mg od).[4]

Pharmacokinetics

Rapidly and completely absorbed after oral administration (bioavailability 95%) with peak levels ≈1–4h. It is 79% bound to plasma proteins, erythrocytes, and also by the vascular wall in smooth vascular muscle due to its high lipid solubility. Indapamide is extensively metabolized in the liver, with 7% of the unchanged drug found in the urine during the 48h following administration. Approximately 70% of a single oral dose is eliminated by the kidneys. Elimination $t_{1/2}$ ≈15–18h.

Practical points

💊 Doses

For hypertension and HF: 1.25–5mg od usually in the morning (or 1.5mg SR)

☺ *Side effects*

(See 📖 Thiazide and related diuretics, p.604)
Hypokalaemia (<3.4mmol/L in 10%); maculopapular rashes

Interactions

(See also 📖 Thiazide and related diuretics, p.604)
There is an increased risk of arrhythmia with torsades de pointes-inducing
drugs (e.g. class Ia, III antiarrhythmics; phenothiazones; butyrophenones
and benzamide antipsychotics; erythromycin; halofantrine, moxifloxacin,
vincamine) particularly with hypokalaemia. Risk of hypokalaemia may also
be increased by mineralocorticoids and amphotericin B.

There is a reduction in efficacy and also acute renal failure reported with
NSAIDs, COX II inhibitors, and high-dose salicylic acid (≥3g/day). There
is also a risk of sudden hypotension and acute renal failure when given
with an ACEI in the presence of sodium depletion, especially with renal
artery stenosis.

Hypotensive effects may be increased by baclofen, imipramine-like antidepressants and neuroleptics, and attenuated by corticosteroids. There is
an increased risk of lactic acidosis with metformin and acute renal failure
with iodinated contrast media.

Cautions/notes

(See 📖 Thiazide and related diuretics, p.604)
Serum electrolytes should be monitored in the 1st week of treatment used
with an ACEI. Indapamide may give positive reaction in doping tests.

Pregnancy and lactation (see 📖 Thiazide and related diuretics, p.604)

Contraindications

(See 📖 Thiazide and related diuretics, p.604)
• Known allergy to sulphonamides
• Severe hepatic failure

References

1 PROGRESS Collaborative Group (2001). Randomised trial of a perindopril-based blood-pressure-
lowering regimen among 6,105 individuals with previous stroke or transient ischaemic attack.
Lancet **358**:1033–41.
2 Beckett NS *et al.*; HYVET Study Group (2008). Treatment of hypertension in patients 80 years of
age or older. *N Engl J Med* **358**:1887–98.
3 Patel A *et al.*; ADVANCE Collaborative Group (2007). Effects of a fixed combination of perindopril and indapamide on macrovascular and microvascular outcomes in patients with type 2
diabetes mellitus (the ADVANCE trial): a randomised controlled trial. *Lancet* **370**:829–40.
4 Gosse P *et al.*, for the LIVE investigators (2000). Regression of left ventricular hypertrophy in
hypertensive patients treated with indapamide SR 1.5mg versus enalapril 20mg: the LIVE study. *J
Hypertens* **18**:1465–75.

Indometacin

Indometacin (indomethacin) is a NSAID.

CV indications

Pericarditis, closure of ductus arteriosus.

Other indications

Severe rheumatoid arthritis, ankylosing spondylitis and osteoarthritis, acute painful shoulder (bursitis and/or tendinitis), and acute gouty arthritis.

Mechanism of action

It is a potent inhibitor of COX-1, the enzyme which catalyzes (from arachidonic acid) the synthesis of prostaglandins known to be among the mediators of inflammation. Indometacin exhibits potent anti-inflammatory, antipyretic, and analgesic properties.

Pharmacokinetics

Indometacin is readily absorbed by oral route (bioavailability 100%), attaining peak plasma concentrations within 2h. It binds (99%) to plasma proteins and is widely distributed (V_d 0.29L/kg), crossing the blood–brain barrier and the placenta. It is metabolized in the liver by demethylation and deacetylation while also undergoing appreciable glucuronidation and enterohepatic circulation. Indometacin and its metabolites are excreted in urine (60%) and faeces. $t_{1/2}$ is 4.5 (3–11)h.

Practical points

Indometacin should be given with food, milk, or antacids to reduce the chance of GI disturbance. Always aim to use the lowest effective dose for the shortest duration possible to minimize undesirable effects, and avoid the use of multiple NSAIDs. Monitor renal function where appropriate.

♪ Doses

25–50mg every 6–8h

☺ Side effects

- *Cardiovascular*: oedema, hypertension, hypotension, tachycardia, hyperkalaemia, chest pain, arrhythmia, palpitations, and cardiac failure
- *GI*: nausea, anorexia, vomiting, gastritis, epigastric discomfort or abdominal pain, constipation, diarrhoea, stomatitis, flatulence, GI ulceration and bleeding, cholestasis, and elevation of LFTs
- Blood dyscrasias, petechiae, epistaxis, ecchymosis, purpura
- *Neurological*: headache, blurred vision, diplopia, vertigo, dizziness, light-headedness, tinnitus, hearing disturbances. It can worsen Parkinson's disease, epilepsy, and psychiatric disorders
- *Hypersensitivity reactions*: asthma, hepatitis, liver necrosis, angio-oedema, photosensitivity, erythema nodosum, rash, exfoliative dermatitis, Stevens–Johnson syndrome
- *Renal*: haematuria, nephrotic syndrome, proteinuria, interstitial nephritis, renal insufficiency
- Skin reactions and photosensitivity

Interactions:

- *ACEIs and ARBs*: co-administration of indometacin diminishes their antihypertensive effects and in some patients with compromised renal function, the combination may result in reversible renal dysfunction.
- *Antihypertensive drugs*: indometacin may reduce the antihypertensive effect of ACEIs, ARBs, diuretics, and β-blockers due partly to inhibition of prostaglandin synthesis.
- *Anticoagulants and antiplatelet drugs*: co-administration with indometacin increases the risk of bleeding.
- *Antivirals*: increased risk of haematological toxicity with zidovudine. Risks of indometacin toxicity with ritonavir; therefore, avoid concomitant use.
- *Bisphosphonates*: indometacin increases the bioavailability of tiludronic acid.
- *Ciclosporin/tacrolimus*: indometacin increases the risk of nephrotoxicity, possibly due to decreased synthesis of renal prostacyclin. Renal function should be carefully monitored.
- *Corticosteroids*: increase the risk of GI bleeding and ulceration produced by indometacin.
- *Cytotoxics*: indometacin may decrease the tubular secretion of methotrexate and thus potentiate toxicity. Increased risk of bleeding when NSAIDs are given with erlotinib.
- *Desmopressin*: indometacin enhances its effects.
- *Digoxin*: indometacin may exacerbate HF, reduce GFR, and increase plasma concentration of cardiac glycoside. Digoxinaemia should be closely monitored.
- *Diuretics*: indometacin can reduce the diuretic, natriuretic, and antihypertensive effects of loop, K⁺-sparing, and thiazide diuretics, due to inhibition of renal prostaglandin synthesis. Increased risk of hyperkalaemia and renal failure when given with K⁺-sparing diuretics.
- Diuretics can increase the risk of nephrotoxicity of NSAIDs.
- *Iloprost*: increased risk of bleeding.
- *Lithium*: indometacin reduces lithium clearance and increases the risk of lithium toxicity.
- *Mifepristone*: manufacturer recommends avoiding NSAIDs until 8–12 days after mifepristone administration.
- *Muscle relaxants*: NSAIDs reduce excretion of baclofen.
- *Muromonab-CD3*: significant rise in incidence of psychosis and encephalopathy in patients also treated with indometacin.
- *NSAIDs*: avoid concomitant use due to the increased possibility of GI and renal toxicity.
- *Probenecid*: may increase plasma levels of indometacin.
- *Indometacin* may enhance the effects of sulphonylureas and phenytoin. Increased risk of dizziness when indometacin is co-administered with diazepam, and increased drowsiness when given with haloperidol.

Cautions/notes

Consider carefully the potential benefits and risks of indometacin before deciding on its use; use the lowest effective dose for the shortest duration consistent with individual patient treatment goals.

NSAIDs are associated with an increased thrombotic risk. Therefore, care is needed in patients who have a history of, or are at risk of, ischaemic heart disease, stroke, and peripheral vascular disease. In conditions predisposing to fluid retention, caution is required since the use of NSAIDs may result in both deterioration of renal function and fluid retention. This also applies to patients with a history of hypertension. Caution is needed in any patient who has, or is at risk of having, impaired renal function.

Indometacin may aggravate the following conditions: inflammatory bowel disease, sigmoid diverticulae or carcinoma, bleeding disorders, psychiatric disorders, epilepsy, parkinsonism, and asthma. Vigilance is needed in patients receiving concomitant medications which could increase the risk of gastric bleeding, such as corticosteroids, anticoagulants such as warfarin, or antiplatelet agents such as aspirin.

Indometacin reduces basal plasma renin activity (PRA) and the elevations of PRA in response to diuretics or volume depletion.

Pregnancy and lactation
There are no adequate and well-controlled studies in pregnant women (pregnancy category C). During the 3rd trimester of pregnancy, indometacin may produce adverse effects (constriction of the ductus arteriosus prenatally, tricuspid incompetence, platelet dysfunction with bleeding, renal dysfunction, PH, GI bleeding, or perforation), and so its use is contraindicated. Furthermore, indometacin inhibits prostaglandin synthesis and delays the onset of labour. It is excreted in the milk and is not recommended for use in nursing mothers.

Contraindications
- Hypersensitivity to indometacin and other NSAIDs
- Patients with peptic ulcer disease, recent GI bleeding, or perforation
- Severe hepatic, renal, and cardiac failure
- 3rd trimester of pregnancy
- Treatment of perioperative pain in the setting of CABG surgery
- Patent ductus arteriosus-dependent heart defect (such as transposition of the great vessels)

Irbesartan

(See also 📖 Angiotensin II (AT$_1$) receptor blockers, p.359)

Angiotensin receptor blocker.

CV indications

(See 📖 Angiotensin II (AT$_1$) receptor blockers, p.359)
1. Treatment of hypertension
2. Treatment of diabetic nephropathy with an elevated serum creatinine and proteinuria (urinary albumin to creatinine ratio ≥300mg/g) in patients with type 2 diabetes and hypertension

Mechanism of action

(See 📖 Renin–angiotensin–aldosterone system inhibitors, p.568 and 📖 Angiotensin II (AT$_1$) receptor blockers, p.359)

Pharmacodynamics

(See 📖 Renin–angiotensin–aldosterone system inhibitors, p.568 and 📖 Angiotensin II (AT$_1$) receptor blockers, p.359)

Hypertension and diabetic nephropathy: 1° composite endpoint (doubling of creatinine, onset of ESRD or death from any cause) was ≈23% and ≈20% lower in hypertensive patients with diabetic nephropathy treated with irbesartan 75mg od (titrated to 300mg od) compared with amlodipine 2.5mg od (titrated to 10mg od) or placebo respectively and followed up for mean of 2.6 years.[1] These differences were not explained by differences in the BPs that were achieved. There were no significant differences in the rates of death from any cause.

HR 0.61 (absolute rate 5.2%) and 0.30 (absolute rate: 9.7%) in time to the onset of diabetic nephropathy (persistent albuminuria, UACR >200mcg/min and ≥30% greater than baseline level) in hypertensive patients with diabetes and microalbuminuria treated with irbesartan 300mg od or 150mg od respectively compared with placebo (absolute rate: 14.9%) and followed up for 24 months.[2] Regression to normoalbuminuria (<20mg/min, or <30mg/day) at the last visit was more frequent in the patients treated with irbesartan 300mg than in the control group (34% vs. 21%, respectively).

After adjustment for the baseline level of microalbuminuria and the achieved BP during the study, the benefits of irbesartan in slowing progression to overt proteinuria were still present: RRR of 44% and 68% for irbesartan 150mg and 300mg vs. the control group, respectively.

Pharmacokinetics

Well absorbed after oral administration (bioavailability ≈60–80%), which is not influenced by food intake. Plasma concentrations peak at ≈2h. Plasma protein binding is ≈96% and V_d≈0.7–1.2L/kg. Metabolized in the liver via glucuronide conjugation and oxidation by the CYP2C9. Irbesartan exhibits linear and dose-proportional pharmacokinetics over the dose range of 10–600mg. Excreted unchanged in urine (20%) and faeces (80%). The terminal elimination $t_{1/2}$ is ≈11–15h.

Practical points

♣ Doses

150–300mg od. No dose adjustment is required in renal or mild–moderate hepatic impairment. A lower starting dose of 75mg should be considered in those >75 years or with volume depletion.

☺ Side effects (see ▢ Angiotensin II (AT$_1$) receptor blockers, p.359)

Interactions (see ▢ Angiotensin II (AT$_1$) receptor blockers, p.359)

Cautions (see ▢ Angiotensin II (AT$_1$) receptor blockers, p.359)

Pregnancy and lactation (see ▢ Angiotensin II (AT$_1$) receptor blockers, p.359)

Contraindications (see ▢ Angiotensin II (AT$_1$) receptor blockers, p.359)

References

1 Lewis EJ et al.; Collaborative Study Group (2001). Renoprotective effect of the angiotensin-receptor antagonist irbesartan in patients with nephropathy due to type 2 diabetes. N Engl J Med **345**:851–60.

2 Parving HH et al.; Irbesartan in Patients with Type 2 Diabetes and Microalbuminuria Study Group (2001). The effect of irbesartan on the development of diabetic nephropathy in patients with type 2 diabetes. N Engl J Med **345**:870–8.

Isosorbide dinitrate

(See also 📖 Nitrates, p.538)

Long-acting nitrate.

CV indications

(See 📖 Nitrates, p.538)

Mechanism of action

(See also 📖 Nitrates, p.538)

Pharmacodynamics

(See also 📖 Nitrates, p.538)

Heart failure: RR ~34% (absolute rate: 25.6% vs. 34.3%) in 2.3-year mortality in patients with chronic HF (established on digoxin and diuretic therapy) treated with ISDN (160mg/day) in combination with hydralazine (300mg/day) as compared with prazosin (20mg/day) or placebo.[1]

28% RR (18% vs. 25%) in mortality in patients treated for 2 years with enalapril (20mg/day) as compared with those in the hydralazine-isosorbide dinitrate arm.[2]

RR ≈44% (absolute rates: 6.2% vs. 10.2%) in mortality and RR 39% in hospitalization associated with an improvement in quality of life in African-American patients with NYHA class III/IV HF treated with ISDN in combination with hydralazine (20mg and 37.5mg tds, respectively) compared with placebo and followed up for a mean of 10 months.[3]

Pharmacokinetics

Absorption of ISDN after PO administration is near complete but bioavailability is highly variable (mean 25%, 10–90%) due to extensive 1st-pass metabolism. ISDN reaches peak plasma level within 1h and presents a V_d of ~2–4L/kg. ISDN is metabolized predominantly in the liver to 2 active metabolites, isosorbide 5-mononitrate (75–85%) and 2-nitrate; also undergoes extra-hepatic metabolism, is excreted in urine and has a plasma $t_{1/2}$ of ~1h.

Practical points

🔑 Doses

Sublingual: 2.5–15mg; onset 5–10 min, but the antianginal effect persists for 1h or longer. The onset of its effect is slower than with GTN, so that it should be used only if the patient is unresponsive or intolerant to GTN.

Spray: 1.25mg/metered dose with 1–3 doses given under tongue, 30s apart; the onset of its effects 1–3min. It may also be administered as a chewable tablet as a single 5mg dose; effects last for up to 2.5h.

PO: 30–120mg tds (with last dose around 6pm); for angina, maximum dose 240mg/day. Extended release formulation: eccentric 40mg bd (in the morning and 7h later).

IV: 1.2–10mg/h by IV infusion. Higher doses (up to 20mg/h) may be required in UA.

Transdermal: 100mg daily as an ointment.

☺ *Side effects* (see 📖 Nitrates, p.538)

Interactions (see 📖 Nitrates, p.538)

Cautions/notes (see 📖 Nitrates, p.538)

Pregnancy and lactation (see 📖 Nitrates, p.538)

Contraindications
(See also 📖 Nitrates, p.538)
Skin allergy.

References

1 Cohn JN *et al.* (1986). Effect of vasodilator therapy on mortality in chronic congestive heart failure. Results of a Veterans Administration Cooperative Study. *N Engl J Med* **314**:1547–52.
2 Cohn JN *et al.* (1991). A comparison of enalapril with hydralazine-isosorbide dinitrate in the treatment of chronic congestive heart failure. *N Engl J Med* **325**:303–10.
3 Taylor AL *et al.* (2004). Combination of isosorbide dinitrate and hydralazine in blacks with heart failure. *N Engl J Med* **351**:2049–57.

Isosorbide-5-mononitrate

(See also 📖 Nitrates, p.538)

Long-acting nitrate.

CV indications

(See 📖 Nitrates, p.538)

Mechanism of action

(See 📖 Nitrates, p.538)

Pharmacodynamics

(See 📖 Nitrates, p.538)

Pharmacokinetics

ISMN is completely absorbed after PO administration, but does not undergo 1st-pass metabolism (100% bioavailability) and so it has predictable clinical effects with minimal intra- and interindividual variation in plasma levels. ISMN is <5% protein bound and presents a V_d of ≈0.6L/kg. Elimination is primarily by denitration and conjugation in the liver, excretion of metabolites mainly in urine. Elimination $t_{1/2}$ ≈5h. Hepatic and renal impairment do not appear to significantly affect the pharmacokinetics of ISMN.

Practical points

🎝 Doses

PO: 10mg bd initial starting dose (increasing to maximum dose 120mg/day in divided doses) in an eccentric dose (doses spaced 7h: 8am and 3pm). Slow-release formulation: 120–240mg od; efficacy up to 12–14h.

☺ **Side effects** (see 📖 Nitrates, p.538)

Interactions (see 📖 Nitrates, p.538)

Cautions/notes (see 📖 Nitrates, p.538)

Pregnancy and lactation (see 📖 Nitrates, p.538)

Contraindications (see 📖 Nitrates, p.538)

Ivabradine

Blocker of the pacemaker hyperpolarization-activated current I_f.

CV indication

Symptomatic treatment of chronic stable angina pectoris in patients with CAD and normal sinus rhythm whose heart rate is >60bpm.

Mechanism of action

The pacemaker funny current (I_f) is a mixed Na^+–K^+ inward current activated by membrane hyperpolarization and modulated by the autonomic nervous system. It appears to regulate diastolic depolarization in the SA node and cardiac pacemaker activity. Ivabradine blocks the I_f current and so reduces heart rate. Consequently, it diminishes the symptoms of angina by reducing cardiac work and myocardial O_2 demands and increasing the diastolic time when coronary perfusion takes place.

Pharmacodynamics

Reduces resting and exercise heart rate by ≈10bpm; so there is less risk of severe SA node depression than with β-blockers. However, ivabradine has no effect on BP, AV nodal conduction, cardiac conduction, and contractility or ventricular repolarization.

Bicycle exercise tolerance has been shown to increase by 40.8s, 27.2s, and 22.5s with 10mg, 5mg, and 2.5mg bd respectively.[1] Non-inferiority studies suggest that ivabradine has similar antianginal efficacy to atenolol[2] or amlodipine.[3]

Ivabradine (5–7.5mg bd) does not reduce the 1° composite endpoint (CV death, admission to hospital for AMI, and hospitalization for new-onset or worsening HF) in patients with CAD, heart rate ≥60bpm, and LVEF ≤ 39%.[4] However, in patients with baseline heart rate >70bpm receiving the current optimal CV therapy, ivabradine reduced the risk of hospitalization for fatal and non-fatal MI (36%) and the risk of coronary revascularization (30%).

Pharmacokinetics

Rapid and almost complete absorption after oral administration (bioavailability 40%), reaching peak plasma level within 1h. Absorption is delayed by food. It binds to plasma proteins by 70%, presents V_d ≈1.3L/kg, is metabolized via CYP3A4, and only 5% is excreted unchanged in urine. Effective $t_{1/2}$ is ≈11h with excretion via faeces and urine.

Practical points

⚡ Doses

5mg bd (starting dose), which can be increased to 7.5mg bd.

Due to limited experience, it is advisable to use a lower starting dose in the elderly. Dose should be down-titrated with resting HR <50/bpm or symptoms of bradycardia.

☺ Common side effects

(>10%): flashing lights (phosphenes)—usually disappear with continued use. (1–10%): 1st-degree AV block, bradycardia; ventricular extrasystoles; headache; blurred vision and dizziness.

Sinus bradycardia was reported as an adverse event in 2.2 and 5.4% in the ivabradine 7.5 and 10mg groups in 43% with atenolol.[2]

Interactions

There are no specific drug–drug interactions with PPIs, ACEIs, ARBs, sildenafil, statins, and dihydropyridine CCBs.

Plasma levels of ivabradine are increased markedly by co-administration with azole antifungals, macrolides, HIV protease inhibitors, and less significantly by co-administration with non-dihydropyridine CCBs and CYP3A4 inhibitors and is therefore not recommended. Intake of grapefruit juice should be restricted.

Inducers of CYP3A4 (e.g. rifampicin, barbiturates, phenytoin, St John's wort) may decrease levels of ivabradine.

Cautions/notes

Ivabradine should be used with caution in:
- Chronic HF
- Mild–moderate hypotension
- Retinitis pigmentosa
- Moderate hepatic or severe renal impairment

Pregnancy and lactation

Animal studies have shown embryotoxicity, teratogenesis and excretion in breast milk with ivabradine (pregnancy category C). Therefore, it is contraindicated during pregnancy and breastfeeding.

Contraindications

- Resting heart rate <60bpm without a pacemaker
- Sick sinus syndrome; 3rd-degree and SA heart block; AF
- AMI; unstable angina
- HF classes NYHA III–IV
- Cardiogenic shock; severe hypotension (BP <90/50mmHg)
- Severe hepatic impairment; combination with potent CYP3A4 inhibitors
- Pregnancy and breastfeeding
- Galactose intolerance; Lapp lactase deficiency; glucose-galactose malabsorption

References

1 Borer JS et al.; Ivabradine Investigators Group (2003). Antianginal and antiischemic effects of ivabradine, an I(f) inhibitor, in stable angina: a randomized, double-blind, multicentered, placebo-controlled trial. *Circulation* **107**:817–23.

2 Tardif JC et al.; INITIATIVE Investigators (2005). Efficacy of ivabradine, a new selective I(f) inhibitor, compared with atenolol in patients with chronic stable angina. *Eur Heart J* **26**:2529–36.

3 Ruzyllo W et al. (2007). Antianginal efficacy and safety of ivabradine compared with amlodipine in patients with stable effort angina pectoris: a 3-month randomised, double-blind, multicentre, noninferiority trial. *Drugs* **67**:393–405.

4 Fox K et al.; BEAUTIFUL Investigators (2008). Ivabradine for patients with stable coronary artery disease and left-ventricular systolic dysfunction (BEAUTIFUL): a randomised, double-blind, placebo-controlled trial. *Lancet* **372**:807–16.

Labetalol

(See also 📖 β-blockers, p.376)

Labetalol combines both selective, competitive α_1-adrenergic blocking and nonselective, competitive β_1- and β_2-adrenergic-blocking activity.

CV indications

(See 📖 β-blockers, p.376)
1. Hypertension in pregnancy
2. Severe hypertension

Mechanism of action

(See 📖 β-blockers, p.376)

Pharmacodynamics

(See 📖 β-blockers, p.376)
Labetalol has membrane-stabilizing properties but at doses much greater than required for α- and β-blockade.

Pharmacokinetics

Labetalol is completely absorbed following PO administration with levels peaking at ≈1–2h. Oral bioavailability is ≈25% compared to IV administration due to extensive 1st-pass metabolism, and is increased by food. Labetalol binds to plasma proteins (90%) and is extensively metabolized in the liver to produce inactive metabolites, excreted in urine (50%, <5% unchanged) and bile, and has a $t_{1/2}$ ≈6–8h. Elimination appears reduced in the elderly.

Practical points

💊 Doses

PO: recommended initial dose is 100mg bd. The maintenance dose is 200–400mg bd. Patients with severe hypertension may require from 1200 to 2400mg per day, with or without thiazide diuretics. A reduced initial dose (50mg bd) is recommended in the elderly.

IV: 50mg bolus; or 15mg/h infusion (up to a maximum of 120–200mg/h).

😕 Side effects (see 📖 β-blockers, p.376)

Interactions (see 📖 β-blockers, p.376)

Cautions/notes (see 📖 β-blockers, p.376)

Pregnancy and lactation

Offspring of mothers treated with labetalol have been found retrospectively to have significantly higher birth weights (3280g vs. 2750g) compared to infants of atenolol-treated mothers.[1] Labetalol crosses the placenta and so should only be used in pregnancy where potential benefits outweigh potential harms (pregnancy category C). Labetalol is also excreted in

breast milk (although without reported adverse effects) and so is not recommended in breastfeeding.

Contraindications (see 📖 β-blockers, p.376)

Reference

1 Lardoux H et al. (1983). Hypertension in pregnancy: evaluation of two beta blockers atenolol and labetalol. *Eur Heart J* **4**(Suppl G):35–40.

Lercanidipine

(See also 📖 Calcium-channel blockers, p.390)

Oral dihydropyridine derivative L-type CCBs.

CV indication

Treatment of hypertension.

Mechanism of action

(See 📖 Calcium-channel blockers, p.390)

Pharmacodynamics

Hypertension: BP reduction after 3 months' treatment with lercanidipine 10mg od in hypertensive patients (mean baseline BP 160/96mmHg) was ~19/12mmHg.[1]

Angina: Lercanidipine 10 and 20mg significantly increased total duration of exercise and time to moderate angina and to onset of ST segment depression ≥1mm.[2]

Pharmacokinetics

Completely absorbed after oral administration, with plasma levels peaking ~1.5–3h after dosing. Due to the high 1st-pass metabolism, the absolute oral bioavailability is around 10%, increasing 4-fold when ingested up to 2h after a high-fat meal, and reduced to 1/3 when administered under fasting conditions; accordingly, lercanidipine should be taken before meals. Plasma levels do not appear directly proportional to dosage (non-linear kinetics), suggesting a progressive saturation of 1st-pass metabolism. It binds to plasma proteins (98%), presents a V_d of 2–2.5L/kg and elimination occurs essentially by biotransformation via CYP3A4 into inactive metabolites (no parent drug is found in the urine or faeces). Despite its short pharmacokinetic plasma $t_{1/2}$ (2–5h) the antihypertensive effect of lercanidipine lasts for 24h due to its high membrane partition coefficient.

Practical points

💊 Doses

10mg od at least 15min before meals (increased to 20mg as required). Dose titration should be gradual, as maximal effects may occur after 2 weeks.

In mild–moderate renal or hepatic dysfunction, the usual recommended dose schedule may be tolerated, but an increase in dose to 20mg od should be approached with caution. Although adjustment of the daily dosage is not required, care should be exercised when initiating treatment in the elderly.

😖 **Side effects** (see 📖 Calcium-channel blockers, p.390)

Interactions (see 📖 Calcium-channel blockers, p.390)

Cautions/notes

Lercanidipine is not recommended in patients with severe hepatic or renal impairment (GFR <30mL/min).

One tablet contains 30mg lactose, therefore should not be administered to patients with Lapp lactase insufficiency, galactosaemia, or glucose-galactose malabsorption syndrome.

Pregnancy and lactation

(See ⌘ Calcium-channel blockers, p.390)

Contraindications

(See ⌘ Calcium-channel blockers, p.390)
- Severe renal or hepatic impairment
- Co-administration with strong inhibitors of CYP3A4 or ciclosporin

References

1 Barrios V *et al.*; Investigators of ELYPSE Study (Eficacia de Lercanidipino y su Perfil de Seguridad) (2002). Antihypertensive efficacy and tolerability of lercanidipine in daily clinical practice. The ELYPSE Study. Eficacia de Lercanidipino y su Perfil de Seguridad. *Blood Press* **11**:95–100.
2 Acanfora D *et al.* (2002). A randomized, double-blind comparison of 10 and 20mg lercanidipine in patients with stable effort angina: effects on myocardial ischemia and heart rate variability. *Am J Ther* **9**:444–53.

Lidocaine

(See also 📖 Antiarrhythmic drugs: classification, p.362)

Sodium-channel blocker with class Ib antiarrhythmic properties.

Mechanism of action

Lidocaine blocks fast Na^+ channels that are responsible for the rapid depolarization (phase 0) of fast-response cardiac action potentials found in nonnodal cardiomyocytes. By inhibiting rapid Na^+ entry into cells, lidocaine decreases the slope of phase 0, amplitude of the action potential, and conduction velocity. Lidocaine binds preferentially to the inactivated Na^+ channels and therefore it acts selectively on ischaemic-depolarized tissues, where it promotes conduction block and suppresses re-entry circuits.

Lidocaine also reduces ventricular automaticity by decreasing the slope of phase 4, via a mechanism unrelated to its action on fast Na^+ channels. Lidocaine also shortens the duration of the action potential and effective refractory period (ERP) in ventricular tissues, possibly through an inhibitory effect of the late Na^+ current.

The shortening is more marked in the Purkinje fibres than in the ventricular muscle, so that lidocaine reduces the dispersion of ventricular refractoriness and the re-entry of cardiac impulses.

Pharmacodynamics

Compared with other class I antiarrhythmics, lidocaine is a relatively weak Na^+-channel blocker. It does not prolong ventricular depolarization (QRS complex) or repolarization (QT intervals), and does not reduce HR, contractility, AV conduction, or BP.

Pharmacokinetics

Lidocaine is rapidly distributed to all body tissues after an initial IV loading dose (V_d 1L/kg), so that a subsequent infusion or repeated doses should be administered to maintain therapeutic blood levels. About 65% is protein bound. About 80% of the dose is metabolized rapidly in the liver via CYP1A2 (and to a minor extent CYP3A4) to the active metabolites monoethylglycinexylidide and glycinexylidide and <10% is found unchanged in the urine. The elimination $t_{1/2}$ is 1.5–2h. Clearance is prolonged in the elderly, in cardiac failure, and in hepatic disease. Therapeutic plasma levels: 1.5–6mcg/mL. At higher doses there is an increase in CNS adverse effects.

Practical points

⚬ Doses

50–100mg IV under ECG monitoring with a rate of 25–50mg/min (2.5–5.0mL 1% solution). A 2nd dose may be given after 5min. No more than 200–300mg of lidocaine should be administered in a 1h period. In recurrent arrhythmia, IV infusions of lidocaine may be administered at the rate of 1–4mg/min (20–50mcg/kg/min) under ECG monitoring. As soon as possible, patients should be changed to an oral antiarrhythmic agent for maintenance therapy.

☻ Common side effects

Cardiovascular: hypotension, CV collapse, bradycardia which may lead to cardiac arrest and arrhythmias

CNS: nausea, light-headedness, drowsiness, dizziness, apprehension, nervousness, euphoria, tinnitus, blurred or double vision, nystagmus, vomiting, sensations of heat, cold, or numbness, twitching, tremors, paraesthesia, convulsions, unconsciousness, respiratory depression and arrest

Interactions

Propranolol, metoprolol, halothane, amiodarone, and cimetidine reduce hepatic clearance. The cardiac depressant effects of lidocaine are additive to those of other antiarrhythmic agents. Lidocaine prolongs the action of suxamethonium.

Cautions/notes

- Constant ECG monitoring is necessary during IV administration. Resuscitative equipment and drugs should be immediately available for the management of severe adverse CV, respiratory, or CNS effects. Hypokalaemia, hypoxia, and disorders of acid–base balance should be corrected before treatment with lidocaine begins.
- Lidocaine IV should be used with caution in patients with epilepsy, liver disease, congestive HF, severe renal disease, marked hypoxia, severe respiratory depression, hypovolaemia, or shock and in patients with any form of heart block or sinus bradycardia.
- Half dose in patients with severe hepatic disease or reduced hepatic blood flow [e.g. cardiogenic shock, severe HF, elderly patients, administration of cimetidine, halothane or hepatically metabolized β-blockers (propranolol, metoprolol)].
- With hepatic enzyme inducers (phenytoin, rifampicin) the dose of lidocaine needs to be increased.

Pregnancy and lactation

Safety has not been established with respect to possible adverse effects on fetal development in pregnancy (pregnancy category B). Lidocaine is excreted in breast milk, may produce fetal acidosis, respiratory depression, apnoea, and bradycardia in children and so should be used with caution in breastfeeding.

Contraindications

- Known hypersensitivity to local anaesthetics of the amide type or to other components of the solution
- Grade 2 or 3 AV block or nodal or intraventricular rhythm (lidocaine may suppress escape foci and produce cardiac arrest)

References

1 Sadowski ZP et al. (1999). Multicenter randomized trial and a systematic overview of lidocaine in acute myocardial infarction. *Am Heart J* **137**:792–8.
2 Gorgels AP et al. (1996). Comparison of procainamide and lidocaine in terminating sustained monomorphic ventricular tachycardia. *Am J Cardiol* **78**:43–6.
3 Ho DS et al. (1994). Double-blind trial of lignocaine versus sotalol for acute termination of spontaneous sustained ventricular tachycardia. *Lancet* **344**:18–23.

Lisinopril

(See also 📖 Angiotensin-converting enzyme inhibitors, p.355)

Orally active ACEI.

Indications

(See 📖 Angiotensin-converting enzyme inhibitors, p.355)

Mechanism of action

(See 📖 Renin–angiotensin–aldosterone system inhibitors, p.568 and 📖 Angiotensin-converting enzyme inhibitors, p.355)

Pharmacodynamics

Post-MI: RRR ≈6% (absolute rate=18.1% vs. 19.3%) in combined endpoint (mortality or development of severe LVF at 6 months) with 6 weeks of lisinopril compared with placebo following AMI.[1]

Heart failure: RRR ≈12% (HR=0.88%) in 2° combined endpoint (all-cause mortality or hospitalization), but not in the risk of death, with high-dose (32.5–35mg od) compared with low-dose lisinopril (2.5–5mg od) in patients with NYHA II–IV HF.[2]

Hypertension: no difference in 1° endpoint of fatal CHD or non-fatal MI (6-year rate ≈11.4%) with lisinopril compared with chlortalidone or amlodipine in hypertensive patients aged >55 years with at least one additional risk factor for CHD after a mean follow-up of 4.9 years.[3]

Diabetic nephropathy: 18% reduction in albumin excretion (absolute difference=2.2mcg/L) with lisinopril 10–20mg od compared with placebo in patients with type 1 diabetes.[4]

Pharmacokinetics

Variable oral bioavailability (10–60%) that is reduced to 16% in HF. Peak plasma concentrations reached in 7h and absorption is not affected by food. Lisinopril is not a prodrug, is not metabolized in the liver, is excreted unchanged in the urine (70%), and can be removed by dialysis. Excretion of lisinopril is reduced with renal impairment, especially with severe impairment (CrCl <30mL/min) when there is a 4.5-fold increase AUC. $t_{1/2}$ ≈12.6h.

Practical points

⚡ Doses

(See also 📖 Angiotensin-converting enzyme inhibitors for initiation under supervision, p.355)

Hypertension: 10mg initially (to maintenance of 20mg od or max 80mg od). Patients with cardiac decompensation or volume depletion should be started on 2.5–5mg od

Heart failure: (see doses for 📖 Angiotensin-converting enzyme inhibitors, p.355) 2.5mg od (increased in intervals ≤10mg/2 weeks to max of 35mg od if tolerated)

IV loop diuretics (furosemide) exhibit a venodilator effect that reduces preload and pulmonary congestion. When given to patients with pulmonary oedema, relief appears within 5–15min (even before diuresis). Loop diuretics are effective when the GFR <30mL/min.

Diuretic resistance: repetitive diuretic use can be associated with a decrease of the diuretic effect because the Na^+ reabsorption increases. This can be due to:

- reduced renal blood flow due to hypovolaemia, low cardiac output, hypotension
- stimulation of the RAAS. Aldosterone can produce distal tubular hypertrophy which reacts by reabsorbing more Na^+ (ACEIs or ARBs should be added to thiazides/loop diuretics)
- increased sympathetic tone (use β-blockers)
- incorrect use of diuretics: excessive doses, poor compliance, use of thiazides when GFR <20mL/min or combination of 2 loop diuretics or 2 thiazides (instead of combining 1 of each type)
- electrolyte imbalance: hyponatraemia, hypokalaemia
- concomitant therapy with drugs that antagonize the effects of the diuretics.

Pharmacokinetics

(See 📖 individual drugs)
They are rapidly absorbed from the GI tract, are highly bound to plasma proteins, and do not pass directly to the glomerular filtrate but are secreted in the proximal convoluted tubule by the organic acid transport mechanism to reach their site of action. Drug absorption by the oral route is impaired in severe HF; under these circumstances, the IV route can be useful. In the nephrotic syndrome, loop diuretics bind to albumin in the tubular fluid and so are less available to act on the $Na^+–K^+–2Cl^-$ symporter (diuretic resistance).

Practical points

⚗ Doses

(See 📖 individual drugs)
They can be given intravenously in urgent situations (e.g. acute pulmonary oedema) or when the intestinal absorption is decreased (e.g. in patients with congestive HF and reduced intestinal perfusion).

☺ Side effects

(>1%): electrolyte disturbances including hypovolaemia (with risk of pre-renal azotemia), hypokalaemia and hyponatraemia; hypochloraemia, metabolic alkalosis, hypocalcaemia and hypomagnesaemia, hyperuricaemia. Urinary retention due to vigorous diuresis in the elderly. Hypokalaemia can be treated by concomitant use of K^+-sparing diuretics or K^+ supplements.

Hypovolaemia and hyponatraemia stimulate renin secretion, leading to angiotensin II and aldosterone formation.

Cardiovascular: postural hypotension and arrhythmias from hypokalaemia, especially in patients taking digoxin.

Others: muscle cramps, paraesthesia; tinnitus, reversible or irreversible loss of hearing (after large doses, prolonged or parental administration; or renal impairment or hypoproteinaemia); blood dyscrasias, marrow suppression, and pancreatitis are uncommon. Photosensitive skin eruptions (furosemide).

Interactions

Hypotensive effects may be exacerbated when given with antihypertensive agents, nitrates, MAOIs, phenothiazines and tricyclic antidepressants (postural hypotension). Conversely, diuretic effects of loop diuretics are antagonized by NSAIDs (especially indometacin and ketorolac) that decrease the renal and vascular responses by inhibiting the formation of renal prostaglandins and corticosteroids.

Hypokalaemia may enhance arrhythmogenic effect of drugs (e.g. digoxin; sotalol; antiarrhythmic agents; drugs that prolong QT interval; and pimozide). Risk of hypokalaemia is increased when used with amphotericin; β-blockers; corticosteroids; tacrolimus; thiazide and related diuretics; theophylline.

Serum K^+ <3.5mmol/L increases CV events by about 4 times over a mean follow-up of 6.7 years.[3] In HF patients, non-K^+-retaining diuretics presented an increased rate of arrhythmic death compared with a K^+-sparing diuretic.[4]

There is an increased risk of toxicity with the following drugs when given with loop diuretics: lithium (due to reduced excretion); ciclosporin; and nephrotoxicity with NSAIDs (especially indometacin and ketorolac).

Ototoxicity with aminoglycosides, polymyxins, vancomycin.

Colestyramine and colestipol decrease their absorption.

Synergic diuretic effect when combined with thiazides or K^+-sparing diuretics (they reduce the hypokalaemia).

Cautions/notes

(See 📖 individual drugs)
Electrolytes, blood urea and creatinine, complete blood counts, and uric acid need to be monitored when using loop diuretics particularly in patients with cardiac disease, diabetes, renal or hepatic impairment and in elderly patients. Should be used with caution in patients receiving nephrotoxic, ototoxic or QT-prolonging drugs.

Pregnancy and lactation (see 📖 individual drugs)

Contraindications
- Anuria, renal failure
- Hypovolaemia, dehyration. In HF without fluid retention, furosemide increases aldosterone levels and produces LV dysfunction
- Severe hyponatraemia or hypokalaemia
- Severe hepatic impairment or coma
- Hypotension
- Sensitivity to sulphonamides (due to cross-sensitivity)

References

1 Greger R (2000). Physiology of sodium transport. *Am J Med Sci* **319**:51–62.

2 Mancia G et al. (2007). 2007 Guidelines for the management of arterial hypertension: The Task Force for the Management of Arterial Hypertension of the European Society of Hypertension (ESH) and of the European Society of Cardiology (ESC). *Eur Heart J* **28**:1462–536.

3 Cohen HW et al. (2001). High and low serum potassium associated with cardiovascular events in diuretic-treated patients. *J Hypertens* **19**:1315–23.

4 Domanski M et al. (2003). Diuretic use, progressive heart failure, and death in patients in the Studied Of Left Ventricular Dysfunction (SOLVD). *J Am Coll Cardiol* **42**:705–8.

Losartan

(See also 📖 Angiotensin II (AT$_1$) receptor blockers, p.359)

Angiotensin receptor blocker.

Indications

(See also 📖 Angiotensin II (AT$_1$) receptor blockers, p.359)

1. Treatment of hypertension
2. Treatment of diabetic nephropathy with an elevated serum creatinine and proteinuria (urinary albumin to creatinine ratio ≥ 300mg/g) in patients with type 2 diabetes and hypertension
3. HF (where intolerant of ACEIs)
4. Reduction of risk of stroke in hypertensive patients with LVH

Mechanism of action

(See also 📖 Renin–angiotensin–aldosterone system inhibitors. p.568 and 📖 Angiotensin II (AT$_1$) receptor blockers, p.359)

Pharmacodynamics

(See also 📖 Renin–angiotensin–aldosterone system inhibitors, p.568 and 📖 Angiotensin II (AT$_1$) receptor blockers, p.359)

Hypertension, diabetes, and LVH: RRR 13% (absolute rate 23.8 vs. 27.9/1000 patient years) in 1° composite endpoint of CV morbidity and mortality (CV death, stroke, or MI) in patients with diabetes, hypertension, and LVH given losartan 50–100mg od (mean dose 79mg) and additional hydrochlorothiazide and other antihypertensives as required to achieve a BP <140/90mmHg compared with atenolol with additional hydrochlorothiazide and other additional antihypertensives as required for mean of 4.8 years.[1] BP fall was significantly greater in the losartan compared to atenolol group (30.2/16.6mmHg vs. 29.1/16.8mmHg).[1] RRR 25% (absolute rate 13 vs. 17.5/1000 patient years) in new-onset diabetes mellitus compared with atenolol.[2]

RRR 24% (absolute rate 39.2 vs. 53.6/1000 patient years) in 1° composite endpoint of CV morbidity and mortality (CV death, non-fatal AMI, or non-fatal stroke) in patients with diabetes, hypertension, and LVH given losartan compared with atenolol for mean of 4.7 years.[3] Mortality from all causes was 63 and 104 in losartan and atenolol groups, respectively. BP fall was similarly greater in the losartan compared to atenolol group (19/11mmHg vs. 17/11mmHg).

Diabetic nephropathy: RRR≈16% (absolute rate: 43.5% vs. 47.1%) in combined 1° endpoint (doubling of baseline creatinine level 25%, end-stage renal disease ESRD 28%, or death) in patients with type 2 diabetes and nephropathy treated with losartan 50–100mg od compared with placebo and followed up for mean of 3.4 years.[4] RRR 32% in first hospitalization for HF, although the composite of morbidity and mortality from CV causes was similar in the 2 groups. The level of proteinuria declined by 35% with losartan vs. placebo. The benefit exceeded that attributable to changes in BP (140 vs. 142mmHg in the losartan and placebo groups).

Heart failure: no significant difference (annual mortality rate: 11.7% vs. 10.4%) in 1° endpoint of all-cause mortality in patients >60 years old, NYHA class II–IV HF and LVEF <40% treated with losartan titrated to 50mg od compared with captopril titrated to 50mg tds followed up for 80 weeks. Losartan was significantly better tolerated with fewer discontinuations.[5]

AMI: no significant difference (RR=1.13, 95% CI: 0.99–1.28; annual mortality rate: 18% vs. 16%) in 1° endpoint of all-cause mortality in patients >50 years old with AMI and LVF treated with losartan titrated to 50mg od compared with captopril titrated to 50mg tds followed up for 2.7 years. Losartan was significantly better tolerated.[6]

Pharmacokinetics
Well absorbed, but undergoes 1st-pass metabolism via CYP2C9 and CYP3A4 to form an active metabolite (bioavailability ≈30%), more potent than losartan, and inactive metabolites. Food reduces the absorption (30–40%). Peak levels of losartan and active metabolite occurred at ≈1 and ≈3–4h, respectively. Losartan binds to plasma proteins (35%), and presents a V_d of ≈0.6L/kg. Terminal $t_{1/2}$ of losartan and its active metabolite are ≈2h and ≈6–9h respectively. Over 95% of the absorbed dose is eliminated in the urine, 40–50% as unchanged drug.

Losartan levels do not appear to be altered with CrCl ≥10mL/ml but are increased in those on dialysis. Levels of active metabolite do not appear altered in renal impairment or dialysis.

Practical points

Doses
Hypertension: 50–100mg od

Heart failure: 12.5mg od (titrated up gradually by 12.5mg to 100mg od if tolerated)

A lower dose should be considered in hepatic impairment and those with intravascular volume depletion.

Side effects
(See also ☐ Angiotensin II (AT₁) receptor blockers, p.359)
(1–10%): nausea, vomiting, musculoskeletal pain.

Interactions (see ☐ Angiotensin II (AT₁) receptor blockers, p.359)
Cautions
(See ☐ Angiotensin II (AT₁) receptor blockers, p.359)

A lower dose should be considered in hepatic impairment.

Pregnancy and lactation (see ☐ Angiotensin II (AT₁) receptor blockers, p.359)

Contraindication
(See also ☐ Angiotensin II (AT₁) receptor blockers, p.359)
• Severe hepatic impairment

References

1 Dahlöf B *et al.*; LIFE Study Group (2002). Cardiovascular morbidity and mortality in the Losartan Intervention For Endpoint reduction in hypertension study (LIFE): a randomised trial against atenolol. *Lancet* **359**:995–1003.

2 Lindholm LH *et al.* (2002). Risk of new-onset diabetes in the Losartan Intervention For Endpoint reduction in hypertension study. *J Hypertens* **20**:1879–86.

3 Lindholm LH *et al.*; LIFE Study Group (2002). Cardiovascular morbidity and mortality in patients with diabetes in the Losartan Intervention For Endpoint reduction in hypertension study (LIFE): a randomised trial against atenolol. *Lancet* **359**:1004–10.

4 Brenner BM *et al.*; RENAAL Study Investigators (2001). Effects of losartan on renal and cardiovascular outcomes in patients with type 2 diabetes and nephropathy. *N Engl J Med* **345**:861–9.

5 Pitt B *et al.* (2005). Effect of losartan compared with captopril on mortality in patients with symptomatic heart failure: randomised trial—the Losartan Heart failure Survival Study ELITE II. *Lancet* **355**:1582–7.

6 Dickstein K *et al.*; OPTIMAAL Steering Committee of the OPTIMAAL Study Group (2002). Effects of losartan and captopril on mortality and morbidity in high-risk patients after acute myocardial infarction: the OPTIMAAL randomised trial. Optimal Trial in Myocardial Infarction with Angiotensin II Antagonist Losartan. *Lancet* **360**:752–60.

Lovastatin

(See also 📖 Statins, p.591)

Oral HMG-CoA reductase inhibitor.

CV indications

1. 1° hypercholesterolaemia, heterozygous familial hypercholesterolaemia or mixed dyslipidaemia, as an adjunct to diet, when response to non-pharmacological treatments is inadequate
2. 1° prevention of coronary events: reduction of CV mortality and morbidity in patients with moderate or severe hypercholesterolaemia and at high risk of a 1st CV event, as an adjunct to diet
3. 2° prevention of cardiovascular events: in patients with clinically evident CHD to reduce the risk of total mortality by reducing coronary death, MI, myocardial revascularization procedures, and stroke/TIA and slow the progression of coronary atherosclerosis

Mechanism of action

(See 📖 Statins, p.591)

Pharmacodynamics

1° hypercholesterolaemia

Reduces elevated LDL-C, total cholesterol, triglycerides and increases HDL-C (Table 9).

Table 9 Effects of lovastatin on lipid profile (adjusted mean % change)

Dose (mg)	Percentage change			
	Total chol	LDL chol	HDL chol	TG
Placebo	−2.0	−1.0	−1.0	+9.0
10	−16.0	−21.0	+5.0	−10.0
20	−19.0	−27.0	+6.0	−9.0
40	−22.0	−31.0	+5.0	−8.0
80	−29.0	−40.0	+9.5	−19.0

1° prevention

37% RRR (3.5% vs. 5.5% absolute rates) in mortality from coronary disease and non-lethal MI, 32% RRR (1.8 vs. 2.6%) in UA, 40% (1.7 vs. 2.9%) in MI (1.7 vs. 2.9%), and 33% (3.2 vs. 4.8%) of undergoing coronary revascularization procedures in patients with normal LDL-C (221mg/dL, 5.71mmol/L). Participants with ≥2 risk factors had RR in both acute major coronary events (43%) and coronary revascularization procedures (7%).[1]

Lovastatin alone[2,3] or in combination with colestipol and nicotinic acid[4,5] slowed the progression of coronary lesions (change in minimum lumen diameter, percentage diameter stenosis), increased the frequency of regression and reduced the incidence of CV events.

Pharmacokinetics

Lovastatin is incompletely absorbed after oral administration and because of extensive hepatic extraction, its bioavailability is low (<5%) and shows considerable interindividual variability. Peak plasma concentrations are reached after 2–3h. Lovastatin is highly bound (>95%) to human plasma proteins, undergoes extensive 1st-pass extraction and metabolism by cytochrome P450 3A4 in the liver, leading to active metabolites and 10% of the dose is eliminated in urine and 80% in faeces. Plasma elimination $t_{1/2}$ is 2–3h.

Practical points

♪ Doses

- 10–80mg od. Elderly patients may require a lower dose. In severe renal insufficiency (CrCl <30 mL/min), doses above 20mg/day should be carefully considered.
- Adolescents (10–17 years of age) with heterozygous familial hypercholesterolaemia: 10–40mg/day.
- For patients taking potent CYP3A4 inhibitors, the dose of lovastatin should not exceed 20mg daily. The dose of lovastatin should not exceed 40mg daily in patients treated with amiodarone or verapamil.

☺ Side effects

(See ☐ Statins, p.591)
Elevations of serum transaminases >3× upper limit occurred in ≤1.5% and myopathy, defined as muscle symptoms plus a CK elevation, in 0.1%.

Interactions (see ☐ Statins, p.591)

Cautions/notes (see ☐ Statins, p.591)

Pregnancy and lactation (see ☐ Statins, p.591)

Contraindications (see ☐ Statins, p.591)

References

1 Downs JR et al. (1998). Primary prevention of acute coronary events with lovastatin in men and women with average cholesterol levels: results of AFPS/TexCAPS. Air Force/Texas Coronary Atherosclerosis Prevention Study. *JAMA* **279**:1615–22.

2 Mack WJ et al. (1996). Lipoprotein subclasses in the Monitored Atherosclerosis Regression Study (MARS). Treatment effects and relation to coronary angiographic progression. *Arterioscler Thromb Vasc Biol* **16**:697–704.

3 Waters D et al. (1995). Effects of cholesterol lowering on the progression of coronary atherosclerosis in women: a Canadian Coronary Atherosclerosis Intervention Trial (CCAIT) substudy. *Circulation.* **92**:2404–10.

4 Brown G et al. (1990). Regression of coronary artery disease as a result of intensive lipid-lowering therapy in men with high levels of apolipoprotein B. *N Engl J Med* **323**:1289–98.

5 Furberg CD et al. (1994). Effect of lovastatin on early carotid atherosclerosis and cardiovascular events. Asymptomatic Carotid Artery Progression Study (ACAPS) Research Group. *Circulation* **90**:1679–87.

Low-molecular-weight heparins

(See also: ▭ Ardeparin, ▭ Dalteparin, p.415, ▭ Enoxaparin, p.446, ▭ Nadroparin, ▭ Tinzaparin)

These agents are about 1/3 of the MW of heparin, and are also heterogeneous in size.

LMWHs present several advantages over UFH: (a) greater bioavailability and a longer plasma $t_{\frac{1}{2}}$, so that they can be given SC in a fixed dose according to body weight; (b) a predictable level of anticoagulation without the need for APTT monitoring; (c) less unspecific binding to plasma or vascular proteins and not inhibited by PF4; (d) greater capacity to release tissue factor-pathway inhibitor; (e) less propensity to stimulate platelet aggregation and less risk of HIT. Therefore, LMWHs are much easier to use than UFH.

In aspirin-treated patients with STEMI who receive thrombolytic therapy, LMWH administered for 4–8 days compared with placebo reduces reinfarction by approximately 1/4 (1.6% vs. 2.2%) and death by 10% and when directly compared with UFH, it reduces reinfarction by 45% (3.0% vs. 5.2%).[1] The benefits of LMWH are seen early and remain evident at 30 days. These data suggest that LMWH should be the preferred antithrombin in this setting.

Cautions/notes

When epidural/spinal anaesthesia or spinal puncture is employed, patients treated with LMWH for prevention of thromboembolic complications are at risk of developing an epidural or spinal haematoma, which can result in long-term or permanent paralysis. The risk is increased by the use of indwelling epidural catheters for administration of analgesia or by the concomitant use of drugs affecting haemostasis (e.g. NSAIDs, platelet inhibitors, other anticoagulants).

Reference

1 van de Werf F et al. (2008). Management of acute myocardial infarction in patients presenting with persistent ST-segment elevation. *EHJ* **29**:2909–45.

Methyldopa

Oral centrally acting antihypertensive.

CV indications

Hypertension.

Mechanism of action

The antihypertensive effect is probably due to its metabolism to α-methylnoradrenaline, which binds to and activates central α_2-adrenergic receptors. These are auto-inhibitory receptors and so their stimulation by methyldopa results in inhibition of the sympathetic nervous outflow and a reduction in BP from a reduction in: (a) heart rate and contractility; (b) peripheral vascular resistances, and (c) plasma renin activity (i.e. inhibition of the RAAS).

Methyldopa causes a net reduction in the tissue concentration of serotonin, dopamine, adrenaline, and noradrenaline.

Pharmacodynamics

Methyldopa reduces both supine and standing BP but has no direct effect on cardiac function and does not reduce GFR, renal blood flow, or filtration fraction.

Methyldopa (750–1500mg od) reduces BP by ≈28/14mmHg and atenolol (150–300mg od) by 27/17mmHg in patients with inadequately controlled hypertension on chlortalidone; the combination on both drugs decreased BP by 38/25mmHg.[1]

27% RR in CV mortality in hypertensive patients treated with hydrochlorothaizide and triamterene following the addition of methyldopa.[2] A meta-analysis of clinical trials has suggested that pregnancies complicated by hypertension treated with antihypertensives including methyldopa may also have a lower risk of developing severe hypertension.[3]

Pharmacokinetics

Oral absorption of methyldopa is variable and incomplete (bioavailability ≈25–50%), reaching peak plasma concentrations at 2–3h. Methyldopa slightly binds to plasma proteins (12%), presents a V_d of 0.5L/kg and is extensively metabolized; approximately 70% of the drug absorbed is excreted in the urine as methyldopa and its mono-O-sulphate conjugate. Plasma $t_{1/2}$ is ≈1.8h. After oral doses, excretion is essentially complete in 36h.

Practical points

♣ Doses

250mg bd–tds initially (adjusted at intervals of no less than 2 days, to a maximum dose of 3g/day). To minimize the sedation, start dosage increases in the evening. Since methyldopa has a relatively short duration of action, after withdrawal BP usually returns to pretreatment levels within 48h.

An appropriate starting dose in the elderly would be 125mg tds, increasing slowly as required, but not to exceed a maximum daily dosage of 2g.

☺ *Side effects*

- *GI:* including nausea, vomiting, stomatitis, sialadenitis, nasal stuffiness; constipation, diarrhoea, mild dryness of mouth, sore or 'black' tongue, pancreatitis
- *Cardiovascular:* bradycardia, aggravation of angina, myocarditis, pericarditis, orthostatic hypotension
- *Haematological:* haemolytic anaemia, bone-marrow depression, leukopenia, granulocytopenia, thrombocytopenia, eosinophilia
- *Nervous system:* sedation (usually transient), depression, headache, paraesthesia, nightmares, parkinsonism, Bell's palsy, involuntary choreoathetotic movements; impaired mental acuity, prolonged carotid sinus hypersensitivity; dizziness, light-headedness, and symptoms of cerebrovascular insufficiency (may be due to lowering of BP)
- *Dermatological:* eczema or lichenoid eruption, toxic epidermal necrolysis
- *Musculoskeletal:* lupus-like syndrome, mild arthralgia with or without joint swelling, myalgia
- *Others:* hyperprolactinaemia, breast enlargement, gynaecomastia, amenorrhoea, lactation, impotence, failure of ejaculation, decreased libido. Asthenia or weakness, oedema (and weight gain) usually relieved by use of a diuretic. Drug-related fever. Liver disorders including hepatitis, jaundice, abnormal LFTs
- Positive Coombs' test, positive tests for antinuclear antibody, LE cells, and rheumatoid factor, abnormal LFTs, rise in blood urea
- *Rare:* fatal hepatic necrosis has been reported

Interactions

- It can potentiate the effects of other antihypertensives. Sympathomimetics, phenothiazines and tricyclic antidepressants may diminish its antihypertensive effects.
- Patients taking methyldopa may require lower doses of anaesthetic agents.
- Bioavailability of methyldopa may be reduced when ingested with ferrous sulphate or ferrous gluconate.
- Increased risk of lithium toxicity.

Cautions/notes

Blood counts and LFTs should be performed at intervals in the first 6–12 weeks or when fever occurs. It may also be helpful to perform a Coombs' test before and ~6–12 months after commencement of therapy due to the possibility of development of a dose-dependent and reversible positive Coombs' test. Methyldopa may also interfere with measurement of urinary uric acid, serum creatinine, aspartate transaminase, cathecholamines (but it does not interfere with the measurement of vanillylmandelic acid), antinuclear antibodies, and rheumatoid factor, depending on method used.

Should be used with extreme caution in patients with previous hepatic disease and patients with hepatic porphyria. Due to renal excretion, patients with impaired renal function may respond to lower doses. Methyldopa is not recommended for the treatment of hypertension associated with phaeochromocytoma.

Occasionally tolerance may occur, usually between the 2nd and 3rd month of therapy. Adding a thiazide or increasing the dosage of methyldopa will frequently restore an effective control of BP.

Pregnancy and lactation

Although methyldopa crosses the placenta, it has been used under close medical supervision for the treatment of hypertension during pregnancy. Published reports indicate that if this drug is used during pregnancy the possibility of fetal harm appears remote (pregnancy category B). Methyldopa appears in breast milk, and breastfeeding mothers must weigh the anticipated benefits against possible risks.

Contraindications

- Active hepatic disease (acute hepatitis and active cirrhosis)
- Depression; concurrent treatment with MAO inhibitors

References

1 Webster J et al. (1977). Atenolol, methyldopa, and chlorthalidone in moderate hypertension. Br Med J **1**(6053): 76–8.

2 Amery A et al. (1985). Mortality and morbidity results from the European Working Party on High Blood Pressure in the Elderly trial. Lancet **1**(8442):1349–54.

3 Abalos E et al. (2007). Antihypertensive drug therapy for mild to moderate hypertension during pregnancy. Cochrane Database Syst Rev CD002252.

Metolazone

(See also 📖 Thiazide and related diuretics, p.604)

Metolazone is a substituted quinazolinone thiazide-like diuretic.

CV and other indications

(See 📖 Thiazide and related diuretics, p.604)

Mechanism of action

(See 📖 Thiazide and related diuretics, p.604)

Pharmacodynamics

Diuresis begins within 1h and persists for 24h, particularly at the higher recommended dosages.

Metolazone is around 10x as potent as hydrochlorothiazide. Metolazone 5mg od is more potent and produces greater BP lowering than bendro-flumethiazide 5mg od.[1] When given in addition to a CCB in hypertensive patients,[2] it reduces BP by 10–15/7–11mmHg. In contrast to other thiazides, metolazone remains effective in renal impairment but with the risk of excessive diuresis. In combination with furosemide produce a profound diuresis.

Metolazone at fixed dose of 10mg od for 3 days given in combination with loop diuretics to patients with NYHA II and IV HF produces, by ≈day 6–7, a median maximum weight loss of ≈5.6 kg; a maximal fall in serum Na^+ and K^+ of ≈3–4mmol/L and ≈0.7mmol/L respectively; and a maximal rise in creatinine of ≈30–40 µmol/L.[3]

Pharmacokinetics

≈65% of the amount ingested becomes available in the bloodstream. Highly bound (95%) to red blood cells and plasma protein. Only a small amount of metolazone is metabolized, and 80% is excreted in the unconverted form in the urine. $t_{1/2}$ is ≈12–14h.

Practical points

⚡ Doses

For hypertension: 2.5–5mg od initially (on alternate days for maintenance)
For oedema: 5–10mg od to a max of 80mg if required

Given its potency, it is advisable to start metolazone at doses much lower than those recommended, especially when given in combination with a loop diuretic.

☺ Side effects

(See 📖 Thiazide and related diuretics, p.604)
Other common side effects include dizziness, headaches, muscle cramps and fatigue.

Interactions (see 📖 Thiazide and related diuretics, p.604)

Cautions/notes

(See also 📖 Thiazide and related diuretics, p.604)
Serum electrolytes, including serum potassium, should be carefully monitored, especially when given with other diuretics.

Pregnancy and lactation (see 📖 Thiazide and related diuretics, p.604)

Contraindications

(See also 📖 Thiazide and related diuretics, p.604)
Anuria, in hepatic coma or pre-coma, and in cases of known allergy and hypersensitivity to metolazone

References

1 Winchester JF et al. (1980). Metolazone and bendroflumethiazide in hypertension: physiologic and metabolic observations. *Clin Pharmacol Ther* **28**:611–18.

2 Lüscher TF, Waeber B (1993). Efficacy and safety of various combination therapies based on a calcium antagonist in essential hypertension: results of a placebo-controlled randomized trial. *J Cardiovasc Pharmacol* **21**:305–9.

3 Channer KS et al. (1994). Combination diuretic treatment in severe heart failure: a randomised controlled trial. *Br Heart J* **71**:146–150.

Metoprolol

(See also 📖 β-blockers, p.376)

Cardioselective β_1-adrenergic receptor antagonist with high lipid solubility and membrane-stabilizing activity.

CV indications

(See 📖 β-blockers, p.376)

Mechanism of action

(See 📖 β-blockers, p.376)

Pharmacodynamics

(See 📖 β-blockers, p.376)

Metoprolol has membrane-stabilizing properties but only at doses much greater than that required for β-blockade.

Hypertension: RRR ≈40% in CV endpoints and RRR ≈43% in mortality in elderly hypertensive patients (70–84 years) treated with metoprolol (mean difference in BP ≈19.1/8.5mmHg) compared with placebo and followed up for ≈4.5 years.[1]

Heart failure: studies with metoprolol succinate controlled-release or extended-release (CR/XL) formulation have shown efficacy of metoprolol in HF. In contrast, metoprolol immediate release (IR, 50mg bd) appears to be associated with relatively increased risk of mortality compared with carvedilol 25mg bd (HR≈0.83) after 58 months in patients with NYHA II–IV and LVEF ≤35%.[2] The reduction of all-cause mortality was consistent across predefined subgroups.

RR≈0.66 (absolute rate: 7.2% vs. 11.0% per patient year of follow-up) in all-cause mortality in patients with NYHA class II–IV and LVEF ≤40% treated with metoprolol (target dose 200mg od of controlled/extended release—CR/XL formulation) and followed up for a mean of ≈1 year.[3] There were fewer sudden deaths (RR 0.59) and deaths from worsening HF (RR 0.51).

RR≈0.42 (absolute rates: 3.4% vs. 8.1%) of death in patients with symptomatic NYHA II–IV HF (on treatment with ACEI, ARB, or both) treated with metoprolol CR added to standard therapy compared to placebo and followed up for 24 weeks.[4] Metoprolol also improves ventricular function and reduces activation of the RAAS.

Post-MI: 36% RRR in mortality (absolute values 8.9% vs. 5.7%) at 90 days in patients with AMI treated with metoprolol (15mg IV + 200mg/day) for 90 days. 35% RRR in the incidence of fatal and non-fatal MI during the next 4–90 days.[5] Furthermore, metoprolol reduces the incidence of VT during AMI.[6]

Pharmacokinetics

Metoprolol tartrate (immediate-release–IR) formulation is almost completely absorbed, but its bioavailability is ≈40–50% due to hepatic 1st-pass metabolism. Protein binding is ≈12% and V_d in steady state is ≈3.5L/kg. Metoprolol undergoes extensive oxidative metabolism in the liver, primarily by the CYP2D6 isoenzyme, into inactive metabolites, and <5% of an oral dose is recovered unchanged in the urine. The oxidative metabolism is under genetic control, so that poor metabolizers (PM) have higher plasma levels; there are marked ethnic differences in the prevalence of the PM phenotype (≈7% of Caucasians and <1% Asian). $t_{1/2}$ ≈3–5h (7.5h in PM and 2.8h in extensive metabolizers), but the effects persists for 12h. The pharmacokinetic properties of metoprolol are unaltered in patients with renal failure; thus, no reduction in dosage is needed in patients with chronic renal failure.

Compared to metoprolol tartrate IR formulation, metoprolol succinate (CR/XL formulation) has lower bioavailability (≈70% compared with IR formulation) and is characterized by lower C_{max}, longer time to peak plasma levels (to ≈8h) and lower peak to trough variation.

Practical points

⚕ Doses
50–100mg bd or tds (max dose 400mg/day) for metoprolol IR formulation

IV: 5mg over 5min; 5min later a 2nd bolus and 5min later a 3rd bolus

Metoprolol CR/XL formulation: 25–100 or 200mg od (doses of 12.5mg od may be initially required in patients with severe HF).

Dose adjustment is not usually required in hepatic impairment except with severe dysfunction.

☻ Side effects (see 📖 β-blockers, p.376)

Interactions

(See 📖 β-blockers, p.376)
CYP2D6 inhibitors (e.g. fluoxetine, paroxetine, bupropion, thioridazine, propafenone, ritonavir, diphenhydramine, hydroxychloroquine, quinidine, terbinafine, cimetidine) may increase plasma concentration of metoprolol. Conversely, enzyme-inducing agents (e.g. rifampicin) can decrease plasma concentration of metoprolol.

Cautions/notes (see 📖 β-blockers, p.376)

Pregnancy and lactation
Metoprolol crosses the placenta and is found in breast milk. Its use is not recommended in pregnancy and breastfeeding (pregnancy category C).

Contraindications (see 📖 β-blockers, p.376)

References
1 Dahlöf B et al. (1991). Morbidity and mortality in the Swedish Trial in Old Patients with Hypertension (STOP-Hypertension). Lancet **338**(8778):1281–5.
2 Poole-Wilson PA et al.; (1994) Carvedilol Or Metoprolol European Trial Investigators (2003). Comparison of carvedilol and metoprolol on clinical outcomes in patients with chronic heart failure in the Carvedilol Or Metoprolol European Trial (COMET): randomised controlled trial. Lancet **362**:7–13.

3 (1999) Effect of metoprolol CR/XL in chronic heart failure: Metoprolol CR/XL Randomised Intervention Trial in Congestive Heart Failure (MERIT-HF). *Lancet* 1999; **353**:2001–7.

4 The RESOLVD Investigators (2000). Effects of metoprolol CR in patients with ischemic and dilated cardiomyopathy: the randomized evaluation of strategies for left ventricular dysfunction pilot study. *Circulation* **101**:378–84.

5 Hjalmarson A et al. (1983). The Göteborg metoprolol trial. Effects on mortality and morbidity in acute myocardial infarction. *Circulation* **67**:126–32.

6 Rydén L et al. (1983). A double-blind trial of metoprolol in acute myocardial infarction. Effects on ventricular tachyarrhythmias. *N Engl J Med* **308**:614–18.

Mexiletine

(See also 📖 Antiarrhythmic drugs: classification, p.362)

Oral and IV administration class Ib antiarrhythmic agent (discontinued in the UK and available by order in the US).

CV indications

Treatment of life-threatening arrhythmias.

Mechanism of action

(See 📖 Lidocaine, p.503)

Pharmacodynamics

(See 📖 Lidocaine, p.503)

Pharmacokinetics

Good oral absorption (bioavailability 85–90%), reaching peak plasma levels within 1–2h. Mexiletine is ≈50–70% protein bound, widely distributed (V_d 5.5–9.5L/kg) throughout the body, metabolized in the liver via CYP2C6 and CYP1A2, with about 15% of the dose being excreted unchanged in urine. Plasma $t_{1/2}$: 5–17h in healthy individuals (19–26h in patients with HF, AMI, or liver disease). Therapeutic plasma levels: 2–5mcg/ml. An increase in the CNS adverse effects has been observed when plasma levels exceed 2mcg/mL.

Practical points

⚡ Doses

A loading dose is required, particularly with IV infusion, to compensate for rapid phase of tissue distribution.

IV: loading dose: 100–250mg at a rate of 12.5mg/min. Then 2mg/kg/h for 3.5h and then 0.5mg/kg/h.

Maintenance dose: infusion of 250mg of mexiletine in 500mL of saline at a rate of 1mL/min, for as long as required or until oral administration is commenced.

PO: loading dose of 400mg followed in 8h by 200–250mg tds (bd in hepatic or severe renal failure). Max dose 900mg/day.

☺ Side effects

(>10%): nausea, vomiting, unpleasant taste, dizziness, heartburn, nausea, nervousness, tremor, diplopia, paraesthesia, nystagmus, lightheadedness.
(1–10%): palpitations, chest pain, bradycardia, transient AV block, ventricular arrhythmias, incoordination, numbness, headache, dyspnoea.

Interactions

Plasma levels of mexiletine may be increased by drugs that inhibit CYP450 (1A2 and 2D6). Consequently, reduced doses of mexiletine may be required during concomitant administration with such drugs (paroxetine, ritonavir). Conversely, doses may need to be increased during co-administration with drugs that induce liver enzymes (phenytoin, rifampicin).

Drugs that acidify or alkalinize urine may increase or decrease excretion of mexiletine respectively. Concurrent administration of mexiletine with warfarin may lead to increased risk of bleeding. Mexiletine increases plasma levels of theophylline. Amiodarone increases the plasma levels of mexiletine.

Concurrent administration of mexiletine with some other antiarrhythmic drugs may lead to an increased effect on conduction and pumping of the heart. Concurrent use of mexiletine and local anaesthetics may also cause toxicity of local anaesthetics.

Cautions/notes
In the following situations, the patient should be carefully monitored:
- sinus node dysfunction, conduction defect, bradycardia, hypotension, or cardiac failure
- moderate to severe hepatic disease and patients with features of impaired liver function

Pregnancy and lactation
Mexiletine freely crosses the placenta and is also expressed in breast milk (pregnancy category C). Therefore, its use should only be considered if deemed essential.

Contraindications
- Patients with previous MI within the preceding 3 months or with LVEF <35% (except for patients with life-threatening ventricular arrhythmias)
- Cardiogenic shock or pre-existing 2nd- or 3rd-degree AV block (if no pacemaker is present)
- Premature infants

Reference
1 Mason JW (1993). A comparison of seven antiarrhythmic drugs in patients with ventricular tachyarrhythmias. Electrophysiologic Study versus Electrocardiographic Monitoring Investigators. *N Engl J Med* **329**(7):452–8.

Moxonidine

Oral centrally-acting I_1-imidazoline-selective receptor agonist.

CV indications

Mild to moderate hypertension.

Mechanism of action

Moxonidine selectively interacts with I_1-imidazoline receptors within the brainstem (in the rostral ventrolateral medulla) to reduce sympathetic nervous activity. Moxonidine also promotes sodium excretion.

Moxonidine reduces adrenaline, noradrenaline, and renin levels, a finding that is consistent with central inhibition of sympathetic tone.

Pharmacodynamics

Moxonidine reduces BP through a fall in systemic vascular resistances and an increase in sodium excretion, while heart rate, cardiac output, stroke volume, and pulmonary artery pressures are not affected. LVH has been found to regress after 6 months' treatment with moxonidine.

BP reduction $\approx$25/13mmHg with 6 weeks' moxonidine 0.6mg od therapy, significantly greater than placebo ($\approx$1/2mmHg) and comparable to enalapril 20mg od.[1]

In animal models moxonidine improves insulin resistance and glucose tolerance and reduces structural renal damage in various models of renal failure.

In patients with NYHA class II–IV HF and reduced ejection fraction, moxonidine SR (1.5mg bd) increased mortality as compared to placebo (5.5 vs. 3.4%); hospitalization rates for HF, AMI, and adverse events were also more frequent in the moxonidine SR group.[2]

Pharmacokinetics

Moxonidine is well absorbed via the GI tract (bioavailability ~90%) and is unaffected by food. Maximum plasma levels are reached in 1h. It is ~7% bound to plasma proteins and its V_d is ~2.5L/kg. Moxonidine is mostly excreted unchanged in the urine (75%), while only about 1% is eliminated via the faeces. The mean elimination $t_{1/2}$ is 2.5h, which is prolonged by renal insufficiency. However, the antihypertensive effect lasts longer than would be expected from its $t_{1/2}$, as moxonidine is suitable for once-daily administration.

Practical points

♣ Doses

Initial dose of 0.2mg in the morning (up to a maximum of 0.6mg in divided doses)

In moderate renal dysfunction (GFR >30mL/min, but <60mL/min), the single dose should not exceed 0.2mg and the daily dose should not exceed 0.4mg. It is contraindicated in GFR <30mL/min.

☻ *Side effects*

(>1%): dry mouth, headache, fatigue, asthenia, dizziness, nausea, sleep disturbances and vasodilatation.

(Others): sedation (<1%), skin reactions, isolated cases of angio-oedema.

The frequency and intensity of these symptoms often decrease in the course of treatment.

Interactions

Hypotensive effects are enhanced with use of other antihypertensives. May potentiate the effect of sedatives and hypnotics.

Cautions/notes

Use with alcohol or tricyclic antidepressants should be avoided. If concomitant treatment with a β-blocker has to be stopped, the β-blocker should be discontinued first, then moxonidine after a few days. Where necessary, moxonidine itself should be withdrawn gradually over 2 weeks.

Pregnancy and lactation

Moxonidine is not teratogenic in animal models. Due to limited therapeutic evidence, it is not recommended in pregnancy (pregnancy category C). It is excreted into breast milk. Due to limited therapeutic evidence, it should not be used in breastfeeding mothers.

Contraindications

- Severe hepatic or renal (GFR <30mL/min) disease
- History of angioneurotic oedema
- Sick sinus syndrome, SA block, 2nd or 3rd AV block, bradycardia, malignant arrhythmias
- Severe HF and/or severe CAD
- Due to limited therapeutic experience, it should not be used in intermittent claudication, Raynaud's syndrome, Parkinson's disease, epileptic disorders, or depression

References

1 Prichard BN *et al.* (2002). Placebo-controlled comparison of the efficacy and tolerability of once-daily moxonidine and enalapril in mild to moderate essential hypertension. *Blood Press* **11**:166–72.
2 Cohn J *et al.* (2003). Adverse mortality effect of central sympathetic inhibition with sustained-release moxonidine in patients with heart failure (MOXCON). *Eur J Heart Fail* **5**:659–67.

Nicorandil

A nitrate derivative of nicotinamide which activates ATP-dependent K^+ channels.

CV indications

1. Prevention and long-term treatment of chronic stable angina
2. Reduction in incidence of ACS in patients with chronic stable angina with previous MI, CABG, or CHD on angiography

Mechanism of action

As an organic nitrate, nicorandil is a NO donor that activates guanylate cyclase, increases cGMP cellular levels, and predominantly relaxes vascular smooth muscle in veins and also causes epicardial coronary vasodilatation. In addition, activation of ATP-dependent K^+ channels results in increased cellular K^+ efflux, membrane hyperpolarization, inhibition of Ca^{2+} entry via L-type Ca^{2+} channels and, consequently, arterial and arteriolar dilatation.

Pharmacodynamics

In animal studies, intracellular hyperpolarization from the opening of ATP-dependent K^+ channels in ischaemic cardiomyocytes also appears to reduce contractility in ATP-depleted cells, and may limit infarct size and hasten recovery from ischaemia-induced injury. However, the clinical significance of these effects is uncertain.

Effects correlate poorly with plasma levels. Overall, nicorandil appears to decrease preload (with a fall of 4.8mmHg in LV end-diastolic pressure and $\approx$5.7mmHg in mPAP at 1h after single 40mg dosing) and afterload (with associated fall in BP), and thereby cardiac work. Improves exercise tolerance by about 1–2min.

Reduces frequency of angina as effectively as other antianginals.

HR $\approx$0.83 (absolute values 15.5% vs. 13.1%) for 1° composite endpoint (CHD death, non-fatal MI or unplanned admission for cardiac chest pain) over a mean of 1.6 years (NNT=42) in patients at high risk of CV events treated with nicorandil (20mg bd) cf placebo in addition to standard therapy.[1] No advantage was seen in 2° endpoint of CHD death or non-fatal MI. (Interpretation of such trial data is difficult as the majority of benefit with nicorandil appeared to be with reduced unplanned admissions; and as there was relatively low prevalence of s prevention treatments such as B-blockers, ACEIs, and statins.)

Pharmacokinetics

Rapid absorption from the gut with high bioavailability ($\approx$75%), reaching peak plasma levels after 0.5–1h. There is minimal 1st-pass effect, and it is bound weakly to plasma proteins (25%); its V_d is 1.0L/kg. It is extensively metabolized in the liver and excreted by the kidney (<5% through the biliary route). $t_{1/2} \approx$1h. The pharmacokinetics are not altered in elderly persons and in patients who have chronic renal impairment or liver insufficiency.

Practical points

♪ Doses
10–30mg bd (for symptomatic treatment of angina)

Doses of 10–20mg bd are usually adequate to control anginal symptoms. Gradual titration from 5mg bd may reduce likelihood of persistent or severe headaches. No dose adjustment appears necessary with age, in renal or hepatic impairment.

☺ Common side effects
(>10%): headaches (up to 36%)
(1–10%): dizziness; nausea and vomiting; flushing; general weakness; rectal bleeding

Headaches appear to be dose dependent and resolve despite continued treatment. Although rare, there have been reports of both oral (occasionally severe) and anal ulcers, which have resolved on discontinuation of nicorandil.

Interactions
No interactions have been observed for β-blockers, CCB, digoxin, or furosemide.

Cautions/notes
Metformin has the potential to close ATP-dependent K^+ channels and hence may antagonize the effects and benefits of nicorandil. PDE-5 inhibitors can cause a marked drop in BP.

Pregnancy and lactation
No data in pregnancy or breastfeeding (pregnancy category B).

Contraindications
- Cardiogenic shock, acute pulmonary oedema or AMI with LV failure and low filling pressures, hypotension, hypovolaemia
- Hypotension, AS
- Concomitant administration with PDE-5 inhibitors (e.g. sildenafil, tadalafil, vardenafil) due to risk of hypotension

Reference
1 The IONA Study Group (2002). Effect of nicorandil on coronary events in patients with stable angina: the Impact Of Nicorandil in Angina (IONA) randomised trial. *Lancet* **359**:1269–75.

Nicotinic acid (niacin)

Nicotinic acid is an antihyperlipidaemic agent.

CV indications

Niacin therapy is indicated as an adjunct to diet when the response to diet and other nonpharmacologic measures alone is inadequate:

- To reduce elevated total cholesterol, LDL-C, ApoB, and triglyceride levels, and to increase HDL-C in patients with 1° hyperlipidaemia (heterozygous familial and nonfamilial) and mixed dyslipidaemia (Fredrickson types IIa and IIb)
- In combination with statins for the treatment of 1° hyperlipidaemia (heterozygous familial and non-familial) and mixed dyslipidaemia (Fredrickson types IIa and IIb) when monotherapy is inadequate
- In patients with a history of MI to reduce the risk of recurrent non-fatal MI
- In patients with a history of CAD and hyperlipidaemia the combination of nicotinic acid with a bile acid-binding resin to slow progression or promote regression of atherosclerotic disease
- In combination with a bile acid-binding resin to reduce elevated total cholesterol and LDL-C levels in adult patients with 1° hyperlipidaemia (type IIa)
- As adjunctive therapy for treatment of adult patients with severe hypertriglyceridaemia (types IV and V hyperlipidaemia) who present a risk of pancreatitis and who do not respond adequately to diet

Mechanism of action

Nicotinic acid acts on G-protein-coupled GPR109A (HM74A or PUMA-G) and GPR109B (HM74) receptors. Stimulation of GPR109A receptors on adipocytes has the following effects:[1]

- reduces triglyceride lipolysis by inhibiting triglyceride lipase which decreases free fatty acid (FFA) mobilization to the liver
- inhibits hepatocyte diacylglycerol acyltransferase 2 (DGAT2), a key enzyme for TG synthesis, resulting in accelerated hepatic ApoB degradation and decreased secretion of VLDL and LDL
- retards the hepatic catabolism of ApoA-I which increases HDL $t_{1/2}$ and concentrations of lipoprotein A-I HDL subfractions, thereby augmenting cholesterol efflux and reverse cholesterol transport
- inhibits the hepatocyte HDL catabolism receptor and the removal of HDL-apoA-I, increasing HDL half-life and concentrations of Lp A-I HDL subfractions, cholesterol efflux and reverse cholesterol transport.

Nicotinic acid also inhibits oxidative stress and vascular inflammatory genes involved in atherosclerosis.

Pharmacodynamics

Nicotinic acid reduces total and LDL-C (10–20%) and triglycerides (30–70%) and increases HDL-C (20–35%).

27% RR reduction (8.9% vs. 12.2%) in non-fatal, recurrent, MI in patients with previous MI treated with nicotinic acid (3g/day) for 5 years as compared to placebo, accompanied by a decrease in total cholesterol (10%) and triglycerides (26%).[2] 10 years later, the group randomized to nicotinic acid presented a significant 11% reduction in total mortality as compared to placebo, which suggested that early reduction in CHD may result in long-term reduction in total mortality.[3]

Statin–niacin combination therapy: in patients with CHD and low HDL-C, 3 years' treatment with simvastatin and nicotinic acid (immediate-release formulation) increases HDL-C (26%) and reduces LDL-C levels (42%).[4] The average stenosis progressed by 3.9% with placebo and regressed by 0.4% with simvastatin–niacin alone. Moreover, the combination produced a 90% RR in 1° event rate (arteriographic evidence of a change in coronary stenosis and the occurrence of death, MI, stroke, or revascularization).

In patients with ApoB levels ≥125mg/dL, CHD, and family histories of vascular disease, intensive lipid-lowering therapy (lovastatin plus colestipol or nicotinic acid plus colestipol) reduced the progression of coronary lesions, increased the frequency of regression, and reduced the incidence of cardiovascular events (death, MI, or revascularization for worsening angina) as compared to monotherapy.[5]

Pharmacokinetics
Nicotinic acid is rapidly absorbed after oral administration, reaching peak plasma levels within 30–60min. Approximately 88% of an oral pharmacologic dose is eliminated by the kidneys as unchanged drug and nicotinuric acid, its 1° metabolite. The plasma elimination $t_{1/2}$ is 20–45min.

Practical points
♣ Doses
Immediate- and sustained-release formulations are available as dietary supplements, while extended-release (ER) nicotinic acid is available only for prescription. Prolonged- and sustained-release nicotinic acid preparations should not be substituted for equivalent doses of IR nicotinic acid.

Extended release: initial dose 375mg od at bedtime to reduce the incidence/severity of side effects. The daily dosage should not be increased by more than 500mg in any 4-week period. Further increases according to the patient's response. Maintenance dose: 1–2g od at bedtime.

A formulation of nicotinic acid/laropiprant (1000mg/20mg) modified-release tablets for patients with dyslipidaemia and 1° hypercholesterolaemia is available. Laropiprant is a potent, selective antagonist of the prostaglandin D2 (PGD2) receptor subtype 1 (DP1). It has no effect on lipid levels, but significantly lowered flushing symptom scores (by approximately 50% or more).[10] The starting dose is 1g nicotinic acid/20mg laropiprant od; after four weeks, it is recommended to reach the maintenance dose of 2000mg/40mg od.

☺ Side effects
The use of nicotinic acid is limited by side effects.

Cardiovascular: AF, arrhythmias, hypotension, orthostasis

GI: dyspepsia (frequent), vomiting, diarrhoea, peptic ulceration, jaundice, abnormal LFTs. Some cases of severe hepatic toxicity, including fulminant hepatic necrosis, have been described. Serum transaminases should be monitored before treatment begins, every 6–12 weeks for the 1st year, and then every 6 months. If the transaminase levels rise to 3× the upper limit of normal, the drug should be discontinued. Hepatotoxicity may be associated with a marked decrease (50%) in LDL-C levels.

Skin: flushing (tolerance develops rapidly over a few weeks), pruritus, hyperpigmentation, acanthosis nigricans, dry skin. The incidence of vasodilatory flushing with prolonged-release formulations is lower than with IR nicotinic acid and it decreases substantially over time as tolerance develops. Flushing and pruritus can be minimized with aspirin or NSAIDs taken 30min prior to nicotinic acid.

Dizziness, headache, paraesthesia; diarrhoea, dyspepsia, nausea, vomiting.

Metabolic: increases glycaemia (~4mg/dL after 6 months), hyperuricaemia, gout.

Rare cases of rhabdomyolysis have been associated when high doses (≥1g/day) of nicotinic acid are co-administered with HMG-CoA reductase inhibitors. Thus, patients receiving this combination should be told to report muscle pain, tenderness, or weakness and should be carefully monitored, and periodic serum CPK and K^+ determinations should be performed.

Interactions
Nicotinic acid potentiates the effects of vasoactive drugs resulting in postural hypotension.

Alcohol or hot beverages (e.g. coffee) may increase flushing and pruritus and should be avoided at the time of drug ingestion.

Cautions/notes
Flushing, pruritus, and GI side effects (dyspepsia) are reduced by slowly increasing the dose of nicotinic acid and avoiding administration on an empty stomach. In general, the incidence of adverse events was higher in women compared to men.

Nicotinic acid should be used with caution in patients with a history of jaundice, hepatobiliary disease, diabetes (it increases insulin resistance and worsens glycaemia), or peptic ulcer or who consume large quantities of alcohol. Frequent monitoring of LFTs and blood glucose should be performed.

Nicotinic acid should be used with caution in patients with UA or in the acute phase of MI, particularly if they are also receiving vasoactive drugs.

Nicotinic acid increases serum uric acid levels; use with caution in patients predisposed to gout.

Nicotinic acid may produce false elevations in some fluorometric determinations of plasma or urinary catecholamines and false-positive reactions (Benedict's reagent) in urine glucose tests.

Pregnancy and lactation
It is not known whether nicotinic acid can cause fetal harm when administered to pregnant women or whether it can affect reproductive capacity (pregnancy category C). Moreover, it is unknown whether this drug is excreted in human milk; it should not be given to nursing mothers.

Contraindications
- Hypersensitivity to any component of this medication
- Active liver diseases or unexplained transaminase elevations
- Active peptic ulcer disease
- Arterial bleeding

References

1 Kamanna VS, Kashyap M (2008). Mechanism of action of niacin. *Am J Cardiol* **101**(suppl):20B-6B.
2 The Coronary Drug Project Research Group (1975). Clofibrate and niacin in coronary heart disease. *JAMA* **231**:360–81.
3 Canner PL *et al.* (1986). Fifteen year mortality in coronary drug project patients: long-term benefit with niacin. *JACC* **8**:1245–55.
4 Brown BG *et al.* (2001). Simvastatin and niacin, antioxidant vitamins, or the combination for the prevention of coronary disease. *N Engl J Med* **345**:1583–92.
5 Brown G *et al.*; Regression of coronary artery disease as a result of intensive lipid-lowering therapy in men with high levels of apolipoprotein B. *N Engl J Med* **323**:1289–98.
6 Blankenhorn DH *et al.* (1987). Beneficial effects of combined colestipol-niacin therapy on coronary atherosclerosis and coronary venous bypass grafts. *JAMA* **257**:3233–40.
7 Cashin-Hemphill L *et al.* (1990). Beneficial effects of colestipol-niacin on coronary atherosclerosis. *JAMA* **264**:3013–17.
8 Taylor AJ (2008). Evidence to support aggressive management of high-density lipoprotein cholesterol: implications of recent imaging trials. *Am J Cardiol* **101**(suppl):36B–43B.
9 Taylor AJ *et al.* (2009). Extended-release niacin or ezetimibe and carotid intima–media thickness. *New Engl J Med* **361**:2113–22.
10 Maccubbin D *et al.* (2009). Flushing profile of E-R niacin/laropiprant versus gradually titrated niacin E-R in patients with dyslipidemia with and without ischemic cardiovascular disease. *Am J Cardiol* **104**:74–81.

Nifedipine

(See also 📖 Calcium-channel blockers, p.390)

Oral dihydropyridine derivative L-type CCB.

CV indications

1. Treatment of hypertension
2. Treatment of chronic stable and vasospastic angina pectoris

Other indications: Raynaud's phenomenon

Mechanism of action

(See also 📖 Calcium-channel blockers, p.390)

Pharmacodynamics

Short-acting preparations of nifedipine can cause a rapid drop in BP, reflex tachycardia, and neurohumoral activation, that may lead to myocardial ischaemia and worsening of patients with ACS. Therefore, they are not suitable for the long-term management of hypertension or angina.

Nifedipine reduced resting SBP at 10 and 20mg daily doses from 140mmHg to 126 and 123mmHg, respectively. Nifedipine also improved exercise testing outcomes increasing the time until 1mm ST depression and the workload at time of 1mm ST depression.[1] Nifedipine reduced the frequency of painful attacks and ischaemic ECG changes, irrespective of the relative contribution from coronary artery spasm or atherosclerosis.

Hypertension: rates of 1° outcome (CV death, MI, HF, stroke) were similar (18.2 vs. 16.5/1000 patient-years) in hypertensive patients (mean baseline BP ~173/99mmHg) treated with nifedipine GITS preparation 30mg od as compared to co-amilozide (hydrochlorothiazide 25mg plus amiloride 2.5mg), and additional antihypertensives as required to achieve a BP 140/90mmHg, and followed up for up to 51 months.[2]

CHD: addition of nifedipine GITS (gastrointestinal therapeutic system) to conventional treatment of angina pectoris has no effect on the major endpoint of death, AMI, refractory angina, new overt HF, debilitating stroke, and peripheral revascularization.[3] However, nifedipine has no effect on the rate of MI but reduces the need for coronary angiography and bypass surgery. A retrospective analysis found a 33% RR in the incidence of stroke and a 30% RR in the incidence of new overt HF in hypertensive patients, without altering all-cause death, CV death, and MI.[4]

HR ~0.89 (95% CI 0.83–0.95) for CV events and procedures in patients with stable CHD treated with nifedipine GITS (30–60mg od) compared to placebo and followed up for a mean of 4.9 years.[5] There were no differences in the occurrence of GI haemorrhage, MI, and suicide.

Common carotid artery intima–media thickness progressed in hypertensive patients treated for 4 years with co-amilozide but not in those treated with nifedipine GITS (30mg od), despite the fact that both treatments produce a similar BP reduction.[6]

Pharmacokinetics

It is important to note that pharmacokinetics vary widely between prepa-rations and brands.

Standard preparation: >90% of a single PO or sublingual dose of nifedipine is absorbed with very rapid onset of action (10–20 minutes). However, it undergoes a significant 1st-pass effect, being extensively metabolized, in the liver by CYP3A4; so oral availability of nifedipine immediate release formulations is ~45–56%. Peak plasma concentrations are achieved 1–2 hrs after enteral administration. Nifedipine binds to plasma proteins (96%), presents a V_d of 0.78 L/kg) and is excreted predominantly in urine but also in faeces (~5–15%). The terminal elimination $t_{1/2}$ is 1.7–3.4 hrs.

Modified-release preparations: they have longer onsets and durations of action as well as lower peak–trough fluctuations in concentrations, such that risks of large BP variations and reflex tachycardia are reduced. For example, nifedipine GITS preparation Adalat LA®, has a bioavailability of 68–86% relative to immediate-release preparations and provides zero-order delivery of nifedipine and plateau levels within 6h which last for up to 24h. By comparison, with Adalat Retard®, peak levels are reached ~1.5–4.2h after administration and there is a terminal $t_{1/2}$ of ~6–11h due to delayed absorption.

Practical points

.⌀ Doses

Different preparations and formulations of nifedipine are not directly interchangeable. Clinical effects vary considerably between them due to differences in pharmacokinetics. Consequently, brands and formulations should be specified when nifedipine is prescribed.

Unmodified immediate-release preparations are not recommended for the long-term management of hypertension or angina due to large variations in BP and reflex tachycardia. Use at 5mg tds (increased to maximum of 20mg tds as required) for Raynaud's phenomenon.

Modified-release preparations: 20–90mg (either od or bd, depending on preparation). Modified-release nifedipine is also available in a combination preparation with the β-blocker atenolol.

☺ Side effects

(See 📖 Calcium-channel blockers, p.390)

Interactions

(See 📖 Calcium-channel blockers, p.390)
Concomitant administration of nifedipine with quinidine decreases the plasma levels of quinidine. Conversely, concomitant administration with digoxin or tacrolimus may lead to increased concentrations of the latter drugs, with dose reductions possibly required.

Cautions/notes

Due to hepatic metabolism, use of nifedipine in liver dysfunction should be carefully monitored, and in severe cases a dose reduction may be necessary. Patients with renal impairment should not require adjustment of dosage.

Nifedipine should be used with caution in patients with LV dysfunction, as deterioration of HF has occasionally been observed with nifedipine when used in high doses in the management of CHD and particularly after an MI. Treatment with short-acting nifedipine may induce an exaggerated fall in BP and reflex tachycardia, which can cause complications such as myocardial and cerebrovascular ischaemia.

For specific modified-release formulations, such as Adalat LA®, tablets should not be broken or chewed. As the outer membrane of the Adalat LA® tablet is not digested, it may appear in faeces and rarely cause bezoars. Therefore, Adalat LA® should be given with caution in patients with obstructive symptoms and not to patients with ileostomies.

Pregnancy and lactation

(See 📖 Calcium-channel blockers, p.390)

Contraindications

(See 📖 Calcium-channel blockers, p.390)
Nifedipine LA preparations are contraindicated in patients with inflammatory bowel disease or Crohn's disease, history of oesophageal and GI obstruction, or any degree of decreased lumen diameter of the GI tract.

References

1 Ekelund LG et al. (1994). Effects of felodipine versus nifedipine on exercise tolerance in stable angina pectoris. Am J Cardiol 73:658–60.
2 Brown MJ et al. (2000). Morbidity and mortality in patients randomised to double-blind treatment with a long-acting calcium-channel blocker or diuretic in the International Nifedipine GITS study: Intervention as a Goal in Hypertension Treatment (INSIGHT). Lancet 356:366–72.
3 Poole-Wilson PA et al.; Coronary disease Trial Investigating Outcome with Nifedipine gastro-intestinal therapeutic system investigators (2004). Effect of long-acting nifedipine on mortality and cardiovascular morbidity in patients with stable angina requiring treatment (ACTION trial): randomised controlled trial. Lancet 364:849–57.
4 Lubsen J et al.; ACTION (A Coronary disease Trial Investigating Outcome with Nifedipine GITS) investigators (2005). Effect of long-acting nifedipine on mortality and cardiovascular morbidity in patients with symptomatic stable angina and hypertension: the ACTION trial. J Hypertens 23:641–8.
5 Poole-Wilson PA et al.; ACTION Investigators (2006). Safety of nifedipine GITS in stable angina: the ACTION trial. Cardiovasc Drugs Ther 20:45–54.
6 Simon A et al. (2001). Differential effects of nifedipine and co-amilozide on the progression of early carotid wall changes. Circulation 103:2949–54.

Nitrates

(See also 📖 Glyceryl trinitrate, p.477, 📖 Isosorbide dinitrate, p.494, and 📖 Isosorbide-5-mononitrate, p.496)

CV indications

1. Angina pectoris (symptomatic relief and prophylaxis)
2. Acute and chronic HF

Mechanism of action

GTN, ISDN, and ISMN are organic nitrates that indirectly release NO following enzymatic denitration. Endothelial NO has several important functions including relaxation of vascular smooth muscle cells (vasodilatation) via the activation of soluble guanylate cyclase and the formation of cyclic GMP that reduces the intracellular Ca^{2+} concentrations, and inhibition of platelet aggregation (antithrombotic) and leukocyte–endothelial interactions (anti-inflammatory).

At low doses, nitrates cause venous and coronary dilatation. Venodilatation promotes pooling of blood in the peripheral veins and decreases venous return to the heart, thereby reducing LV end-diastolic pressure (preload) and myocardial oxygen demands (MVO_2); the reduction of intraventricular pressure and volume also indirectly increases subendocardial blood flow. Nitrates also vasodilate large epicardial arteries and arterioles with a diameter >100μm, producing a redistribution of blood flow from epicardial to endocardial regions, and reduce coronary tone, suppressing coronary vasospasm especially at epicardial sites. All these effects alleviate symptoms of angina pectoris.

At higher doses, nitrates produce arterial vasodilatation, reducing systemic vascular resistances (afterload), BP and MVO_2; at these doses, they can produce reflex tachycardia that can overcome the decrease in MVO_2.

Like NO, nitrates inhibit platelet aggregation.

Pharmacodynamics

In stable angina, nitrates improve exercise tolerance, time to onset of symptoms, and time to ST depression during exercise testing. Due to pharmacokinetics, only short-acting nitrates should be used in the management of acute angina attack.

At high doses, nitrates reduce both pre- and afterload, improve haemodynamics (decrease LV filling pressure and PCWP without compromising stroke volume or increasing MVO_2) and exercise tolerance, and relieve pulmonary congestion when added to standard therapy in patients with acute and chronic HF, particularly in patients with ACS. The effect on cardiac output depends on pretreatment pre-/afterload, and the ability of the heart to respond to baroreceptor-induced increases in sympathetic tone.

Oral and IV nitrates failed to reduce mortality in patients with ACS (UA, NSTEMI, or STEMI).[1] In these patients, the goal of nitrates is to relieve pain and to manage associated acute HF or severe hypertension.

Pharmacokinetics
(See 📖 individual drugs)
Nitrates are rapidly absorbed from the skin, mucous membranes, or GI tract and undergo enzymatic denitration to release NO.

Practical points

⚡ *Dose* (see 📖 individual drugs)

☺ *Common side effects*
(≥10%): headache. Co-administration of aspirin reduces headaches and protects from coronary events.

(0.1–10%): dizziness, facial flushing, nausea, vomiting; lightheadness, postural hypotension, tachycardia, bradycardia (after AMI), syncope, halitosis (sublingual formulations).

(Others): postprandial hypotension, syncope, blurred vision, contact dermatitis (patients receiving GTN in ointments or patches) and methaemoglobinaemia (very rarely). In patients with cor pulmonale, the vasodilator effect of nitrates may produce venous mixture and may decrease arterial O_2 tension.

Interactions
(Due to pharmacodynamics)
Concomitant administration with the following agents can lead to an additive hypotensive effect: β-blockers, CCBs, ACEIs, diuretics, PDE-5 inhibitors (e.g. sildenafil, tadalafil, vardenafil), alcohol, neuroleptics, and tricyclic antidepressants.

Because the hypotension associated with GTN overdose is due to venodilatation and hypovolaemia, therapy should be directed to increase central fluid volume.

Life-threatening hypotension can occur if nitrates are used in conjunction with PDE-5 inhibitors; nitrates may be started 24h after sildenafil or vardenafil and 48h after tadalafil.

Nitrates, β-blockers, and CCBs are combined in many patients with angina pectoris. These 3 groups of drugs decrease myocardial O_2 demands; nitrates and CCBs also increase coronary blood flow, and β-blockers suppress the tachycardia induced by nitrates.

Cautions/notes
Long-acting nitrates with slow onset of action should not be used to treat acute anginal attacks.

The efficacy of repeated nitrate administration is limited by the appearance of tolerance, but the vasodilator response recovers quickly after a short (8–24h) nitrate-free interval. Thus, tolerance can be avoided by intermittent dosing, leaving ~8–24h dose-free intervals. Tolerance can be attributed to: (a) impaired activation of nitrates leading to a decrease in the release of NO, due to inhibition of mitochondrial aldehyde dehydrogenase (GTN) or cytochrome P450 reductase (isosorbide mono- and dinitrates);

(b) the release of free radicals (peroxinitrite, superoxide) that inhibit endothelial NO synthase, NO availability, and the formation of cGMP producing endothelial dysfunction; (c) reduced guanilyl cyclase activity; and (d) increased release of vasoconstrictor factors (catecholamines, angiotensin II and endothelin-1) that counteract the vasodilator effect of nitrates.

Nitrate withdrawal following large doses of long-acting nitrates can cause rebound angina symptoms.

GTN should be kept in airtight containers. Nitrate sprays are inflammable.

Pregnancy and lactation
Safety of nitrates in pregnancy and breastfeeding has not been established (pregnancy category C). Nitrates should be given to a pregnant woman only if clearly needed.

Contraindications
- Constrictive cardiomyopathy and pericarditis; cardiac tamponade; hypertrophic cardiomyopathy; AS; MS
- Hypotension (SBP <90mmHg)
- Acute inferior MI with RV involvement because the decrease in pre-load may aggravate hypotension
- Concomitant treatment with PDE-5 inhibitors (e.g. sildenafil, tadalafil, and vardenafil)
- Severe anaemia

Reference
1 GISSI-3 Study Group (1994). GISSI-3: Effects of lisinopril and transdermal glyceryl trinitrate singly and together on 6–week mortality and ventricular function after acute myocardial infarction. *Lancet* **343**:1115–22.

Omega-3 fatty acids (ethyl esters)

The omega-3 series polyunsaturated fatty acids, eicosapentaenoic acid (EPA), and docosahexaenoic acid (DHA), are essential fatty acids.

CV indications

1. As an adjunct to diet to reduce very high (≥500mg/dL) triglyceride levels in adult patients with type IV hyperlipidaemia and with statin therapy for type IIb hypercholesterolaemia
2. Adjuvant treatment in 2° prevention after MI, added to standard therapy

Mechanism of action

Omega-3 fatty acids reduce the synthesis of triglycerides in the liver by several mechanisms: (a) reduction of substrate availability as EPA and DHA are poor substrates for the enzymes responsible for triglyceride synthesis; (b) decrease in activity of triglyceride-synthesizing enzymes (diacylgylcerol acyltranferase, phosphatidic acid phosphohydrolase, and hormone-sensitive lipase; (c) increase in peroxisomal β-oxidation of fatty acids in the liver and stimulate ApoB degradation.

Omega-3 fatty acids also inhibit platelet aggregation and produce vasodilatation, antiarrhythmic, and anti-inflammatory effects.

Pharmacodynamics

Diets leading to high consumption of long-chain omega-3 fatty acids are associated with low prevalence of CHD in epidemiological studies. One meta-analysis found that fish consumption is inversely associated with fatal CHD and that mortality from CHD may be reduced by eating fish once per week or more,[1] while another meta-analysis concluded that long-chain and shorter-chain omega-3 fatty acids do not have a clear effect on total mortality, combined CV events, or cancer.[2]

2° *prevention:* 15% RR in the 1° endpoint of death, non-fatal MI, and non-fatal stroke, 20% RR in all-cause mortality, and 45% RR in sudden death in patients with a recent MI (<3 months) treated for 3.5 years with 850mg of omega-3 fatty acid ethyl esters (as EPA and DHA) as compared with the control group.[3]

19% RR (2.8% vs. 3.5%) in any major coronary event (including sudden cardiac death, fatal and non-fatal MI, and other non-fatal events including UA, angioplasty, stenting, or CABG) in Japanese patients with a total cholesterol ≥6.5 mmol/L treated for 5 years with 1800mg of EPA daily with statin or statin only.[4] UA and non-fatal coronary events were also significantly reduced in the EPA group. Post-treatment LDL-C levels decreased 25% in both groups.

Hypertriglyceridaemia: Omacor® (a drug composed of ethyl esters of EPA ~465mg and DHA ~375mg) significantly reduced mean triglyceride (45%), total cholesterol (15%), VLDL (32%) and LDL-C (31%), and increased HDL-C (13%) levels in patients with severe hypertriglyceridaemia (5.65–22.60mmol/L).[5]

Pharmacokinetics

Omega-3 fatty acids are absorbed when administered as ethyl esters orally, and induce an increase in serum phospholipid EPA content (increases in DHA content are less marked). Omega-3 fatty acids can be: (a) transported to the liver where they are incorporated into various lipoproteins and then channelled to the peripheral lipid stores; (b) incorporated in cell membrane phospholipids and can then act as precursors for various eicosanoids; and (c) oxidized to meet energy requirements.

Practical points

⚖ *Doses*

- *Post-MI:* 1 capsule (containing EPA ethyl ester 460mg and DHA ethyl ester 380mg) daily
- *Hypertriglyceridaemia:* 2 capsules daily, and if adequate response not reached, may be increased to 4 daily

☻ *Side effects*

Common: dyspepsia, nausea, abdominal pain, GI disorders, gastritis, hypersensitivity, dizziness, dysgeusia, fever, flu symptoms, skin rashes

Moderate elevation of transaminases has been reported in patients with hypertriglyceridaemia.

Interactions

High doses (4g daily) of omega-3 fatty acids prolong the bleeding time, so that patients receiving anticoagulant therapy should be monitored periodically.

Monitoring of hepatic function is required in hepatic impairment, especially with the high dose.

Cautions/notes

The capsules may be taken with food to avoid GI disturbances.

Pregnancy and lactation

Potential risk unknown (pregnancy category C). Should not be used during pregnancy and lactation unless clearly necessary.

Contraindications

Hypersensitivity to the active substance or any of the excipients.

References

1 He K et al. (2004). Accumulated evidence on fish consumption and coronary heart disease mortality: a meta-analysis of cohort studies. *Circulation* **109**:2705–11.
2 Hooper L et al. (2006). Risks and benefits of omega 3 fats for mortality, cardiovascular disease, and cancer: systematic review. *BMJ* **332**:752–60.
3 GISSI-Prevenzione Investigators (1999). Dietary supplementation with n-3 polyunsaturated fatty acids and vitamin E after myocardial infarction: results of the GISSI-Prevenzione trial. Gruppo Italiano per lo Studio della Sopravvivenza nell'Infarto miocardico. *Lancet* **354**:447–55.
4 Yokoyama M et al. (2007). Effects of eicosapentaenoic acid on major coronary events in hypercholesterolaemic patients (JELIS): a randomised open-label, blinded endpoint analysis. *Lancet* **369**: 1090–8.
5 Harris WS et al. (1997). Safety and efficacy of Omacor in severe hypertriglyceridaemia. *J Cardiovasc Risk* **4**:385–91.

Perindopril

(See 🕮 Angiotensin-converting enzyme inhibitors, p.355)

Orally active ACEI (prodrug).

Indications

(See 🕮 Angiotensin-converting enzyme inhibitors, p.355)

Mechanism of action

(See also 🕮 Renin–angiotensin–aldosterone system inhibitors, p.568 and 🕮 Angiotensin-converting enzyme inhibitors, p.355)

Pharmacodynamics

Hypertension, stroke, and cardiovascular risk

RRR ≈28% (absolute rate 10% vs. 14%) in 1° endpoint of stroke and RRR 26% in 2° endpoint of major vascular event with perindopril 4mg od with additional indapamide 1.25mg as required for 4 years compared with placebo in patients with previous stroke or TIA.[1] Combination therapy reduced BP (12/5mmHg) and stroke risk (43%); single-drug therapy reduced BP (5/3mmHg) without reduction in the risk of stroke.

RRR ≈30% (absolute rate 12.4% vs. 17.7%) in 1° endpoint of stroke (NNT≈94) and RRR 21% in 2° endpoint of all-cause mortality (NNT≈40) in hypertensive patients ≥80 years old treated with indapamide 1.25mg od and additional perindopril 2–4mg od as required to achieve SBP <150mmHg (mean BP fall 29.5/12.9mmHg) compared with placebo (mean BP fall 14.5/6.8mmHg) after 1.8 years.[2]

RRR 10% in non-fatal MI and fatal CHD after 5.5 years in the amlodipine-perindopril (5–10mg/4–8mg/day) group compared to atenolol-bendro-flumethiazide arm (50–100/1.25–2.5mg/day).[3] Amlodipine-perindopril-based regimen reduced RRR 24% fatal and non-fatal stroke, 16% total CV events and procedures, 19% all-cause mortality and 30% incidence of developing diabetes as compared to the atenolol-based regimen.

CHD: RRR ≈20% (absolute rate 8.0% vs. 9.9%) in 1° outcome of CV death, non-fatal MI, or successful cardiac arrest with perindopril 8mg od for 4.2 years compared with placebo in patients with stable CHD without apparent HF.[4]

Diabetes: RRR≈9% (absolute rate 15.5% vs. 16.8%) in 1° composite endpoint of all macro- and microvascular events (CV death, non-fatal MI, or stroke, new or worsening renal or eye disease), and RRR≈18% (absolute rate 3.8% vs. 4.6%) in 2° endpoint of CV death with perindopril 4mg od in fixed-dose combination with indapamide 1.25mg (average difference in BP vs. placebo ≈5.6/2.2mmHg) compared with placebo after a mean of 4.5 years in patients with diabetes and ≥1 additional CV risk factor.[5]

Pharmacokinetics

Perindopril is a prodrug that is rapidly absorbed after oral administration (bioavailability 65%). Peak concentrations reached within 1h. The plasma

$t_{1/2}$ of perindopril is ≈1h. ≈27% of administered perindopril reaches the bloodstream as the active metabolite perindoprilat that reaches peak concentrations within 3–4h. Ingestion of food decreases conversion to perindoprilat and hence bioavailability. Consequently, perindopril should be administered orally in the morning before a meal.

There is a linear relationship between the dose of perindopril and its plasma exposure. Perindoprilat is ≈20% protein-bound, is eliminated in the urine (70%), and its terminal $t_{1/2}$ is ≈17h, reaching steady-state within 4 days. Elimination of perindoprilat is decreased in the elderly and in patients with heart or renal failure. Dosage adjustment in renal insufficiency is desirable depending on creatinine clearance. Dialysis clearance of perindoprilat is 70mL/min.

Practical points

♣ Doses
(See also 📖 Angiotensin-converting enzyme inhibitors for initiation under supervision, p.355)

Hypertension, diabetes, and CV risk: 2mg od (to increase to maximum of 8mg if required)

Heart failure: 2mg od (to increase at intervals of 2 weeks to maximum of 4mg/day in divided doses if tolerated)

Dose changes in hepatic impairment are generally not required as although clearance is reduced, activation of prodrug is similarly reduced. Doses should be reduced in patients with renal impairment:

Creatinine clearance	Maximum dose
>60mL/min	4mg/day
30–60mL/min	2mg/day
15–30mL/min	2mg on dialysis days
Haemodialysis	2mg on day of dialysis

☺ **Common side effects** (see 📖 Angiotensin-converting enzyme inhibitors, p.355)

Interactions (see 📖 Angiotensin-converting enzyme inhibitors, p.355)

Cautions/notes (see 📖 Angiotensin-converting enzyme inhibitors, p.355)

Pregnancy and lactation (see 📖 Angiotensin-converting enzyme inhibitors, p.355)

Contraindications (see 📖 Angiotensin-converting enzyme inhibitors, p.355)

References

1 PROGRESS Collaborative Group (2001). Randomised trial of a perindopril-based blood-pressure-lowering regimen among 6,105 individuals with previous stroke or transient ischaemic attack. *Lancet* **358**:1033–41.

2 Beckett NS *et al.*; HYVET Study Group (2008). Treatment of hypertension in patients 80 years of age or older. *N Engl J Med* **358**:1887–98.

3 Dahlöf B *et al.*; ASCOT Investigators (2005). Prevention of cardiovascular events with an anti-hypertensive regimen of amlodipine adding perindopril as required versus atenolol adding ben-droflumethiazide as required, in the Anglo-Scandinavian Cardiac Outcomes Trial-Blood Pressure Lowering Arm (ASCOT-BPLA): a multicentre randomised controlled trial. *Lancet* **366**:895–906.

4 Fox KM *et al.*; EURopean trial On reduction of cardiac events with Perindopril in stable coronary Artery disease Investigators (2003). Efficacy of perindopril in reduction of cardiovascular events among patients with stable coronary artery disease: randomised, double-blind, placebo-controlled, multicentre trial (the EUROPA study). *Lancet* **362**:782–8.

5 Patel A *et al.*; ADVANCE Collaborative Group (2007). Effects of a fixed combination of perindopril and indapamide on macrovascular and microvascular outcomes in patients with type 2 diabetes mellitus (the ADVANCE trial): a randomised controlled trial. *Lancet* **370**:829–40.

Phenoxybenzamine

(See also 📖 Alpha₁-adrenoreceptor blockers, p.342)

Non-selective, irreversible, α-adrenergic receptor antagonist.

CV indications

1. Treatment of hypertension (and sweating) associated with phaeochromocytoma
2. Preoperative preparation for surgery of phaeochromocytoma

Mechanism of action

Phenoxybenzamine is a non-selective, irreversible α-adrenergic receptor antagonist. It forms a permanent covalent bond with adrenergic receptors, preventing adrenaline and noradrenaline from binding. This decreases peripheral vascular resistance and BP.

Pharmacodynamics

Due to its pharmacological properties of irreversible blockade, phenoxybenzamine has been traditionally used in the management of phaeochromocytoma.

Pharmacokinetics

Approximately 20–30% of oral dose is absorbed. Onset of action is gradual over several hours, with effects persisting for 3–4 days after a single oral dose. The $t_{1/2}$ of phenoxybenzamine after oral administration is not clear but is ≈24h after IV administration. Phenoxybenzamine is metabolized hepatically and excreted in urine and bile. Small amounts and activity remain for several days, possibly due in part to its stable covalent bonding.

Practical points

🥄 Doses

PO: 10mg od. Usual dose 20–40mg tds 1–2 weeks before surgical removal of phaeochromocytoma

IV: 1mg/kg daily over 2h

☺ Side effects

Postural hypotension with dizziness and compensatory tachycardia. Inhibition of ejaculation, nasal congestion, GI disturbances, drowsiness, dizziness and weakness.

Cautions/notes

Use with caution in patients in whom a BP fall or tachycardia is undesirable (e.g. elderly, HF, CVD, renal disease). Use of phenoxybenzamine can result in significant tachycardia which can be controlled with a cardioselective β-blocker. In patients with a phaeochromocytoma, β-blockers must never be used prior to adequate α-blockade (for 1 week) to avoid a hypertensive crisis. Avoid intake of alcohol or other sedating medications to prevent excessive drowsiness and dizziness.

Pregnancy and lactation

Phenoxybenzamine is carcinogenic in rats, has little evidence of safety in pregnancy, and so should not be used in pregnancy unless essential (pregnancy category B). It is also excreted in breast milk and can cause hypotension in newborn and should be avoided in breastfeeeding.

Contraindications
(See 📖 Alpha$_1$-adrenoreceptor blockers, p.342)
• History of CVA, immediately post MI (usually 4–6 weeks)

Pravastatin

(See also 📖 Statins, p.591)

Oral HMG-CoA reductase inhibitor.

CV indications

1. 1° hypercholesterolaemia or mixed dyslipidaemia, as an adjunct to diet, when response to non-pharmacological treatments is inadequate
2. 1° prevention of coronary events in hypercholesterolic patients without clinically evident CHD to reduce the risk of MI, myocardial revascularization procedures, and cardiovascular mortality, as an adjunct to diet
3. 2° prevention of CV events to reduce the risk of total mortality by reducing coronary death, the risk of MI, myocardial revascularization procedures, stroke, and TIA and slow the progression of coronary atherosclerosis
4. Post-transplantation: reduction of post-transplantation hyperlipidaemia in patients receiving immunosuppressive therapy following solid organ transplantation

Mechanism of action

(See 📖 Statins, p.591)

Pharmacodynamics

1° hypercholesterolaemia

Reduces elevated LDL-C, total cholesterol, triglycerides, and increases HDL-C (Table 10).[1]

Table 10 Effects of pravastatin on lipid profile (adjusted mean % change from baseline)

Dose (mg)	Percentage change			
	Total chol	LDL chol	HDL chol	TG
Placebo	−2.6	−3.7	+0.5	−4.3
5	−14.3	−19.2	+5.2	−14.1
10	−16.2	−22.4	+6.6	−14.9
20	−23.9	−32.4	+2.4	−11.4
40	−25.1	−34.1	+11.7	−23.9

1° prevention

31% RRR (7.9% vs. 5.5% absolute rates) in mortality from coronary disease and non-lethal MI, 32% RRR (1.6% vs. 2.3% absolute rates) in death from all CV causes, 24% RRR in total mortality after risk factors were considered, comparing 40mg daily pravastatin vs. placebo over an average duration of 4.9 years in patients aged 45–64 years with moderate to severe hypercholesterolaemia (LDL-C 4.0–6.0mmol/L) and with no history of MI.[2]

2° prevention
24% RRR (15.9% vs. 12.3% absolute rates) in major CHD events, 22% RRR (11.0% vs. 14.1% absolute rates) in total mortality, 24% RRR (12.3% vs. 15.9%) in CHD mortality or non-fatal MI, comparing 40mg daily pravastatin (40mg/daily) vs. placebo over an average of 5.6 years in patients aged 31–75 years, with normal to elevated serum cholesterol levels (total cholesterol 4.0–7.0mmol/L) and with variable triglyceride levels of up to 5.0mmol/L and with a history of MI or UA pectoris.[3]

Pravastatin 40mg daily was inferior to atorvastatin 80mg daily in the reduction of LDL-C and clinical events.[4]

2° prevention: 24% RRR (10.2% vs. 13.2% absolute rates) in coronary events (CHD mortality or nonfatal MI), 27% RRR (14.1% vs. 18.8% absolute rates) in revascularization procedures and 32% RRR (4.5% vs. 6.0% absolute rates) in stroke or TIA, comparing pravastatin (40 mg/day) vs. placebo over an average of 4.9 years in patients aged 21 to 75 years, with normal total cholesterol levels, who had experienced a MI in the preceding 3 to 20 months.[5]

Elderly patients: RRR 34% for CHD death and RRR 15% for the 1° endpoint (a composite of coronary death, non-fatal MI, and fatal or non-fatal stroke) in elderly (70–82 years) patients with, or at high risk of developing, CVD and stroke, treated for 3.2 years with pravastatin 40mg/day as compared with placebo.[6] RRR 19% for CHD death and non-fatal MI, but pravastatin had no effect on stroke risk or cognitive function or disability.

Pharmacokinetics
Rapidly absorbed with ≈66% undergoing 1st-pass metabolism. Absolute bioavailability is ≈17% with serum levels peaking 1–1.5h after ingestion. Pravastatin is ≈50% bound to plasma proteins (V_d is ≈0.5L/kg). The major degradation product of pravastatin is the 3-α-hydroxy isomeric metabolite, which has 1/10th to 1/40th the HMG-CoA reductase inhibitor activity of the parent compound. Following oral administration, 20% of the initial dose is eliminated in the urine and 70% in the faeces. Elimination $t_{1/2}$ is 1.5–3h.

Peak pravastatin values are markedly increased in cirrhotic patients.

Practical points

⚗ Doses
10–40mg od
- *Hypercholesterolaemia*: 10–40mg od
- *Cardiovascular prevention*: in all preventive morbidity and mortality trials, the only studied starting and maintenance dose was 40mg daily
- *Dosage after transplantation*: starting dose of 20mg od in patients receiving ciclosporin, with or without other immunosuppressive therapy (up to 40mg under close supervision)
- The recommended dose is 20mg in children 8–13 years of age, and 40mg in adolescents 14–18 years of age

☺ Side effects
(See 📖 Statins, p.591)

None of reported side effects occurred at a rate in excess of 0.3% in the pravastatin group compared to the placebo group. Myalgia occurred in 1.4%, muscle weakness in 0.1%, and the incidence of CK level >3× and >10× upper limit of normal is 1.6% and 1.0% respectively (all rates comparable to placebo).

Elevations of serum transaminases have been reported, and marked abnormalities of ALT and AST (>3× upper limit) occurred at similar frequency (≤1.2%) in both pravastatin and placebo groups.

Interactions
(See 📖 Statins, p.591)
There is no interaction between pravastatin and cimetidine, digoxin, or warfarin.

Cautions/notes
(See 📖 Statins, p.591)
Moderate to severe renal or significant hepatic impairment: starting dose 10mg daily is recommended. Not been evaluated in homozygous familial hypercholesterolaemia, and is not suitable when hypercholesterolaemia is due to elevated HDL-C.

Combination with fibrates is not recommended.

Pregnancy and lactation (see 📖 Statins, p.591)

Contraindications (see 📖 Statins, p.591)

References

1 Jones PH et al. (1991). Once-daily pravastatin in patients with primary hypercholesterolemia: a dose-response study. Clin Cardiol **14**:146–51.
2 Shepherd J et al. (1995). Prevention of coronary heart disease with pravastatin in men with hypercholesterolemia. West of Scotland Coronary Prevention Study Group. N Engl J Med **333**: 1301–7.
3 Keech A et al. (2003). Secondary prevention of cardiovascular events with long-term pravastatin in patients with diabetes or impaired fasting glucose: results from the LIPID trial. Diabetes Care **26**:2713–21.
4 Cannon CP et al. (2004). Comparison of Intensive and Moderate Lipid Lowering with Statins after Acute Coronary Syndromes (PROVE IT-TIMI 22). N Engl J Med **350**: 1495–504.
5 Sacks FM et al. (1996). The effect of pravastatin on coronary events after myocardial infarction in patients with average cholesterol levels. Cholesterol and Recurrent Events Trial investigators. N Engl J Med **335**:1001–9.
6 Shepherd J et al.; PROSPER study group (2002). PROspective Study of Pravastatin in the Elderly at Risk. Pravastatin in elderly individuals at risk of vascular disease (PROSPER): a randomised controlled trial. Lancet **360**:1623–30.
7 Jukema JW et al. (1995). Effects of Lipid Lowering by Pravastatin on Progression and Regression of Coronary Artery Disease in Symptomatic Man With Normal to Moderately Elevated Serum Cholesterol Levels. The Regression Growth Evaluation Statin Study (REGRESS). Circulation **91**:2528–40.
8 Pitt B et al. (1995). Pravastatin Limitation of Atherosclerosis in the Coronary Arteries (PLAC I): Reduction in Atherosclerosis Progression and Clinical Events. J Am Coll Cardiol **26**:1133–9.
9 Crouse JR et al. (1992). Pravastatin, Lipids, and Atherosclerosis in the Carotid Arteries: Design Features of a Clinical Trial with Carotid Atherosclerosis Outcome (PLAC II). Controlled Clinical Trials **13**:455–9.
10 Salonen R et al. (1995). Kuopio Atherosclerosis Prevention Study (KAPS). A population-based primary preventive trial of the effect of LDL lowering on atherosclerotic progression in carotid and femoral arteries. Research Institute of Public Health, University of Kuopio, Finland. Circulation **92**:1758.

Prazosin

(See also 📖 Alpha$_1$-adrenoreceptor blockers, p.342)

Selective postsynaptic competitive α$_1$-adrenoreceptor blocker.

CV indications

(See 📖 Alpha$_1$-adrenoreceptor blockers, p.342)
1. Congestive HF
2. Hypertension
3. Raynaud's phenomenon

Mechanism of action

(See 📖 Alpha$_1$-adrenoreceptor blockers, p.342)

Pharmacodynamics

(See 📖 Alpha$_1$-adrenoreceptor blockers, p.342)
Prazosin reduces peripheral vascular resistances, but unlike other β-blockers it reduces BP without changes in heart rate, cardiac output, renal blood flow, PRA or GFR. In patients with heart failure prazosin reduces LV filling pressure and cardiac impedance and increases cardiac output. However, it is ineffective in prolonging survival in patients with HF.[1]

Pharmacokinetics

Oral bioavailability 60%, reaching peak plasma concentrations within 1–2h after oral administration. Plasma $t_{1/2}$ is ≈2–3h in normotensive and hypertensive individuals. Prazosin is highly bound to plasma protein (97%), extensively metabolized in the liver (by demethylation and conjugation), and excreted mainly via bile and faeces (<10% in urine). Renal blood flow and GFR are not impaired by long-term oral administration, and thus prazosin can be used safely in patients with impaired renal function.

Practical points

🔅 Doses

Hypertension: 0.5–5mg od (maximum: 20mg od)
Heart failure: 0.5mg bd–qds (maximum: 4mg/day in divided doses)

Lower doses of 0.5mg may be considered as starting doses in renal and hepatic impairment.

☺ Common side effects

(See 📖 Alpha$_1$-adrenoreceptor blockers, p.342)
(1–10%): depression, nervousness; blurred vision; constipation, diarrhoea, dry mouth, vomiting; rash

Others: syncope, nasal congestion

Orthostatic hypotension is more pronounced after the 1st dose.

Interactions

(See 📖 Alpha$_1$-adrenoreceptor blockers, p.342)
Use with other antihypertensives (CCBs, diuretics or β-blockers) may produce substantial fall in BP. May produce false positives in some tests of noradrenaline metabolites (vanillylmandelic acid, VMA; and methoxyhydroxyphenyl glycol, MHPG).

Cautions/notes
(See 📖 Alpha₁-adrenoreceptor blockers, p.342)
Prazosin is not recommended in HF 2° to mechanical obstruction (e.g. valvular stenoses; pulmonary embolism; restrictive pericardial disease). A significant fall in BP may occur in HF patients who have already received aggressive diuretic or vasodilator therapy. Thus, careful assessment and adjustment of fluid balance and diuretic therapy may be required. Clinical efficacy may decline with time on treatment (tachyphylaxis) and this is often overcome with increased doses.

Pregnancy and lactation
No teratogenic effects have been reported in human pregnancy. Use with a β-blocker and also other antihypertensives in small numbers of severely hypertensive mothers was not associated with fetal abnormalities. However, safety in pregnancy remains undocumented (pregnancy category C). Prazosin is also excreted in breast milk. Thus, caution should be used in either pregnancy or breastfeeding.

Contraindications
(See 📖 Alpha₁-adrenoreceptor blockers, p.342)

Reference

1 Cohn JN et al. (1986). Effect of vasodilator therapy on mortality in chronic congestive heart failure. Results of a Veterans Administration Cooperative Study. *N Engl J Med* **314**:1547–52.

Procainamide

(See also 📖 Class Ia antiarrhythmic drugs, p.403)

IV sodium-channel blocker with class Ia antiarrhythmic properties (only available by order in the US).

CV indications

1. Ventricular arrhythmias, especially after MI
2. Atrial tachycardias

Mechanism of action

(See 📖 Class Ia antiarrhythmic drugs, p.403)

Pharmacodynamics

Compared with other class I antiarrhythmics, procainamide is a moderate sodium-channel blocker and causes comparatively less depression of cardiac contractility. Procainamide slows heart rate and prolongs the PR, QRS and QT intervals of the ECG. As with other class Ia drugs, there is a potential—albeit weaker—anticholinergic effect, most prominent in the SA and AV nodes (due to vagal innervation).

Procainamide is also a peripheral vasodilator at supratherapeutic doses.

Pharmacokinetics

Following oral administration it is rapidly absorbed (bioavailability 85%), reaching peak plasma levels in 1.5–2h. Procainamide undergoes plasma protein binding (15%) and also binds to heart, lung, and renal tissue. Consequently, V_d is large (2L/kg). Elimination $t_{1/2}$ is ≈2.5–5h (longer in renal insufficiency and in elderly). Procainamide is partly metabolized in hepatocytes to the active metabolite N-acetylprocainamide (NAPA); 16–21% of an administered dose in 'slow acetylators' and 24–33% in 'fast-acetylators'. It is predominantly (60%) excreted unchanged in urine (6–50% as NAPA) by active tubular secretion as well as by glomerular filtration. Therapeutic plasma levels: 3–8mcg/mL.

Practical points

💊 Doses

For acute treatment: 100mg every 5min (at a rate of 10–20mg/min) until arrhythmia is suppressed or a maximum of 1g is given.

For chronic treatment: infuse 500–600mg at a constant rate during 25–30min and then change to infusion maintenance at 2–4mg/min.

😊 Common side effects

(>10%): lupus like syndrome (particularly in slow-acetylators) that limits oral use to 6 months

(1–10%): anorexia, nausea, diarrhoea, bitter metallic taste, (with PO procainamide); blood dyscrasias: leukopenia or agranulocytosis (0.5%). Proarrhythmic effects, heart block and bradycardia

Due to pharmacokinetics, elimination may be decreased with increased age, renal, and hepatic impairment. Thus, doses may need to be reduced.

Interactions

Amiodarone increases plasma concentrations of procainamide. In addition, procainamide elimination may be reduced by trimethoprim, cimetidine, and propranolol, and increased by alcohol. Consequently, doses may need to be altered accordingly. There is no interaction with digoxin.

Risk of bradycardia, intracardiac blockade, and proarrhythmia when given with class I and III antiarrhythmic drugs. Risk of torsades de pointes when given with QT-prolonging drugs.

Procainamide may enhance effects of other antiarrhythmic and antihypertensive agents and inhibit the effects of sulphonamides and neuromuscular blocking agents. Caution is required when procainamide is used in combination with captopril due to reports of neutropenia and/or Stevens–Johnson syndrome and in combination with anticholinergic agents, due to potential of enhanced antivagal effects on sinus rate and AV conduction.

Cautions/notes
- IV administration should be undertaken with BP and ECG monitoring and procainamide discontinued if hypotension occurs or if excessive widening of QRS, an increasing PR interval, or other features of cardiotoxicity occur. Caution is also required in patients with chronic HF, ACS, cardiogenic shock, or cardiomyopathy due to risk of reduced myocardial contractility.
- Accumulation may occur with severe renal or hepatic impairment. Electrophysiological actions may be affected by electrolyte imbalance.
- Procainamide may worsen symptoms of asthma and myasthenia gravis due to reduction in acetylcholine release.

Pregnancy and lactation
Procainamide crosses the placenta and its safety has not been established in pregnancy (pregnancy category C). It is excreted in breast milk and so should be avoided in breastfeeding.

Contraindications
- High-degree AV block or bifascicular block
- Torsades de pointes
- Hypotension, HF
- Severe renal failure
- Hypersensitivity: in patients sensitive to procaine or other ester-type local anaesthetics
- SLE

Propafenone

(See also 📖 Antiarrhythmic drugs: classification, p.362)

Class Ic antiarrhythmic drug.

CV indications

1. Prophylaxis and treatment of ventricular arrhythmias
2. Prophylaxis and treatment of paroxysmal supraventricular tachyarrhythmias, including PAF/AF and paroxysmal re-entrant tachycardias involving the AV node or accessory bypass tracts, when standard therapy has failed or is contraindicated

Mechanism of action

(See 📖 Flecainide, p.466)

Pharmacodynamics

Propafenone has moderate β-blocking and L-type Ca^{2+}-channel antagonistic activity with uncertain clinical relevance. However, high daily doses (900–1200mg) may trigger a sympatholytic (antiadrenergic) effect. In clinical trials, resting heart rate decreases of ≈8% were noted at the higher end of the therapeutic plasma concentration range. ECG changes are a slight prolongation of PR and QRS intervals while the QTc interval remains unaffected as a rule. A clinically relevant reduction of LV function is to be expected only in patients with pre-existing poor ventricular function. There appears to be a close relationship between plasma concentrations and AV conduction times.

Propafenone (300mg od) is of value in the prophylaxis of both paroxysmal supraventricular tachycardia and paroxysmal AF[1] and is also a drug of choice for cardioversion of AF to sinus rhythm.[2] In selected, risk-stratified patients with recurrent AF, out-of-hospital self-administration of propafenone (pill-in-the-pocket approach) is feasible and safe, with a high rate of compliance by patients, a low rate of adverse effects and a marked reduction in emergency room visits and hospital admissions.[3]

Pharmacokinetics

Propafenone is nearly completely absorbed but undergoes an extensive 1st-pass effect, so that oral bioavailability is 5–30%. T_{max} is ≈2–3h. More than 95% is bound to plasma proteins and is extensively distributed (V_d 2.5–4L/kg). Extensive 1st-pass hepatic metabolism produces 2 main active metabolites which have antiarrhythmic activity comparable with propafenone, but are present in concentrations <20%. The elimination of propafenone and its metabolites is through urine (<1% of unchanged propafenone; 38% of metabolites) and faeces (53% of metabolites). Therapeutic plasma levels: 0.2–3mcg/mL.

There are 2 genetically determined pathways of metabolism for propafenone with >90% of patients rapidly and extensively metabolizing the drug (by CYP2D6, 3A4, and 1A2) with an elimination $t_{1/2}$ of ≈2–10h. In <10% of whites, CYP2D6 is genetically absent, so that its metabolism is slower and elimination $t_{1/2}$ is ≈10–32h. A slow-release preparation is also available and has a slower onset of action with reduced bioavailability (necessitating higher doses).

Practical points

♨ *Doses*
- *Adults*: 150–300mg tds (increasing at a minimum of 3day intervals to 300mg bd and if necessary, to a maximum of 300mg tds)
- *IV*: 2mg/kg followed by an infusion of 2mg/min
- *Elderly*: may respond to a lower dose
- *Liver dysfunction*: a reduction in the recommended dose may be necessary
- *Renal dysfunction*: should be administered cautiously

Therapy should be initiated under hospital conditions and dose should be determined under ECG monitoring and BP control.

☺ *Common side effects*
(>10%): dizziness, nausea and vomiting, unusual taste

(1–10%): arrhythmia, HF, VT, weakness, intraventricular conduction delay, fatigue, dyspnoea, headache, ataxia, tremor, rash, blurred vision, constipation, dyspepsia, joint pain

In atrial flutter, propafenone may induce 1:1 conduction and increased ventricular rate may appear.

Interactions
Propafenone can potentially lead to conduction abnormalities and potential arrhythmias when used with amiodarone; increased risk of lidocaine-related CNS side effects. Drugs that prolong the QT interval (e.g. cisapride, bepridil, tricyclic antidepressants) and antiarrhythmic agents (class Ia and III, e.g. amiodarone, quinidine) can increase the risk of life-threatening cardiac arrhythmias when given with propafenone.

SA and AV node depression when combined with verapamil or diltiazem. Conduction defects may increase when combined with class Ia antiarrhythmics.

Propafenone increases the effects of digoxin, oral anticoagulants (reduce the dose of warfarin), propranolol, and metoprolol. It may also increase effects of ciclosporin, theophylline, and desipramine.

Drugs that inhibit CYP2D6, CYP1A2, and CYP3A4 (ketoconazole, quinidine, tropisetron, dolasetron, mizolastine, venlafaxine, erythromycin, and grapefruit juice) may lead to increased levels of propafenone hydrochloride. Consequently, patients should be monitored closely and doses adjusted accordingly when propafenone is administered with such drugs. Effects of propafenone may also be increased by concomitant use of cimetidine, paroxetine, fluoxetine, and local anaesthetic-type agents, and decreased by rifampicin.

Cautions/notes
- Each patient should be evaluated clinically and electrocardiographically prior to and during therapy, to determine whether the response to propafenone supports continued treatment. Patients with structural heart disease may be predisposed to serious adverse effects. Care should be exercised in the treatment of patients with obstructive airways disease or asthma (due to its β-blocking effect).

- The weak negative inotropic effect of propafenone may assume importance in patients predisposed to cardiac failure. Due to altered sensitivity and thresholds, appropriate adjustments may be required for pacemakers.
- Blurred vision, dizziness, fatigue, and postural hypotension may affect the patient's speed of reaction and impair the individual's ability to operate machinery or motor vehicles.
- Propafenone should not be used in combination with ritonavir (at doses of 800–1200mg/day).

Pregnancy and lactation

Should not be used during pregnancy and lactation (pregnancy category C).

Contraindications

(See 📖 Flecainide, p.466)
- Structural heart disease (CAD, LVF), severe COPD, asthma, severe liver dysfunction, or marked hypotension
- Myasthenia gravis (may be worsened)

References

1 UK Propafenone PSVT Study Group (1995). A randomized, placebo-controlled trial of propafenone in the prophylaxis of paroxysmal supraventricular tachycardia and paroxysmal atrial fibrillation. *Circulation* **92**:2550–7.
2 Fuster V *et al.* (2006). ACC/AHA/ESC 2006 Guidelines for the Management of Patients with Atrial Fibrillation. *Circulation* **114**:e257–4.
3 Alboni P *et al.* (2004). Outpatient treatment of recent-onset atrial fibrillation with the 'pill-in-the-pocket' approach. *N Engl J Med* **351**:2384–91.

Prostanoids

Prostacyclin (PGI_2) and thromboxane A_2 are major arachidonic acid metabolites. PGI_2 is produced by endothelial cells. PGI_2 binds to IP receptors, activates adenylyl cylase, and increases the cellular levels of cAMP, producing a potent arteriolar vasodilatation (reducing systemic and pulmonary vascular resistances) and inhibition of platelet aggregation and growth of vascular smooth muscle cells. Prostacyclin synthase is decreased in pulmonary arteries in PAH, resulting in a decrease in PGI_2, and therefore the balance is shifted to thromboxane A_2, a potent vasoconstrictor that promotes vascular smooth muscle proliferation and platelet aggregation.

Prostanoids (analogues of PGI_2): see also 📖 Epoprostenol, p.451, 📖 Treprostinil, p.619, 📖 Iloprost, p.486

Quinidine

(See also 📖 Class la antiarrhythmic drugs, p.403)

Class la antiarrhythmic drug.

CV indications

1. Pharmacological conversion of symptomatic atrial flutter or fibrillation to sinus rhythm (almost totally replaced by class Ic and III agents)
2. Maintenance of sinus rhythm AF
3. Suppression of recurrent ventricular arrhythmias

Mechanism of action

In atrial and ventricular muscle and in Purkinje fibres, quinidine inhibits the I_{Na}; thereby, it decreases excitability and slows conduction velocity and increases the effective refractory period relative to the duration of the action potential in these tissues. In Purkinje fibres, it reduces the slope of phase-4 depolarization and shifts the threshold voltage to less negative values; these effects reduce the automaticity of cardiac ectopic pacemakers. Quinidine also raises the fibrillation thresholds of the atria and ventricles. Because of these effects, quinidine has a wide spectrum of activity against re-entrant as well as ectopic atrial and ventricular tachyarrhytmias. It slows conduction and increases refractoriness in the retrograde fast pathway limb of AV nodal tachycardias and over the accessory pathway, slowing the ventricular response to AF in patients with WPW syndrome.

Quinidine prolongs the QT interval due to the prolongation of the reactivation of the I_{Na} and the blockade of several K^+ currents. This effect may lead to increased ventricular automaticity and polymorphic VTs, including torsades de pointes. Quinidine also has negative inotropic effects.

Quinidine inhibits α-adrenergic receptors, producing vasodilatation and hypotension, and exerts anticholinergic effects. This vagolytic activity may cause sinus tachycardia and facilitate AV conduction to increase ventricular rate in atrial flutter or fibrillation.

ECG effects: bradycardia, prolongation of the PR and QT intervals and widening of the QRS complex

Pharmacokinetics

The absolute oral bioavailability of quinidine (sulphate/gluconate) is 70–80%, but this varies widely (45–100%) between patients, reaching peak plasma levels within 1–3h. It binds to plasma proteins (85%), its V_d is 2.7L/kg (3–5L/kg in patients with cirrhosis) and it is metabolized (50–90%) in the liver (via CYP3A4) to hydroxylated active metabolites. About 20% of the dose is excreted unchanged in the urine. Plasma $t_{1/2}$ is ~6h, but increased in elderly and in pacients with hepatic insufficiency. Therapeutic plasma concentrations 2–6mg/L.

Pharmacodynamics

Quinidine was compared in 6 clinical trials (published between 1970 and 1984) to non-treatment or placebo for the maintenance of sinus rhythm after cardioversion from chronic AF.[1] Quinidine was consistently more efficacious in maintaining sinus rhythm, but a meta-analysis found that mortality in the quinidine-treated patients (2.9%) was significantly greater than in those not treated with active drug (0.8%).[2]

Quinidine has been compared with flecainide, mexiletine, propafenone, and tocainide in patients with a variety of ventricular arrhythmias (mainly frequent ventricular premature beats and non-sustained VT).[3] In these studies, the mortality in the quinidine group was greater than in the comparator group. When the studies were combined in a meta-analysis, quinidine was associated with a statistically significant 3-fold relative risk of death.

Practical points

,5 Doses
300mg or 400mg every 6h (1.2–1.6g/day). Reduce dose in liver disease patients

☺ Common side effects
Diarrhoea (33%), nausea (18%), headache (13%), dizziness (8%), light-headedness, fatigue, and vomiting; bradycardia, conduction block, palpitation, tachyarrhythmias, torsades de pointes, HF

Hypersensitivity reactions include fever, skin rash, angio-oedema, thrombocytopenia, agranulocytosis, hypotension, hepatitis, and lupus erythematosus.

Interactions
- Drugs that alkalinize the urine (carbonic-anhydrase inhibitors, sodium bicarbonate, thiazide diuretics) reduce renal elimination of quinidine.
- Quinidine levels are increased by co-administration of amiodarone, verapamil, or cimetidine, and decreased by co-administration of nifedipine. Co-administration of quinidine with β-blockers, diltiazem, or verapamil increases the risk of hypotension and decreases cardiac contractility.
- In some studies, propranolol appears to increase peak serum levels and decreases the V_d and the total clearance of quinidine. Diltiazem and verapamil decrease the clearance and increase the $t_{1/2}$ of quinidine.
- Quinidine plasma levels rise when ketoconazole (or grapefruit juice) is co-administered, probably because they inhibit CYP3A4-mediated metabolism of quinidine to 3-hydroxyquinidine. Therefore this combination should be avoided. Hepatic elimination of quinidine can be accelerated by co-administration of CYP3A4-inducer drugs (phenobarbital, phenytoin, rifampicin, ketoconazole).
- Quinidine slows the elimination of digoxin and simultaneously reduces digoxin's apparent V_d. As a result, serum digoxin levels may be doubled, and thus digoxin doses usually need to be reduced.
- Quinidine potentiates the anticoagulant effect of warfarin; reduce the anticoagulant dose and monitor the INR.
- Perhaps by competing for pathways of renal clearance, quinidine increases serum levels of procainamide. Serum levels of haloperidol are increased when quinidine is co-administered.

- Quinidine's anticholinergic, vasodilating, and negative inotropic actions may be additive to those of other drugs with these effects, and antagonistic to those of drugs with cholinergic, vasoconstricting, and positive inotropic effects.
- Quinidine potentiates the actions of depolarizing (succinylcholine) and nondepolarizing (pancuronium) neuromuscular blocking agents.

Cautions/notes

Quinidine toxicity is best prevented by serial measurements of the QRS and QTc intervals of the ECG. The dose should be reduced or therapy discontinued if the QRS duration widens by 30%, or if total QRS duration exceeds 140ms, or if QTc or QTU prolongation is >500ms, or the patient develops tachycardia, symptomatic bradycardia, or hypotension.

Treatment of acute quinidine toxicity includes stopping quinidine, reducing plasma K^+ levels if elevated, and acidifying urine to increase drug renal excretion. Torsades de pointes or severely disorganized conduction may require correction of serum K^+ levels, magnesium sulphate infusion, cardioversion, or temporary atrial or ventricular overdrive pacing.

By its anticholinergic effects, quinidine shortens the refractoriness of the AV node, with a resultant paradoxical increase in ventricular rate in patients with atrial flutter/AF. This hazard may be decreased if AV nodal drugs (digoxin, diltiazem, verapamil, β-blockers) are given prior to initiation of quinidine therapy.

Pregnancy and lactation

There are no adequate and well-controlled studies in pregnant women (pregnancy category C). Quinidine is present in human milk at levels slightly lower than those in maternal serum, so that its administration should be avoided in lactating women.

Contraindications

- Ventricular tachyarrhythmias associated with or caused by QT prolongation or when QT-prolonging drugs are prescribed
- Patients whose cardiac rhythm is dependent upon a junctional or idioventricular pacemaker in the absence of a function artificial pacemaker
- Myasthenia gravis
- Severe hepatic impairment
- Patients who are allergic to the drug, or who have developed thrombocytopenic purpura during prior therapy with quinidine or quinine

References

1 Coplen SE et al. (1990). Efficacy and safety of quinidine therapy for maintenance of sinus rhythm after cardioversion. A meta-analysis of randomized control trials. *Circulation* **82**:1106–16.
2 Nichol G et al. (2002). Meta-analysis of randomized controlled trials of the effectiveness of antiarrhythmic agents at promoting sinus rhythm in patients with atrial fibrillation. *Heart* **87**:535–43.
3 Morganroth J, Goin JE (1991). Quinidine-related mortality in the short-to-medium-term treatment of ventricular arrhythmias. A meta-analysis. *Circulation* **84**:1977–83.

Ramipril

(See also 📖 Angiotensin-converting enzyme inhibitors, p.355).
Orally active ACEI (prodrug).

Indications

(see 📖 Angiotensin-converting enzyme inhibitors, p.355).
Ramipril has additional indications specifically for:
1. reducing risk of MI, stroke, CV death, or need for revascularization procedures in patients ≥55 years with clinical evidence of CVD (previous MI, UA, or multivessel CABG, or multivessel PTCA), stroke, or PVD
2. reducing risk of MI, stroke, CV death, or need for revascularization procedures in diabetic patients ≥55 years who have 1 or more of the following risk factors: hypertension (SBP >160mmHg or DBP >90mmHg); high total cholesterol (>5.2mmol/L), low HDL (<0.9mmol/L), current smoker, microalbuminuria, and clinical evidence of previous vascular disease.

Mechanism of action

(See 📖 Renin–angiotensin–aldosterone system inhibitors, p.568 and 📖 Angiotensin-converting enzyme inhibitors, p.355)

Pharmacodynamics

Hypertension and cardiovascular risk: RRR≈22% (absolute rate 14.0% vs. 17.8%) in composite 1° endpoint of MI (20%), stroke (33%), or CV death (26%) with ramipril 10mg od for 5 years compared with placebo in patients ≥55 years at high risk of CVD (previous CHD, stroke, or PVD) or diabetes with an additional risk factor.[1] RRR≈26% in death from CV causes, 15% in revascularization procedures, 38% in cardiac arrest, 23% in HF, and 16% in complications related to diabetes.

AMI and heart failure: RRR≈27% (absolute rate 17% vs. 23%) in 1° outcome of all-cause mortality with ramipril 2.5–5mg od commenced 3–14 days post-MI compared with placebo in patients with clinical features of LVF post-MI after a mean of 15 months.[2] RRR≈36% (absolute rate 27.5% vs. 38.9%) in all-cause mortality with ramipril (target dose of 5mg bd) commenced 3–14 days post-MI compared with placebo in patients with clinical features of LVF post-MI after a mean of 59 months.[3]

Diabetes and diabetic nephropathy: RRR≈25% in composite 1° endpoint (MI: 22%; stroke: 33%; or CV death: 37%) and RRR≈25% in 2° endpoint of development of overt nephropathy and ~24% for total mortality with ramipril 10mg od with ramipril (2.5–5mg od) compared with placebo after 4.5 years in patients ≥55years with diabetes and CVD or an additional risk factor.[4]

Nephrophathy: in patients with chronic nephropathy and high risk of rapid progression to end-stage renal failure, ramipril (1.25–5mg/day) reduced the rate of GFR decline more than expected from BP reduction.[5] A treatment period ≥36 months eliminated the need for dialysis.

RRR 36% slower decline in GFR and RRR 48% of the clinical endpoints in patients treated with ramipril (2.5 to 10mg/day) than with amlodipine

(5 and 10mg/day) over 3 years in African-American individuals with hypertensive renal disease (GFR of 20–65 mL/min per 1.73 m^2) and proteinuria >300mg/d).[6]

Pharmacokinetics

Ramipril is a prodrug. Following oral administration ramipril is rapidly absorbed (bioavailability ~30%), reaching peak plasma concentrations within 1h. Absorption does not appear to be delayed with food. Peak plasma concentrations of its active metabolite, ramiprilat, are reached within 2–4h; steady-state plasma concentrations are reached after 4 days. Ramiprilat is 60% protein bound and its $t_{1/2}$ after multiple once-daily administration of ramipril is 13–17h for 5–10mg ramipril and markedly longer for lower doses. Ramipril is almost completely metabolized and metabolites are excreted mainly via urine (60%; <2% unchanged) and faeces (40%).

Practical points

⚖ Doses

(See 📖 Angiotensin-converting enzyme inhibitors for initiation under supervision, p.355)

Hypertension and cardiovascular risk: 1.25–2.5mg od (titrated to maximum of 10mg).

Heart failure: 2.5mg od in patients stabilized on diuretics (to be doubled in intervals 1–2 weeks to max of 10mg/day in divided doses if tolerated).

Post-MI: 2.5mg od in hospital within 3–10 days of MI (to be gradually increased to 5mg bd). Treatment should be withdrawn if 2.5mg bd is not tolerated.

Diabetic nephropathy: 2.5mg od initially to usual dose 10–20mg od.

Doses should be reduced in patients with renal impairment: usual doses for those with a CrCl >30mL/h; 1.25mg od initial dose (to max maintenance of 5mg od) with clearance <30mL/h; and 1.25mg in those with severe renal impairment (CrCl <10mL/h) but maintenance not to exceed 2.5mg od.

Doses should be reduced in the elderly. In hepatic impairment, initial doses should be 1.25mg, under medical supervision, and higher doses used with caution. A reduced initial dose (e.g. 1.25mg) should also be considered for those who may be sodium- or fluid-depleted in whom hypotension is of particular risk.

☺ Common side effects (see 📖 Angiotensin-converting enzyme inhibitors, p.355)

Interactions (see 📖 Angiotensin-converting enzyme inhibitors, p.355)

Cautions/notes
(see 📖 Angiotensin-converting enzyme inhibitors, p.355)
As ramipril is a prodrug, it should be used with caution in hepatic impairment.

Pregnancy and lactation (see 📖 Angiotensin-converting enzyme inhibitors, p.355)

Contraindications (see 📖 Angiotensin-converting enzyme inhibitors, p.355)

References

1 Yusuf S et al. (2000). Effects of an angiotensin-converting-enzyme inhibitor, ramipril, on cardiovascular events in high-risk patients. The Heart Outcomes Prevention Evaluation Study Investigators. N Engl J Med **342**:145–53.

2 The Acute Infarction Ramipril Efficacy (AIRE) Study Investigators (1993). Effect of ramipril on mortality and morbidity of survivors of acute myocardial infarction with clinical evidence of heart failure. Lancet **342**:821–8.

3 Hall AS et al. (1997). Follow-up study of patients randomly allocated ramipril or placebo for heart failure after acute myocardial infarction: AIRE Extension (AIREX) Study. Acute Infarction Ramipril Efficacy. Lancet **349**:1493–7.

4 (2000). Effects of ramipril on cardiovascular and microvascular outcomes in people with diabetes mellitus: results of the HOPE study and MICRO-HOPE substudy. Lancet **355**:253–9.

5 Ruggenenti P et al. (1998). Renal function and requirement for dialysis in chronic nephropathy patients on long-term ramipril: REIN follow-up trial. Gruppo Italiano di Studi Epidemiologici in Nefrologia (GISEN). Ramipril Efficacy in Nephropathy. Lancet **352**:1252–6.

6 Agodoa LY et al.; African American Study of Kidney Disease and Hypertension (AASK) Study Group (2001). Effect of ramipril vs amlodipine on renal outcomes in hypertensive nephrosclerosis: a randomized controlled trial. JAMA **285**:2719–28.

Ranolazine

Selective late I_{Na} inhibitor.

CV indication

Add-on therapy in patients with symptomatic chronic refractory angina inadequately controlled or intolerant to 1st-line anti-anginals.

Mechanism of action

Ranolazine appears to selectively inhibit the late cardiac inward Na^+ current. Most cardiac Na^+ channels open transiently, within milliseconds, but then rapidly inactivate following depolarization. However, a small percentage of Na^+ channels either fail to inactivate properly (i.e. fail to close), or close and then reopen during the plateau phase, carrying the so-called persistent or late Na^+ current (late I_{Na}) that facilitates the entry of Na^+ during the plateau phase of the action potential. The late I_{Na} increases in pathological conditions, e.g. ischaemia, HF, some types of the congenital LQTS.

In ischaemic tissue, there appears to be a marked increase in intracellular Na^+ levels that is possibly due to an increase in the late I_{Na} and decreased Na^+ efflux. It has been postulated that this increase in late I_{Na} leads to elevated intracellular Ca^{2+} levels through the reverse mode of the $Na^+–Ca^{2+}$ exchanger. Ischaemia-induced disruption of cellular Na^+ and Ca^{2+} homeostasis can result in contractile (increased diastolic tension, reduced contractility and coronary blood supply), and metabolic (decrease ATP formation) and electrophysiologic disturbances (arrhythmias).

Pharmacodynamics

Studies suggest that ranolazine is associated with decreases in mean heart rate by <2bpm and SBP by <3mmHg and a dose- and concentration-dependent increase in QTc interval (~2–7msec).

In chronic stable angina patients, ranolazine (500, 1000, and 1500mg bd) increases exercise duration, time to onset of angina, and time to 1mm ST-segment depression at trough (12h after dose) and peak (increased with increased dose).[1]

It reduces frequency of angina (2.9 vs. 3.3 episodes/week) in patients with chronic stable angina with ≥3 episodes of angina/week (mean=5.6 episodes/week) established on amlodipine 10mg od treated with ranolazine 1g bd compared to placebo and followed up for 6 weeks.[2] Ranolazine (750mg or 1000mg bd) also increases time to onset of angina and also to 1mm ST depression during modified Bruce exercise testing in patients with CHD and exertional angina treated for 12 weeks with once-daily atenolol (50mg), diltiazem (180mg), or amlodipine (5mg) compared with placebo.[3]

It reduces 2° endpoint of risk of recurrent ischaemia (HR=0.87; absolute rates: 13.9% vs. 16.1%) in patients with ACS receiving standard therapy treated with ranolazine 1g bd compared with placebo and followed up for median of ≈1 year.[4] No significant difference in the 1° composite endpoint (risk of CV death, MI, or recurrent ischaemia) was seen between ranolazine and placebo.

In these patients, treatment with ranolazine resulted in significantly lower incidence of arrhythmias as assessed by Holter monitoring. Drug-treated patients had fewer episodes of VT ≥8 beats (5.3% vs. 8.3%), SVT (44.7% vs. 55%), new onset AF (1.7% vs. 2.4%), or pauses >3s (3.1% vs. 4.3%) as assessed by Holter monitoring performed for the 1st 7 days after randomization.[5]

Finally, in patients with diabetes mellitus treated with ranolazine, HbA_{1c} declined from 7.5 to 6.9 at 4 months compared with placebo and ranolazine reduced recurrent ischaemia.[6] In patients without diabetes mellitus at baseline, the incidence of new fasting glucose >110mg/dL or $HbA_{1c} \geq 6\%$ was reduced by ranolazine (31.8% vs. 41.2%).

Pharmacokinetics

Oral bioavailability of ranolazine extended-release (ER) is 30–55% and peak plasma levels are reached within 2–6h. Ranolazine binds to serum proteins (62%), presents a V_d of 2.3L/kg, and is rapidly and extensively metabolized in the liver primarily via CYP3A4 pathway and to a lesser extent by CYP2D6 (10–15%). Approximately 75% is excreted in urine and 25% in faeces, with <5% excreted unchanged; $t_{1/2}$ of ~12h.

Practical points

.♣ Doses

500mg bd (which can be increased to 1g bd).

Doses of 1500mg have been shown to be associated with unacceptable side effects. Due to risk of increased exposure, careful dose titration is recommended in renal and hepatic impairment, in the elderly, and when used concomitantly with CYP3A4 and P-glycoprotein (P-gp) inhibitors.

☺ Side effects

(≥2.0%): constipation, diarrhoea, dyspepsia, abdominal pain, nausea; dizziness, headache; angina, palpitations, chest pain; nasopharyngitis; asthenia.

Others: increased QTc, reduction in T-wave amplitude and notched T waves, bradycardia; increased blood creatinine and urea; palpitations, tinnitus, vertigo, abdominal pain, dry mouth, vomiting, peripheral oedema, dyspnoea.

Interactions

Ivabradine plasma concentrations may rise with use of CYP3A inhibitors (e.g. azole antifungals such as ketoconazole, diltiazem, verapamil, macrolide antibiotics, HIV protease inhibitors, grapefruit juice). Conversely, concentrations may be decreased with CYP3A inducers (e.g. rifampicin, phenobarbital, phenytoin, carbamazepine, St John's wort).

Drug interactions may occur with co-administration of P-gp inhibitors (e.g. ritonavir, ciclosporin) and P-gp substrates (e.g. digoxin, simvastatin). The dose of P-gp substrate drugs may need to be reduced.

Modest increases in plasma concentrations are seen with use of CYP2D6 inhibitors (e.g. paroxetine), and interactions may occur with CYP2D6 substrates (e.g. tricyclic antidepressants, antipsychotics).

Risk of ventricular arrhythmia may be increased when used concomitantly with QT-prolonging drugs: class Ia (e.g. quinidine) and class III (e.g. sotalol) antiarrhythmic agents, antipsychotics (e.g. thioridazine, ziprasidone), antidepressants (e.g. imipramine, amitriptyline), erythromycin, and antihistamines (e.g. terfenadine, mizolastine).

There are no interactions with warfarin, atenolol, or amlodipine.

Cautions/notes

A population-based analysis of combined data from patients and healthy volunteers demonstrated that the slope of the plasma concentration-QTc relationship was estimated to be 2.4 msec per 1000 ng/ml, which is approximately equal to a 2- to 7-msec increase over the plasma concentration range for ranolazine 500 to 1000 mg twice daily. Therefore, caution should be observed when treating patients with a history of congenital or a family history of long QT syndrome, in patients with known acquired QT interval prolongation, and in patients treated with drugs affecting the QTc interval.

Pregnancy and lactation

The potential effects of ranolazine on fertility, fetal development, and lactation have not been adequately studied and, therefore, its use in these circumstances is avoided (pregnancy category C).

Contraindications

- Pre-existing QT prolongation, co-administration of QT-prolonging drugs
- Severe renal disease (creatinine clearance <30mL/min)
- Severe or moderate hepatic impairment
- Co-administration of potent CYP3A inhibitors (e.g. itraconazole, keto-conazole, HIV protease inhibitors, clarithromycin)
- Concomitant use with class I or class III (except amiodarone) anti-arrhythmics
- Previous history of VT

References

1 Chaitman BR et al. for the Monotherapy Assessment of Ranolazine in Stable Angina (MARISA) Investigators (2004). Anti-ischemic effects and long-term survival during ranolazine monotherapy in patients with chronic severe angina. J Am Coll Cardiol 43:1375–82.
2 Stone PH et al. (2006). Anti-anginal efficacy of ranolazine when added to treatment with amlo-dipine: the ERICA (efficacy of ranolazine in chronic angina) trial. J Am Coll Cardiol 48: 566–75.
3 Chaitman BR et al. (2004). Effects of ranolazine with atenolol, amlodipine, or diltiazem on exercise tolerance and angina frequency in patients with severe chronic angina: a randomised controlled trial. JAMA 291:309–16.
4 Morrow DA et al.; MERLIN-TIMI 36 Trial Investigators (2007). Effects of ranolazine on recurrent cardiovascular events in patients with non-ST-elevation acute coronary syndromes: the MERLIN-TIMI 36 randomized trial. JAMA 297:1775–83.
5 Scirica BM et al. (2007). Effect of ranolazine, an antianginal agent with novel electrophysiological properties, on the incidence of arrhythmias in patients with non ST-segment elevation acute coronary syndrome: results from the Metabolic Efficiency With Ranolazine for Less Ischemia in Non ST-Elevation Acute Coronary Syndrome Thrombolysis in Myocardial Infarction 36 (MERLIN-TIMI 36) randomized controlled trial. Circulation 116:1647–52.
6 Morrow DA et al. (2009). Evaluation of the glycometabolic effects of ranolazine in patients with and without diabetes mellitus in the MERLIN-TIMI 36 Randomized Controlled Trial. Circulation 119:2032–9.
7 Moss A et al. (2008). Ranolazine shortens repolarization in patients with sustained inward sodium current due to type-3 long-QT syndrome. J Cardiovasc Electrophysiol 19:1289–93.

Renin–angiotensin–aldosterone system inhibitors

There are 3 main categories of drugs that inhibit the RAAS:
- ACEIs (see 📖 Angiotensin-converting enzyme inhibitors, p.355)
- ARBs (see 📖 Angiotensin II AT$_1$ receptor blockers, p.359)
- Direct renin inhibitors (DRIs) (see 📖 Aliskiren, p.340)
- Aldosterone antagonists (see 📖 p.339)

CV indications

(See 📖 individual drug categories)

Mechanism of action

The RAAS is a major hormone cascade that is fundamental to the regulation of BP and sodium homeostasis, as well as in the structure and function of the CV system. Renin is an aspartic protease that catalyses the 1st- and rate-limiting step in the RAAS cascade. It is released acutely from the juxtaglomerular apparatus within the kidney in response to: (a) a decrease in renal blood flow, as in ischaemia or hypotension; (b) β_1 adrenergic receptor stimulation; and (c) sodium depletion or sodium diuresis. Once released, renin cleaves circulating angiotensinogen peptide to generate the inactive pro-hormone, angiotensin I.[1] Angiotensin I in turn is converted to yield the active hormone angiotensin II within the lungs and a variety of local tissues by ACE[1] and also by several non-ACE pathways.[2]

Angiotensin II is the active component of the RAAS and acts at multiple sites producing: arteriolar and venous vasoconstriction (that increases peripheral vascular resistances and preload/afterload) and endothelial dysfunction, increases the sympathetic tone and oxidative stress (increases NADPH oxidase activity), stimulates the release of aldosterone, endothelin-1 and vasopressin, and produces proliferative (hypertrophy, hyperplasia) and profibrotic (interstitial fibrosis), pro-inflammatory, and pro-arrhythmic effects. In the kidney, angiotensin II produces a vasoconstriction of the efferent glomerular arteriole, increases intraglomerular pressure and glomerular growth, and fibrosis as well as Na$^+$ reabsorption in the proximal tubule. Angiotensin II increases heart rate, contractility, and myocardial O$_2$ demands. Finally, it increases platelet aggregation and inhibits the fibrinolytic system (increases PAI-1 and decreases tPA). Thus, angiotensin II and aldosterone have been implicated in the development of many of the complications of hypertension and CVD.[3–5] Consequently, inhibition of the RAAS with an ACEI, ARBs, DRIs, and aldosterone antagonist reduces BP and can improve outcome in hypertension and various CVDs.

Pharmacodynamics

(See 📖 individual drug categories)
Both ACEIs and ARBs produce arteriolar vasodilatation, which decreases peripheral vascular resistances, BP pressure, and afterload, decreases

sympathetic tone and reduces the release of aldosterone (promoting Na^+ excretion and K^+ retention) and vasopressin, and also exert antiproliferative (decrease LVH, vascular hyperplasia), antioxidant, anti-inflammatory, and antiarrhythmic effects.

ACEIs and ARBs are effective in hypertensive patients with LVH and decrease vascular remodelling. They are indicated in hypertensives with HF or LV dysfunction, post-MI, asthma/CPOD, diabetes, hyperlipidaemia, depression, aortic coarctation, hyperuricaemia, proteinuria, and ischaemic heart disease. However, ACEIs and ARBs are less effective as monotherapy in black hypertensive males.

ACEIs and ARBs improve outcome and CV events in hypertension, HF, AMI, coronary heart disease, diabetes, and diabetic nephropathy.[5,6] Available evidence suggests that blockade of the RAAS with either ACEIs or ARBs reduces BP similarly in hypertensive patients.[6] In patients with HF, ACEIs decrease preload, improving signs and symptoms of pulmonary congestion, and afterload, increasing cardiac output, functional capacity, and coronary, skeletal muscle, and kidney blood flow, inhibit neurohumoral activation, and produce natriuresis. They reduce symptoms, improve haemodynamics, slow progression of the disease, and decrease LV remodelling, hospitalizations, and mortality.

Renoprotection: in patients with diabetic nephropathy, ACEIs and ARBs produce a preferential vasodilatation of efferent glomerular arterioles, reducing intraglomerular pressure and protecting against progressive glomerulosclerosis. ACEIs slow the progression of type 1 diabetes with microalbuminuria[7] and ARBs slow the progression of nephropathy caused by type 2 diabetes independent of reduction in BP.[8,9]

Aliskiren, a direct renin inhibitor, is relatively new. Trials are currently ongoing to determine if RAAS blockade with aliskiren confers similar benefits.

References

1 Danser AH (1996). Local renin-angiotensin systems. *Mol Cell Biochem* **157**:211–16.
2 Hollenberg NK *et al.* (1998). Pathways for angiotensin II generation in intact human tissue: evidence from comparative pharmacological interruption of the renin system. *Hypertension* **32**:3873–92.
3 Dzau VJ (2001). Theodore Cooper Lecture: tissue angiotensin and pathobiology of vascular disease: a unifying hypothesis. *Hypertension* **37**:1047–52.
4 Paul M *et al.* (2006). Physiology of local renin-angiotensin systems. *Physiol Rev* **86**:747–803.
5 Schmieder RE *et al.* (2007). Renin-angiotensin system and cardiovascular risk. *Lancet* **369**:1208–19.
6 Turnbull F; Blood Pressure Lowering Treatment Trialists' Collaboration (2003). Effects of different blood-pressure-lowering regimens on major cardiovascular events: results of prospectively-designed overviews of randomised trials. *Lancet* **362**:1527–35.
7 Lewis EJ *et al.* for the Collaborative Study Group (1993). The effect of angiotensin-converting enzyme inhibition on diabetic nephropathy. *N Engl J Med* **229**:1456–62.
8 Brenner BM *et al.*; RENAAL Study Investigators (2001). Effects of losartan on renal and cardiovascular outcomes in patients with type 2 diabetes and nephropathy. *N Engl J Med* **345**:861–9.
9 Parving HH *et al.*; Irbesartan in Patients with Type 2 Diabetes and Microalbuminuria Study Group (2001). The effect of irbesartan on the development of diabetic nephropathy in patients with type 2 diabetes. *N Engl J Med* **345**:870–8.

Rivaroxaban

Novel, orally active, direct factor Xa inhibitor.

CV indication

Short-term prevention of VTE in patients undergoing orthopaedic surgery (total hip or knee replacement surgery).

Mechanism of action

Factor Xa directly converts prothrombin to thrombin through the pro-thrombinase complex, a reaction leading to fibrin clot formation and activation of platelets by thrombin.

Rivaroxaban is a direct, specific and selective inhibitor of factor Xa, therefore prolonging clotting times and reducing the formation of thrombin, an essential component to the development of thrombus formation. This high selectivity allows the drug to inhibit free factor Xa, prothrombinase activity, and clot-associated factor Xa, giving it the ability not only to prevent clots from forming, but also to possibly break down clots already present. Inhibition of factor Xa interrupts the intrinsic and extrinsic pathway of the blood coagulation cascade, inhibiting both thrombin formation and development of thrombi. However, it does not have significant direct effects on thrombin, platelets, or antithrombin activity. The mechanism of action of rivaroxaban is beneficial in the prevention and treatment of thromboembolic diseases.

Pharmacodynamics

There are strong correlations between the inhibition of factor Xa and plasma concentrations as well as plasma concentrations and prothrombin time, with no need for dose adjustments and routine coagulation monitoring. Maximum inhibition of factor Xa occurs within 1–4h after administration and ranges from 20 to 61% for the 5–80mg doses.

Absolute RR 2.6% (1.1% vs. 3.7%)[1] and 7.3% (2.0% vs. 9.3%)[2] in the 1° endpoint of asymptomatic DVT, non-fatal symptomatic DVT, non-fatal pulmonary embolism or all-cause mortality in patients undergoing hip replacement surgery treated for 5 weeks[1] and 10–14 days[2] respectively with rivaroxaban (10mg daily given after surgery) as compared to enoxaparin (40mg SC od given before surgery).

Absolute RR 9.2% (9.6% vs. 18.9%)[3] and 3.2% (6.9% vs. 10.1%)[4] in any DVT, non-fatal pulmonary embolism, or death from any cause within 17 days after surgery in patients undergoing knee replacement surgery treated with rivaroxaban (10mg daily, beginning 6–8h after surgery) compared to SC enoxaparin (40mg od, beginning 12h before surgery).

A pooled analysis of data from these studies showed that rivaroxaban was more effective than enoxaparin in reducing the incidence of the composite of symptomatic VTE and all-cause mortality at 2 weeks after elective hip and knee surgery (OR 0.44), and at the end of the planned medication period (OR 0.38), without increasing major bleeding.[5]

Pharmacokinetics

Oral bioavailability of rivaroxaban ranges from 80 to 100%, reaching peak plasma concentrations within 2–4h. The presence of food increases maximum concentration, time to maximum concentration, and AUC. Maximum inhibition of factor Xa (20–61%) occurs within 1–4h for the 5–80mg doses. After multiple doses of rivaroxaban, dose-proportional increases in AUC are observed. It has also been noted that once the drug reaches steady state, there is no significant accumulation of the drug. Rivaroxaban binds to plasma proteins (92–95%), its V_d is 0.65L/kg and it is metabolized (75% of the dose) via CYP (3A4 and 3A5, 18%; 2J2, 14%) and CYP-independent mechanisms. Rivaroxaban is also a substrate for the active transport proteins P-gp and BCRP ('breast cancer resistance protein'). Rivaroxaban is eliminated through both renal (66%) and biliary (28%) excretion, and 36% is excreted as unchanged drug in the urine. Drug elimination demostrate 1st-order kinetics and is impaired (and AUC increased) with advancing age, renal impairment (most trials excluded patients with creatinine clearances below 30mL/min), hepatic impairment (Child–Pugh A or B), and in the presence of strong CYP3A4 inhibitors. Terminal $t_{1/2}$ is 7–11h.

Practical points

⚫ *Doses*

Prophylaxis of VTE following knee replacement surgery, adult over 18 years: 10mg od for 2 weeks starting 6–10h after surgery

Prophylaxis of VTE following hip replacement surgery, adult over 18 years: 10mg od for 5 weeks starting 6–10h after surgery

☺ *Side effects*

Common: headache, post-procedural haemorrhage (including postoperative anaemia and wound haemorrhage), thrombocythaemia, GI (nausea, constipation, diarrhoea, dyspepsia, dry mouth, vomiting), and tachycardia

Less common: asthenia, fatigue, hypotension, oedema, urinary tract infection, increased levels of transaminases, insomnia, renal impairment, pain in extremities, pruritus

Interactions

Rivaroxaban is a substrate of CYP3A4 and P-gp, so its plasma levels increase when co-administered with inhibitors of CYP3A4 and/or P-gp, including azole-antimycotics (fluconazole, voriconazole, ketoconazole, posaconazole), HIV inhibitors (indinavir, lopinavir, ritonavir), or macrolides (erythromycin, clarithromycin). In contrast, the AUC of the drug decreases when co-administered with CYP3A4 inducers (rifampicin, carbamazepine, St John's wort).

No drug interaction with digoxin, NSAIDs, ranitidine/antacids or atorvastatin

Cautions/notes

The haemorrhagic risk is increased in patients with: congenital or acquired bleeding disorders, concomitant use of drugs that increase risk of bleeding, uncontrolled severe hypertension, active or recent GI ulceration, vascular retinopathy, recent intracranial or intracerebral haemorrhage, intraspinal or intracerebral vascular abnormalities, recent brain, spinal, or ophthalmologic surgery, anaesthesia with postoperative indwelling epidural catheter (risk of paralysis—monitor neurological signs and wait at least 18h after rivaroxaban dose before removing catheter and do not give next dose until at least 6h after catheter removal), hepatic (Child–Pugh B) and renal impairment (CrCl <30mL/min), and strong inhibitors of CYP3A4.

Pregnancy and lactation

Rivaroxaban passes through the placenta and in animal models produces reproductive toxicity. Thus, it is contraindicated in pregnant woman (pregnancy category C). No data are available in breastfeeding women.

Contraindications

- Clinically significant active bleeding
- Hepatic disease associated with coagulopathy and clinically relevant bleeding risk
- Impaired haemostasis
- Patients with CrCl <15mL/min
- Pregnant and breastfeeding women

References

1 Eriksson BI et al. (2008). Rivaroxaban versus enoxaparin for thromboprophylaxis after hip arthroplasty. N Engl J Med 358:2765–75.
2 Kakkar AK et al. (2008). Extended duration rivaroxaban versus short-term enoxaparin for the prevention of venous thromboembolism after total hip arthroplasty: a double-blind, randomised controlled trial. Lancet 372:31–9.
3 Lassen MR et al. (2008). Rivaroxaban versus enoxaparin for thromboprophylaxis after total knee arthroplasty. N Engl J Med 358:2776–86.
4 Turpie AG et al. (2009). Rivaroxaban versus enoxaparin for thromboprophylaxis after total knee arthroplasty (RECORD 4): a randomised trial. Lancet 373:1673–80.
5 Eriksson BI et al. (2009). Oral rivaroxaban for the prevention of symptomatic venous thromboembolism after elective hip and knee replacement. J Bone Joint Surg Br 91:636–44.

Rosuvastatin

(See also 📖 Statins, p.591)

Oral HMG-CoA reductase inhibitor.

CV indications

1. 1° hypercholesterolaemia (type IIa including heterozygous familial hyper-cholesterolaemia) or mixed dyslipidaemia (type IIb) as an adjunct to diet when response to diet and other non-pharmacological treatments is inadequate
2. Homozygous familial hypercholesterolaemia, as an adjunct to diet and other lipid-lowering treatments (e.g. LDL apheresis) or if such treatments are not appropriate
3. Hypertriglyceridaemia

Mechanism of action

(See 📖 Statins, p.591)

Pharmacodynamics

Reduces elevated LDL-C, total cholesterol, triglycerides and ApoB, as well as increasing HDL-C and ApoA-I (Table 11).[1]

Table 11 Levels of lipid lowering with rosuvastatin (adjusted mean % change from baseline)

Dose (mg)	Percentage change						
	Total chol	LDL chol	HDL chol	TG	HDL-C	ApoA	ApoB
Placebo	−2	−4	−3	−1	4	4	−2
5	−31	−43	−38	−35	14	7	36
10	−35	−51	−42	−10	14	7	−41
20	−40	−56	−46	−23	10	7	−49
40	−46	−63	−54	−28	10	2	−54

Hypercholesterolaemia: slowed the rate of progression of the maximum carotid intima–media thickness for the 12 carotid artery sites comparing rosuvastatin 40mg daily vs. placebo (by −0.0145mm/year) in patients between 45 and 70 years of age and at low risk for coronary heart disease (Framingham risk <10% over 10 years), with a mean LDL-C of 4.0mmol/L, but with subclinical atherosclerosis. However, the population studied is low risk for CHD and does not represent the target population for 40mg.[2]

In patients with coronary artery lesions with baseline >25% stenosis, treatment with rosuvastatin 40mg/day at 24 months reduced by 6.8% the mean change in per cent atheroma volume (PAV) and the most diseased 10mm subsegment by −6.1 mm[3,3] For the 1° efficacy parameter of PAV, 63.6% of patients showed regression and 36.4% showed progression. For the change in the 10mm subsegment with the greatest disease severity, 78.1% of patients demonstrated regression and 21.9% showed progression.

Homozygous familial hypercholesterolaemia: effective in reducing LDL-C, in a population that has not usually responded to lipid-lowering medication. Mean reduction from baseline with 6 weeks of rosuvastatin 80mg was 19.1% for LDL-C, 17.6% total cholesterol, and 11.4% ApoB (part of a crossover trial with 80mg atorvastatin, resulting in 18.0%, 17.9%, and 11.7% reductions, respectively).[4]

Pharmacokinetics

Oral bioavailability is ≈20% and peak plasma concentrations are reached within 3–5h. Rosuvastatin is ≈90% bound to plasma proteins, its V_d is ≈1.9L/kg, and it undergoes limited hepatic metabolism (10% of the dose). Approximately 90% of the dose is excreted unchanged in the faeces and ≈5% excreted unchanged in urine. Elimination $t_{1/2}$ is ≈19 (13–20)h. Systemic exposure increases in proportion to dose. There are no changes in pharmacokinetic profile after multiple daily doses.

Practical points

⚡ Doses

10mg daily (5mg in Asian patients) at any time of day, with or without food

- Dose adjustments can be made after 4 weeks.
- The maximum dose of 40mg should only be considered in patients with severe hypercholesterolaemia at high CV risk (in particular those with familial hypercholesterolaemia), who do not achieve their treatment goal on 20mg, and in whom routine follow-up will be performed—specialist supervision recommended.
- For patients of advanced age or with severe renal impairment (CrCl <30mL/min/1.73 m^2), the starting dose is 5mg daily (do not exceed 10mg once daily).

☺ Side effects

(See 📖 Statins, p.591)

Increases in serum transaminases to >3× the ULN occurred in 1.1% (0.5% of patients treated with placebo).

Proteinuria, detected by dipstick testing and mostly tubular in origin, has been observed in patients treated with higher doses, in particular 40mg. In most cases it was transient or intermittent, and has not been shown to be predictive of acute or progressive renal disease.

Interactions

(See 📖 Statins, p.591)

- Rosuvastatin increases the INR in patients receiving coumarin anticoagulants. Appropriate monitoring of INR is desirable in patients taking coumarin anticoagulants, before starting rosuvastatin, and frequently during early therapy.
- Concomitant aluminium/magnesium antacids reduce rosuvastatin concentration; therefore dose 2h after rosuvastatin.

- Co-administration of ciclosporin or gemfibrozil with rosuvastatin results in reduced clearance; reduce the dose of rosuvastatin.
- When co-administered with fenofibrate there is no increase in the AUC of rosuvastatin or fenofibrate.

Cautions/notes
(See 📖 Statins, p.591)
Dose adjustment for renal impairment:
- CrCl of <60mL/min: starting dose 5mg, and 40mg dose is contraindicated
- CrCl <30mL/min: contraindicated.

Hepatic impairment:
- in patients with Child–Pugh B disease, C_{max} and AUC were increased 100% and 21%, respectively; and is contraindicated in patients with active liver disease.

Asian subjects:
- an approximate 2-fold elevation in median exposure (AUC and C_{max}) is observed in Asian subjects when compared with a Caucasian control group. Recommended start dose is 5mg, and 40mg dose contraindicated.

Patients with predisposing factors to myopathy:
- recommended start dose is 5mg, and the 40mg dose is contraindicated.

Pregnancy and lactation (see 📖 Statins, p.591)

Contraindications
(See 📖 Statins, p.591)
- Severe renal impairment: CrCl <30mL/min
- Myopathy
- Concomitant ciclosporin
- The 40mg dose is contraindicated in patients with predisposing factors for myopathy/rhabdomyolysis

References
1 Olsson et al. (2001). Effect of rosuvastatin on low-density lipoprotein cholesterol in patients with hypercholesterolemia. *Am J Cardiol* **88**:504–8.
2 Crouse JR 3rd et al.; METEOR Study Group (2007). Effect of rosuvastatin on progression of carotid intima–media thickness in low-risk individuals with subclinical atherosclerosis: the METEOR Trial. *JAMA* **297**:1344–53.
3 Nissen SE et al. (2006). Effect of very high-intensity statin therapy on regression of coronary atherosclerosis: the ASTEROID trial. *JAMA* **295**:1556–65.
4 Marais AD et al. (2008). A dose-titration and comparative study of rosuvastatin and atorvastatin in patients with homozygous familial hypercholesterolaemia. *Atherosclerosis* **197**:400–6.

Sildenafil

Orally active, potent, and selective cyclic guanosine monophosphate (cGMP)-specific phoshodiesterase type 5 (PDE-5) inhibitor.

CV indications

To improve symptoms and exercise capacity in patients with 1° PAH WHO class III.

Other indications

Treatment of erectile dysfunction.

Mechanism of action

NO mediates vascular smooth muscle relaxation by increasing intracellular cGMP levels. Within pulmonary vascular smooth muscle cells and the corpus cavernosum of the penis, cGMP is rapidly degraded by PDE-5 isoenzyme.

PAH is associated with impaired release of NO because of reduced expression of NO synthase in the vascular endothelium of pulmonary arteries and an upregulation of PDE-5 activity in the pulmonary vasculature. Inhibition of PDE-5 increases cGMP levels, which may mediate the antiproliferative and vasodilating effects of endogenous NO in the pulmonary vasculature and in the corpus cavernosum of the penis.

Pharmacodynamics

Sildenafil reduces mean right arterial pressure (RAP, 3mmHg), pulmonary (PVR, −11.2%) and systemic vascular resistances (SVR, −7.2%) and improves functional class and exercise capacity (45m in 6-min walk distance) after 12 weeks.[1]

Pharmacokinetics

Oral absorption is rapid (bioavailability ≈40%), reaching peak plasma levels within 30–120min. Drug absorption is reduced when taken with a high-fat meal. Protein binding is 96% and V_d is large (1.3L/kg). It is hepatically metabolized by CYP450 3A4 (major pathway) and also 2C9. Excreted as active and inactive metabolites in faeces (80% of administered oral dose) and in the urine (13%); $t_{1/2} \approx$ 3–4h.

Practical points

⚫ Doses

20mg tds (for symptomatic treatment of PAH). Studies have not shown benefit at higher doses up to 80mg tds.

Age >65, and hepatic and renal impairment (CrCl <30mL/min) are associated with decreased clearance of sildenafil. Hence, doses may need to be decreased to 20mg bd in such patients, if recommended doses are not tolerated.

☺ Common side effects

(>10%): flushing; headache, diarrhoea, dyspepsia
(1–10%): alopecia, night sweats, pyrexia, fluid retention, hypotension, nasal congestion, upset stomach

Potency of sildenafil for PDE-6 (which is found within the retina and involved in the phototransduction pathway) is about 1/10th. Consequently, patients may also experience visual disturbances, including photophobia, blurred vision, and increased sensitivity to light and blue/green tingeing at higher doses.

Rare: sudden vision loss caused by non-arteritic anterior ischaemic optic neuropathy (NAION), priapism, severe hypotension, MI, arrhythmias, increased intraocular pressure, and sudden hearing loss.

Interactions
Concomitant use of sildenafil and antihypertensive drugs increases the risk of hypotension. Combination with an α_1-blocker may lead to low BP; this effect does not occur if they are taken at least 4h apart.

Co-administration with powerful CYP450, 3A4, and 2C9 inhibitors (e.g. erythromycin, clarithromycin, telithromycin, ketoconazole, itraconazole; ritonavir, nelfinavir, fluoxetine, sertraline, amiodarone, ciclosporin) or cimetidine results in increased sildenafil plasma levels; co-administration with rifampicin decreases plasma levels of sildenafil.

Precautions
Assess CV status before use; caution with LV outflow obstruction and/or conditions aggravated by hypotension (i.e. aortic stenosis, HOCM, etc).

Pregnancy and lactation
Sildenafil is safe in pregnancy (pregnancy category B).

Contraindications
- Documented hypersensitivity
- Concurrent or intermittent use of organic nitrates in any form
- Severe hepatic impairment; recent stroke or MI; severe hypotension (BP<90/50mmHg)

Reference
1 Galie N et al. (2005). Sildenafil citrate therapy for pulmonary arterial hypertension. *N Engl J Med* **353**:2148–57.

Simvastatin

(See also 📖 Statins, p.591)

Oral HMG-CoA reductase inhibitor.

CV indications

1. 1° hypercholesterolaemia/mixed dyslipidaemia, as adjunct to diet, when response to diet and other non-pharmacological treatments is inadequate
2. Homozygous and heterozygous familial hypercholesterolaemia as an adjunct to diet and other lipid-lowering treatments (e.g. LDL apheresis) or if such treatments are not appropriate
3. Adolescent patients with heterozygous familial hypercholesterolaemia (HeFH)
4. 2° prevention of CVD in patients with either normal or increased cholesterol levels

Mechanism of action

(See 📖 Statins, p.591)

Pharmacodynamics

Hypercholesterolaemia: in a meta-analysis of 72 clinical trials (4906 participants), simvastatin at 5, 10, 20, 40, and 80mg produced reductions in LDL-C (standardized to pre-treatment LDL-C of 4.8mmol/L) of 23%, 27%, 32%, 37%, and 42% respectively.[1]

2° prevention: 30% RRR (8.2% vs. 11.5% absolute rates) in risk of death, 42% in RRR (5.0% vs. 8.5% absolute rates) in CHD death, 34% RRR (15.9% vs. 22.6% absolute rates) in major coronary events, 28% RRR (11.3% vs. 17.1% absolute rates) in coronary revascularizations, and 28% RRR in fatal plus non-fatal cerebrovascular events (combined stroke and TIAs), comparing simvastatin 20–40mg daily vs. placebo, over median duration of 5.4 years, in patients with CHD and baseline total cholesterol 212–309mg/dL (5.5–8.0mmol/L).[2]

RRR 13% for total and RRR 18% for CHD mortality in patients (aged 40–80 years) with CHD, other occlusive arterial disease, or diabetes treated for 5 years with simvastatin 40mg/day or placebo.[3] There were highly significant reductions of about one-quarter in the first event rate for non-fatal MI or coronary death, for non-fatal or fatal stroke, and for coronary or non-coronary revascularization. For the first occurrence of any of these major vascular events, there was a definite 24% (95% CI 19–28) reduction in the event rate. The proportional reduction in the event rate was similar in each subcategory of participants studied.

In hypercholesterolaemic patients with CHD, simvastatin (20mg/day) significantly slowed the progression of lesions and decreased the proportion of patients with new lesion occlusions.[4]

A significant reduction in vessel aortic and carotid wall area was already observed after 18 months' treatment with simvastatin (20 or 80mg/day) in newly diagnosed hypercholesterolaemic patients with asymptomatic aortic and/or carotid atherosclerotic plaques. Patients reaching mean on-treatment LDL-C ≤ 100mg/dL had larger decreases in plaque size.[5]

Pharmacokinetics

Simvastatin is well absorbed and undergoes extensive hepatic 1st-pass extraction, dependent on the hepatic blood flow, and so the availability of the drug to the general circulation is low (<5%). Maximum plasma concentration of active inhibitors is reached ~1–2h after administration, and is unaffected by food intake. Protein binding of simvastatin and its β-hydroxyacid active metabolite is >95%. The major metabolites of simvastatin present in human plasma are the β-hydroxyacid and 4 additional active metabolites. Following an oral dose, 13% is excreted in the urine and 60% in the faeces. $t\frac{1}{2}$=3–4h.

Practical points

⚐ Doses

The dosage range is 5–80mg daily (in the evening).

- Adjustments of dosage, if required, should be made at intervals of not <4 weeks.
- The 80mg dose is only recommended in patients with severe hypercholesterolaemia and high risk for cardiovascular complications.

Hypercholesterolaemia: usual starting dose is 10–20mg daily. Patients who require a large reduction in LDL-C may be started at 20–40mg/day.

Homozygous familial hypercholesterolaemia: the recommended dosage is 40mg od or a daily dose of 80mg in 3 divided doses of 20mg, 20mg, and an evening dose of 40mg, and should be used as an adjunct to other lipid-lowering treatments (e.g. LDL apheresis) in these patients.

Cardiovascular prevention: the usual dose is 20–40mg in the evening in patients at high risk of coronary heart disease (with or without hyperlipidaemia).

Also available in combination with ezetimibe (10mg of ezetimibe with 20, 40 or 80mg of simvastatin).

☻ Side effects

(See 📖 Statins, p.591)
Persistent increases (to more than 3× the ULN) in serum transaminases have occurred in 1% of patients. The incidence of myopathy was ≈0.02%, 0.08% and 0.53% at 20, 40, and 80mg/day.

Interactions

(See 📖 Statins, p.591)
Simvastatin modestly potentiated the effect of coumarin anticoagulants, and discontinuation or downtitration may result in a decrease in INR. Appropriate monitoring of INR is desirable.

Cautions/notes

(See 📖 Statins, p.591)
Patients titrated to the 80mg dose should receive an additional liver function test prior to titration, 3 months after titration to the 80mg dose, and

periodically for the 1st year. Dosages above 10mg/day should be carefully considered in severe renal insufficiency (CrCl <30mL/min) and, if necessary, implemented cautiously. Chinese patients should not receive the highest dose of simvastatin when taking ≥1g/day of niacin.

Pregnancy and lactation
(See 📖 Statins, p.591)

Contraindications
(See 📖 Statins, p.591)
Concomitant administration of potent CYP3A4 inhibitors (e.g. itraconazole, ketoconazole, HIV protease inhibitors, erythromycin, clarithromycin, telithromycin, and nefazodone).

References

1 Law MR et al. (2003). Quantifying effect of statins on low density lipoprotein cholesterol, ischaemic heart disease, and stroke: systematic review and meta-analysis. *BMJ* **326**:1423.

2 Scandinavian Simvastatin Survival Study Group (1994). Randomised trial of cholesterol lowering in 4444 patients with coronary heart disease: the Scandinavian Simvastatin Survival Study (4S). *Lancet* **344**:1383–9.

3 Heart Protection Study Collaborative Group (2002). MRC/BHF Heart Protection Study of cholesterol lowering with simvastatin in 20,536 high-risk individuals: a randomised placebo-controlled trial. *Lancet* **360**:7–22.

4 (1994). Effect of simvastatin on coronary atheroma: the Multicentre Anti-Atheroma Study (MAAS). *Lancet* **344**:633–8.

5 Corti R et al. (2005). Effects of aggressive versus conventional lipid-lowering therapy by simvastatin on human atherosclerotic lesions: a prospective, randomized, double-blind trial with high-resolution magnetic resonance imaging. *J Am Coll Cardiol* **46**:106–12.

Sitaxentan

This is a relatively selective antagonist of the ET_A receptor.

CV indications

Treatment of PAH to improve exercise capacity and symptoms in patients with grade III and IV functional status.

Mechanism of action

Pharmacodynamics

Sitaxentan improves exercise capacity (33–35m) and functional class after 12 weeks.[1]

Pharmacokinetics

High oral bioavailability (70–95%). It is highly bound to plasma proteins (99%) and is metabolized in the liver via CYP 2C9 (and 3A4 and 2C19 to a lesser extent) and excreted by urine (60%) and faeces (49%). $t_{1/2}$ ~10 h.

Practical points

⅊ Dose

100mg orally od

Cautions/notes

Similar to bosentan (see p.385)

- The incidence of elevated hepatic transaminases (>3× ULN) was 6% for placebo, 5% for sitaxentan 50mg, 3% for sitaxentan 100mg, and 11% for bosentan.[1]
- In a pilot study, sitaxentan was associated with fatal hepatitis when used at higher doses.[2]
- Sitaxentan inhibits CYP2C9 P450 enzyme, the principal hepatic enzyme involved in the metabolism of warfarin and increases the INR or prothrombin time.

Contraindications

Similar to bosentan (📖 see p.385)

References

1 Barst RJ et al. (2004). Sitaxentan therapy for pulmonary arterial hypertension. Am J Respir Crit Care Med **169**:441–7.

Sodium nitroprusside

IV direct NO donor.

CV indications

1. Immediate reduction of BP of patients with hypertensive crisis
2. Acute HF
3. Controlled hypotension in anaesthesia to reduce bleeding during surgery

Mechanism of action

Sodium nitroprusside is a non-organic nitrate that acts as a direct NO donor. Endothelial NO has several important functions including relaxing vascular smooth muscle (vasodilatation) through the activation of soluble guanylate cyclase and formation of cyclic AMP. NO also inhibits platelet aggregation (antithrombotic) and leucocyte–endothelial interactions (anti-inflammatory), and exhibits antiproliferative properties. Thus, by mimicking the actions of endogenous NO, sodium nitroprusside causes dilatation of peripheral arteries and veins. Venodilatation decreases venous return to the heart, thereby reducing LV end-diastolic pressure (preload) and PCWP (preload). Arteriolar relaxation reduces systemic vascular resistance (afterload) and BP, and increases heart rate, with variable effects on cardiac output. In hypertensive patients, sodium nitroprusside induces renal vasodilatation, without changes in renal blood flow or GFR.

Pharmacodynamics

Sodium nitroprusside is a very potent antihypertensive agent with a very rapid onset of action (within 1–2min after starting the infusion), but changes in BP dissipate rapidly after the infusion is discontinued. Its effects on pre- and post-load can improve LV performance when given in severe hypertension, with a relative reduction ~20% in end-systolic volume.[1] Due to its potency and onset of action, its use in severe hypertension can lead to compensatory mechanisms that may cause reflex tachycardia and volume expansion through the activation of the RAAS.[2] In addition, a significant reduction in regional blood flow (coronary steal) can occur in patients with CHD.[3]

The hypotensive effect of sodium nitroprusside is associated with reduced blood loss in a variety of major surgical procedures.

Progressive tachyphylaxis to the hypotensive effects of sodium nitroprusside has been described but the mechanism remains unknown.

Pharmacokinetics

IV infusion of sodium nitroprusside produces an almost immediate reduction in BP; thus, BP begins to rise immediately when the infusion is slowed or stopped and returns to pre-treatment levels within 1–10min. It is eliminated entirely as metabolites in the urine, principally thiocyanate which has an elimination $t_{1/2}$ of 2.7–7 days (longer in patients with decreased renal function and hyponatraemia).

Sodium nitroprusside is cleared by an intra-erythrocyte reaction with haemoglobin to form cyanomethaemoglobin and cyanide ion, resulting in a circulatory $t_{1/2}$ of ≈2–3min. Cyanide ions largely react with thiosulphate to produce thiocyanate, which is excreted in urine, and some cyanide is removed as expired hydrogen cyanide; cyanide ions not removed by these pathways are enzymatically converted to thiocyanate by the mitochondrial enzyme thiosulphate-cyanide sulphurtransferase and may cause toxicity through the inhibition of oxidative phosphorylation.

Practical points

♪ Doses

Dosage varies between individuals, hence there is a need for titration. The solutions are made in saline (avoid alkaline solutions) and should be used as soon as possible under continuous monitoring to avoid excessive hypotension.

Hypertensive crises: the initial dose of ~0.3mcg/kg/min (uptitrated to 0.5–8mcg/kg/min as required). The maximal dose (10mcg/kg/min) should never last for more than 10min. In hypertensive patients receiving concomitant antihypertensive medication, smaller doses might be required.

Heart failure: the initial dose of 10–15mcg/min (uptitrated to 10–200mcg/min as required).

Due to an increased risk of cyanide poisoning, doses of sodium nitroprusside should be reduced in renal impairment. Risk of toxicity may also be reduced by protecting it from light (and so minimizing degradation), and by not exceeding a dose equivalent to 2mcg/kg/min (over a maximum of 48h).

☺ Side effects

Headache, dizziness, drowsiness, palpitations, nausea, vomiting, abdominal pain, apprehension, diaphoresis, and retrosternal discomfort have been noted when the reduction in BP is too rapid. In acute HF, sodium nitroprusside may cause a coronary steal syndrome. These symptoms disappear when the rate of infusion is decreased or the infusion is temporarily discontinued and do not reappear with continued slower rate of administration.

Other: rash, hypothyroidism, decreased platelet aggregation, flushing, venous streaking, irritation at the infusion site, pulmonary hypoxia (from increased ventilation–perfusion mismatch), cyanide toxicity (changed mental status, convulsions, lactic acidosis, and venous hyperoxaemia) and thiocyanate toxicity (tinnitus, miosis, hyperreflexia at serum levels of 1mmol/L). To maintain steady-state thiocyanate levels <1mmol/L, a prolonged infusion of sodium nitroprusside should not exceed a dose of 3mcg/kg/min (1mcg/kg/min in anuric patients). Thiocyanate interferes with iodine uptake by the thyroid.

Cyanide toxicity is treated with sodium nitrite (10mL of 3% solution over 2–5 min) followed by an infusion of sodium thiosulphate (12.5g in 50mL of 5% glucose over 10min).

At high doses, nitroprusside can lead to methaemoglobin formation through dissociation of cyanomethaemoglobin and by direct oxidation of haemoglobin by the released nitroso group. Treatment of methaemoglobinaemia is 1–2mg/kg of methylene blue.

Interactions
Potentiates hypotensive effects of other antihypertensives and some anaesthetic agents.

Cautions/notes
(Also see 'Pharmacodynamics')
Sodium nitroprusside needs careful continuous monitoring and it should be protected from light with aluminum foil or opaque materials to minimize degradation and should only be administered by IV infusion by a controlled infusion device that allows precise measurement of flow rates.

Because its hypotensive effect is very rapid in onset and in dissipation, small variations in infusion rate can lead to wide, undesirable variations in BP. Thus, it should be infused through a volumetric infusion pump.

Infusions may be continued for several days (normally should not exceed 3 days), but care must be taken to ensure that the blood cyanide concentrations do not exceed 100mcg/100mL and blood thiocyanate concentrations 100mcg/mL. Risk of toxicity is increased in renal impairment.

Elderly patients appear to be more sensitive to the hypotensive effects of the drug, and should be administered with caution in this age group. Like other vasodilators, sodium nitroprusside can cause increases in intracranial pressure.

Pregnancy and lactation
Sodium nitroprusside crosses the placental barrier with fetal cyanide levels dose related to maternal levels of nitroprusside. It is not known whether sodium nitroprusside can cause fetal harm when administered to a pregnant woman and so use in pregnancy only if clearly needed. It is not known if sodium nitroprusside is distributed in breast milk; therefore, it should be used with caution in breastfeeding mothers.

Contraindications
- Hypotension (SBP <90mmHg)
- Acute HF associated to reduced peripheral vascular resistances (i.e. high-output HF observed in endotoxic sepsis)
- Severe obstructive valvular disease or obstructive cardiomyopathy
- Inadequate cerebral circulation and compensatory hypertension (i.e. aortic coarctation or arteriovenous shunting)
- Severe vitamin B_{12} deficiency, hepatic and renal insufficiency and Leber's optic atrophy (due to the metabolites cyanide and thiocyanide)

References

1 Hackman BB et al. (1992). Comparative effects of fenoldopam mesylate and nitroprusside on left ventricular performance in severe systemic hypertension. *Am J Cardiol* **69**:918–22.
2 White WB, Halley SE (1989). Comparative renal effects of intravenous administration of fenoldopam mesylate and sodium nitroprusside in patients with severe hypertension. *Arch Intern Med* **149**:870–4.
3 Mann T et al. (1978). Effect of nitroprusside on regional myocardial blood flow in coronary artery disease. Results in 25 patients and comparison with nitroglycerin. *Circulation* **57**:732–8.

Sotalol

(See also 📖 β-blockers, p.376)

Non-selective $β_1$-adrenergic receptor antagonist with high lipid solubility and membrane-stabilizing activity that has class II and III antiarrhythmic activity.

CV indications

(See 📖 β-blockers, p.376)

In contrast to other β-blockers, sotalol has specific indications limited to the following:

- supraventricular arrhythmias
- ventricular arrhythmias
- maintenance of sinus rhythm following cardioversion of atrial flutter or AF

Mechanism of action

(See also 📖 β-blockers, p.376).

In addition to acting as a β-blocker with related class II antiarrhythmic activity, sotalol also has additional class III antiarrhythmic activity through the blockade of the rapid component of the delayed rectifier K^+ current (I_{Kr}) responsible for phase 3 of the cardiac action potential and so may be effective in the management of arrhythmias (especially re-entrant tachycardias), by delaying repolarization, prolonging the cardiac action potential, and increasing the effective refractory period.

Pharmacodynamics

(See also 📖 β-blockers, p.376)

Sotalol is a racemic mixture of dextro- and levo-isomers. Although both isomers present class III antiarrhythmic activity, the l-isomer is almost exclusively responsible for its β-blocking effects and related class II antiarrhythmic activity. However, sotalol does not possess membrane-stabilizing or intrinsic sympathomimetic activity. β-blocking effects occur with oral doses as low as 25mg, but class III effects are seen at higher doses. It is effective in maintaining sinus rhythm and controlling ventricular rate but there is limited evidence that it is efficacious in converting recent-onset or persistent AF.

Atrial fibrillation: RR≈19% (absolute rates: 67% vs. 83%) of AF recurrence or death in patients with persistent AF successfully cardioverted and treated with sotalol 160mg bd compared with placebo and followed up for 266 days.[1]

Rates of spontaneous cardioversion in patients with persistent AF treated with sotalol (24.2%) appear comparable to those treated with amiodarone (27.1%) and greater than with placebo (0.8%).[2] Including electrical cardioversion at 28 days, the total rate of cardioversion with sotalol was 79.9%, comparable to amiodarone (79.8%) and greater than placebo (68.2%). Median time to recurrence of AF was 74 days with sotalol compared to 487 days with amiodarone and 6 days with placebo; in patients with CHD, the median time to recurrence was 569 days with amiodarone therapy and 428 days with sotalol.

Pharmacokinetics

Sotalol is completely absorbed from the GI tract (bioavailability 90–100%), reaching peak plasma concentrations after ~2–3h. It does not bind to plasma proteins, is not metabolized, and presents a V_d of 1.5–2.5L/kg. Excretion is predominantly (70%) via the kidney in the unchanged form, and it has a $t_{1/2}$~7–18h.

Practical points

⑂ *Doses*

Initial dose: 80mg in single or divided doses
Maintenance: 160–320mg/day in 2 doses

Doses should be reduced in renal impairment (½ dose with CrCl 30–60mL/min; and ¼ dose with clearance 10–30mL/min) and in geriatric patients.

☺ *Side effects* (see 🕮 β-blockers, p.376)

Interactions (see 🕮 β-blockers, p.376)

Cautions/notes
(See 🕮 β-blockers, p.376)

Co-administered with QT-prolonging drugs increases the risk of torsades de pointes

Pregnancy and lactation
(See 🕮 β-blockers, p.376)

Use of sotalol is not recommended in pregnancy and breastfeeding (pregnancy category B)

Contraindications
(See 🕮 β-blockers, p.376)

Patients with acquired/congenital LQTS

References

1 Fetsch T *et al.*; Prevention of Atrial Fibrillation after Cardioversion Investigators (2004). Prevention of atrial fibrillation after cardioversion: results of the PAFAC trial. *Eur Heart J* **25**:1385–94.
2 Singh BN *et al.*; Sotalol Amiodarone Atrial Fibrillation Efficacy Trial (SAFE-T) Investigators (2005). Amiodarone versus sotalol for atrial fibrillation. *N Engl J Med* **352**:1861–72.

Spironolactone

(See also 📖 Aldosterone antagonists, p.339)

Competitive aldosterone receptor antagonist (K^+-sparing diuretic).

CV indications

1. NYHA stage III–IV congestive cardiac failure
2. 1° hyperaldosteronism (diagnosis and treatment of Conn's syndrome) or oedemas associated with 2° hyperaldosteronism caused by liver cirrhosis with portal hypertension, nephrotic syndrome, vasculorenal hypertension)

Other indications

Resistant hypertension combined with thiazides or loop diuretics to avoid hypokalaemia, especially low-renin hypertension; hypokalaemia; treatment of the Bartter syndrome.

Mechanism of action

Spironolactone is a specific antagonist of aldosterone and so prevents aldosterone-dependent synthesis of epithelial Na^+ channels and consequently, Na^+–K^+ exchange in the distal convoluted renal tubule. Thus, spironolactone promotes natriuresis and hence BP lowering, as well as K^+ retention. It is believed that the beneficial effects of spironolactone in HF may be related to blockade of deleterious effects of aldosterone which include an increase in Na^+ and water retention and in sympathetic tone, cardiac hypertrophy, fibrosis, and necrosis, reduced vascular compliance, endothelial dysfunction, and vasoconstriction, and promotion of cardiac arrhythmias.

Pharmacodynamics

Hypertension: spironolactone has a gradual onset and a prolonged action. Reduces BP (by ≈17/10mmHg) at doses of 50mg bd in patients with mild–moderate hypertension.[1] It has a gradual and prolonged action. It is indicated in patients with CHF, post-MI, 1° and 2° hyperaldosteronism.

RRR 30% (~35% absolute rate) for 1° endpoint of death over a mean of 24 months (mean dose of 26mg od) cf placebo (≈43% absolute rate) in patients with NYHA III–IV chronic HF.[2] RRR 35% for 2° endpoint of hospitalization for HF cf placebo, as well as an improvement in NYHA functional classification.[2]

Heart failure: spironolactone is indicated in patients with: (a) recent or current symptoms despite ACEIs (or ARBs), diuretics, digoxin, and β-blockers; (b) chronic, severe systolic HF; and (c) systolic HF after MI.[3]

Pharmacokinetics

Oral bioavailability 80–90%, reaching peak plasma levels in 2–3h. Protein binding 90%. Metabolized to active sulphur-containing metabolites (80%) and canrenone (20%). Plasma $t_{1/2}$ of spironolactone is short (1.3h) but longer for its metabolite canrenone (13–24h). Thus, the duration of diuresis is up to 35h. Elimination of metabolites is through urine and faeces.

Practical points

♣ Doses

Hyperaldosteronism: 25–200mg od (to a max of 400mg od)

For HF: 25–50mg od. Assess K^+ within 1 week, if <5mEq/L, 25mg od. If K^+ reaches 5.5mEq/L, the drug should be discontinued.

Added to thiazides or loop diuretics increases diuresis and serum potassium remains within the normal range.

Spironolactone may be used long term in patients with hyperaldosteronism at the lowest dose determined for each patient.

☻ Common side effects

(1–10%): gynaecomastia, painful breasts, hyperkalaemia, GI upset.

Others: hyponatraemia, menstrual disorders, testicular atrophy, headaches, ataxia, metabolic acidosis, allergies.

Spironolactone has anti-androgenic activity through binding to androgen receptor and preventing interaction with dihydrotestosterone. Such activity may underlie its side effects (gynaecomastia, menstrual disorders, and testicular atrophy), which are related to dose and duration of treatment, being usually reversible. If the patient develops gynaecomastia, triamterene or amiloride can replace the drug.

Interactions

Spironolactone decreases renal excretion of digoxin and increases its plasma concentrations. Spironolactone increases the plasma concentrations of lithium and potentiates the effects of antihypertensives.

Concomitant use of ACEIs, ARBs, other K^+-sparing diuretics, β-blockers, and K^+ supplements can precipitate serious hyperkalaemia, particularly in renal impairment.

Aspirin and NSAIDs may attenuate the effects of spironolactone. Indometacin combined with spironolactone may precipitate acute renal failure.

Cautions/notes

Plasma creatinine and electrolytes should be closely monitored, particularly in the elderly, and those with renal and hepatic impairment. Hyperkalaemia may occur with renal impairment or excessive K^+ intake.

Pregnancy and lactation

Avoid in pregnancy due to risk of feminization of fetus (observed in animal studies) (pregnancy category C). Spironolactone expresses in breast milk and can therefore affect breastfeeding babies.

Contraindications

- Anuria; deteriorating or severely impaired renal function. Avoid the drug if there is evidence of renal failure or when serum creatinine >1.3mg/dL
- Hyperkalaemia (>5.5 mEq/L); Addison's disease
- Concurrent treatment with other K^+-sparing diuretics; K^+ supplements

References

1 Pitt B et al. (1999). The effect of spironolactone on morbidity and mortality in patients with severe heart failure. *N Engl J Med* **341**:709–17.
2 Weinberger MH et al. (2002). Eplerenone, a selective aldosterone blocker, in mild-to-moderate hypertension. *Am J Hypertens* **15**:709–16.
3 Nieminen MS et al.; for the ESC Committee for Practice Guideline (CPG) (2005). Executive summary of the guidelines on the diagnosis and treatment of acute heart failure: the Task Force on Acute Heart Failure of the European Society of Cardiology. *Eur Heart J* **26**:384–416.

Statins

Statins are HMG-CoA (3-hydroxy-3-methyl-glutaryl-CoA) reductase inhibitors, e.g. atorvastatin, fluvastatin, lovastatin, pravastatin, rosuvastatin, simvastatin.

CV indications

1. Hypercholesterolaemia and mixed dyslipidaemias
2. 1° prevention in patients at high risk of CV events
3. 2° prevention in patients with previous CV events

Mechanism of action

HMG-CoA reductase is the rate-limiting enzyme that converts HMG-CoA to mevalonate, a precursor for cholesterol. Statins are selective and competitive inhibitors of hepatocyte HMG-CoA reductase, hence effecting a modest reduction in intracellular cholesterol synthesis. This results in an increase in the number of LDL receptors on cell surfaces and enhanced receptor-mediated catabolism and clearance of circulating LDL-C. At present, it is uncertain whether a variety of pleiotropic effects associated with statins (including effects on plaque stability, endothelial function, inflammatory process, platelet activation, and the coagulation) may also contribute to the therapeutic effects of statins in CV disease.

Pharmacodynamics

The effects of statins on total cholesterol and LDL-C reduction are variable and largely dose dependent[1] (see Fig. 1). Respective statins also have differential effects on triglyceride and HDL-C.

LDL-C-lowering effects of statins are proportional to pre-treatment levels. Consistent with epidemiological data, each 1mmol/L (40mg/dL) reduction in LDL-C concentration by statin therapy is associated with a fall in major vascular events (MI, coronary death, coronary revascularization, or stroke) of around 20% (RR 0.79, 95% CI 0.77–0.81) and in mortality rate of around 12% (RR 0.88, 95% CI 0.84–0.91).[2] These benefits are broadly similar across a wide range in levels of baseline CV risk.

In contrast to these relative benefits, absolute benefits are directly related to baseline levels of CV risk such that there are 'diminishing returns' for statin therapy as baseline risk falls. Thus, for instance, for a 1mmol/L reduction in LDL-C concentration, the NNT to avoid a major vascular event is 40 for 1° compared to 21 for 2° prevention.[2]

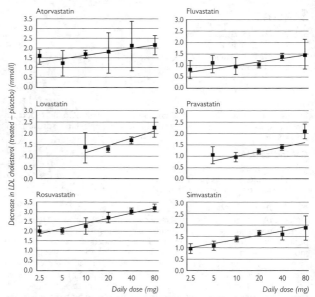

Fig. 1 Estimated effects of statins at various doses, standardized to a pre-treatment LDL-C of 4.8mmol/L. Reproduced from Law, et al. (meta-analysis of 164 clinical trials), with permission from BMJ publishing Group Ltd.[1]

A meta-analysis of trials (TNT, IDEAL, PROVE IT-TIMI-22, and A-to-Z [Aggrastat-to-Zocor]) comparing intensive vs. moderate statin therapy in 27,548 patients with chronic angina and ACS suggests that intensive therapy provides a 16% RR in coronary death or MI, 16% RRR of coronary death or any CV event, 18% RR in stroke, and a trend toward decreased CV mortality (12%).[3] No difference was observed in total or non-CV mortality, but a trend toward decreased CV mortality (OR 12%) was observed. Thus, intensive lipid lowering with high-dose statin therapy provides a significant benefit over standard-dose therapy for preventing predominantly non-fatal CV events.

A meta-analysis of 42 RCTs found a significant reduction of ischaemic stroke (RR 0.84; 95% CI 0.79–0.91) and associated mortality (RR 0.88; 95% CI 0.83–0.93) that cannot be related to the degree of LDL-C reduction.[4]

Some effects of statins are independent from LDL-C reduction. These pleiotropic effects include improvement of endothelial function, inhibition of platelet aggregation, reduction of fibrinogen, anti-inflammatory, antioxidant, antiproliferative, immunodepressant, antithrombotic, and antiarrhythmic effects.

Pharmacokinetics
(See 📖 individual drugs)

Practical points

🎣 Doses
(See 📖 individual drugs)

Statins are more effective when given with the evening meal, as cholesterol synthesis occurs mainly at night.

😣 Side effects
Common (>1%): abdominal pain, dyspepsia, nausea, flatulence, constipation, diarrhoea, insomnia, headache, dizziness, asthenia, allergic reactions,
rash. Central side effects are less frequent with fluvastatin and pravastatin.

Other side effects that vary between individual drugs and which are largely
dose-related include:
- hepatic: elevated serum transaminase levels
- muscular: elevated serum CPK (of which a proportion reported
  muscle pain, tenderness, or weakness); and rhabdomyolysis (~1 per
  100,000 patient-years), with or without renal insufficiency.

Interactions
Risk of dose-related side effects including rhabdomyolysis is increased
when administered concomitantly with medications that may increase the
plasma concentration of statins, such as:
- strong inhibitors of CYP3A4: ciclosporin, erythromycin, clarithromycin,
  telithromycin, itraconazole, ketoconazole, nefazodone, niotinic acid
  (≥1g/day), gemfibrozil and other fibrates, and HIV-protease inhibitors
- the risk of myopathy may also be increased with the concomitant use
  of ezetimibe
- alternative therapies, dose reduction, or temporary suspension of
  statin therapy should be considered where co-administration of these
  medications is only for a few days

Concomitant administration with CYP3A4 inducers (carbamazepine,
phenytoin, griseofulvin, rifampicin) reduces plasma levels of statins.

Reduce the dose when given in patients taking amiodarone or verapamil.

Lipid-lowering effects on total and LDL-C are enhanced when combined
with cholesterol-lowering resins, but should be given either 1h before or
at least 4h after the resin.

Cautions/notes
Prior to therapy, patients should be on a cholesterol-lowering diet and a
lipid profile performed to assess total cholesterol, HDL-C, and triglyceride levels; and 2° causes of hypercholesterolaemia should be excluded/
treated.

Dose adjustment may be required in moderate to severe renal and hepatic
dysfunction (see 📖 individual drug for specifics).

Monitoring of LFTs is recommended prior to therapy and in patients who develop any signs or symptoms suggestive of liver injury:
- stopping or reducing the dose of statins should be considered in transaminase elevations to ≥3× ULN or ≥100 IU
- patients who develop increased transaminase levels should be monitored until resolution.

Monitoring for muscular disorders:
- Treatment with statins has been associated with myalgia, myopathy, and, very rarely, rhabdomyolysis.
- Myopathy must be considered in unexplained muscle symptoms such as pain or tenderness, muscle weakness, or muscle cramps, and CPK levels should be measured.
- CPK should not be measured following strenuous exercise or in the presence of any plausible alternative cause of CPK increase as this makes value interpretation difficult.
- Statins should be prescribed with caution in patients with predisposing factors for rhabdomyolysis (renal impairment, hypothyroidism, personal or familial history of hereditary muscular disorders, previous history of muscular toxicity with a statin or fibrates, previous history of liver disease, and/or high alcohol consumption; age>70 years).
- If CPK levels are significantly elevated (>5× ULN), statins should be discontinued and levels remeasured within 5–7 days to confirm the results.

Pregnancy and lactation
Statins have caused problems to the fetus in pregnant women who have mistakenly taken the medicine (pregnancy category X). Therefore, they should be avoided in women of child-bearing potential not using appropriate contraception. They are also excreted in the mother's milk. An interval of 1 month should be allowed from stopping treatment to planned conception.

Contraindications
- Active liver disease or unexplained persistently elevated serum transaminases >3× ULN
- Pregnancy and breastfeeding
- Rare hereditary problems of galactose intolerance, Lapp lactose deficiency, or glucose-galactose malabsorption
- Concomitant administration of certain medications (see 📖 individual drug for specifics)
- Hypersensitivity to any component of this medication

References
1 Law MR *et al.* (2003). Quantifying effect of statins on low density lipoprotein cholesterol, ischaemic heart disease, and stroke: systematic review and meta-analysis. *BMJ* **326**:1423–7.

2 Cholesterol Treatment Trialists (CTT) Collaborators (2005). Efficacy and safety of cholesterol-lowering treatment: prospective meta-analysis of data from 90 056 participants in 14 randomised trials of statins. *Lancet* **366**:1267–78.

3 Cannon CP *et al.* (2006). Meta-analysis of cardiovascular outcomes trials comparing intensive versus moderate statin therapy. *J Am Coll Cardiol* **48**:438–45.

4 O'Regan C *et al.* (2008). Statin therapy in stroke prevention: a meta-analysis involving 121,000 patients. *Am J Med* **121**:24–33.

Streptokinase

(See also 📖 Thrombolytic agents, p.608)

Thrombolytic agent (47kDa) produced by β-haemolytic streptococci.

CV indications

1. Thrombolytic treatment of AMI within 12 hours of onset, with persistent ST-segment elevation or recent left bundle branch block (in the absence of contraindications if 1° PCI cannot be performed)
2. Thrombolytic treatment in the acute pulmonary embolism: when the pulmonary embolism is accompanied by unstable haemodynamics
3. Treatment of DVT
4. Treatment of arterial thrombosis or embolism
5. Treatment of occlusion of arteriovenous cannulae

Mechanism of action

Streptokinase (SK) forms a complex in the plasma with plasminogen to form an activator complex that converts unbound plasminogen to the proteolytic enzyme, plasmin. IV infusion of SK is followed by increased fibrinolytic activity, which decreases plasma fibrinogen levels for 24–36h; the decrease in plasma fibrinogen is associated with decreases in blood viscosity, and red blood cell aggregation. Depending upon the dosage/duration of infusion of SK, the thrombin time will decrease to less than twice the normal control value within 4h, and return to normal by 24h.

Pharmacodynamics

2 very large randomized and placebo-controlled studies involving almost 30,000 patients with MI have demonstrated that a 60min IV infusion of 1,500,000 IU of SK significantly reduces mortality following a MI:

- in the *GISSI* trial the reduction in mortality was time dependent. There was a 47% reduction in mortality among patients treated within 1h of the onset of chest pain, a 23% reduction among patients treated within 3h, and a 17% reduction among patients treated between 3 and 6h. There was also a reduction in mortality in patients treated between 6 and 12h, but the reduction was not statistically significant[1]
- in the *ISIS-2* study the reduction in mortality was also time dependent but the reduction was still significant when treatment was started 5–24h after symptom onset: 33% for the combined therapy with aspirin plus SK and 17% SK alone.[2]

SK administered by the intracoronary route has resulted in thrombolysis usually within 1h, and results in improvement of cardiac function and reduction of mortality. LVEF was increased in patients treated with intracoronary SK when compared to patients treated with conventional therapy.

Pharmacokinetics

IV infusion of SK is followed by increased fibrinolytic activity, which decreased plasma fibrinogen levels for 24–36h. This effect disappears within a few hours after discontinuation but a prolonged thrombin time may persist for up to 24h. The plasma $t_{1/2}$ of streptokinase is ≈23min. The complex plasminogen–streptokinase is inactivated, in part, by antistreptoccocal antibodies. The clearance is mediated primarily by the liver (<5% in urine).

Practical points
♪ Doses

In myocardial infarction:
- IV infusion: 1,500,000 U within 60min
- Intracoronary infusion: 20,000 U by bolus followed 2000 IU/min for 60min

In acute pulmonary embolism:
- Loading dose: 250,000 U/30min
- Infusion IV: 100,000 U/h over 12–24h (72h if concurrent DVT is suspected)

Deep vein thrombosis:
IV bolus of 250,000 U followed by a maintenance drip at 100,000 U/h. The drip is continued for 1–3 days

Peripheral arterial disease:
5,000–10,000 U/h intra-arterially

In CVAD_c:
Slowly instil 250,000 U of SK in 2mL of solution into each occluded limb of the cannula. Clamp off the cannula limb(s) for 2h, and then aspirate the contents of the cannula limb(s), flush with saline, and reconnect the cannula

☺ Common side effects
- Bleeding: major bleeding 0.3–0.5% (however rates as high as 16% have been reported if anticoagulants were used); minor bleeding 3.9%. Serious haemorrhage calls for discontinuation of SK, followed by administration of clotting factors or a proteinase inhibitor (aprotinin: 200,000–1 million KIU, followed by 50,000 KIU/h IV until bleeding stops)
- Hypotension (<5%) and bradycardia due to the formation of plasmin that generates kinins
- Allergic reactions: minor breathing difficulty to bronchospam, peri-orbital swelling or angioneurotic oedema, urticaria, flushing, headache, or nausea. Anaphylactic shock is very rare (0–0.1%). tPA is indicated in patients allergic to SK and in those having SK within a period of 12 months
- Fever and shivering (1–4%)
- Transient elevations of serum transaminases
- Others: cholesterol embolism, chest pain, non-cardiogenic pulmonary oedema, polyneuropathy, pulmonary embolism

Interactions
(See 📖 Alteplase, p.344)

Cautions/notes
(See 📖 Alteplase, p.344)

The effect of SK is blocked by antibodies which appear a few days after the initial dose. At least 1 year must elapse before SK is used again.

Pregnancy and lactation
(See 📖 Alteplase, p.344)

Contraindications
(See 📖 Alteplase, p.344)

- Major recent streptococcal infection (antistreptococcal infection causes SK resistance)
- Previous treatment with SK, because of the antibodies' diminished efficacy

References

1 Gruppo Italiano per lo Studio della Streptochi-nasi nell'Infarto Miocardico (GISSI) (1987). Long-term effects of intravenous thrombolysis in acute myocardial infarction: final report of the GISSI study. *Lancet* **2**:871–4.

2 ISIS Steering Committee (1987). Intravenous streptokinase given within 0–4 hours of onset of myocardial infarction reduced mortality in ISI-2. *Lancet* **1**:501.

Tadalafil

Orally active, potent, and selective cGMP-specific PDE-5 inhibitor.

CV indications

To improve symptoms and increase exercise capacity in patients with 1° PAH (WHO class I).

Other indications

Treatment of erectile dysfunction.

Mechanism of action (see 📖 Sildenafil, p.576)

Pharmacodynamics

Tadalafil reduces mean RAP (3mmHg), PVR (−11.2%), and SVR (−7.2%) and improves functional class and exercise capacity (44m in 6MWT) after 16 weeks.[1]

Pharmacokinetics

Tadalafil is rapidly absorbed after oral administration (bioavailability 88%), reaching peak plasma concentration after 2h. Food has no effect on the rate and extent of absorption. It binds to plasma proteins (94%), presents a V_d of 0.9L/kg, and is metabolized by P450 CYP3A4 (>80%), with minor contributions by CYPs 2C8, 2C9, 2C19, and 2D6. It is excreted mainly in faeces (61% of the dose) and to a lesser extent in urine (36%). Mean $t_{1/2}$ is 17.5h in healthy subjects. Steady-state plasma concentrations are attained within 5 days of od dosing.

Practical points

⚕ Doses 40mg PO qds

CrCl 51–80mL/min: 20mg qds initially; may increase to 40mg qds based on individual tolerability. CrCl <30mL/min and on haemodialysis: avoid use.

Mild-to-moderate hepatic impairment (Child–Pugh class A or B): 20mg qds initially. Severe hepatic impairment (Child–Pugh class C): avoid use

Use with strong CYP3A4 inhibitors (e.g. ritonavir): 20mg qds initially; may increase to 40mg PO qds based on individual tolerability

☺ Common side effects

(See 📖 Sildenafil, p.576)

It may cause prolonged or painful erection; may cause back pain or myalgias.

Interactions (see 📖 Sildenafil, p.576)

Pregnancy and lactation (see 📖 Sildenafil, p.576)

Contraindications (see 📖 Sildenafil, p.576)

Cautions (see 📖 Sildenafil, p.576)

Contraindications (see 📖 Sildenafil, p.576)

Reference

1 Galiè N et al.; Pulmonary Arterial Hypertension and Response to Tadalafil (PHIRST) Study Group (2009). Tadalafil therapy for pulmonary arterial hypertension. *Circulation* **119**:2894–903.

Telmisartan

(See also 📖 Angiotensin II (AT$_1$) receptor blockers, p.359)

Angiotensin receptor blocker.

Indication

(See 📖 Angiotensin II (AT$_1$) receptor blockers, p.359)

Treatment of hypertension.

Reduction of cardiovascular morbidity in patients with (i) manifest athero-thrombotic cardiovascular disease (history of coronary heart disease, stroke, or peripheral arterial disease); or, (ii) type 2 diabetes mellitus with documented target organ damage.

Mechanism of action

(See 📖 Renin–angiotensin–aldosterone system inhibitors, p.568 and 📖 Angiotensin II (AT$_1$) receptor blockers, p.359)

Pharmacodynamics

(See 📖 Renin–angiotensin–aldosterone system inhibitors, p.568 and 📖 Angiotensin II (AT$_1$) receptor blockers, p.359)

Hypertension, diabetes, and high CV risk: no difference (RR 1.01, 95% CI: 0.94–1.09; absolute rates: 16.5% vs. 16.7%) in 1° composite endpoint (CV death, MI, stroke, or hospitalization for HF) in patients with vascular disease or high-risk diabetes without HF treated with telmisartan 80mg od compared with ramipril 10mg od followed up for median of 56 months.[1] No differences in the 1° endpoint were observed in the combination-therapy group (RR 0.99, 95% CI: 0.92–1.07). Compared with ramipril monotherapy, the combination of telmisartan and ramipril was associated with greater BP lowering (2.4/1.6mmHg), increased risk of hypotensive symptoms (4.8% vs. 1.7%, P<0.001), syncope (0.3% vs. 0.2%, P=0.03), and renal dysfunction (13.5% vs. 10.2%).[2] Thus, the combination of telmisartan and ramipril was associated with more adverse events without an increase in benefit.

No difference (HR 1.0, 95% CI: 0.92–1.09; absolute rates: 13.5% vs. 13.5%) in 1° composite endpoint (dialysis, doubling of serum creatinine, and death) in patients aged ≥55 years with established atherosclerotic vascular disease or with diabetes with end-organ damage treated with telmisartan 80mg od compared with ramipril 10mg od followed up for median of 56 months.[3] However, the primary composite endpoint was increased with combination therapy (HR 1.09, 95% CI: 1.01–1.18). The secondary renal outcome (dialysis or doubling of serum creatinine) was similar with telmisartan and with ramipril but more frequent with combination therapy. eGFR declined least with ramipril compared with telmisartan or combination therapy. The increase in urinary albumin excretion was less with telmisartan or with combination therapy than with ramipril. Thus, although combination therapy reduces proteinuria to a greater extent than monotherapy, it worsens major renal outcomes overall.

Pharmacokinetics

Telmisartan is rapidly absorbed (bioavailability≈50%), reaching peak plasma levels after 1–2h. Extensively (≈99.5%) protein bound with V_d≈34L, telmisartan is hepatically metabolized by conjugation to inactive metabolites and almost exclusively (98%) excreted in faeces. No linear kinetics, C_{max} and AUC increased at higher doses. Terminal $t_{1/2}$ is 24h.

Practical points

Doses

20–40mg od (titrated to maximum of 80mg/daily)

Doses >40mg od should not be used in hepatic impairment and a starting dose of 20mg is recommended in severe renal impairment or dialysis.

Side effects (See also 📖 Angiotensin II (AT$_1$) receptor blockers, p.359)

Interactions

(See also 📖 Angiotensin II (AT$_1$) receptor blockers, p.359)

Telmisartan increases digoxin plasma levels (20–40%).

Cautions (See also 📖 Angiotensin II (AT$_1$) receptor blockers, p.359)

Pregnancy and lactation (See also 📖 Angiotensin II (AT1) receptor blockers, p.359)

Contraindications

(See also 📖 Angiotensin II (AT$_1$) receptor blockers, p.359)

• Severe hepatic impairment; biliary obstructive disorders

References

1 Mann JF et al.; ONTARGET investigators (2008). Renal outcomes with telmisartan, ramipril, or both, in people at high vascular risk (the ONTARGET study): a multicentre, randomised, double-blind, controlled trial. *Lancet* **372**:547–53.
2 ONTARGET Investigators, Yusuf S et al. (2008). Telmisartan, ramipril, or both in patients at high risk for vascular events. *N Engl J Med* **358**:1547–59.
3 Mann JF et al.; ONTARGET investigators (2008). Renal outcomes with telmisartan, ramipril, or both, in people at high vascular risk (the ONTARGET study): a multicentre, randomised, double-blind, controlled trial. *Lancet* **372**:547–53.

Tenecteplase (TNKase)

(See also 📖 Thrombolytic agents, p.608)

TNKase (70kDa) is a genetically engineered, triple combination mutant (Thr103Asn and Asn117Gln, both within the kringle 1 domain; Lys296-His297–Arg298–Arg299 to Ala in the protease domain) of native tPA.

CV indications

Thrombolytic treatment of AMI with persistent ST elevation or recent LBBB, diabetes, and HF within 6h after the onset of AMI symptoms.

Mechanism of action

TNKase binds to the fibrin component of the thrombus and selectively converts thrombus-bound plasminogen to plasmin, which degrades the fibrin matrix of the thrombus. Tenecteplase has a higher fibrin specificity, longer plasma $t_{1/2}$ (so that it can be given as a single bolus injection) and greater resistance to inactivation by its endogenous inhibitor (PAI-1) compared to native tPA.

Pharmacodynamics

The *ASSENT-2 trial*, a large-scale mortality trial in patients with onset of chest pain within 6h of randomization and STEMI or left bundle branch on ECG showed that TNKase was therapeutically equivalent to front-loaded alteplase in reducing mortality (6.2% for both treatments) at 30 days in patients administered the drugs <4h of onset, but it is superior in patients treated after 4h (7% vs. 9.2%). Rates of intracranial bleeding were similar, but TNKase was associated with a significantly lower incidence of non-intracranial major bleedings (4.7% vs. 5.9%).[1]

The *ASSENT-4 PCI trial* evaluated patients with MI pre-treatment with full dose TNKase and heparin administered prior to PCI compared with 1° PCI alone. The trial was prematurely terminated for higher mortality in the facilitated PCI group receiving TNKase.[2]

Pharmacokinetics

After administration as a single bolus TNKase exhibits a biphasic disposition from the plasma with an initial $t_{1/2}$ of 20–24min and a terminal phase $t_{1/2}$ of 90–130min. Liver metabolism and excretion. No clinically relevant antibody formation was detected at 30 days.

Practical points

⚬⅃ Doses

IV administration: TNKase should be administered on the basis of body weight. Maximum dose of 10,000 units (50mg). See Table 12.

Table 12 Tenecteplase posology

Patients' weight (kg)	TNKase (U)	TNKase (mg)	Volume of reconstituted solution (mL)
<60	6000	30	6
≥60 to <70	7000	35	7
≥70 to <80	8000	40	8
≥80 to <90	9000	45	9
≥90	10000	50	10

☺ *Common side effects*
- Minor bleeding (21.8%): haematoma (12.3%), urinary tract (3.7%), puncture site (including cardiac catheterization site) (3.6%), pharyngeal (3.1%), GI tract (1.9%), epistaxis (1.5%), other (1.3%)
- Major bleeding (4.7%): haematoma (1.7%), GI tract (1%)
- Allergic-type reactions (<1%): anaphylaxis (<0.1%), angio-oedema, laryngeal oedema, rash, and urticaria
- CV effects: cardiogenic shock, arrhythmias, AV block, pulmonary oedema, HF, cardiac arrest, recurrent myocardial ischaemia, myocardial reinfarction, myocardial rupture, cardiac tamponade, pericarditis, pericardial effusion, MR, thrombosis, embolism, and electromechanical dissociation
- Others: nausea, vomiting, hypotension, and fever

Interactions
(See 📖 Alteplase, p.344)

Cautions/notes
Tenecteplase is not recommended for use in children (<18 years).

It is not necessary to adjust tenecteplase dose in patients with hepatic or severe renal insufficiency.

If serious bleeding occurs:
- stop concomitant heparin administration
- administration of protamine should be considered if heparin has been administered within 4h before the onset of bleeding
- transfusion of cryoprecipitate, fresh frozen plasma, and platelets should be considered (target fibrinogen level of 1g/L)
- antifibrinolytic agents are available as a last alternative

Pregnancy and lactation
Animal studies have shown a high risk of vaginal bleeding, presumably from the placenta, and of pregnancy loss; thus the benefit of treatment has to be evaluated against the potential risks (pregnancy category C). Breast milk should be discarded within the first 24h after thrombolytic therapy.

Contraindications
(See 📖 Alteplase, p.344)

Hypersensitivity to the active substance tenecteplase and to any of the excipients

References

1 Assessment of the Safety and Efficacy of a New Thrombolytic (ASSENT-2) Investigators (1999). Single-bolus tenecteplase compared with front-loaded alteplase in acute myocardial infarction: The ASSENT-2 double-blind randomized trial. *Lancet* **354**:716–22.
2 Assessment of the Safety and Efficacy of a New Treatment Strategy with Percutaneous Coronary Intervention (ASSENT-4 PCI) investigators (2006). Primary versus tenecteplase-facilitated percutaneous coronary intervention in patients with ST-segment elevation acute myocardial infarction (ASSENT-4 PCI): randomised trial. *Lancet* **367**:569–78.

Thiazide and related diuretics

Class of diuretics derived from benzothiadiazine. (See also 📖 Bendro-flumethiazide, p.374, 📖 Chlortalidone, p.401, 📖 Indapamide, p.487, and 📖 Metolazone, p.520)

CV indications

1. Hypertension
2. Oedema associated with congestive HF, hepatic cirrhosis, various forms of renal dysfunction (nephrotic syndrome, acute glomerulonephritis, and CRF) and corticosteroid and oestrogen therapy
3. Severe resistant oedema (in combination with loop diuretics)

Other indications

Treatment of Dent's disease, prevention of recurrent stone formation in idiopathic hypercalciuria, nephrogenic diabetes insipidus

Mechanism of action

Thiazides bind to the Cl^- site of the Na^+–Cl^- co-transporter in the distal convoluted tubules and inhibit its action, causing natriuresis and diuresis. As a result of increased delivery of Na^+ to the distal segment of the distal tubule, K^+ and H^+ loss are increased there due partly to stimulation of the aldosterone-sensitive Na^+ pump and partly due to activation of the RAAS caused by natriuresis and fall in BP. Consequently, thiazide diuretics can cause hypokalaemia with hypochloraemic alkalosis. Excretion of uric acid is decreased. Thiazides also increase Ca^{2+} reabsorption in the proximal tubule and decrease urinary Ca^{2+} excretion and so are useful in preventing calcium-containing kidney stones. This effect is associated with a positive Ca^{2+} balance and an increase in bone mineral density and reductions in fracture rates attributable to osteoporosis. Additionally, thiazides directly stimulate osteoblast differentiation and bone mineral formation, further slowing the course of osteoporosis.

Pharmacodynamics

(See 📖 individual drugs)

They are the preferred diuretics in treating hypertension. The mechanism of the antihypertensive effect is unknown, but it may be related to a decrease in blood volume caused by diuresis, negative Na^+ balance, and a direct arteriolar vasodilatation (probably related to the activation of vascular smooth muscle K^+ channels).

1st choice in elderly and African origin hypertensives and in patients with CHF, but the response in younger whites is less; if a diuretic is not the 1st choice it is logical to add a thiazide if goal BP is not achieved.[1]

Thiazides increase the risk of new-onset diabetes and the risk increases when combined with β-blockers.[2] Patients who develop diabetes during treatment have cardiac morbidity intermediate between diabetic subjects and, in the longer follow-up, equal risks.[3]

Diuresis: loop diuretics deliver a greater fraction of filtered Na^+ to the site of action of thiazides in the distal tubule, so that their combination produces a synergistic diuretic effect. The diuresis induced by thiazides decreases in renal failure (serum creatinine >2mg/dL or about 180µmol/L; GFR <20mL/min).

Thiazides reduce the urine volume in patients with diabetes insipidus by interfering with the production of hypotonic fluid in the distal tubule, and, thus, they reduce free water clearance.

Thiazides increase proximal tubular reabsorption of calcium and may decrease the risk of hip fractures in the elderly, but protection disappears when discontinued.[4]

Pharmacokinetics

(See 📖 individual drugs)

They are well and rapidly absorbed by the oral route to produce diuresis in 1–2h and they are excreted in the urine mainly by tubular secretion, for which they compete with uric acid.

Practical points

💊 Doses

(See 📖 individual drugs)

High doses of thiazides doses are associated with metabolic side effects. In hypertension, combination with ACEIs/ARBs may be preferable to increasing the dose of thiazides. In CHF, combination with a loop diuretic produces considerable diuretic advantage.

😊 Common side effects

- GI effects: anorexia, gastric irritation
- Hydroelectrolyte disturbances: dehydration, hypovolaemia, hypokalaemia, hypomagnesaemia, hyponatraemia; hypercalcaemia; hypochloraemic alkalosis
- CV: postural hypotension, arrhythmias from hypokalaemia
- Central: dizziness, vertigo, paraesthesia, headache
- Metabolic: hyperuricaemia and gout. Hyperglycaemia, increased insulin requirement; latent diabetes may become manifest. Increased serum cholesterol, LDL-C and triglycerides
- Immunological: cholestatic jaundice, pancreatitis, blood dyscrasias, interstitial nephritis
- Others: rashes; photosensitivity; erectile dysfunction

Interactions

Thiazides may potentiate the effects of other antihypertensive agents and non-depolarizing neuromuscular blockers (e.g. tubocurarine). Risk of hyponatraemia is increased when used with carbamazepine and amphotericin. Risk of hypokalaemia may be increased with loop diuretics, β-agonists, ACTH, corticosteroids, xanthines, acetazolamide, carbenoxolone, and reboxetine.

Hypokalaemia caused by thiazides may increase the toxicity of antiarrhythmics (e.g. amiodarone, digoxin, disopyramide, flecainide), increase the risk of ventricular arrhythmias when combining with QT-prolonging drugs, and antagonize the effects of some antiarrhythmics (e.g. lidocaine, mexiletine).

Serum K^+ <3.5mmol/L increases CV events by about 4× over a mean follow-up of 6.7 years.[5] In HF patients, non-K^+-retaining diuretic was associated with an increased rate of arrhythmic death compared with a K^+-retaining diuretic.[6]

Risk of lithium toxicity is increased because thiazides decrease lithium renal clearance. There is also an increased risk of nephrotoxicity and ototoxicity when used with cisplatin; and hypercalcaemia with vitamin D preparations.

There is an increased risk of 1st-dose hypotension with α-blockers. Postural hypotension associated with treatment may be exacerbated by alcohol, opioids, and barbiturates, and also tricyclic antidepressants, MAO inhibitors, baclofen, or tizanidine. Conversely, diuretic effects of thiazides may be attenuated by concomitant use of NSAIDs, oestrogen-containing OCPs.

Glucocorticoids cause salt retention and antagonize the diuretic effect of thiazides. NSAIDs inhibit the diuretic response.

Thiazides increase the risk of new-onset diabetes. They increase serum glucose levels and may inhibit the release of insulin induced by oral hypoglycaemic agents.

Colestyramine and colestipol decrease their absorption.

Synergic diuretic effect when combined with loop diuretics or K^+-sparing diuretics (they reduce the risk of hypokalaemia).

Cautions/notes
Electrolytes should be monitored, particularly with high doses or in renal impairment. Risk of hypokalaemia is increased in the elderly, malnourished, polymedicated, cirrhotic patients, CHD, and HF patients. With the exception of metolazone, thiazide and thiazide-like diuretics become ineffective when the GFR falls to <30mL/min. In hepatic impairment, hypokalaemia caused by thiazides may precipitate coma and so should be avoided. Thiazides can also exacerbate diabetes, SLE, and gout, and increase the risk of hypomagnesaemia in alcoholic cirrhosis.

Hypovolaemia and hyponatraemia stimulate renin secretion, leading to angiotensin II and aldosterone formation. This may limit the antihypertensive effect of thiazides.

Marked diuresis can produce hypovolaemia and postural hypotension, particularly in the elderly.

Pregnancy and lactation
Thiazides cross the placental barrier, appear in breast milk, and can cause fetal or neonatal abnormalities (thrombocytopenia, jaundice), hypovolaemia, and decrease placental perfusion. Therefore, they should be avoided in pregnancy (pregnancy category B). Amounts excreted in breast milk are likely to be too small to be harmful. Large doses may suppress lactation.

Contraindications

- Refractory hypokalaemia, hyponatraemia, hypercalcaemia
- Symptomatic hyperuricaemia
- Addison's disease
- Severe renal or hepatic impairment
- Hypersensitivity to thiazides or sulphonamides
- Pregnancy and breastfeeding
- Ventricular arrhythmias, co-administration with antiarrhythmic drugs

References

1 Mancia G *et al*. (2007). 2007 Guidelines for the management of arterial hypertension: The Task Force for the Management of Arterial Hypertension of the European Society of Hypertension (ESH) and of the European Society of Cardiology (ESC). *Eur Heart J* **28**:1462–536.

2 Lam SK *et al*. (2007). Incident diabetes in clinical trials of antihypertensive drugs. *Lancet* **369**:1513–14.

3 Aksnes TA *et al*. (2007). Impact of new-onset diabetes mellitus on cardiac outcomes in the Valsartan Antihypertensive Long-term Use Evaluation (VALUE) trial population. *Hypertension* **50**:467–73.

4 Schoofs MW *et al*. (2003). Thiazide diuretics and the risk of hip fracture. *Ann Intern Med* **139**:476–82.

5 Cohen HW *et al*. (2001). High and low serum potassium associated with cardiovascular events in diuretic-treated patients. *J Hypertens* **19**:1315–23.

6 Domanski M *et al*. (2003). Diuretic use, progressive heart failure, and death in patients in the Studied Of Left Ventricular Dysfunction (SOLVD). *J Am Coll Cardiol* **42**:705–8.

Thrombolytic agents

(See also 📖 Alteplase, p.344, 📖 Streptokinase, p.595, and 📖 Tenecteplase, p.601)

The term acute coronary syndromes encompasses a spectrum of unstable coronary artery disease, including UA and 2 forms of MI: NSTEMI and STEMI. Annually in the USA, about 1 million people suffer an AMI and AMI remains fatal in >33% of patients. AMI is caused by occlusion of the infarct-related coronary artery by thrombosis overlying a fissured or ruptured atheromatous plaque. After coronary occlusion, myocardial cell death begins in about 20min and the area supplied by the occluded artery becomes necrotic within 4–6h.

When the coagulation cascade and the platelet aggregation are activated, the fibrinolytic system is also activated via several endogenous plasminogen activators, such as tissue plasminogen activator (tPA) or urokinase-type plasminogen activator. These activators are serine proteases that diffuse into the thrombus where they promote the formation within the coagulum of plasmin from its precursor plasminogen. Plasmin produces fibrin degradation products and lysis of the clot. Plasmin lyses not only fibrin contained in a clot but also fibrinogen, factors II, V, and VIII, and in the circulation is inactivated by plasmin inhibitors, including PAI-1.

Thrombolytic (fibrinolytic) agents given within the first 4h of onset of symptoms in patients with STEMI produce the lysis of intracoronary thrombi, reopen the occluded artery, increase myocardial salvage (reduce infarct size), preserve LV function, and reduce mortality. The benefit is greatest within the first 2h and then falls off dramatically after 4h. Therefore, thrombolytic agents should be administered as soon as possible after an AMI if no contraindication exists.

Thrombolytic agents are divided into 2 categories: (1) fibrin-specific agents such as alteplase and tenecteplase (TNKase), which produce limited plasminogen conversion in the absence of fibrin, and (2) non-fibrin-specific agents such as streptokinase (SK), which catalyse systemic fibrinolysis. tPA has several advantages over IV SK and is more effective than SK in producing higher early patency of infarcted related vessels. The thrombolysis can be inhibited with tranexamic acid and aprotinin; both drugs can be used to treat conditions in which there is bleeding or a risk of bleeding.

Tirofiban

Non-peptide glycoprotein IIb/IIIa receptor antagonist.

CV indications

Prevention of STEMI in patients with UA in whom the last episode of chest pain occurred <12h ago and who have ECG changes and/or elevated cardiac enzymes. (See 📖 Management of ST elevation myocardial infarction (STEMI), p.48).

Mechanism of action

(See 📖 Eptifibatide, p.453)

Pharmacodynamics

The *PRISM-PLUS study* evaluated the efficacy of tirofiban in patients with UA or acute non-Q wave MI. The incidence of all-cause death, new MI, or refractory ischaemia was significantly lower in the tirofiban-plus-heparin group than in the heparin-alone group at 7, 30, and 180 days.[1]

The RESTORE trial evaluated tirofiban in patients undergoing coronary interventions within 72h of an ACS.[2] Tirofiban reduced (RRR 16%) the 1° composite endpoint (death from any cause, MI, coronary bypass surgery due to angioplasty failure or recurrent ischaemia, repeat target-vessel angioplasty for recurrent ischaemia, and insertion of a stent due to actual or threatened abrupt closure of the dilated artery) at 30 days vs. placebo. However, 2 days after angioplasty, the tirofiban group had a 38% relative reduction in the composite endpoint and at 7 days there was a 27% relative reduction, largely because of a reduction in non-fatal MI and the need for repeat angioplasty. Major bleeding, including transfusion, was not significantly different between the 2 groups.

In the *TARGET trial* abciximab was tested in comparison with tirofiban in patients with recent NSTEMI. Abciximab was superior to tirofiban in reducing the risk of death, non-fatal MI, or urgent revascularization at 30 days, primarily by reducing non-fatal MI (7.6 vs. 6.0%).[3] There were no significant differences in the rates of major bleeding complications or transfusions, but tirofiban was associated with a lower rate of minor bleeding episodes and thrombocytopenia. However, at 6 and 12 months, there was significant difference in 1° outcomes between abciximab and tirofiban.[4,5]

Pharmacokinetics

The effect of tirofiban is observed with 30min loading infusion. Platelet function returns to baseline 4–8h after discontinuation.

It binds to plasma proteins (60%) and presents a V_d of 0.18–0.25L/kg, a $t_{1/2}$ of 1.5–2h, and renal (65%) and biliary (25%) excretion.

Practical points

🥄 Doses

Initial infusion: 0.4mcg/kg/min for 30min
Maintenance infusion: 0.1mcg/kg/min for 48h. The total duration of treatment should not exceed 108h

😞 *Common side effects*

- Bleeding: major (1.4%), minor (10.5%)
- Nausea (1.7%), fever (1.5%) and headache (1.1%)
- Slow heart rate, leg pain, dizziness

Interactions

(See 📖 Abciximab, p.330)

Cautions/notes

- In severe kidney failure (CrCl <30mL/min), the dosage should be reduced by 50%.
- Tirofiban is not recommended in children.
- In view of suspected increase of risk of bleeding, tirofiban is not recommended in the following conditions:
  - traumatic cardiopulmonary resuscitation, organ biopsy, or lithotripsy within the past 2 weeks
  - severe trauma or major surgery >6 weeks but <3 months previously
  - active peptic ulcer within the past 3 months
  - uncontrolled hypertension (>180/110mmHg)
  - acute pericarditis
  - active or a known history of vasculitis
  - suspected aortic dissection
  - haemorrhagic retinopathy
  - occult blood in the stool or haematuria
  - thrombolytic therapy—concurrent or <48h
  - concurrent use of drugs that increase the risk of bleeding

Pregnancy and lactation

(See 📖 Abciximab, p.330)

Contraindications

- Hypersensitivity to the active substance or to any of the excipients
- Thrombocytopenia during earlier use of a GP IIb/IIIa receptor antagonist
- Evidence of GI bleeding, gross GU bleeding, or other active abnormal bleeding
- Bleeding within the previous 30 days of treatment
- History of stroke within 30 days or any history of haemorrhagic stroke
- Concomitant use of another parenteral GP IIb/IIIa inhibitor
- Aortic dissection
- Known history of intracranial disease (neoplasm, arteriovenous malformation, aneurysm)
- Malignant hypertension
- Major surgery or severe trauma within past 6 weeks
- History of bleeding diathesis
- Thrombocytopenia (<100,000 cells/mm^3)
- Prothrombin time >1.3× control or INR ≥1.5
- Severe liver failure

References

1 The Platelet Receptor Inhibition in Ischemic Syndrome Management in Patients Limited by Unstable Signs and Symptoms (PRISM-PLUS) study investigators (1998). *N Engl J Med* **338**: 1488–97.

2 The RESTORE investigators (1997). Effects of platelet glycoprotein IIb/IIIa blockade with tirofiban on adverse cardiac events in patients with unstable angina or acute myocardial infarction undergoing coronary angioplasty. *Circulation* **96**:1445–53.
3 Topol E (2001). Comparison of two platelet glycoprotein IIB/IIIA inhibitors, tirofiban and abciximab, for the prevention of ischemic events with percutaneous coronary revascularization. *N Engl J Med* **244**:1888–94.
4 Moliterno DJ et al. for the TARGET Investigators (2002). Outcomes at 6 months for the direct comparison of tirofiban and abciximab during percutaneous coronary revascularisation with stent placement: The TARGET follow-up study. *Lancet* **360**:355–60.
5 Mukherjee D et al. for the TARGET Investigators (2005). Mortality at 1 year for the direct comparison of tirofiban and abciximab during percutaneous coronary revascularization: do tirofiban and ReoPro give similar efficacy outcomes at trial 1-year follow-up. *Eur Heart J* **26**:2524–8.

Tolvaptan

Vasopressin V2 receptor antagonist (see also 📖 Vasopressin antagonists, p.627).

CV indications

1. Euvolaemic and hypervolaemic hyponatraemia in patients with HF, cirrhosis, or syndrome of inappropriate antidiuretic hormone
2. Tolvaptan is being evaluated for the treatment of acute descompensated HF and hyponatraemia
3. Tolvaptan is also being studied for the treatment of autosomal dominant polycystic kidney disease

Mechanism of action

Arginine vasopressin (AVP, antidiuretic hormone) is a nonapeptide hormone released from the neurohypophysis in response to increases in plasma osmolarity, hypovolaemia, hypotension, and angiotensin II. AVP stimulates 3 types of receptors. Stimulation of V2 receptors, expressed on the basolateral membrane of the renal collecting ducts, increases the synthesis of aquaporin-2 water-channel-containing vesicles that are inserted into the apical cell membrane and increase water reabsorption. This water reabsorption decreases serum osmolarity, contributing to the development of dilutional hyponatraemia (serum Na^+ concentration, <135mmol/L), and increases LV end-diastolic volume and pressure. Elevated levels of AVP are present in HF and contribute to the development of fluid retention and hyponatraemia.

Pharmacodynamics

V2 receptor antagonists are termed aquaretics, not saliuretics, because they produce a marked increase in solute-free water excretion and, thus, elevate serum Na^+ concentrations in patients with acute heart failure and hyponatraemia. Unlike loop diuretics, V2 receptor antagonists do not activate the RAAS.

The *ACTIV in CHF trial* examined tolvaptan vs. placebo added to standard therapy on change in body weight at 24h and worsening HF at 60 days after randomization.[1] Tolvaptan increased urine output, reduced body weight, oedema, and furosemide use during hospitalization, and normalized serum Na^+ in hyponatraemic patients, but no differences were observed in rates of rehospitalization over the 60-day follow-up period vs. placebo.

The *EVEREST trial* was designed to further assess the short- and long-term safety and efficacy of tolvaptan.[2,3]

• The short-term studies demonstrated that tolvaptan (30mg/day), when added to standard HF therapy, improves some of the signs and symptoms (dyspnoea, oedema) of HF, reduces body weight, and normalizes serum Na^+ throughout hospitalization.[2]
• The long-term trial evaluated patients who received tolvaptan or placebo for ≥60 days. Tolvaptan shows a good safety profile with no deleterious effects on serum electrolytes, BP, or renal function.[3]

Overall, this study demonstrated that long-term tolvaptan therapy had no effect, either favourable or unfavourable, on all-cause mortality, CV mortality, or subsequent hospitalization for worsening HF.
- In patients with euvolaemic or hypervolaemic hyponatraemia (serum sodium concentration, <135mmol/L), tolvaptan (15–60mg od) increases serum Na^+.[4]

Pharmacokinetics

Tolvaptan presented good oral availability (40%), reached peak plasma concentrations after 2–3h, and presented a non-linear dose–response curve, probably due to rate-limited intestinal absorption. Tolvaptan binds (99%) to plasma proteins and is extensively metabolized in the liver via CYP3A4 (renal excretion is <1%). Terminal $t_{1/2}$ 6–9h.

Practical points

♣ Doses

Oral: tolvaptan has been studied in doses of 30, 60, and 90mg/day for HF and 15, 30, and 60mg/day for hyponatraemia.

☺ Common side effects

- Thirst, dry mouth (4.2–13%), polyuria (3.3%), headache (≥10%)
- Hypernatraemia: rare
- CV effects: postural hypotension, tachycardia (0.01–0.1%), postprandial hypotension, syncope
- Others: dizziness, flushing, nausea, vomiting, constipation

Interactions

With drugs that are metabolized in the liver through CYP3A4 enzyme:
- antibiotics: erythromicin, rifabutin, rifampicin
- antifungals: fluconazole, itraconazole, ketoconazole
- antihistaminics: terfenadine, astemizole, loratadine
- antiarrhythmics: verapamil, diltiazem, nifedipine, amiodarone
- oral anticoagulants
- oral contraceptives
- antiepiletics: phenytoin, valproate, gabapentin, carbamazepine

Cautions/notes

Tolvaptan therapy does not affect BP, heart rate, renal function, or serum potassium.

Pregnancy and lactation

Safety of nitrates in pregnancy and breastfeeding has not been established (pregnancy category C). Use in these situations is not recommended.

Contraindications

Hypersensitivity to tolvaptan and any of the other components

References

1 Gheorghiade M *et al.;* for the Acute and Chronic Therapeutic Impact of a Vasopressin Antagonist in Congestive Heart Failure (ACTIV in CHF) Investigators (2004). Effects of tolvaptan, a vasopressin antagonist, in patients hospitalized with worsening heart failure: a randomized controlled trial. *JAMA* **291**:1963–71.

2 Gheorghiade M *et al.;* Efficacy of Vasopressin Antagonism in Heart Failure Outcome Study With Tolvaptan (EVEREST) Investigators (2007). Short-term clinical effects of tolvaptan, an oral

vasopressin antagonist, in patients hospitalized for heart failure: the EVEREST Clinical Status Trials. *JAMA* **297**: 1332–43.

3 Konstam MA et al.; Efficacy of Vasopressin Antagonism in Heart failure Outcome Study With Tolvaptan (EVEREST) Investigators (2007). Effects of oral tolvaptan in patients hospitalized for worsening heart failure: the EVEREST Outcome Trial. *JAMA* **297**:1319–31.

4 Schrier RW et al.; SALT Investigators (2006). Tolvaptan, a selective oral vasopressin V2-receptor antagonist, for hyponatremia. *N Engl J Med* **355**:2099–112.

Torasemide

(See also 📖 Loop diuretics, p.507)

Long-acting loop diuretic.

CV indications

(See 📖 Loop diuretics, p.507)

Essential hypertension.

Others

(See 📖 Loop diuretics, p.507)

Mechanism of action

(See 📖 Loop diuretics, p.507)

Pharmacodynamics

(See 📖 Loop diuretics, p.507)

Produces less renal K^+ excretion than other loop diuretics, probably due to an anti-aldosteronic effect.

Hypertension: torasemide appears to have a BP-lowering effect at low doses. BP lowering is in the region of 11/7mmHg with doses of 5–10mg od. Peak concentrations within 1–2h after PO administration and diuresis last approximately 6–8h.[1]

Heart failure: torasemide reduced mortality rate (2.2% vs. 4.5%) and improved NYHA class in patients with NYHA class II–III CHF who received diuretic therapy with torasemide 10mg/day orally vs. patients who received furosemide 40mg/day orally or other diuretics in addition to standard CHF therapy for 12 months. Abnormally low serum K^+ levels were observed in fewer torasemide (12.9%) than furosemide/other diuretics patients (17.9%).[2]

Pharmacokinetics

It has high reliability and predictability compared with furosemide. Well absorbed with a bioavailablity of ≈90%. It is ≈99% protein-bound, with a V_d ≈0.22L/kg; and undergoes extensive hepatic metabolism with only 20% of the parent drug excreted unchanged in the urine. Elimination $t_{1/2}$ of about 3.5h (cirrhosis 7–8h).

Practical points

🥄 Doses

5–10mg od for hypertension

10–20mg od (PO, IV) for CHF and peripheral oedema

5mg od to a maximum of 40mg od for oedema

☺ **Common side effects** (see 📖 Loop diuretics, p.507)

Interactions (see 📖 Loop diuretics, p.507)

Cautions/notes

(See 📖 Loop diuretics, p.507)

Hypokalaemia, hyponatraemia, hypovolaemia, and disorders of micturition must be corrected before treatment. On long-term treatment with torasemide, regular monitoring of the electrolyte balance, glucose, uric acid, creatinine, and lipids in the blood is recommended.

Pregnancy and lactation

There are no data available on pregnancy or excretion in breast milk. In pregnancy, torasemide may be relatively safe (pregnancy category B).

Contraindications (see 📖 Loop diuretics, p.507)

References

1 Roca-Cusachs A et al.; Torasemide-PR in Hypertension Clinical Trial Investigators Group (2008). Clinical effects of torasemide prolonged release in mild-to-moderate hypertension: a randomized noninferiority trial versus torasemide immediate release. *Cardiovasc Ther* **26**:91–100.

2 Cosin J, D'ez O; TORIC investigators (2002). Torasemide in chronic heart failure: results of the TORIC study. *Eur J Heart Fail* **4**(4):507–13.

Trandolapril

(See also 📖 Angiotensin-converting enzyme inhibitors, p.355)

Orally active ACEI (prodrug).

Indications

(See 📖 Angiotensin-converting enzyme inhibitors, p.355)

Mechanism of action

(See also 📖 Renin–angiotensin–aldosterone system inhibitors, p.568 and 📖 Angiotensin-converting enzyme inhibitors, p.355)

Pharmacodynamics

Heart failure: RRR ≈20% (absolute rate 34.7% vs. 42.3%) in 1° outcome of all-cause mortality; RRR 22% in death from CV causes; RRR 24% in sudden death; and RRR 29% in 2° endpoint of progression to severe HF with trandolapril (1–2mg od) compared with placebo in patients 3–7 days post-MI with LVEF <35% after 24–50 months.[1]

Hypertension: composite 1° endpoint of death from CV causes, MI, or coronary revascularization over 4.8 years was not significantly different with trandolapril 4mg od compared with placebo (21.9% vs. 22.5%) in patients with hypertension, stable CAD, and normal or slightly reduced LV function.[2]

In hypertensive patients with CAD after 24 months, the verapamil–trandolapril-based strategy was as clinically effective as the atenolol–hydrochlorothiazide-based strategy.[3]

In subjects with type 2 diabetes and hypertension but with normo-albuminuria, the use of trandolapril (2mg/day) plus verapamil (SR 180mg/day) and trandolapril alone decreased the development of persistent microalbuminuria (overnight albumin excretion ≥20mcg/min) to a similar extent, while the effect of verapamil alone was similar to that of placebo.[4]

Pharmacokinetics

Trandolapril is a prodrug that is rapidly absorbed after oral administration. Bioavailability is ≈40–60% and absorption not affected by food. Plasma concentrations peak ≈30min after administration and thereafter disappear rapidly. Trandolapril is hydrolysed to trandolaprilat, a specific ACEI, reaching peak plasma concentrations after 3–8h; after repeated daily administration of trandolapril, steady state of trandolaprilat is reached in ≈4 days. Trandolaprilat binds to plasma proteins (>80%), presents a V_d ≈0.2L/kg and is excreted as trandolaprilat in urine (33%) and faeces (66%). The effective $t_{1/2}$ of trandolaprilat is between 15–23 hrs.

Practical points

💊 Doses

(See 📖 ACEIs for initiation under supervision, p.355)

0.5mg od (to increase gradually to maximum of 4mg od if required)

Treatment should be initiated at 0.5mg in hepatic impairment under close supervision. Maximum doses should be also reduced in patients with renal impairment:

Creatinine clearance	Maximum dose
10–70mL/min	Usual doses
<10mL/min	2mg/day (under close supervision)

☻ *Common side effects* (see 📖 Angiotensin-converting enzyme inhibitors, p.355)

Interactions (see 📖 Angiotensin-converting enzyme inhibitors, p.355)

Cautions/notes
(See also 📖 Angiotensin-converting enzyme inhibitors, p.355)
As trandolapril is a prodrug, it should be used with caution in hepatic impairment.

Pregnancy and lactation (see 📖 Angiotensin-converting enzyme inhibitors, p.355)

Contraindications (see 📖 Angiotensin-converting enzyme inhibitors, p.355)

References

1 Køber L et al. (1995). A clinical trial of the angiotensin-converting-enzyme inhibitor trandolapril in patients with left ventricular dysfunction after myocardial infarction. *N Engl J Med* **333**:1670–6.
2 Braunwald E et al.; PEACE Trial Investigators (2004). Angiotensin-converting-enzyme inhibition in stable coronary artery disease. *N Engl J Med* **351**:2058–68.
3 Pepine CJ et al.; INVEST Investigators (2003). A calcium antagonist vs a non-calcium antagonist hypertension treatment strategy for patients with coronary artery disease. The International Verapamil-Trandolapril Study (INVEST): a randomized controlled trial. *JAMA* **290**:2805–16.
4 Ruggenenti P et al. (2004). Preventing microalbuminuria in type 2 diabetes. *N Engl J Med* **351**: 1941–51.

Treprostinil

(See also 📖 Prostanoids, p.558)

Synthetic prostacyclin analogue (member of the eicosanoid family).

CV indications

1. SC treprostinil for use in WHO functional class II, III, and IV PAH
2. IV treprostinil in PAH patients in whom SC infusion is not tolerated

Mechanism of action

Treprostinil is a stable analogue of prostacyclin at room temperature that can be administered as a continuous SC or IV infusion via a pump.

Pharmacodynamics

In a 12-week RCT, SC treprostinil improved symptoms and increased exercise capacity (16m in the 6MWT).[1] In an open-label, uncontrolled trial, IV treprostinil increased exercise capacity (82m).[2] Exercise endurance was maintained in patients who completed the transition from IV epoprostenol to IV treprostinil.[3]

Pharmacokinetics

SC bioavailability 100%, reaching steady-state level after 10h at the dose of 10ng/kg/min for 72h. It binds to plasma proteins (91%), its V_d is 0.2L/kg, and it is excreted in urine (79%) and faeces (13%). The elimination $t_{1/2}$ is 4.5h following IV and SC administration. Thus, IV- and SC-administered treprostinil are bioequivalent at steady state.

Practical points

⚡ Dose

Initial dose: 1.25ng/kg/min SC via continuous infusion; the dose may increase by 1.25ng/kg/min for the first 4wk, then by 2.5ng/kg/min thereafter, depending on clinical response; if initial dose not tolerated, decrease to 0.625ng/kg/min. Do not discontinue abruptly (potential for severe rebound PH and death).

Subsequent dose: most patients derive optimal benefit with 25–40ng/kg/min; doses exceeding 40ng/kg/min after 1 year of therapy are not uncommon; IV dosing is similar to that used in SC delivery.

It may be administered as supplied by a continuous SC infusion or after dilution (with sterile water or a 0.9% NaCl solution) by continuous IV infusion via a small infusion pump that the patient must wear at all times.

☺ Side effects

- Pain, irritation or erythema at the site of the SC infusion in 85% of patients.[1] Headache, hypotension, nausea, vomiting and diarrhoea
- Other common side effects: see 📖 Epoprostenol, p.451

Interactions (see 📖 Epoprostenol, p.451)

Precautions

(See 📖 Epoprostenol, p.451)
The overall infection rate is significantly greater than that of epoprostenol, with a higher rate of Gram-negative bacteraemia.[4] Given the complexity of administration of both IV and SC treprostinil, administration should be limited to centres with experience with this agent.

Abrupt interruption of the treprostinil infusion can lead to worsening of PH symptoms, and should be avoided.

It is not known whether treprostinil is excreted in breast milk. Caution is advised when administering this medication to nursing women (pregnancy category C).

Contraindications (see 📖 Epoprostenol, p.451)

References

1 Simonneau G et al. (2002). Continuous subcutaneous infusion of treprostinil, a prostacyclin ana- logue, in patients with pulmonary arterial hypertension: a double-blind, randomized, placebo- controlled trial. *Am J Respir Crit Care Med* **165**:800–4.
2 Tapson VF et al. (2006). Safety and efficacy of IV treprostinil for pulmonary arterial hypertension: a prospective, multicenter, open-label, 12–week trial. *Chest* **129**:683–8.
3 Gomberg-Maitland M et al. (2005). transition from intravenous epoprostenol to intravenous treprostinil in pulmonary hypertension. *Am J Respir Crit Care Med* **172**:1586–9.
4 Doran A et al. (2008). Guidelines for the prevention of central venous catheter-related blood- stream infections with prostanoid therapy for pulmonary arterial hypertension. *Adv Pulm Hypertens* **7**:245–8.

Trimetazidine

Metabolic antianginal agent (3-ketoacyl CoA thiolase (3-KAT) inhibitor).

CV indications
1. Long-term symptom control in chronic refractory angina
2. Patients with ACS requiring percutaneous intervention and those with ischaemic cardiomyopathy.

Other indications
Symptomatic treatment of Menière's disease, vertigo, and tinnitus; treatment of chorioretinal ischaemic disorders

Mechanism of action
Trimetazidine selectively inhibits the long-chain 3-KAT mitochondrial enzyme which catalyses the final step of fatty acid oxidation. Consequently, trimetazidine decreases fatty acid oxidation, and, as a result, promotes glucose oxidation, which improves ATP production with lesser oxygen utilization. During cardiac ischaemia, trimetazidine acts as a metabolic anti-anginal agent. It is possible that part of its antianginal properties may be derived from various cytoprotective mechanisms including the prevention of calcium overload and acidosis.

Pharmacodynamics

A Cochrane review (involving 23 studies and 1378 patients) has suggested that trimetazidine reduces the frequency of weekly angina attacks by 40% (−1.44 episodes/week mean difference, 95% CI: −2.10–0.79) in addition to a statistically significant reduction in nitroglycerin usage and time to 1mm ST-segment depression when compared with placebo.[1]

Preliminary open-label studies have also suggested that the addition of trimetazidine to conventional therapy compared with placebo may improve functional class and LV function in patients with HF.[2]

Because it does not decrease BP, trimetazidine may replace nitrates in patients with erectile dysfunction.

It improves LV function, insulin sensitivity, and glucose control in idiopathic dilated or ischaemic cardiomyopathy patients.[3]

Pharmacokinetics

Well absorbed after oral administration (bioavailability 90%), reaching peak plasma levels at ~2–3h. Poorly bound to plasma proteins (20%) and $t_{1/2}$ ~5–6.5h. Primarily excreted in urine.

Practical points
Dose
20mg tds
(35mg bd for modified-release formulation)

☺ Side effects
Heartburn, nausea, vomiting, dry mouth, hot flushes, diarrhoea, weakness, muscular cramps, dizziness, depression, sedation, drowsiness, palpitations, visual disturbances, anorexia.

Interactions
No reported drug interactions of trimetazidine with β-blockers, CCBs, nitrates, heparin, hypolipidaemic agents, or digoxin have been reported.

Cautions/notes
Dose reduction may be required in patients with impaired renal clearance.

Pregnancy and lactation
No demonstrated teratogenic effects. However, safety in pregnancy and during breastfeeding has not been sufficiently evaluated. Therefore, its use is not recommended under these circumstances.

Contraindications
Pregnancy and breastfeeding

References
1 Ciapponi A et al. (2005). Trimetazidine for stable angina. *Cochrane Database Syst Rev* **I4**:CD003614.
2 Fragasso G et al. (2006). A randomized clinical trial of trimetazidine, a partial free fatty acid oxidation inhibitor, in patients with heart failure. *J Am Coll Cardiol* **4**:992–8.
3 Tuunanen H et al. (2008). Trimetazidine, a metabolic modulator, has cardiac and extracardiac benefits in idiopathic dilated cardiomyopathy. *Circulation* **118**:1250–8.

Unfractionated heparin

(See also 📖 Heparin, p.479)

Parental anticoagulant, with rapid and short duration of action.

CV indications

(See 📖 Heparin, p.479)

Mechanism of action

(See 📖 Heparin, p.479)

Pharmacodynamics

In AMI, UFH is given together with thrombolysis or 1° angioplasty. In patients with UA, dose-adjusted heparin added to aspirin helps to prevent MI.[1] Although no placebo-controlled trials have been performed, UFH is indicated in PCIs because of risk of acute thrombotic closure.

Main advantages as compared to LMWH are that the anticoagulant effects rapidly disappear by stopping IV infusion and can be reversed by protamine sulphate and it is safer in renal failure.

Pharmacokinetics

(See 📖 Heparin, p.479)

Practical points

·§ Doses

IV: 60–70 IU/kg bolus up to 5000 IU, followed by an infusion of 12–15 IU/kg/h (maximum 1000 IU/24h) in 0.9% saline solution. Doses should be adjusted according to APPT, with monitoring at 6, 12, and 24h.

Intermittent IV injection: initial dose of 10,000 IU; then 5000–10,000 IU every 4–6h either undiluted or in 0.9% NaCl solution.

SC: 5000 IU by deep injection. Then 8000–20,000 IU every 8–12h. A different site should be used for each injection to prevent the development of haematoma. The anticoagulant effect is delayed for approximately 1h and peak plasma levels occur at approximately 3h.

Surgery of the heart and blood vessels: 150 IU/kg up to 300 IU/kg for procedures lasting <60min, or 400 IU/kg for those estimated to last >60min.

Low-dose heparin prophylaxis prior to and after surgery to reduce the incidence of postoperative DVT: 5000 IU SC 2h before surgery and 5000 IU every 8–12h thereafter for 7 days or until the patient is fully ambulatory.

☺ Common side effects

(See 📖 Heparin, p.479)

Interactions

(See 📖 Heparin, p.479)

Digoxin, tetracyclines, or antihistamines may partially counteract the anti-coagulant action of heparin sodium. In heparinized patients, IV GTN may decrease the APPT time with subsequent rebound effect upon discontinuation of GTN; careful monitoring of APPT and adjustment of heparin dosage are recommended under these conditions.

Cautions/notes
(See 📖 Heparin, p.479)

When an oral anticoagulant is started in patients already receiving heparin sodium, baseline and subsequent determinations of prothrombin time (PT) must be determined at a time when heparin activity is too low to affect the test (~5h after the last IV bolus; 24h after the last SC dose). If continuous IV heparin infusion is used, PT can usually be measured at any time. To ensure continuous anticoagulation, full heparin therapy must continue for several days after the PT has reached the therapeutic range; heparin therapy may then be discontinued without tapering.

When UFH is given after fibrinolytic therapy in patients with ACS, it should be discontinued immediately after the PCI.

Pregnancy and lactation
(See 📖 Heparin, p.479)

The high doses (20,000 IU daily) needed to reduce the risk of thrombosed maternal valves may cause osteoporosis when used for >5 months.

Contraindications
(See 📖 Heparin, p.479)

Reference
1 Bassand JP et al. (2007). Guidelines for the diagnosis and treatment of non-ST-segment elevation acute coronary syndromes. *Eur Heart J* **28**:1598–660.

Valsartan

(See also 📖 Angiotensin II (AT$_1$) receptor blockers, p.359)

Angiotensin receptor blocker.

CV indications

(See also 📖 Angiotensin II (AT$_1$) receptor blockers, p.359)
1. Treatment of hypertension
2. Symptomatic HF (NYHA class II–IV) when ACEI is not tolerated
3. LV failure or LV dysfunction following MI

Mechanism of action

(See also 📖 Renin–angiotensin–aldosterone system inhibitors, p.568 and 📖 Angiotensin II (AT$_1$) receptor blockers, p.359)

Pharmacodynamics

(See also 📖 Renin–angiotensin–aldosterone system inhibitors, p.568 and 📖 Angiotensin II (AT$_1$) receptor blockers, p.359)

Hypertension: no significant difference (absolute rates: 25.5 vs. 24.7/1000 patients years) in 1° endpoint (CV death and morbidity) in untreated hypertensive patients at high risk of CV events treated with valsartan (160mg od) compared with amlodipine (10mg od) and followed up for a mean of 42 months.[1] BP reduction was greater in the amlodipine compared with valsartan group (BP 4.0/2.1mmHg lower in amlodipine than valsartan group after 1 month; 1.5/1.3mmHg after 1 year).

RRR 39% in CV morbidity and mortality in Japanese patients treated for hypertension, CHD, HF, or a combination of these disorders for 3.1 years with valsartan (40–160mg per day) compared with conventional treatment (but not including ARBs). This difference was mainly attributable to a decrease in stroke and transient ischaemic attacks, angina pectoris, and HF in those given valsartan that could not be explained by a difference in BP control.[2]

AMI and heart failure: HR 1.00 in 1° endpoint of all-cause mortality in patients with AMI treated with valsartan compared with captopril during a mean follow-up of 24.7months.[3] Combination therapy with valsartan and captopril did not result in greater survival but there was an increased rate of adverse effects.

RRR≈13% in combined 1° endpoint (death and HF-related morbidity) in patients with NYHA class II–IV HF treated with valsartan 160mg bd or placebo in addition to standard HF therapy and followed up for mean of 23 months.[4] No overall difference in mortality was seen.

There is no evidence that valsartan provides added benefits when it is used with an adequate dose of an ACEI.[3]

Pharmacokinetics

Mean absolute bioavailability is ≈23%, reaching peak plasma concentrations within 2–4h. Valsartan is 94–97% protein bound but not extensively distributed in tissues, with a $V_d \approx 0.25$L/kg. Primarily excreted unchanged in faeces (83%) and also urine (17%), with a terminal $t_{\frac{1}{2}} \approx 6$–9h.

Practical points

♪ Doses

40–80mg od (titrated to maximum of 320mg od)

No dose adjustment is required in renal impairment where CrCl >10mL/L or mild–moderate hepatic impairment.

☺ **Side effects** (see 📖 Angiotensin II (AT$_1$) receptor blockers, p.359)

Interactions

(See also 📖 Angiotensin II (AT$_1$) receptor blockers, p.359)
Valsartan increases digoxinaemia (20–50%).

Cautions (see 📖 Angiotensin II (AT$_1$) receptor blockers, p.359)

Pregnancy and lactation (see 📖 Angiotensin II (AT1) receptor blockers, p.359)

Contraindications

(See also 📖 Angiotensin II (AT$_1$) receptor blockers, p.359)

Severe hepatic impairment; biliary cirrhosis, cholestasis

References

1 Julius S et al.; VALUE trial group (2004). Outcomes in hypertensive patients at high cardiovascular risk treated with regimens based on valsartan or amlodipine: the VALUE randomised trial. *Lancet* **363**:2022–31.
2 Mochizuki S et al.; Jikei Heart Study group (2007). Valsartan in a Japanese population with hypertension and other cardiovascular disease (Jikei Heart Study): a randomised, open-label, blinded endpoint morbidity-mortality study. *Lancet* **369**:1431–9.
3 Pfeffer MA et al.; Valsartan in Acute Myocardial Infarction Trial Investigators (2003). Valsartan, captopril, or both in myocardial infarction complicated by heart failure, left ventricular dysfunction, or both. *N Engl J Med* **349**:1893–906.
4 Cohn JN, Tognoni G; Valsartan Heart failure Trial Investigators (2001). A randomized trial of the angiotensin-receptor blocker valsartan in chronic heart failure. *N Engl J Med* **345**:1667–75.

Vasopressin antagonists

(See also 📖 Tolvaptan, p.612)

AVP (antidiuretic hormone) is a nonapeptide hormone that plays a key role in the control of body water content through its action on the distal convoluted and collecting tubules of the nephron. AVP is released from the neurohypophysis in response to increases in plasma osmolarity, hypovolaemia, hypotension, and angiotensin II, and stimulates 3 typical G-protein-coupled receptors. Stimulation of V1A receptors increases intracellular Ca^{2+} concentrations ($[Ca^{2+}]_i$) and cardiac contractility, and produces vasoconstriction, platelet aggregation, and vascular and myocardial hypertrophy and remodelling. Stimulation of V1B receptors in the anterior pituitary increases adrenocorticotropin release. Stimulation of V2 receptors, expressed on the basolateral membrane of the renal collecting ducts, increases the synthesis of aquaporin-2 water-channel-containing vesicles that are inserted into the apical cell membrane and increase water reabsorption. This water reabsorption decreases serum osmolarity, contributing to the development of dilutional hyponatraemia (serum Na^+ concentration, <135mmol/L) and increases LV end-diastolic volume and pressure.

Elevated levels of AVP are present in HF and adversely affect LV function by increasing peripheral vascular resistances and systemic and pulmonary congestion, and contribute to the development of fluid retention and hyponatraemia.

V2 (lixivaptan, mozavaptan, tolvaptan) or dual V1A/V2 receptor antagonists (conivaptan) have been approved for the treatment of hyponatraemia due to inappropriate AVP secretion, HF, and cirrhosis with ascites.

Verapamil

(See also 📖 Calcium-channel blockers, p.390)

A phenylalkylamine (non-dihydropyridine) L-type CCB, available in oral and IV preparations. It is also a class IV antiarrhythmic agent.

CV indications

1. Treatment of hypertension
2. Treatment of chronic stable and vasospastic angina pectoris
3. Prophylaxis of paroxysmal SVT and control of ventricular rate in atrial flutter/AF
4. (Selected preparations) Secondary prevention of re-infarction after an acute MI in patients without heart failure, and not receiving diuretics (apart from low-dose diuretics when used for indications other than heart failure), and where beta-blockers are not appropriate

Mechanism of action

(See also 📖 Calcium-channel blockers, p.390)

Pharmacodynamics

Verapamil reduces the mean sitting systolic BP by ~10.7%[1] and (when titrated up to 480mg/day) improves ETT (symptom-limited ETT time, time to moderate angina, and time to 1mm ST depression) compared to placebo.[2]

Hypertension and CHD: no significant difference (absolute rates: 9.9% vs. 10.2%) in 1° combined endpoint (all-cause mortality, non-fatal MI, or CVA) in hypertensive patients with documented CHD treated with verapamil SR-based therapy compared to atenolol-based therapy (with addition of trandolapril and hydrochlorothiazide as required), and followed up for a mean of 2.7 years.[3]

Atrial fibrillation: HR ~1.15 (95% CI: 0.99–1.34; absolute rate=23.8 vs. 21.3% at 5 years) in total mortality in patients with AF and high risk of death or stroke treated by rate control with drugs including verapamil compared to rhythm control using other antiarrhythmic agents.[4] Recurrence of AF or death is reduced in patients who have undergone successful electrical cardioversion treated with verapamil in combination with quinidine (absolute rate=65% vs. 83%) compared to placebo; and comparable to those treated with sotalol.[5]

Verapamil reduces afterload and myocardial contractility, improving LV diastolic function in patients with idiopathic hypertrophic subaortic stenosis.[6] In patients with severe LV dysfunction (e.g. PCWP >20mmHg or ejection fraction <30%), verapamil can deteriorate ventricular function.

In supraventricular arrhythmias, verapamil has been replaced by adenosine and esmolol. It is not effective in ventricular arrhythmias except in those associated with ischaemia.

Pharmacokinetics

Pharmacokinetic properties of different modified-release preparations may vary. Approximately 90% of verapamil is absorbed following oral administration and is subject to extensive hepatic 1st-pass metabolism. Bioavailability (20–30%) is not affected by food but there is considerable inter-individual variation in plasma concentrations. The time to maximal concentration is ~1.2h and ~7.6h with the immediate-release and modi-fied-release preparations, respectively. Verapamil binds to plasma proteins (90%) and is extensively metabolized in the liver; norverapamil is an active metabolite that has 20% of the effect of verapamil. Approximately 70% of the dose is excreted as metabolites in the urine (<1% unchanged) and 20% in the faeces. The $t_{1/2}$ of verapamil is ~4h, and increases in the elderly, in AF, and in hepatic insufficiency (up to 14h).

Practical points

🔆 *Doses*

Dosing varies depending on type of preparation and manufacturer. The list is a guide to daily doses:

- *PO*: hypertension: 120mg/day up to a maximum of 480mg/day od or tds if required
- *Angina*: 240–360mg/day, and may be increased to a maximum of 480mg daily if required
- *Supraventricular arrhythmia*: 120–480mg daily
- *Rate control in patients with atrial flutter/AF*: 5–10mg IV over 2min monitoring BP and ECG; a further 5mg may be given after 5–10min. *Maintenance dose*: 120–360mg daily in divided doses
- *2° prevention of re-infarction*: Treatment is to be started at least 1 week after an AMI. Daily dose of 360mg, to be taken in divided doses

Verapamil is also available as a combination preparation with trandolapril.

😊 *Side effects*

(See 📖 Calcium-channel blockers, p.390)

(~10%): constipation (particularly in the elderly)

(1–10%): fatigue, headache, dizziness; bradycardia, 1st-degree AV block; oedema; nausea, paraesthesia, flushing

Rare: gynaecomastia, reversible hepatic impairment, paraesthesia, gingival hyperplasia, erythromelalgia, hyperprolactinaemia

At high doses or with prior myocardial damage: bradyarrhythmias, 2nd- and 3rd-degree AV block, transient asystole, hypotension, HF

Interactions

(See 📖 Calcium-channel blockers, p.390)

It is also a moderate inhibitor of CYP3A4; therefore caution is required when given with drugs that modulate its activity (atorvastatin, lovastatin, simvastatin, ketoconazole, theophylline, midazolam, ciclosporin, carbamazepine, grapefruit juice).

Verapamil is also an inhibitor of P-gp that decreases the clearance of digoxin and increases its plasma levels (50–75%); thus, the maintenance dose of digoxin should be reduced to avoid the risk of bradycardia or AV block.

Hypotension and bradycardia have been described in patients treated with verapamil receiving telithromycin.

Verapamil increases the risk of lithium toxicity.

The combination of verapamil with β-blockers can be beneficial in some patients with chronic stable angina or hypertension. This combination, however, may produce additive negative effects on heart rate, AV conduction, and/or cardiac contractility and, therefore, it should be used under close supervision. To avoid pharmacokinetic interactions, verapamil should be combined with hydrophilic β-blockers (atenolol, nadolol).

The combination of verapamil with class I antiarrhythmic agents or inhaled anaesthetics may lead to additive negative inotropic effects and prolongation of AV conduction, and should be avoided. Verapamil increases quinidine plasma levels.

Verapamil may increase blood alcohol concentrations and prolong its effects and may also potentiate the activity of neuromuscular blocking agents (decrease the dose of verapamil and/or of the neuromuscular-blocking agent).

Cautions/notes
(See 📖 Calcium-channel blockers, p.390)

Verapamil is extensively metabolized in the liver, and the dose should be reduced and carefully titrated in patients with hepatic dysfunction. Elderly patients show enhanced bioavailability, and therapeutic control may require only lower doses.

Abrupt withdrawal of verapamil may produce rebound angina.

Pregnancy and lactation
(See 📖 Calcium-channel blockers, p.390)

Contraindications
(See 📖 Calcium-channel blockers, p.390)
- 2nd- and 3rd-degree AV block, sick sinus syndrome, SA block, or severe sinus bradycardia without pacemaker
- AF or atrial flutter associated with an accessory pathway
- Severe LV dysfunction
- Hypotension (SBP <90mmHg) or cardiogenic shock

References

1 Singh BN et al. (1986). Calcium antagonists and beta blockers in the control of mild to moderate systemic hypertension, with particular reference to verapamil and propranolol. Am J Cardiol **57**:99D–105D.

2 Frishman WH et al. (1999). Comparison of controlled-onset, extended-release verapamil with amlodipine and amlodipine plus atenolol on exercise performance and ambulatory ischemia in patients with chronic stable angina pectoris. Am J Cardiol **83**:507–14.

3 Pepine CJ et al.; INVEST Investigators (2003). A calcium antagonist vs a non-calcium antagonist hypertension treatment strategy for patients with coronary artery disease. The International Verapamil-Trandolapril Study (INVEST): a randomized controlled trial. JAMA **290**:2805–16.

4 Wyse DG et al.; Atrial Fibrillation Follow-up Investigation of Rhythm Management (AFFIRM) Investigators (2002). A comparison of rate control and rhythm control in patients with atrial fibrillation. N Engl J Med **347**:1825–33.

5 Fetsch T et al.; Prevention of Atrial Fibrillation after Cardioversion Investigators (2004). Prevention of atrial fibrillation after cardioversion: results of the PAFAC trial. Eur Heart J **25**:1385–94.

6 Bonow RO (1985). Effects of calcium-channel blocking agents on left ventricular diastolic function in hypertrophic cardiomyopathy and in coronary artery disease. Am J Cardiol **55**:172B–178B.

Warfarin

Oral coumarin anticoagulant.

CV indications

1. DVT prophylaxis
2. Treatment of DVT and pulmonary embolism
3. Prophylaxis and treatment of thromboembolic complications associated with AF and/or cardiac valve replacement
4. Management of TIAs
5. Reduction of the risk of death, recurrent MI, and thromboembolic events (e.g. stroke or systemic embolization) after MI
6. Arterial thromboembolism prophylaxis with mechanical prosthetic heart valves

Mechanism of action

Warfarin inhibits the vitamin K-dependent synthesis of biologically active forms of the calcium-dependent clotting factors II, VII, IX, and X, as well as the anticoagulant proteins C and S. The precursors of these factors require the carboxylation of their glutamic acid residues by γ-carboxy-glutamic acid residues to allow the coagulation factors to bind to phospholipid surfaces on the vascular endothelium, thereby accelerating blood coagulation. This reaction requires reduced vitamin K and is catalysed by the γ-glutamyl carboxylase; the carboxylation is coupled to the oxidation of vitamin K to its epoxide. Vitamin K epoxide is regenerated to vitamin K, reduced by the vitamin K epoxide reductase complex-1 (VKORC-1).

Warfarin directly inhibits VKORC-1, reduces the levels of reduced vitamin K, and induces the hepatic synthesis of partially decarboxylated proteins with reduced coagulant activity. After a loading dose of warfarin, the appearance of its anticoagulant effect requires the degradation of functional clotting factors and the synthesis of non-functioning factors. The factor with the shortest $t_{1/2}$ is factor VII ($t_{1/2}$ ~6h) and that with the longest $t_{1/2}$ is factor II ($t_{1/2}$ ~60h). The anticoagulant effect of warfarin can be overcome by low doses of vitamin K1 (phytomenadione).

Pharmacodynamics

The anticoagulant effect of warfarin is dose dependent. It occurs within 24h after drug administration, but peaks after 72–96h and persists for 2–5 days. Large loading doses do not shorten the time to achieve a full therapeutic effect but cause rapid falls in protein C levels, which may precipitate paradoxical thrombosis in the first few days of warfarin therapy.

Warfarin is monitored by using the PT or the better standardized INR. Thus, a normal person will have an INR of 1.

Efficacy in reducing risk of clot formation and embolism (e.g. prevention of stroke in AF) is best with an INR between 2 and 3 (see table 14, p.633); it diminishes sharply with INR <2 and is absent with INR <1.5.[1] Conversely, risk of bleeding (e.g. intracranial bleeding) increases significantly when INR >4 and in patients aged >75 years.[2]

Atrial fibrillation: 62% RR (95% CI: 48–72%) in all stroke in patients with AF (mean age ~69 years) treated with dose-adjusted warfarin compared to placebo (see Table 13).[3] 64% RR of stroke in a meta-analysis of 29 CTs in patients with AF treated for 1.5 years with adjusted-dose warfarin (22% RR in patients treated with antiplatelet agents).[4] 39% RR (95% CI: 22–52%) of stroke in patients treated with dose-adjusted warfarin as compared to antiplatelet therapy.[4] The risk of intracranial bleeding was doubled with dose-adjusted warfarin in patients with AF (absolute rate: 0.2%/year) compared with aspirin.[4]

Table 13 Stroke reduction with warfarin compared with aspirin in AF[3]

	Annual stroke rate with aspirin (%)	NNT for 1 year to prevent 1 stroke with warfarin	Number of strokes saved with warfarin (/year/1000)
1° prevention			
Low risk	1	250	4
Medium risk	3	83	12
High risk	6	42	24
2° prevention	10	25	40

Myocardial infarction: 24% RR in total mortality, 55% RR in CVAs, and 34% RR in recurrent MI in patients within 30 days of a MI treated for 37 months with warfarin (INR 2.8–4.8) as compared with placebo.[5] Serious bleeding was noted in 0.6% of the warfarin-treated patients per year.

29% RR in the composite of death, non-fatal MI, or thromboembolic stroke in patients with STEMI treated with the combination of warfarin (INR 2–2.5) and aspirin (75mg/day); the combination was significantly more effective than 160mg/daily aspirin (19% RR) but not than warfarin alone with a target INR of 2.8–4.2 (12% RR).[6] Major, non-fatal bleeding was observed in 0.62% of patients per treatment-year in both groups receiving warfarin and in 0.17% of patients receiving aspirin.

Pharmacokinetics

Warfarin is a racemic mixture of *R*- and *S*-enantiomers. The *S*-enantiomer has 2–5× the anticoagulation activity of the *R*-enantiomer, but its clearance is faster. Warfarin is completely absorbed following PO administration (bioavailability 98%), reaching peak plasma levels within 4–9h. Warfarin is highly bound to plasma proteins (~97%) and presents a small V_d (0.14L/kg). Warfarin is transported to the liver where it is metabolized by cytochrome P450 (CYP1A1, CYP1A2, and CYP3A4 metabolize *R*-warfarin and CYP2C9 metabolizes *S*-warfarin) to inactive hydroxylated metabolites, and by VKORC-1 to warfarin alcohols with minimal anticoagulant activity; these metabolites are excreted mainly in urine. The $t_{1/2}$ of *R*-warfarin ranges from 37 to 89h, and that of *S*-warfarin from 21 to 43h.

The CYP2C9*2 and *3 alleles encoding for the enzyme are associated with decreased S-warfarin clearance. Individuals with these common alleles require lower maintenance doses, have longer times to dose stabilization and are at a higher risk of serious and life-threatening bleeding complications.[7] Variants of the VKROC-1, which can lead to reduced susceptibility to antagonism by vitamin K, may explain up to 30% of dose variation in warfarin doses and also relative resistance to warfarin in some individuals.[8]

Practical notes

Dose

Therapy can be initiated with a dose of 2–5mg/day for 5 days checking the INR daily until it reaches the therapeutic range (see Table 14); then 3 times weekly for 2 weeks. Most patients are satisfactorily maintained at a dose of 2–10mg daily (mean 4–5mg daily), the doses being adjusted according to the INR. Patients with hepatic HF, renal insufficiency, malnutrition (lead to vitamin K deficiency), liver disease, or an increased risk of bleeding require lower doses; myxoedema has the opposite effect. Asians require lower doses, while African-Americans require higher doses.

Table 14 Therapeutic recommendations for warfarin. Prescribers should familiarize themselves with local guidelines

Disease	INR range
DVT/pulmonary embolism	2.0–3.0
AF	2.0–3.0
Post-MI	2.0–3.0
Mechanical prosthetic heart valves	2.5–3.5

Side effects

Haemorrhage from any tissue or organ even when the INR is within the therapeutic range; this is a consequence of the anticoagulant effect. Bleeding can be treated with vitamin K_1 (5–10mg PO or IV over 30min). In patients where vitamin K is contraindicated (carriers of prosthetic valves), that do not respond to vitamin K or there is a life-threatening bleeding, the treatment should be fresh frozen plasma or a concentrate of clotting factors (II, IX, and X).

Haemorrhagic necrosis, systemic atheroemboli, and cholesterol microemboli including purple toe syndrome.

Others: alopecia, rash, diarrhoea, jaundice, hepatic dysfunction, nausea, vomiting, pancreatitis, fall in haematocrit; agranulocytosis. Long-term warfarin treatment (>1 year) may produce osteoporotic fractures, more frequent in males.

Skin necrosis may occur in patients treated with high doses of warfarin after cardiopulmonary bypass, particularly in patients with protein C deficiency. Since warfarin reduces protein C levels, it exacerbates this deficiency and predisposes to thrombosis in small vessels in adipose tissue. The treatment is fresh frozen plasma (providing protein C), IV heparin, and temporary discontinuation of warfarin.

Interactions

The following groups of drugs can inhibit the metabolism and so can enhance the effects and risk of bleeding when administered concomitantly with warfarin:

- antiarrhythmics: amiodarone (inhibits metabolism of warfarin), propafenone; quinidine
- antibiotics: carbenicillin, chloramphenicol; ciprofloxacin, co-trimoxazole, erythromycin, mofloxacin, moxalactam, metronidazole, sulphonamides
- antidiabetic agents: chlorpropamide, tolbutamide
- antiepileptics: sodium valproate
- azole antifungals: fluconazole, itraconazole, ketoconazole
- antiulcer drugs: cimetidine, omeprazole
- herbal medicines: danshen, dong quai (*Angelica sinensis*), garlic, Ginkgo biloba, and ginseng
- hormone antagonists: bicalutamide, toremifene, tamoxifen, and flutamide
- leucotriene antagonists: zafirlukast, zileuton
- lipid-lowering agents: statins (especially pravastatin, lovastatin) and fibrates
- NSAIDs: inhibit the synthesis of prothrombin and platelet aggregation, exert proulcerogenic effects, and displace warfarin from plasma proteins
- uricosuric agents: allopurinol, sulfinpyrazone
- others: alcohol (acute ingestions); capecitabine disulfiram, isoniazid, tamoxifen, thyroid hormones

Other drugs that can enhance the effects of warfarin when used concomitantly due in part to the respective mechanisms include:

- additive effects: heparins, NSAIDs, platelet antiaggregation inhibitors, fibrinolytics
- inhibition of vitamin K activity: cephalosporins (including cefuroxime, cefalexin, cefaclor); high-dose penicillins—possibly due to decreased synthesis of vitamin K by GI flora
- others: venlafaxine, SSRIs, mirtazapine, and tricyclic antidepressants. Entacapone, imatinib, fluorouracil and ifosfamide, bicalutamide, flutamide, iloprost, testosterone, and anabolic steroids

Conversely, other drugs can induce the metabolism of warfarin, so it may be necessary to increase the dose:

- carbamazepine, rifampicin, alcohol (chronic ingestion); phenytoin; barbiturates; St John's wort; griseofulvin
- other drugs that can reduce the anticoagulant effects of warfarin: azothioprine, griseofulvin, mercaptopurine; aminoglutethimide, danazol, oestrogens and progestogens and retinoids.
- resins, laxatives, sulfacrate and orlistat can reduce the absorption of warfarin.

In addition, ingestion of vitamin K and foods rich in vitamin K (e.g. Brussels sprouts, liver, spinach, chickpeas, broccoli, watercress) can antagonize the anticoagulant effect of warfarin and it may be necessary to increase the dosage of warfarin. Cranberry juice enhances the anticoagulant effect of warfarin.

Protein-bound drugs can increase the effects of warfarin by interfering with its protein binding, and include: NSAIDs, sulphonamides, and sulphonylureas.

Warfarin can increase the plasma levels of hypoglycaemic agents (chlorpropamide and tolbutamide) and anticonvulsants (phenytoin and phenobarbital).

Cautions/notes

Due to mechanisms of metabolism and excretion, caution is needed with warfarin in patients with hepatic and/or renal impairment. Frequency of monitoring of INR should be increased with changes in clinical status, or in medication (including over-the-counter medications), or intercurrent illness.

Due to shorter $t_{1/2}$ of the proteins S and C (8h and 30h, respectively) relative to vitamin K-dependent clotting factors, warfarin can promote an initial prothrombotic state which may be exaggerated with deficiencies in underlying levels of protein S or C and can lead to haemorrhagic necrosis.

Warfarin should be started at least 4 days before UFH is discontinued, to allow for the synthesis of non-functioning clotting factors; UFH can be discontinued when the INR reaches the therapeutic range for 48h.

Pregnancy and lactation

Warfarin is contraindicated in women who are, or may become, pregnant, because it passes through the placenta, is teratogenic, and may cause fatal fetal haemorrhage in utero (pregnancy category X). The teratogenic effect is greatest in the 1st trimester, while the risk of fetal haemorrhage is most dangerous in the last trimester. If a patient becomes pregnant, use UFH or LMWH; they should be discontinued 12h before labour induction and restarted postpartum, together with warfarin for 4–5 days; during treatment APTT or anti-Xa levels should be regularly monitored. Warfarin is excreted into breast milk at extremely low concentrations and is therefore considered compatible with breastfeeding.

Contraindications

- Haemorrhagic tendencies or blood dyscrasias
- Bleeding tendencies associated with active ulceration or overt bleeding: GI, GU, or respiratory tracts; cerebrovascular haemorrhage; aneurysms—cerebral, dissecting aorta; pericarditis; bacterial endocarditis
- Recent or contemplated surgery
- Severe hypertension
- Pregnancy, threatened abortion
- Impaired hepatic or renal function

- Unsupervised patients with senility, history of falls, dementia, or other lack of patient cooperation
- Diagnostic or therapeutic procedures with potential for uncontrollable bleeding

References

1 Hylek EM *et al.* (1996). An analysis of the lowest effective intensity of prophylactic anticoagulation for patients with nonrheumatic atrial fibrillation. *N Engl J Med* **335**:540–6.

2 Hylek EM, Singer DE (1994). Risk factors for intracranial hemorrhage in outpatients taking warfarin. *Ann Intern Med* **120**:897–902.

3 Hart RG *et al.* (1999). Antithrombotic therapy to prevent stroke in patients with atrial fibrillation: a meta-analysis. *Ann Intern Med* **131**:492–501.

4 Hart RG *et al.* (2007). Meta-analysis: antithrombotic therapy to prevent stroke in patients who have nonvalvular atrial fibrillation. *Ann Intern Med* **146**:857–67.

5 Smith P *et al.* (1990). The effect of warfarin on mortality and reinfarction after myocardial infarction. *N Engl J Med* **323**:147–52.

6 Hurlen M *et al.* (2002). Warfarin, aspirin, or both after myocardial infarction. *N Engl J Med* **347**: 969–74.

7 Higashi MK *et al.* (2002). Association between CYP2C9 genetic variants and anticoagulation-related outcomes during warfarin therapy. *JAMA* **287**:1690–8.

8 Rieder MJ *et al.* (2005). Effect of VKORC1 haplotypes on transcriptional regulation and warfarin dose. *N Engl J Med* **352**:2285–93.

Non-cardiac drugs affecting the heart

Anaesthetics (commonest drugs only)

Cardiovascular effects and incidence of side effects is classified as: very common ($\geq 1/10$), common ($\geq 1/100$ and $<1/10$), uncommon ($\geq 1/1000$ and $<1/100$), rare ($\geq 1/10,000$ and $<1/1000$), very rare ($<1/10,000$ and isolated reports) (see Table A.1).

Table A.1 Anaesthetics

Drug name/class/indication	Cardiovascular effects and incidence	Special recommendations for use/notes
Thiopental (barbiturate) *Induction of anaesthesia*	Reduced cardiac output/myocardial depression causing hypotension Prolongation of QT interval	*Caution:* severe CVD, hypertension. May precipitate acute circulatory failure in CVD, particularly constrictive pericarditis. Reduce dose in metabolic conditions, myxoedema, hyperkalaemia, shock, dehydration, elderly
Ketamine *Induction of anaesthesia, analgesia*	*Common:* temporary elevation in pulse (can be >100bpm) and BP. Median peak in BP rise is 20–25% Arrhythmias also reported as well as hypotension and bradycardia	*Contraindications:* where rise in BP would constitute a serious hazard *Caution:* monitor in patients with hypertension and cardiac disease
Propofol *Induction and sedation agent*	*Common:* myocardial depression, hypotension, bradycardia. *Very rare:* pulmonary oedema. Cases of metabolic alkalosis, rhabdomyolysis, hyperlipidaemia and cardiac failure have been reported in both adults and children when maximum concentrations exceeded	For sedation in ITU maximum concentration of 4mg/kg/h. Not licensed for sedation in those aged <16 years Lacks vagal activity so relative vagal overactivity can occur, with profound bradycardia and asystole reported Effect on QTc unclear but may reduce QTc
Etomidate *Induction of anaesthesia*	Hypotension due to loss of peripheral vascular resistance. At higher doses decreased cardiac output. *Rare:* cardiac arrhythmias, bradycardia, tachycardia. *Very rare:* AV	Less used in anaesthesia and ITU due to nausea and vomiting and adrenal suppression

Table A.1 (Contd.)

Drug name/class/indication	Cardiovascular effects and incidence	Special recommendations for use/notes
Alfentanil *Potent opioid analgesic with rapid onset and marked respiratory depression. Aid to induction of anaesthetic*	*Common*: hypotension through loss of vascular tone. *Uncommon*: bradycardia, asystole, arrhythmias, hypertension, tachycardia	Bradycardia should be treated with atropine
Fentanyl *Analgesia and aid to induction of anaesthetic*	*Common*: vasodilatation. *Uncommon*: bradycardia, tachycardia, arrhythmias. *Rare*: circulatory depression	*Caution*: in patients with bradyarrhythmias, hypotension, hypovolaemia
Remifentanil *Opioid analgesic agent with very short $t_{\frac{1}{2}}$ (10–15min), general anaesthesia. Specifically targets μ receptor*	*Common*: hypotension, bradycardia *Very rare*: severe bradycardia followed by asystole	*Caution*: elderly, hypovolaemic, debilitated, hypotensive or those receiving antihypertensives. Very potent respiratory depressant, apnoea universal with high doses but consciousness maintained
Isoflurane, sevoflurane, desflurane, enflurane *Inhalational anaesthesia*	**Isoflurane**: mild negative inotropic effect, marked decrease in systemic vascular resistance leading to a decrease in mean arterial pressure/hypotension. Causes a reflex tachycardia. Decreases coronary vascular resistance hence in presence of fixed coronary stenosis may cause coronary steal syndrome. However, commonly used during cardiac surgery at low concentrations and high flow rates. Cardiovascular side effects reduced when less than 1.0 MAC (minimum active concentration) are used. *Occasionally reported*: arrhythmias, tachycardia, hypotension	All inhalational agents are shown to prolong QTc. Order of prolongation sevoflurane > halothane > isoflurane. Isoflurane may even shorten QTc (desflurane unknown) All cause dose-dependent cardiorespiratory depression **Sevoflurane**: has little effect on the heart rate and does not sensitize the myocardium to circulating catecholamines. Does not cause 'coronary steal' so ideal choice for patients with ischaemic heart disease *(degree of hypotension may provide an indication of depth of anaesthesia)*

Sevoflurane: causes a decrease in myocardial contractility and mean arterial pressure. *Very common:* bradycardia, hypotension. *Common:* tachycardia, hypertension. *Uncommon:* complete heart block, AF, arrhythmias, ventricular and supraventricular extrasystoles

Desflurane: sympathetic tone well preserved, does not sensitize the myocardium to circulating catecholamines. *Common:* bradycardia, hypertension, nodal arrhythmia, tachycardia via indirect autonomic effect. *Uncommon:* bigeminy, ECG abnormality, myocardial ischaemia, vasodilatation. Postmarketing reports indicate negative inotropism/ventricular hypokinesia, ventricular failure

Enflurane: mild negative inotropic effect, marked decrease in systemic vascular resistance leading to a decrease in mean arterial pressure/hypotension. Causes a reflex tachycardia. Decreases coronary vascular resistance. Sensitizes the myocardium to circulating catecholamines

Table A.1 (Contd.)

Drug name/class/indication	Cardiovascular effects and incidence	Special recommendations for use/notes
Halothane	Sensitizes the heart to adrenaline predisposing to cardiac arrhythmias. Bradycardia due to vagal stimulation. Depression of cardiac contractility causing hypotension due to inhibition of calcium ion flux within myocardial cells	No longer licensed in USA
Suxamethonium *Depolarizing neuromuscular-blocking drugs*	*Common:* bradycardia, tachycardia, skin flushing. *Uncommon:* hypertension, hypotension. *Rare:* ventricular arrhythmias, cardiac arrest	The action of suxamethonium on the heart may cause cardiac arrhythmias including cardiac arrest. Those taking digoxin are more prone to cardiac arrhythmias. Suxamethonium causes K⁺ release from cell and hyperkalaemia, usually transient
Naloxone *Opioid antagonist Reversal of opioid overdose*	*Common:* tachycardia. *Uncommon:* bradycardia, arrhythmia. *Rare:* on induction of anaesthesia. VT/VF cardiac arrest	Too sudden reversal can cause cardiac arrhythmia, hypertension, and cardiac arrest
Benzodiazepines (midazolam, diazepam, lorazepam, temazepam etc) *Anxiety, pre-medication, sedation, termination of seizures*	*Class effect: Uncommon:* hypotension **Midazolam:** severe CV effects have occurred, bradycardia, hypotension, vasodilatation, cardiac arrest. Life-threatening reactions are more likely in the >60 age group **Lorazepam:** *Rare:* hypertension	*Caution:* extreme care when administering (mainly IV) to very ill, elderly or those with limited pulmonary reserve due to risk of apnoea and/or cardiac arrest. Rapid withdrawal of prolonged therapy can lead to symptoms of tachycardia, palpitations, mild hypertension, and orthostatic hypotension besides other non-CV symptoms

Local anaesthesia toxicity—cardiac uses mentioned elsewhere

Generally CV system effects are depressant; Hypotension, bradycardia, myocardial depression, and cardiac arrest. CNS effects can be excitatory or depressant but usually manifest as nervousness, tremor, blurred vision, nausea and vomiting, followed by drowsiness, convulsions, coma, and possibly respiratory arrest

Systemic toxicity usually manifests with CNS and CV symptoms Raised plasma concentrations occur mainly from accidental intravascular injection, excessive dosage, or rapid absorption

Table A.2 Antibiotics

Drug name/class/indication	Cardiovascular effects and incidence	Special recommendations for use/notes
β-lactam (ertapenem) *Inhibits bacterial cell wall synthesis following attachment to the penicillin-binding proteins*	Side effects noted in those aged over 18 years *Uncommon:* sinus bradycardia, hypotension, chest pain. *Rare:* arrhythmia, tachycardia, syncope, hypertension, AF	
Macrolides (erythromycin, azithromycin, clarithromycin, roxithromycin, telithromycin) *Appear to inhibit protein synthesis in susceptible organisms by reversible binding to 50S ribosomal subunit of the 70S ribosome. Some metabolites also have antibacterial action*	Erythromycin: prolonged QT has rarely been reported in patients receiving IV erythromycin Azithromycin: palpitations, hypotension, arrhythmias, VT, torsades de pointes and prolonged QT Clarithromycin: *Rare:* prolonged QT, VT, torsades de pointes Telithromycin: *Uncommon:* palpitations. *Rare:* atrial arrhythmias, hypotension, bradycardia. *Unknown frequency:* prolonged QT, VT, torsades de pointes Roxithromycin: *Unknown frequency:* prolonged QT, VT, torsades de pointes	Macrolides: due to potential to prolong QT care should be taken with coronary heart disease, history of ventricular arrhythmias, bradycardia <50ppm, low K^+ or Mg^{2+}, administration of drugs that prolong QT or CYP34A inhibitors Erythromycin: *Caution with drugs known to prolong the QT. Contraindicated with certain specific drugs known to prolong QT* (astemizole, terfenadine, cisapride) Clarithromycin: *Contraindicated when patient is receiving either cisapride, pimozide, or terfenadine due to raised drug levels and QT prolongation* Telithromycin and roxithromycin: *Contraindicated in those with congenital or acquired LQTS and in those with a family history of LQTS if not excluded by an ECG*

Vancomycin
Inhibition of cell-wall biosynthesis. In addition, vancomycin may alter bacterial cell-membrane permeability and RNA synthesis

Hypotension. Local phlebitis at the site of injection hence recommended to go through central line

Symptoms can be reduced with slow IV infusion. Bradycardia noted in animal studies in large doses

Daptomycin
Binds to cell membranes and causes depolarization. Result is rapid inhibition of protein, DNA, and RNA synthesis

Uncommon: hypertension, hypotension, SVT, extrasystoles

Quinupristin with dalfopristin
Inhibit bacterial protein synthesis

Uncommon: chest pain, palpitations, tachycardia, hypotension, phlebitis

Drugs that are metabolized by cytochrome P450 3A4 enzyme system and are known to prolong the QT should be avoided

Sulphonamides (co-trimoxazole)
Competitively inhibits the utilization of para-aminobenzoic acid in the synthesis of dihydrofolate by the enzyme dihydropteroate synthase in the bacterial cell

Co-trimoxazole: allergic myocarditis reported

Table A.2 (Contd.)

Drug name/class/indication	Cardiovascular effects and incidence	Special recommendations for use/notes
Rifampicin *Interacts with bacterial DNA-dependent RNA polymerase*		Potent enzyme inducer of P450 system resulting in decreased plasma levels of many drugs. In overdose: hypotension, sinus tachycardia, ventricular arrhythmias. Seizures and cardiac arrest were reported in some fatal cases
Dapsone	*Uncommon:* tachycardia	*Caution with CVD*
Quinolones (ciprofloxacin, gemifloxacin, gatifloxacin, levofloxacin, moxifloxacin, norfloxacin, oxofloxacin, sparfloxacin) *Inhibits topoisomerase II (a bacterial DNA gyrase)*	**Ciprofloxacin:** *Rare:* hypotension, syncope, vasodilatation, tachycardia. *Unknown:* ventricular arrhythmias, prolonged QT, torsades de pointes **Moxifloxacin:** causes QT prolongation by 6ms ± 26ms. Common when hypokalaemia present. *Uncommon:* palpitations, tachycardia, AF, angina, vasodilatation. *Rare:* ventricular tachyarrhythmias, syncope, hypertension, hypotension. *Very rare:* unspecified arrhythmias, torsades de pointes, cardiac arrest **Norfloxacin:** *Very rare:* prolonged QTc, ventricular arrhythmias including torsades de pointes **Sparfloxacin:** *Common:* prolonged QTc. *Rare:* bradycardia, tachycardia, VT and ventricular arrhythmias including torsades de pointes **Gemifloxacin, gatifloxacin, levofloxacin:** *Rare:* tachycardia. *Unknown frequency:* prolonged QTc, possible risk of ventricular arrhythmias including torsades de pointes	**Fluoroquinolones:** *Caution* in patients with known risk factors for prolonged QT interval, e.g. drugs that prolong QT, congenital or acquired long QT, electrolyte imbalances, elderly, cardiac disease, such as HF, myocardial infarct, bradycardia **Ciprofloxacin:** associated with QT prolongation, *caution* in treating those at risk of torsades de pointes **Moxifloxacin:** *Contraindicated* in congenital and acquired prolonged QT, and with other drugs that prolong the QT. Clinically significant bradycardia, previous history of symptomatic arrhythmia, and significant HF with reduced ejection fraction. *Caution* in patients undergoing proarrhythmic conditions such as myocardial ischaemia If arrhythmias develop during treatment the drug should be stopped

Norfloxacin: *Caution* in patients with hypokalaemia, significant bradycardia, or undergoing concurrent treatment with class Ia or class III antiarrhythmics. *Caution* in acquired or congenital QT prolongation and in concomitant use of drugs that prolong the QT

Sparfloxacin: *Contraindicated* in congenital and acquired prolonged QT, and with antiarrhythmic drugs amiodarone, sotolol, and bepridil. Advise avoidance with any drugs that prolong QT, bradycardia, AV conduction defects, low K^+, or Mg^{2+}

650 APPENDIX **Non-cardiac drugs affecting the heart**

Antifungals

Very common (≥1/10), common (≥1/100 and <1/10), uncommon (≥1/1000 and <1/100), rare (≥1/10,000 and <1/1000), very rare (<1/10,000 and isolated reports) (see Table A.3).

Table A.3 Antifungals

Drug name/class/ indication	Cardiovascular effects and incidence	Special recommendations for use/notes
Amphotericin (AmBisome®, amphotericin B) *Thought to act by binding to ergosterol, a fungal membrane sterol not found in animal cells, resulting in a change in membrane permeability, allowing leakage of a variety of small molecules*	**AmBisome®**: *Common:* chest pain/tightness, tachycardia, hypotension, vasodilatation. *Not known:* cardiac arrest, arrhythmias **Amphotericin B**: *Rare:* tachycardia, hypertension, hypotension. *Very rare:* cardiac arrest, hypokalaemia (often severe)	Mammalian cell membranes also contain sterols, and it has been suggested that the damage to human cells and fungal cells caused by amphotericin B may share common mechanisms
Triazole antifungals (fluconazole, itraconazole, posaconazole, voriconazole) *Highly specific inhibitors of fungal cytochrome P4503A.*	**Fluconazole**: QT prolongation, torsades de pointes **Voriconazole**: *Very common:* oedema. *Common:* chest pain. *Uncommon:* VF, ventricular arrhythmia, syncope, supraventricular arrhythmia, SVT, sinus tachycardia, bradycardia, QTc prolongation on ECG. *Rare:* torsades de pointes, VT, complete heart block, bundle branch block, nodal rhythm	**Itraconazole, voriconazole**: HF CSM advice **Triazole antifungals** have been associated with QT prolongation. They should be used with *caution* in those with congenital or acquired prolonged QT, bradycardia, existing symptomatic arrhythmias, and cardiomyopathy particularly when HF present, and with medications known to prolong the QT (either metabolized or not through CY34A)
Flucytosine (a fluorinated pyrimidine) *Acts as a competitive inhibitor of uracil metabolism* *Inhibits thymidylate synthase and DNA synthesis*	*Uncommon:* myocardial toxicity, cardiac arrest, ventricular dysfunction	

Antivirals

Very common (≥1/10), common (≥1/100 and <1/10), uncommon (≥1/1000 and <1/100), rare (≥1/10,000 and <1/1000), very rare (<1/10,000 and isolated reports) (see Table A.4).

Table A.4 Antivirals

Drug name/class/ indication	Cardiovascular effects and incidence	Special recommendations for use/notes
Antiretroviral treatment *HIV infection* *Protease inhibitors and nucleoside reverse transcriptase inhibitors (stavudine especially in combination with didanosine), lesser extent zidovudine*		Lipodystrophy syndrome: insulin resistance, dyslipidaemia, fat redistribution
Protease inhibitors *HIV infection* **(amprenavir, atazanavir, darunavir, indinavir, lopinavir, nelfinavir, ritonavir, saquinavir)**	**Atazanavir:** dose-related asymptomatic prolongation of PR interval noted in clinical studies. Use with *caution* with pre-existing conduction disturbance (2nd- and higher-degree AV block, QT prolongation), or drugs that affect conduction. *Uncommon:* hypertension, syncope, chest pain. *Rare:* oedema, palpitations **Darunavir:** *Uncommon:* MI, angina pectoris, prolonged QT, sinus bradycardia, tachycardia, palpitations **Lopinavir and ritonavir:** asymptomatic prolonged PR interval (11.6–24.4ms mean increase) in some healthy adult subjects. *Rare:* 2nd- and 3rd-degree heart block in those with structural heart disease or those taking drugs known to prolong the PR. *Uncommon:* palpitations, pulmonary oedema, MI	**Darunavir, lopinavir, ritonavir:** inhibit cytochrome CYP3A. Drugs which are cleared through this system and can therefore build up to high and dangerous plasma levels are *contraindicated* (amiodarone, bepridil, quinidine, systemic lidocaine, simvastatin) **Lopinavir and ritonavir:** *Caution:* with drugs known to prolong the PR or QT interval. May increase plasma digoxin levels

Table A.4 (Contd.)

Drug name/class/indication	Cardiovascular effects and incidence	Special recommendations for use/notes
Other antiretrovirals (maraviroc) *Entry inhibitor (also known as fusion inhibitor)* *HIV infection*	**Maraviroc**: *Common*: Postural hypotension, *Uncommon*: myocardial ischaemia, MI	*Caution* in those with CVD
Aciclovir *Synthetic acyclic purine nucleoside analogue with in vitro and in vivo inhibitory activity against the following: for treatment and prophylaxis against HSV-1, HSV-2, varicella zoster virus (VZV) and Epstein–Barr virus (EBV) highly selective, can also be used for cytomegalovirus (CMV)*	*Uncommon*: hypotension, palpitations	
Ganciclovir, foscarnet *Viral DNA polymerase inhibitors* *Treatment of CMV infection*	**Ganciclovir**: *Uncommon*: arrhythmias, hypotension **Foscarnet**: electrolyte disturbances (hypokalaemia, hypomagnesaemia, hypocalcaemia, hypophosphataemia. Abnormal ECG (1%); hypertension (4%); hypotension (2%); ventricular arrhythmias	
Ribavirin *Nucleoside antimetabolite drug* *Treatment of respiratory syncytial virus*	*Rare*: SVT when used in patients treated with peginterferon alfa-2a for hepatitis C. *Common*: tachycardia, palpitations, peripheral oedema. *Uncommon*: hypertension. *Rare*: endocarditis, MI, congestive HF, angina, SVT, AF, pericarditis	Those with pre-existing cardiac disease (MI, congestive cardiac failure, arrhythmias) should be closely monitored. Recommend ECG prior to treatment

Antimalarials and antiparasitics

Very common (≥1/10), common (≥1/100 and <1/10), uncommon (≥1/1000 and <1/100), rare (≥1/10,000 and <1/1000), very rare (<1/10,000 and isolated reports) (see Table A.5).

Table A.5 Antimalarials and antiparasitics

Drug name/class/indication	Cardiovascular effects and incidence	Special recommendations for use/notes
Artemether with lumefantrine *Treatment of falciparum malaria*	**Artemether, lumefantrine:** *Very common:* palpitations. *Common:* QT prolongation (seen in both adults and children)	*Contraindicated* in patients taking drugs metabolized through cytochrome CYP2D6 (e.g. flecainide, metoprolol etc). History or family history of congenital prolongation of the QTc or condition/drugs known to prolong QTc. History of symptomatic cardiac arrhythmias, bradycardia, or congestive cardiac failure (CCF) when accompanied by reduced ejection fraction
Chloroquine *Chemoprophylaxis and treatment of malaria*	Hypotension (by IV route) and ECG changes at high doses, cardiomyopathy long-term high-dose therapy. *Unknown frequency:* fatal arrhythmias (torsades de pointes) at high doses	**Chloroquine** and **hydroxychloroquine** increase the risk of cardiac arrhythmias (ventricular arrhythmias, bradycardias, and cardiac-conduction defects) when given to patients taking amiodarone
Mefloquine *Prophylaxis and treatment of falciparum malaria*	**Mefloquine:** circulatory disturbance (hypotension, syncope, hypertension, flushing), chest pain, tachycardia/palpitations, bradycardia, irregular pulse, and other transient cardiac conduction disturbance	*Contraindicated* with halofantrine due to potentially fatal prolongation of the QTc. Clinically significant QTc prolongation not found with **mefloquine** alone. Theoretical risk of QTc prolongation with antiarrhythmic agents, β-blockers, Ca^{2+}-channel antagonists, antihistamines, tricyclic antidepressants, and phenothiazines
Proguanil/atovaquone *Prophylaxis and treatment of falciparum malaria*	**Proguanil/atovaquone:** *Uncommon:* palpitations. *Unknown:* tachycardia	

Table A.5 (Contd.)

Drug name/class/indication	Cardiovascular effects and incidence	Special recommendations for use/notes
Quinine *Prophylaxis and treatment of malaria*	Hypotension, QT prolongation (level of prolongation related to peak plasma concentrations), cardiac arrhythmias including VT and torsades de pointes	Avoid CYP3A4 inhibitors *Contraindicated* in those with acute or acquired prolongation of QT Use with caution in those with AF due to paradoxical increase in ventricular rate or other serious heart disease Potentiates the effects of digoxin in plasma by up to 100%. Increases plasma concentration of flecainide
Halofantrine *Resistant malaria*	Chest pain, palpitations, postural hypotension, QT prolongation, torsades de pointes, cardiac arrhythmias	ECG monitoring recommended before and during treatment. The drug should therefore not be given to patients with QT prolongation or those taking QT-prolonging drugs. It should not be combined with mefloquine No longer licensed in USA
Sodium stibogluconate *Treatment of leishmaniasis*	Dose-related prolongation of QT interval. Fatal cardiac arrhythmias at higher doses. Other ECG abnormalities; reduction in T-wave amplitude, T-wave inversion	ECG monitoring recommended before and during treatment. If not available, serious consideration of risk/benefit should be made *Caution* in CVD, ventricular arrhythmias, and prolonged QT
Pentamidine isetionate Pneumocystis pneumoniae, *leishmaniasis,* Trypanosoma gambiense	Fatalities due to severe hypotension and cardiac arrhythmias noted during administration. Torsades de pointes, QT prolongation	Use with *caution* in CVD, ventricular arrhythmias, bradycardia (<50bpm). Anything that prolongs QTc. Cardiac monitoring if QTc >500ms during administration. Use alternative agent if QTc >550ms. Give lying down, correction of electrolyte abnormalities (Mg^{2+}, K^+) prior to administration

Endocrinology

Very common ($\geq 1/10$), common ($\geq 1/100$ and $<1/10$), uncommon ($\geq 1/1000$ and $<1/100$), rare ($\geq 1/10,000$ and $<1/1000$), very rare ($<1/10,000$ and isolated reports) (see Table A.6).

Table A.6 Endocrinology

Drug name/class/indication	Cardiovascular effects and incidence	Special recommendations for use
Levothyroxine sodium *Treatment for thyroid deficiency*	Tachycardia, palpitations, cardiac arrhythmias, anginal pain, cardiac hypertrophy	*Extreme caution* with CVD, angina, MI, HF. Start with low dose and titrate up slowly
Corticosteroids	Palpitations, hypertension, oedema, HF. Very rare: intracranial hypertension with papilloedema (mainly in children, usually after withdrawal), thromboembolism	*Caution* with hypertension, recent MI (ventricular rupture reported), congestive cardiac failure
Tibolone, ethinylestradiol *Hormone-replacement therapy in postmenopausal women*	**Tibolone/ethinylestradiol:** possible increase in CV morbidity in 1st year. Increased risk of stroke in 1st year	*Contraindicated* in any form of thromboembolic disease arterial (MI, angina, TIA, stroke), and venous (deep vein thrombosis (DVT), pulmonary embolism)
Testosterone	Hypertension, oedema	Use with caution in hypertension
Danazol	Oedema, hypertension, palpitations, tachycardia. Thrombotic events such as venous sagittal sinus thrombosis and arterial thrombosis reported, thromboembolism, MI	
Anabolic steroids (nandrolone) *Osteoporosis with and without fractures*	Cardiac hypertrophy, oedema, sudden death	*Caution* in cardiac failure. May occasionally cause sodium and water retention

Posterior pituitary hormones and antagonists

Vasopressin agonists
(vasopressin, desmopressin, terlipressin)

Vasopressin: angina/myocardial ischaemia, decreased cardiac output, arrhythmias, oedema, hypertension, QT prolongation, torsades de pointes
Terlipressin: increased BP (3%), bradycardia (0.4%), isolated reports MI, LVF

Vasopressin: *Caution with vascular disease, CAD*
Desmopressin: *Contraindicated in cardiac insufficiency and other cardiac conditions treated with diuretics*

Bisphosphonates (disodium pamidronate, alendronic acid, risedronate, zoledronic acid)
Osteoporosis, Paget's disease of the bone, bone pain and osteolytic lesions, hypercalcaemia of malignancy

Uncommon: hypertension, hypotension, increased incidence of AF in women

Bromocriptine
Ergot derivative
Inhibits release of prolactin
Treatment of Parkinson's disease

Uncommon: hypotension, orthostatic hypotension. *Rare:* pericardial effusion, constrictive pericarditis, tachycardia, bradycardia, arrhythmia

Contraindicated: hypertension, non-life-threatening conditions with history of coronary artery disease or serious cardiac condition
Monitor for dyspnoea, persistent cough, chest pain, cardiac failure, abdominal pain/tenderness
Cardiac failure can be a presentation of constrictive pericarditis and valvular fibrosis

Gonadorelin analogues
Analogues of gonadotrophin-releasing hormone
Evaluating the functional capacity and response of the gonadotrophs of the anterior pituitary

Rare: palpitations, tachycardia (often as part of a hypersensitivity reaction), hypertension, flushing

Table A.6 (Contd.)

Drug name/class/indication	Cardiovascular effects and incidence	Special recommendations for use
Metyrapone *Competitive inhibitor of steroid 11β-hydroxylase in the adrenal cortex used in the diagnosis of adrenal insufficiency* *Hydroxylation in the adrenal cortex resulting in inhibition of cortisol production*	Occasional dizziness and hypotension reported	
Aminoglutethimide *Inhibits the enzymatic conversion of cholesterol to Δ5-pregnenolone, resulting in a decrease in the production of adrenal glucocorticoids, mineralocorticoids, oestrogens, and androgens*	*Uncommon:* hypotension/orthostatic hypotension, tachycardia	
Somatomedins **Mecasermin** *Recombinant human insulin-like growth factor-I*	Found on investigation: *Common:* cardiac murmur, abnormal echocardiogram, cardiomegaly, ventricular hypertrophy, atrial hypertrophy, tachycardia, paroxysmal tachycardia, mitral valve incompetence, tricuspid valve incompetence, chest discomfort	CV examination, ECG and echo pre- and post-treatment recommended. If found to be abnormal or symptomatic, regular follow-up is required, during and post treatment
Agalsidase *Recombinant human α galactosidase A. For treatment of Fabry disease*	*Common:* tachycardia, palpitations, hypertension, flushing, bradycardia, hypotension *Rare:* cardiomegaly	In advanced Fabry disease, patients may have compromised cardiac function so may be at higher risk from transfusion reactions and side effects

Thiazolidinediones (rosiglitazone, pioglitazone) *Treatment of type II diabetes mellitus particularly in overweight patients. Bind to peroxisome proliferator-activated receptors*	Dose-dependent fluid retention When **rosiglitazone** is combined with **metformin** and **sulphonylurea** the combination commonly results in HF as a side effect. The same occurs with **pioglitazone** and **insulin**	*Contraindications:* HF or history of HF (NYHA I–IV) due to exacerbation by fluid retention, acute coronary syndrome (STEMI, NSTEMI, unstable angina). The use of **rosiglitazone** may be associated with increased risk of serious myocardial ischaemic events
Vitamin D **Ergocalciferol**	Late signs of hypercalcaemia; hypertension, tachyarrhythmias	Generally symptoms come from hypercalcaemia due to excessive consumption of ergocalciferol
Ginkgo biloba	Hypotension, bradycardia	

Obstetrics and gynaecology

Very common (≥1/10), common (≥1/100 and <1/10), uncommon (≥1/1000 and <1/100), rare (≥1/10,000 and <1/1000), very rare (<1/10,000 and isolated reports) (see Table A.7).

Table A.7 Obstetrics and gynaecology

Drug name/class/indication	Cardiovascular effects and incidence	Special recommendations for use/notes
Prostaglandins and oxytocics (oxytocin) *Induction of labour, post caesarean section/termination*	**Oxytocin:** *Very common:* when given as a bolus can cause acute short-lived hypotension and flushing with reflex tachycardia. *Common:* tachycardia, bradycardia. *Uncommon:* arrhythmias, hypertension	**Gemeprost:** *Caution in those with CV insufficiency.* Potentially fatal CV accidents reported in patients taking prostaglandins including gemeprost (MI, coronary artery spasm, severe hypotension)
Gemeprost *Softening and dilation of cervix, therapeutic termination of pregnancy*	**Gemeprost:** chest pain, palpitations reported. *Very rare:* coronary artery spasm, severe hypotension with subsequent MI	**Ergometrine:** ergot alkaloid. *Contraindicated in hypertension, occlusive vascular disorders, Prinzmetal's variant angina, severe cardiac failure.* Can cause widespread vasoconstriction and coronary artery spasm
Ergometrine *Active management of 3rd stage of labour, post partum haemorrhage*	**Ergometrine:** those with coronary artery disease or Prinzmetal's variant angina can develop angina and MI caused by coronary	**Dinoprostone/carboprost:** *Contraindicated in active cardiac disease*
Dinoprostone *Oxytocic agent for termination of pregnancy, missed abortion*	vasospasm. Cardiac arrhythmias, palpitations, bradycardia, chest pain, and coronary artery spasm with very rare reports of MI reported. Hypertension, dyspnoea and pulmonary oedema also reported	**Carboprost:** *Caution in hypotension, hypertension, CVD*
Carboprost *Postpartum haemorrhage*	**Dinoprostone:** hypertension, transient vasovagal symptoms reported. Cardiac arrest reported (unknown context ? hypersensivity reaction)	Decreased arterial oxygen saturation noted with use (relationship unknown) Monitor and give supplemental oxygen as necessary
Carbetocin *Uterine atony following caesarean section under epidural/ spinal*		Prostaglandins (E2) in this class can cause an SIADH (syndrome of inappropriate antidiuretic hormone) effect so causing salt and water retention **Carbetocin:** *Contraindicated in serious CV disorders*

Table A.7 (Contd.)

Drug name/class/indication	Cardiovascular effects and incidence	Special recommendations for use/notes
	Carboprost: *Uncommon:* hypertension, dyspnoea and pulmonary oedema, dizziness. *Very rare:* CV collapse reported **Carbetocin:** *Very common:* hypotension, flushing. *Common:* chest pain, dyspnoea. *Reported:* severe hypertension noted following caudal block anaesthesia	
Drugs for erectile dysfunction, prostaglandin E1, (alprostadil) *Also used for maintaining ductus arteriosus patency*	**Alprostadil:** *Common:* hypertension. *Uncommon:* vasodilatation, hypotension, extrasystole	
Phosphodiesterase type-5 inhibitors (sildenafil, tadalafil, vardenafil) *Erectile dysfunction*	**Sildenafil:** *Uncommon:* palpitations, tachycardia, chest pain. *Rare:* MI, AF, CVA, syncope, hypertension, hypotension. *Unknown:* TIA, ventricular arrhythmia, unstable angina, sudden cardiac death **Tadalafil:** *Common:* flushing, palpitations. *Uncommon:* hypotension, hypertension, tachycardia, chest pain. *Rare:* MI, stroke, TIA, syncope. *Unknown:* ventricular arrhythmia, unstable angina, sudden cardiac death	Serious cardiac events have been reported mainly in those with pre-existing CV risk factors. These include MI, unstable angina, sudden cardiac death, ventricular arrhythmia, hypertension, hypotension, TIA, cerebrovascular haemorrhage Should not be used in men for whom sexual activity is inadvisable **Nitrates must not be taken within 48h of PDE-5 inhibitors**

Vardenafil: prolongs QT by 8–10ms depending on dose, additive effect with other medication known to prolong QT. *Uncommon:* hypertension, hypotension, palpitations, tachycardia, dyspnoea. *Rare:* syncope, angina, myocardial ischaemia. *Unknown:* MI

Sildenafil: *Contraindicated:* with nitrates due to additive effect on hypotension (class effect). Recent MI, stroke, hypotension (BP <90/50). *Caution:* in those taking α-blockers due to hypotension (class effect). Caution in those with fixed cardiac output (class effect)

Tadalafil: *Contraindicated:* MI within 90 days, NYHA grade 2 or above in last 6 months, unstable angina, stroke in last 6 months, uncontrolled hypertension, hypotension (<90/50mmHg)

Vardenafil: as above, avoid use in those with risk factors for prolonged QT including medication and known prolonged QT

Mifepristone

Antiprogestogenic steroid. Medical termination of pregnancy, softening and dilation of cervix

Uncommon: hypotension

Avoid in prosthetic heart valves and history of endocarditis

Myometrial relaxants

Atosiban

Uncomplicated premature labour

Atosiban: *Common:* tachycardia, hot flush, hypotension

Table A.7 (Contd.)

Drug name/class/indication	Cardiovascular effects and incidence	Special recommendations for use/notes
Combined oral contraceptives	Hypertension, oedema, palpitations, venous deep thrombosis, pulmonary embolism, MI	Reasons to immediately stop include: sudden severe chest pain, 'stomach pain' or breathlessness (possibility of MI or pulmonary embolism (PE)). BP above 160mmHg systolic or 100mmHg diastolic, unexplained leg swelling (possibility of DVT) *Cautions:* risk factors for arterial disease, risk factors for venous thromboembolic event (VTE)
Hormone replacement therapy (HRT) (combined formulations)	Increased risk of coronary heart disease with combined HRT if started >10 years after menopause	Reasons to immediately stop include: sudden severe chest pain, 'stomach pain' or breathlessness (possibility of MI or PE), BP above 160mmHg systolic or 100mmHg diastolic, unexplained leg swelling (possibility of DVT)
Progestogen only contraceptives	Tendency to VTE, hypertension, palpitations, oedema	Suitable for those who are smokers, hypertensive, diabetic, and who have valvular heart disease and age >50 years *Contraindicated* in patients with DVT and PE
Indometacin (NSAID) *Closure of patent ductus arteriosus, rheumatoid arthritis, gout*	Reports of oedema, hypertension, hypotension, tachycardia, chest pain, arrhythmia, palpitations, cardiac failure	*Contraindicated:* severe HF

Antimigraine drugs

Very common (≥1/10), common (≥1/100 and <1/10), uncommon (≥1/1000 and <1/100), rare (≥1/10,000 and <1/1000), very rare (<1/10,000 and isolated reports) (see Table A.8).

Table A.8 Antimigraine drugs

Drug name/class/ indication	Cardiovascular effects and incidence	Special recommendations for use/notes
Antimigraine drugs (eletriptan, frovatriptan, naratriptan, rizatriptan, sumatriptan, zolmitriptan). 5-HT$_{1D}$ receptor agonists	5-HT$_1$ receptor agonists have been associated with coronary vasospasm. In rare cases, myocardial ischaemia or infarction have been reported with 5-HT$_1$ receptor agonists including in patients without any underlying CVD *Class effect:* chest pain, sensations of heaviness, tightness and pressure, dyspnoea, throat tightness. If thought that symptoms are coming from the CV system treatment should stop immediately and evaluation be carried out **Eletriptan:** *Common:* palpitations, tachycardia. *Uncommon:* bradycardia, syncope, hypertension **Frovatriptan:** *Uncommon:* palpitations, tachycardia. *Rare:* bradycardia **Naratriptan:** *Uncommon:* bradycardia, tachycardia, palpitations. *Very rare:* coronary artery vasospasm, transient ECG changes, angina, MI **Rizatriptan:** *Common:* palpitations, tachycardia, hypertension. *Rare:* myocardial ischaemia, infarction, CVA (mainly reported in patients with risk factors for CAD) **Sumatriptan:** *Common:* transient increase in BP after treatment. *Very rare:* bradycardia, tachycardia, palpitations, cardiac arrhythmias, transient ischaemic ECG changes, coronary artery vasospasm, angina, MI, hypotension **Zolmitriptan:** *Common:* palpitations. *Uncommon:* tachycardia, transient increase in BP. *Very rare:* angina pectoris, coronary vasospasm, MI	**Eletriptan, frovatriptan, naratriptan, sumatriptan, zolmitriptan:** *Caution in conditions which predispose to coronary artery disease, in postmenopausal women and men who are heavy smokers or undergoing use of nicotine substitution therapy. Contraindicated in ischaemic heart disease, previous MI, coronary vasospasm including Prinzmetal's angina, uncontrolled hypertension, WPW or arrhythmias associated with accessory pathway, TIA and stroke. **Rizatriptan:** as above but further caution in bundle branch block, diabetes, hypertension, and strong family history of CAD*

Ergot alkaloids (ergotamine tartrate) *Partial agonist of 5-HT$_{1D}$ receptor*	Due to its coronary vasoconstrictor effects it can cause myocardial ischaemia and infarction even in the absence of coronary disease and paraesthesias. *Rare:* bradycardia, tachycardia, increase in BP; ergotism and absent pulse due to intense arterial vasoconstriction. *Very rare:* myocardial ischaemia and infarction, often associated with coronary artery spasm	*Contraindications:* coronary heart disease, coronary artery spasm, uncontrolled hypertension. Patients should be warned about symptoms of myocardial ischaemia. If used for many years they may cause fibrotic changes in pleura and retroperitoneum and rarely in cardiac valves. Overdose causes 'ergotism'; intense arterial vasoconstriction mainly in peripheral vasculature but can also affect other tissues, e.g. renal, cerebral, coronary. Symptoms: numbness, cyanosis absent pulse, coma, nausea and vomiting, drowsiness, confusion, tachycardia, hypotension, convulsions, shock, coma
Cyproheptadine hydrochloride (also used as sedating antihistamine) **Methysergide** *5-HT$_2$ receptor antagonist* *Prophylaxis of migraine headaches*	**Cyproheptadine hydrochloride**: hypotension, palpitations, tachycardia, extrasystoles, anaphylactic shock **Methysergide**: *Very rare:* fibrosis of pericardium and heart valves if treated for <6 months. Risk becomes rare with long-term use. Arterial spasm—renal causing transient hypertension, coronary causing angina which rapidly resolves with drug withdrawal. Isolated reports of MI particularly in prior CAD and additional vasoconstrictor use. Increased risk of left-sided cardiac valve dysfunction	**Cyproheptadine hydrochloride**: *Caution:* CVD, hypertension due to atropine-like effect **Methysergide**: *Contraindications:* progressive atherosclerosis, CAD, inadequately controlled hypertension, valvular heart disease. Overdose: tachycardia, vasoconstriction. Fibrotic manifestations are often reversible, retroperitoneal fibrosis is less reversible

Analgesics including morphine-like drugs and non-steroidal anti-inflammatory drugs

Very common (≥1/10), common (≥1/100 and <1/10), uncommon (≥1/1000 and <1/100), rare (≥1/10,000 and <1/1000), very rare (<1/10,000 and isolated reports) (see Table A.9).

Table A.9

Drug name/class/ indication	Cardiovascular effects and incidence	Special recommendations for use/notes
Co-proxamol (dextropropoxyphene and paracetamol)	Can cause arrhythmia and conduction delay in overdose. Late signs are circulatory collapse, myocardial depression, and pulmonary oedema	No longer licensed as safety concerns due to rapid death in overdose. Can still be prescribed to patients who find change to alternative analgesic unacceptable
Opioid analgesics (pentazocine, diamorphine hydrochloride, meptazinol, methadone hydrochloride (see opioid dependence), **morphine salts, oxycodone hydrochloride, pethidine hydrochloride, tramadol hydrochloride)**	Class effect: *Very common*: hypotension. *Common*: bradycardia, tachycardia, palpitations, vasodilatation and postural hypotension. *Uncommon*: hypertension **Pentazocine**: hypertension, syncope **Diamorphine hydrochloride**: circulatory depression, shock and cardiac arrest reported although this would only be found in severe overdose or an already compromised patient **Fentanyl**: *Common*: vasodilatation. *Rare*: arrhythmias. *Very rare*: shock and asystole **Methadone**: risk of torsades de pointes **Oxycodone hydrochloride**: *Uncommon*: SVT **Tramadol hydrochloride**: *Rare*: hypertension, tachycardia, hypotension and syncope **Morphine**: bradycardia, hypotension, palpitations, syncope, tachycardia	Class effect: *Caution* in severe cor pulmonale due to respiratory depression **Pentazocine**: *Caution* after MI due to increased heart rate and BP, also caution in arterial or pulmonary hypertension and cardiac arrhythmias **Meptazinol**: safety not established for use in MI **Morphine salts, pethidine**: *Caution* with cardiac arrhythmia

Non-steroidal anti-inflammatory drugs

Very common (≥1/10), common (≥1/100 and <1/10), uncommon (≥1/1000 and <1/100), rare (≥1/10,000 and <1/1000), very rare (<1/10,000 and isolated reports) (see Table A.10).

Table A.10 NSAIDs

Drug name/ class/ indication	Cardiovascular effects and incidence	Special recommendations for use/notes
NSAIDs general	NSAIDs (including COX-2 selective) are associated with an increase in BP and peripheral oedema (*common* to *very common*)	All NSAIDs cause fluid retention and so should be avoided or used with *caution* in severe HF. Some NSAIDs, particularly when used long term and at high doses, may be associated with a small risk of arterial thrombotic events, e.g. MI, stroke
Ibuprofen, naproxen (see also **indometacin**) *Analgesics* *Thought to act as competitive inhibitors of COX-1*	When co-administered attenuates aspirin's anti-platelet effect **Naproxen**'s effect is greater than ibuprofen and $t_{1/2}$ longer	Attenuates aspirin's ability to irreversibly inhibit thromboxane production Regular NSAID + aspirin use is associated with an increase in MI relative risk compared to aspirin alone[1]
Mefenamic acid *Dysmenorrhoea, menorrhagia* **Etodolac, diclofenac, meloxicam** *Pain and inflammation in rheumatoid arthritis (RA)/ osteoarthritis (OA)*	**Mefenamic acid**: *Rare*: palpitations, hypotension, syncope **Etodolac**: *Common*: palpitations, flushing, syncope, vasculitis (allergic). Causal relationship not established: arrhythmias, MI, CVA **Diclofenac**: *Very rare*: palpitations, chest pain, cardiac failure/congestive HF, MI **Meloxicam**: *Uncommon*: palpitations	**Diclofenac**: particularly at high doses (150mg daily) and in long-term treatment may be associated with a small increased risk of arterial thrombotic events, for example, MI or stroke **Meloxicam**: *Contraindicated* in severe HF. *Caution* in uncontrolled hypertension, established ischaemic heart and peripheral vascular disease, HF. Also in those with risk factors for CVD before initiating long-term therapy

Table A.10 (Contd.)

Drug name/ class/ indication	Cardiovascular effects and incidence	Special recommendations for use/notes
COX-2 inhibitors ketorolac, parecoxib (*post-operative pain*), celecoxib, etoricoxib	**Ketorolac**: bradycardia, chest pain, flushing, palpitations, pulmonary oedema **Parecoxib**: *Common:* hypotension. *Uncommon:* bradycardia. *Rare:* tachycardia **Celecoxib**: *Common:* MI (data from the APC and PreSAP trials). *Uncommon:* HF, palpitations, tachycardia. *Not known:* arrhythmias **Etoricoxib**: *Common:* palpitations. *Uncommon:* AF, congestive HF, non-specific ECG changes, MI, stroke, TIA. *Very rare:* hypertensive crisis	**Ketorolac**: *Caution* increased bleeding time so *contraindicated* pre- and intraoperatively and in patients receiving aspirin **Parecoxib** and **etoricoxib**: *Contraindicated:* NYHA II–IV HF, established ischaemic heart disease, peripheral vascular disease, or cerebrovascular disease. Inadequately controlled hypertension (etoricoxib only), i.e. BP persistently >140/90mmHg **(Parecoxib** only): *Contraindicated* post CABG. *Caution:* significant risk factors for CVD. Use shortest course possible Absolute risk increase for MI and CVA unlikely to exceed 1% per year based on existing data

Reference

1 Kurth T *et al.* (2003). Inhibition of clinical benefits of aspirin on first MI by nonsteroidal antiinflammatory drugs. *Circulation* **108**:1191–5.

Non-steroidal anti-inflammatory drugs and exacerbation of established heart failure

Thought to exacerbate HF by several mechanisms.

Increase in afterload due to systemic vasoconstriction, this effect may antagonize the offloading effect of ACEIs and hence reduce their beneficial effects.

Increased afterload further impairs myocardial contractility and cardiac output, thereby reducing renal blood flow. This causes a rebound effect (via increased antidiuretic hormone (ADH), angiotensin II, as well as noradrenaline secretion) of salt and water reabsorption by the kidney in an attempt to increase blood flow. Hyponatraemia ensues due to dilution with water and the cycle repeats as cardiac output decreases. Risk for hospitalization is dependent on NSAID consumption the week prior to admission.[1]

This effect is seen with both selective and non-selective NSAIDs. Of all those assessed in trials, celecoxib seems to be the safest when compared to the others.[2]

NSAIDs are frequently used in patients with HF and are associated with increased risk of death and CV morbidity.[3]

NSAIDs increase the risk of developing HF in patients with a history of hypertension, diabetes, or renal failure.[4] Existing CHF may worsen after use of NSAIDs by inhibition of diuretic therapy and by adverse renal effects, especially in elderly patients with renal impairment and CV comorbidity and with a history of heavy diuretic use. Furthermore, it has been shown that there is a dose-dependent increase in risk of death and increased risk of hospitalization because of MI and HF.[4]

NSAIDs inhibit the synthesis of renal prostaglandins I2 and E2 and they can cause sodium and water retention and blunt the response to diuretics.

Naproxen is probably the best tolerated, but it still increases fluid retention.[3]

Patients with HF should, if possible, avoid using NSAIDs, and if they do need to use one, they should take an agent that is more COX-1 selective, in as low a dosage and for as short a period as possible.[3,4]

References

1 Page J, Henry D (2000). Consumption of NSAIDs and the development of congestive heart failure in elderly patients: an underrecognized public health problem. *Arch Intern Med* **160**(6):777–84.
2 Hudson M et al. (2005). Differences in outcomes of patients with congestive heart failure prescribed celecoxib, rofecoxib, or non-steroidal anti-inflammatory drugs: population based study. *BMJ* **330**:1370.
3 Gislason GH et al. (2009). Increased mortality and CV morbidity associated with use of nonsteroidal anti-inflammatory drugs in chronic HF. *Arch Intern Med* **169**:141–9. [This reference includes both COX-1 and COX-2 inhibitors]
4 Scott PA et al. (2008). Non-steroidal anti-inflammatory drugs and cardiac failure: meta-analyses of observational studies and randomised controlled trials. *Eur J Heart Fail* **10**:1102–7.

COX-2 inhibitors and cardiovascular risk

Selective COX-2 inhibitors cause a reduction in prostacyclin production by vascular endothelium with little/no inhibition of platelets (they do not block thromboxane A_2 production). It is thought that the reduction in prostacyclin by the endothelium could increase its risk of damage, and hence platelet aggregation occurs at the site.

Specific drugs

Rofecoxib

Withdrawn from the market in 2004 and marked NSAIDs as a risk factor in CV events. Trial results showed that for every 139 patients treated in a year one extra event will occur (stroke, MI).[1] Risk was increased with higher doses.

Valdecoxib

Withdrawn from the market in 2005 following data showing an increased risk of CV event post CABG surgery and an increased risk of Stevens–Johnson syndrome.[2]

Celecoxib

Trial data have shown an increased risk of stroke and MI with increasing doses of celecoxib (RR 2.6 and 3.6 with 200mg *and* 400mg bd respectively).[3]

Lumiracoxib

Assessed in TARGET trial where lumiracoxib was compared to NSAIDs naproxen and ibuprofen. No significant difference was found between the groups.[4]

Etoricoxib

Assessed in the MEDAL study which compared etoricoxib and diclofenac in 34,701 arthritis (OA and RA) patients. It showed 320 and 323 CV events in the etoricoxib and diclofenac group respectively. Fewer complicated GI side effects in the etoricoxib group.[5]

References

1 Bresalier RS *et al.* (2005). Cardiovascular events associated with rofecoxib in a colorectal adenoma chemoprevention trial. *N Engl J Med* **352**:1092–102.
2 Ott E *et al.* (2003). Efficacy and safety of the cyclooxygenase 2 inhibitors parecoxib and valdecoxib in patients undergoing coronary artery bypass surgery. *J Thoracic Cardiovasc Surg* **125**:1481–92.
3 Bertagnolli MM *et al.* (2006). Celecoxib for the Prevention of Sporadic Colorectal Adenomas. *N Engl J Med* **355**:873–84.
4 Farkouh ME *et al.*; TARGET Study Group (2004). Comparison of lumiracoxib with naproxen and ibuprofen in the Therapeutic Arthritis Research and Gastrointestinal Event Trial (TARGET), cardiovascular outcomes: randomised controlled trial. *Lancet* **364**:675–84.
5 Cannon CP *et al.* (2006). MEDAL Steering Committee. Cardiovascular outcomes with etoricoxib and diclofenac in patients with osteoarthritis and rheumatoid arthritis in the Multinational Etoricoxib and Diclofenac Arthritis Long-term (MEDAL) programme: a randomised comparison. *Lancet* **368**:1771–81.

Haematological drugs

Very common (≥1/10), common (≥1/100 and <1/10), uncommon (≥1/1000 and <1/100), rare (≥1/10,000 and <1/1000), very rare (<1/10,000 and isolated reports) (see Table A.11).

Table A.11 Haematological drugs

Drug name/class/indication	Cardiovascular effects and incidence	Special recommendations for use/notes
Iron dextran *Iron-deficiency anaemia*	**Iron dextran:** *Rare:* arrhythmia, tachycardia	
Erythropoietin *Hematopoietic growth factors*	Hypertension that can cause encephalopathy, arrhythmias, congestive HF, thrombocytosis, MI, chest pain, oedema	In chronic renal failure there is an increased risk of death, serious CV events and vascular access thrombosis when erythropoiesis-stimulating agents are given when the haemoglobin (Hb) is >12g/dL Erythropoietins are *contraindicated* for increasing Hb prior to orthopaedic surgery in those with pre-existing hypertension, CVD, coronary, carotid and peripheral arterial disease, recent MI
Darbepoetin *EPO deficient states*	*Very common:* hypertension	As above
Drugs used in platelet disorders (anagrelide) *Essential thrombocythaemia*	**Anagrelide:** *Common:* palpitations, tachycardia. *Uncommon:* CHF, hypertension, arrhythmias (AF, SVT, VT), syncope. *Rare:* angina, MI, cardiomegaly, cardiomyopathy, pericardial effusion, vasodilatation, postural hypotension, and pulmonary hypertension	**Anagrelide:** *Caution:* in known or suspected heart disease. Recommend pre- and during treatment CV exam, ECHO and ECG. Inhibitor of cyclic AMP phosphodiesterase III. Has positive inotropic effect

Malignant disease and immunosuppression

Very common (≥1/10), common (≥1/100 and <1/10), uncommon (≥1/1000 and <1/100), rare (≥1/10,000 and <1/1000), very rare (<1/10,000 and isolated reports) (see Table A.12).

Table A.12 Malignant disease and immunosuppression

Drug name/class/indication	Cardiovascular effects and incidence	Special recommendations for use/notes
Anthracyclines (doxorubicin, daunorubicin, epirubicin, idarubicin, mitoxantrone) *Act by insertion into DNA causing DNA fragmentation, inhibition of polymerases, and a decrease in DNA, RNA, and protein synthesis. Acute leukaemias, Hodgkin's and non-Hodgkin's lymphomas, paediatric malignancies and some solid tumours etc*	Noted non-specific ECG changes (class effect), T-wave flattening, ST depression, and benign arrhythmias. Generally ECG changes are not an indication to stop treatment. Phlebitis when given intravenously. **Doxorubicin:** *Common:* LV dysfunction, ventricular arrhythmias. *Uncommon:* SVT related to drug administration, HF. *Rare:* pericarditis. Cardiotoxicity: see below. **Daunorubicin:** cardiotoxicity, see below. Usually appears within 16 months, may be irreversible and fatal. **Epirubicin:** cardiotoxicity several weeks after discontinuation of treatment	Risk of cardiotoxicity reduced by weekly low-dose administration. Liposomal formulations are also available which may reduce cardiotoxicity. Drugs should not be mixed and matched as accumulated dose of anthracycline is cause of cardiotoxicity rather than any one drug. Avoid concomitant use of trastuzumab as shown to increase cardiotoxicity. If used should be 24 weeks apart. ECG and ECHO advised before treatment to document function. Doxorubicin dose usually limited to maximal accumulated dose of 450mg/m². Toxicity can occur at lower doses if other risk factors present (see below). **Doxorubicin:** *Contraindicated:* Recent MI and severe arrhythmias. **Daunorubicin:** *Contraindicated:* CVD. **Epirubicin:** Maximal accumulated dose 900mg–1g/m², only exceed in extreme caution as risk of cardiotoxicity increases dramatically

Idarubicin: ECG changes as above. *Common:* tachycardia, bradycardia, tachyarrhythmias, VT, premature ventricular beats, asymptomatic reduction of LVEF, congestive HF. *Uncommon:* MI, non-specific ST changes. *Very rare:* pericarditis, myocarditis, AV and bundle branch block. Cardiotoxicity usually 2–3 months after discontinuation but late effects also noted

Mitoxantrone: HF months to years after discontinuation of treatment. Other side effects as above

Idarubicin: maximal accumulated dose 400mg/m^2 (orally). *Contraindicated:* recent MI, severe arrhythmia, myocardial insufficiency

Mitoxantrone: maximal accumulated dose 160mg/m^2

Alkylating agents (busulfan, cyclophosphamide platinum compounds)

Act by insertion into DNA causing DNA fragmentation, thus interfere with cell replication. Damage DNA thus interfere with cell replication

Busulfan: *Very common:* tachycardia, hypertension, hypotension, thrombosis, vasodilatation. *Common:* arrhythmia, AF, cardiomegaly, pericardial effusion, pericarditis. *Uncommon:* ventricular extrasystoles, bradycardia, femoral artery thrombosis, capillary leak syndrome. Cardiac tamponade at high doses in thalassaemia

Cyclophosphamide: ST-T wave changes, pericarditis, supraventricular arrhythmias. May cause cardiotoxicity especially at high doses

Etramustine: congestive HF, ischaemic heart disease, MI, hypertension, thromboembolism

Platinum compounds: oedema, tachycardia, bradycardia, hypotension, HF

Etramustine: *Caution:* CVD, coronary artery disease, congestive HF

Platinum compounds: may need the administration of corticosteroids or H$_1$ antihistamines

Table A.12 (Contd.)

Drug name/class/indication	Cardiovascular effects and incidence	Special recommendations for use/notes
Antimetabolites (capecitabine/ tegafur, cladribine, cytarabine, fludarabine, fluorouracil, gemcitabine, pemetrexed, methotrexate) *Act by preventing normal cell division by incorporating into nuclear material and irreversibly combining with cellular enzymes. Methotrexate is a folic acid antagonist*	**Capecitabine:** *Uncommon:* angina/unstable angina, myocardial ischaemia, AF, arrhythmias, tachycardia, palpitations, hypertension, hypotension, peripheral coldness, flushes **Cladribine:** *Common:* oedema, tachycardia, heart murmur **Clofarabine:** *Common:* tachycardia, pericardial effusion, pericarditis usually without haemodynamic compromise **Cytarabine:** *Very rare:* pericarditis **Fludarabine:** *Rare:* HF, arrhythmia **Fluorouracil:** reports of ECG abnormalities, breathlessness, chest pain/angina. *Rare:* MI; chest pain due to coronary spasm **Gemcitabine:** *Rare:* MI **Pemetrexed:** *Uncommon:* CV and cerebrovascular events, MI, angina, TIA, stroke **Methotrexate:** pericarditis, pericardial effusion, hypotension, and thromboembolic events (including arterial thrombosis, cerebral thrombosis, DVT, retinal vein thrombosis, thrombophlebitis, and pulmonary embolus)	**Capecitabine:** *Caution:* cardiotoxicity reported with **fluoropyrimidine**-based therapy—angina, MI, dysrhythmias, cardiogenic shock, sudden death and ECG changes. May be more common if prior history of CAD present **Fluorouracil:** *Caution:* History of heart disease and in those who experience chest pain during administration **Gemcitabine:** *Caution:* CVD **Pemetrexed:** *Caution:* CVD, especially when given with another cytotoxic agent **Methotrexate:** incidence and severity of adverse reactions related to dose and frequency of administration
Topotecan *Topoisomerase I inhibitor*	Hypotension	

Etoposide

Semisynthetic derivative of podophyllotoxin. Podophyllotoxins inhibit mitosis by blocking microtubular assembly

Inhibits topoisomerase II

Etoposide: *Uncommon:* arrhythmia, MI, hypo/hypertension

Vinca alkaloids

Anti-mitotic/microtubule agent

Vinca alkaloids: *Uncommon:* coronary vasospasm and myocardial ischaemia

Chemotherapy regimens including vinca alkaloids when given to patient with previous medastinal radiotherapy have been associated with CAD and MI. Mechanism not established

Arsenic trioxide

Acute promyelocytic leukaemia

Arsenic trioxide: *Very common:* QT prolongation. *Common:* hypokalaemia. *Uncommon:* cardiac failure, VT (torsades de pointes), ventricular extrasystoles, hypotension, chest pain, pericardial effusion, tachycardia, AF/flutter

Prior to and during therapy, electrolytes should be tightly controlled (K⁺ >4mmol/L, Mg²⁺ >0.7mmol/L)

QT prolongation: during clinical trials 40% of patients had at least 1 QTc >500ms. Occurred between weeks 1 and 5 after medication given. Returned to baseline by week 8. *Caution:* discontinue any QTc-prolonging drugs if possible. ECG at baseline followed by ECG ×2 week minimum. If syncope, or rapid or irregular heart beat develops immediate hospitalization and monitoring is required. Correct any low Mg²⁺, K⁺, Ca²⁺ and discontinuation of trioxide until QTc <460ms

Table A.12 (Contd.)

Drug name/class/indication	Cardiovascular effects and incidence	Special recommendations for use/notes
Bevacizumab *Inhibitor of vascular endothelial growth factor*	**Bevacuzumab:** *Very common:* hypertension (increase in baseline BP of up to 34%). *Common:* congestive cardiac failure, SVT. (Decline in LV function varies from asymptomatic to CHF requiring hospitalization)	*Caution:* hypertension and CVD Prior radiotherapy to left chest wall, anthracycline or other cardiotoxic therapy, previous CVD thought to contribute as risk factor for severe CV effects/CHF Those with worse CHF in clinical studies had metastatic breast cancer + other risk factors mentioned under special recommendations
Bortezomib *Treatment of multiple myeloma*	Hypotension and orthostatic hypotension occasionally causing syncope and often requiring treatment. New onset of decreased LVEF, exacerbation of HF. Isolated cases of QT prolongation reported	*Contraindicated* in diffuse infiltrative pericardial disease. *Caution* in patients treated with antihypertensive drugs and HF
Trastuzumab *Metastatic breast cancer*	*Common:* hypertension, hypotension, vasodilatation, decreased LVEF, HF, supraventricular tachyarrhythmia, cardiomyopathy, palpitation. *Uncommon:* bradycardia, pericarditis	Use associated with cardiotoxicity, risk greatest when used with anthracyclines. Due to long $t_{\frac{1}{2}}$ (28.5 days) trastuzumab may persist in the circulation for up to 24 weeks HERA trial excluded the following conditions so treatment in such conditions cannot be recommended: history of CHF, uncontrolled arrhythmias, angina requiring treatment, significant valvular disease, evidence of transmural infarction on ECG, poorly controlled hypertension

Drug	Cardiac effects	Monitoring / cautions
		All patients for treatment with trastuzumab should undergo baseline cardiac assessment, history, exam, ECG, ECHO ± MRI Formal cardiological assessment should be considered for those in whom there are CV concerns *Caution* in symptomatic HF, hypertension or coronary artery disease and in those with LVEF ≤55% If during treatment LVEF drops 10 points from baseline and to below 50%,trastuzumab should be suspended and repeat ECHO performed within approximately 3 weeks. If no improvement, discontinue treatment
Gemtuzumab *Acute myelogenous leukemia*	Hypotension, hypertension, tachycardia	
Protein kinase inhibitors (dasatinib, imatinib, lapatinib, nilotinib, sorafenib, sunitinib) **Dasatinib** *Chronic myeloid leukaemia* **Imatinib** *Chronic myelogenous leukaemia* **Lapatinib** *Breast cancer* **Nilotinib** *GI stromal tumors*	All these compounds can prolong the QT interval and may produce cardiac arrhythmias **Dasatinib:** *Common:* congestive HF, cardiac dysfunction, pericardial effusion, arrhythmia, palpitations. *Uncommon:* MI, QTc prolongation, pericarditis, ventricular arrhythmia (VT), angina, cardiomegaly. *Rare:* cor pulmonale, myocarditis, ACS **Imatinib:** *Uncommon:* palpitations, tachycardia, congestive cardiac failure, peripheral and pulmonary oedema. *Rare:* arrhythmia (including AF), cardiac arrest, MI, angina, pericardial effusion. *Unknown:* pericarditis, cardiac tamponade	**Dasatinib:** *Caution:* with any cause of QTc prolongation. Recommend correcting electrolytes and stopping any drugs which can prolong QT. Not tested on patients with significant CVD. Increased side effects seen with increased dose **Imatinib:** cardiac events were more commonly observed in those with transformed chronic myeloid leukaemia (CML) than chronic CML **Sorafenib:** not tested on those with recent MI or unstable CAD

Table A.12 (Contd.)

Drug name/class/indication	Cardiovascular effects and incidence	Special recommendations for use/notes
Soratinib *Renal-cell carcinoma* **Sunitinib** *Renal and gastrointestinal cancer* *Tyrosine kinase inhibitors for chronic myeloid leukaemia*	**Nilotinib:** *Rare:* prolonged QT, torsades de pointes **Sorafenib:** *Common:* hypertension. *Uncommon:* myocardial ischaemia and infarction, congestive cardiac failure, hypertensive crisis **Sunitinib:** *Very common:* hypertension. *Common:* decreased ejection fraction. *Uncommon:* cardiac failure, CHF, LV failure. *Rare:* prolonged QT, torsades de pointes **Lapatinib:** QT prolongation	**Sunitinib:** *Caution:* where any cause of prolonged QT present. A decrease in LVEF of ≥ 20% and below level of normal limit was seen in 2–4% of patients depending on cancer and clinical trial
Docetaxel, paclitaxel *Stabilize microtubule structure* *Treatment of multiple types of cancer*	**Docetaxel:** *Common:* arrhythmia, myocardial ischaemia. *Uncommon:* cardiac failure	**Docetaxel:** HF observed in patients who are also taking trastuzumab (particularly following anthracycline therapy) Should undergo baseline cardiac assessment pre therapy and then every 3 months after initiation. No direct relationship found between cardiac toxicity and paclitaxel; however, CV events commonly found in those treated
Alfuzosin *α₁ receptor antagonist used to treat benign prostatic hyperplasia*	*Common:* hypotension/orthostatic hypotension. *Uncommon:* tachycardia, palpitations, syncope, chest pain, oedema. *Very rare:* new onset, aggravation or recurrence of angina pectoris in pre-existing CAD. QT prolongation	*Contraindicated:* history of orthostatic hypotension

Tamoxifen
Antagonist for the oestrogen receptor in breast tissue. Used in treatment of breast cancer

Uncommon: QT prolongation, oedema, thromboembolism. *Rare:* elevation of serum triglyceride levels

Trastuzumab
Metastatic breast cancer

Common: hypertension, hypotension, vasodilatation, decreased LVEF, heart failure, supraventricular tachyarrhythmia, cardiomyopathy, palpitation. *Uncommon:* bradycardia, pericarditis, HF class II–VI observed in patients receiving **trastuzumab** therapy alone or in combination with paclitaxel or docetaxel, and particularly following anthracycline-containing chemotherapy. This may be associated with death

The safety of continuation or resumption of **trastuzumab** in patients who experience cardiotoxicity has not been prospectively studied. However, most patients who developed heart failure in the pivotal trials improved with standard medical treatment (diuretics, cardiac glycosides, β-blockers and/or ACE inhibitors). The majority of patients with cardiac symptoms and evidence of a clinical benefit of **trastuzumab** treatment continued on weekly therapy with **trastuzumab** without additional clinical cardiac events)

Use associated with cardiotoxicity, risk greatest when used with anthracyclines. Due to **trastuzumab**'s long half-life of 28.5 days, **trastuzumab** may persist in the circulation for up to 24 weeks

HERA trial excluded the following conditions so treatment in such conditions cannot be recommended: history of CHF, uncontrolled arrhythmias, angina requiring treatment, significant valvular disease, evidence of transmural infarction on ECG, poorly controlled hypertension

All patients for treatment with **trastuzumab** should undergo baseline cardiac assessment, history, exam, ECG, ECHO +/– MRI. Further assessment should be 3 monthly during treatment and at 6, 12, and 24 months after cessation of treatment for early breast cancer patients

Formal cardiological assessment should be considered where there are cardiovascular concerns

Caution in symptomatic heart failure, hypertension or coronary artery disease, in those with LVEF ≤55%. If during treatment LVEF drops 10 points from baseline *and* to below 50%, **trastuzumab** should be suspended and repeat ECHO performed within approximately 3 weeks. If no improvement discontinue treatment

Anthracycline cardiotoxicity

Types of toxicity: arrhythmias; myocardial necrosis causing a dilated cardiomyopathy; damage to coronary arteries causing vasospasm or occlusion and culminating in ischaemia and/or infarction.

Complications can be seen acutely (during administration), soon after administration (days to weeks), and months to years later.

Toxicity is related to the cumulative dose received by the patient (strongest factor), and various other risk factors. These are previous CVD, age (children and those >70 years in higher-risk group), use of other cardiotoxic agents, in particular paclitaxel and trastuzumab. Prior irradiation to the chest (e.g. left breast cancer) and haemopoietic cell transplantation where cyclophosphamide and total body irradiation is employed. Radiation to the heart is thought to cause endothelial cell damage and compromise to coronary blood flow.

Mechanism of injury

Cardiac myocyte injury is thought to occur through production of oxygen free radicals which cause peroxidation of lipid membranes leading to vacuolation and myocyte replacement by fibrous tissue.[1] This can occur sporadically throughout the heart or only affect one area or ventricle. Hence cardiac septal biopsy may not pick up the damage.

Acute toxicity

Rare and usually resolves within a week. Unknown relationship to long-term damage. Clinically a pericarditis/myocarditis picture with ECG changes, ventricular dysfunction, and increased BNP levels in the blood. In a small RCT the use of valsartan blocked all effects of acute toxicity.[2]

Early toxicity

Typically HF occurs 3 months after last dose of anthracycline and is not related to ECG changes seen during or after therapy. Highly dependent on accumulative dose, occurs in 4% of those receiving 500–550mg/m^2 of doxorubicin, 18% with 551–600mg/m^2, and 36% with >600mg/m^2.[3] Mortality in those affected can approach 60% but has decreased with aggressive medical therapy (β-blockade and ACEI). Diuretics and digoxin also noted to be of some benefit. The acute ECG changes are usually reversible, unrelated to total dose, return to baseline readings within a few months, and usually are not an indication to discontinue the drug.

Late toxicity

HF can occur over a decade after the last dose. Typical picture is of non-ischaemic dilated cardiomyopathy. Patient groups primarily affected are post-childhood malignancy and elderly women who receive anthracyclines as part of adjuvant chemotherapy. There is a dose-dependent cardiomyopathy (0.4–9% of all patients), which has a high mortality. Risk factors include total dose, schedule, older age, pre-existing cardiac disease, prior mediastinal radiotherapy, prior anthracyclines, and hypertension. In adults with risk factors, cardiac function monitoring (echocardiogram or MUGA scan) should be performed before treatment and periodically throughout treatment.

Symptoms described: persistent tachycardia, SOB, oedema of lower limbs, minor changes on ECG.

References

1 Singal PK, Deally CM, Weinberg LE (1987). Subcellular effects of adriamycin in the heart: a concise review. *J Mol Cell Cardiol* **19**:817–28.
2 Nakamae H *et al.* (2005). Notable effects of angiotensin II receptor blocker, valsartan, on acute cardiotoxic changes after standard chemotherapy with cyclophosphamide, doxorubicin, vincristine, and prednisolone. *Cancer* **104**:2492–8.
3 Von Hoff DD *et al.* (1977). Daunomycin-induced cardiotoxicity in children and adults. A review of 110 cases. *Am J Med* **62**:200–8.

Immunosuppression

Very common (≥1/10), common (≥1/100 and <1/10), uncommon (≥1/1000 and <1/100), rare (≥1/10,000 and <1/1000), very rare (<1/10,000 and isolated reports) (see Table A.13).

Table A.13 Immunosuppression

Drug name/class/indication	Cardiovascular effects and incidence	Special recommendations for use/notes
Ciclosporin, tacrolimus *Calcineurin inhibitors*	**Ciclosporin:** *Very common:* hypertension **Tacrolimus:** *Common:* ischaemic coronary artery disease, tachycardia. *Uncommon:* ventricular arrhythmias, cardiac arrest, HF, cardiomyopathies, ventricular hypertrophy, SVTs, palpitations, abnormal ECG, QT prolongation. *Rare:* pericardial effusion	**Tacrolimus:** increased risk of cardiac complications seen when other cardiac risk factors present; hypertension, pre-existing heart disease, corticosteroid usage. Regular ECG and ECHO recommended pre- and post-transplant when treated with tacrolimus. Most cases of LV or septal hypertrophy are reversible and occurred with higher than normal recommended dose. May prolong QT but no substantial evidence for causing torsades de pointes
Sirolimus *Macrocyclic lactone*	*Common:* tachycardia. *Uncommon:* pericardial effusion (can be haemodynamically significant)	
Monoclonal antibodies (rituximab, alemtuzumab, *RA and non-Hodgkin's lymphoma;* **daclizumab,** *immunosuppression for transplantation)* **Daclizumab** *IgG1 monoclonal antibody which binds to the p55 alpha or Tac subunit of the IL-2 receptor found on activated lymphocytes*	**Rituximab:** *Common:* MI, arrhythmia (AF, tachycardia), hypertension, hypotension. *Uncommon:* LV failure, SVT, VT, bradycardia, angina, myocardial ischaemia. *Unknown:* HF, severe cardiac events **Alemtuzumab:** *Very common:* hypotension. *Common:* bradycardia, tachycardia, hypertension, cyanosis, abnormal ECG. *Uncommon:* cardiac arrest, MI, angina, AF, SVT, extrasystoles, orthostatic hypotension **Daclizumab:** *Common:* peripheral oedema, chest pain, hypertension, hypotension, tachycardia. *Uncommon:* fluid overload	Hypotension during infusion may require antihypertensives being withheld 12h prior to infusion **Rituximab:** main side effects noted in those with pre-existing CVD. MI, HF, and severe cardiac events noted also during infusion. *Caution:* CVD **Alemtuzumab:** *Caution:* CVD, antihypertensive use. MI and cardiac arrest noted during infusion in this population

Table A.13 (Contd.)

Drug name/class/indication	Cardiovascular effects and incidence	Special recommendations for use/notes
		Daclizumab: when combined with ciclosporin, mycophenolate mofetil, and corticosteroids for cardiac transplantation may be associated with an increase in mortality mainly due to increase in severe infections
Interferon alfa and beta	**Interferon alfa:** *Uncommon:* arrhythmias (AV block), palpitations, hypertension, hypotension. *Rare:* cardiorespiratory arrest, MI, CHF, pulmonary oedema, cyanosis **Interferon alfa and beta:** *Not known and Rare* respectively: cardiomyopathy, CHF, palpitations, arrhythmias, tachycardia	**Interferon alfa:** *Contraindicated:* severe pre-existing cardiac disease or history of cardiac illness. Likely that self-limiting toxicities during infusion may exacerbate pre-existing cardiac conditions
Glatiramer acetate *Synthetic polypeptides used for reducing frequency of relapses or MS*	**Glatiramer:** *Very common:* palpitations, vasodilatation. *Common:* tachycardia. *Uncommon:* extrasystoles	**Glatiramer:** should explain to patient that vasodilatation (flushing), chest pain, dyspnoea, palpitations/tachycardia may occur within minutes of an injection. Majority of symptoms are transient and resolve spontaneously. If severe stop medication and seek emergency advice
Lenalidomide and **thalidomide** *Immunomodulating drug with anti-neoplastic, anti-angiogenic and pro-erythropoietic properties*	**Lenalidomide:** *Common:* AF, palpitations, hypertension, hypotension. *Uncommon:* CHF, pulmonary oedema, heart valve insufficiency, atrial flutter, arrhythmia, ventricular trigeminy, bradycardia, tachycardia, prolonged QT **Thalidomide:** *Common:* cardiac failure, bradycardia	**Lenalidomide:** increase digoxin levels **Thalidomide:** *Caution:* with substances known to induce torsades de pointes, β-blockers, or anticholinesterase agents due to potential for thalidomide to cause bradycardia

Etanercept
TNFα inhibitor

HF, hypertension, hypotension, myocardial ischaemia/infarction, chest pain, syncope

Contraindicated: HF

Gold salts
(gold sodium aurothiomalate)
RA

Hypotension, bradycardia

Caution: hypotension

Hormone analogues

Very common (≥1/10), common (≥1/100 and <1/10), uncommon (≥1/1000 and <1/100), rare (≥1/10,000 and <1/1000), very rare (<1/10,000 and isolated reports) (see Table A.14).

Table A.14 Hormone analogues

Drug name/class/ indication	Cardiovascular effects and incidence	Special recommendations for use/notes
Antiandrogens (bicalutamide) **Gonadotrophin-releasing hormone analogues (buserelin, goserelin, leuprorelin)** *Prostate cancer*	**Bicalutamide**: *Common:* hot flushes, hypertension, hypotension. *Uncommon:* angina, HF **Buserelin**: hypertension, palpitations	
Somatostatin analogues (octreotide) *Neuroendocrine tumours*	**Octreotide**: isolated bradycardia, QT prolongation, and risk of ventricular arrhythmias	

Respiratory system

Very common (≥1/10), common (≥1/100 and <1/10), uncommon (≥1/1000 and <1/100), rare (≥1/10,000 and <1/1000), very rare (<1/10,000 and isolated reports) (see Table A.15).

Table A.15 Respiratory system

Drug name/class/indication	Cardiovascular effects and incidence	Special recommendations for use/notes
Selective β₂ adrenoceptor agonists (e.g. formoterol fumarate, salbutamol, salmeterol, terbutaline sulphate) *Bronchodilators*	*Common:* palpitations, tachycardia, hypotension. *Rare:* arrhythmias including AF, SVT, and extrasystole. *Unknown:* myocardial ischaemia. High doses: ventricular tachyarrhythmias, sudden death	*Caution in the presence of CVD,* arrhythmias, susceptibility to QT-interval prolongation
Antimuscarinic bronchodilators (ipratropium bromide, tiotropium)	**Ipratropium bromide:** *Uncommon:* tachycardia. *Rare:* palpitations, SVT, AF. **Tiotropium:** *Rare:* tachycardia, palpitations. *Unknown:* SVT, AF	
Theophylline (theophylline, aminophylline) *Bronchodilator effects may be mediated by inhibition of cyclic nucleotide phosphodiesterase which results in increased concentrations of intracellular cAMP*	Side effects usually occur when theophylline blood levels exceed 20mcg/mL. Excessive doses may cause hypotension, tachycardia, arrhythmias (usually SVTs). In overdose, life-threatening arrhythmias can develop. Theophylline stimulates the myocardium and reduces venous pressure in congestive HF, leading to marked increase in cardiac output	*Caution should be exercised in patients* with cardiac arrhythmias and other CVD. Plasma theophylline concentration increased in HF, pulmonary oedema, and cor pulmonale. Effect on the myocardium may result from intracellular translocation of ionized calcium

Histamine H₁ receptor antagonists

Antihistamines

(astemizole, azelastine, terfenadine, diphenhydramine)

Uncommon: hypotension, tachycardia, palpitations. *Unknown*:

Azelastine: hypertension, tachycardia. AF, palpitations, chest pain

Loratadine: *Uncommon*: tachycardia, SVT, palpitations, hypertension, hypotension, syncope

Astemizole: withdrawn from licence due to QT prolongation and serious cardiac arrhythmias including torsades de pointes

Terfenadine: removed from licence in 1998 due to serious adverse cardiac events, QT prolongation and arrhythmias, including torsades de pointes

Non-sedating antihistamines (**mizolastine, loratadine**)

Symptomatic relief of allergy, hayfever and urticaria

Diphenhydramine: *Contraindicated* in severe hypertension or CAD

Mizolastine: *Contraindicated* in clinically significant cardiac disease or a history of symptomatic arrhythmias, suspected or known QT prolongation, or QT-prolonging drugs, significant bradycardia

Sedating antihistamines (chlorphenamine, clemastine, cyproheptadine hydrochloride (also used in prophylaxis of migraine)**, promethazine hydrochloride, alimemazine tartrate)**

Symptomatic relief of allergy, hayfever and urticaria H₁ antagonist, may have significant antimuscarinic activity

Chlorphenamine, clemastine, cyproheptadine hydrochloride, promethazine hydrochloride: palpitations, tachycardia, arrhythmias, extrasystoles, hypotension

Alimemazine tartrate: atrial and ventricular arrhythmias and AV block

Use with *caution* in patients with severe CAD

Cyproheptadine hydrochloride: *Caution*: CVD, hypertension due to atropine-like effect

Table A.15 (Contd.)

Drug name/class/indication	Cardiovascular effects and incidence	Special recommendations for use/notes
Respiratory stimulants (doxapram hydrochloride) *Stimulate peripheral chemoreceptors and at higher doses central receptors in the medulla*	Sinus tachycardia, bradycardia, extrasystoles, ventricular tachycardia and VF, mild to moderate increase in BP due to increase in cardiac output. Higher BP rise in those who are hypovolaemic compared to normovolaemic. Lowered T-waves, chest pain, chest tightness. Increased release of catecholamines noted	*Contraindicated* with significant CV impairment, uncompensated HF, severe coronary artery disease, severe hypertension. *Caution* with impaired cardiac reserve

Central nervous system

Very common (≥1/10), common (≥1/100 and <1/10), uncommon (≥1/1000 and <1/100), rare (≥1/10,000 and <1/1000), very rare (<1/10,000 and isolated reports).

Antipsychotic drugs (Table A.16)

Antipsychotic drugs produce conduction defects, including AV block (this is clear with phenothiazines, butyrophenones (haloperidol, droperidol), and particularly with thioxanthenes (chlorprothixene, flupentixol, thiothixene, zuclopenthixol).

Table A.16 Antipsychotic drugs

Drug name/class/indication	Cardiovascular effects and incidence	Special recommendations for use/notes
Typical antipsychotic drugs		
Act by blocking dopamine D_2 receptors. May also affect cholinergic, α-adrenergic, histaminergic, and serotonergic receptors	*Class effects: Uncommon:* dose-related hypotension. *Rare to very rare* (depending on specific drug): QT prolongation, ventricular arrhythmias (including VF and VT), torsades de pointes, and cardiac arrest	For the majority of antipsychotic drugs, caution is advised in patients with CVD, bradycardia, 2nd-3rd-degree AV block, a family history of sudden death or QT prolongation, a history of QT prolongation ventricular arrhythmias or torsades de pointes, and those prone to postural hypotension
Prochlorperazine		
Nausea and vomiting, dizziness and vertigo, anxiety, schizophrenia, and psychotic disorders	**Chlorpromazine:** ECG abnormalities reported usually benign, including widened QT interval, ST depression, U-waves, and T-wave changes. Atrial arrhythmias including AV block, torsades de pointes	ECG abnormalities can be related to dose, IV administration, and worsened with electrolyte disturbance such as hypokalaemia
Promazine hydrochloride		
Psychomotor agitation	**Droperidol:** hypotension resulting from peripheral α adrenoceptor blockade, QT prolongation, torsades de pointes	*Avoid concomitant use of QT-prolonging drugs*
Sulpiride		
Acute and chronic schizophrenia	**Haloperidol:** *Rare:* orthostatic hypotension, tachycardia, bradycardia, HF, arrhythmias, QT prolongation, and torsades de pointes	It is recommended that all patients on antipsychotic drugs have baseline ECG prior to commencing treatment. ECG monitoring is recommended and dose reduction performed if ECG abnormality or prolonged QTc has developed (if >500ms drug should be stopped)
Trifluoperazine		
Anxiety and agitation, paranoid schizophrenia	**Mesoridazine:** QT prolongation and torsades de pointes	
Zuclopenthixol acetate		
Treatment of psychoses especially schizophrenia		Calcium, potassium, and magnesium should also be monitored

Pericyazine: ECG abnormalities as with other antipsychotics but ST depression also reported as well as sudden death

Pimozide: hypotension. *Very rare*: QT prolongation and risk of torsades de pointes in patients with no prior risk factors. *Contraindicated* in patients with cardiac disease and in presence of other QT-prolonging drugs

Prochlorperazine: ECG changes include QT prolongation, ST depression, U-wave and T-wave changes. Atrial arrhythmias, AV block, and VT which may result in VF or cardiac arrest have been reported and are possibly dose related. Pre-existing cardiac disease, old age, hypokalaemia, and concurrent tricyclic antidepressant use may predispose. Cases of sudden death reported, some possibly cardiac related effects due to presumed QT prolongation and torsades de pointes

Sulpiride: hypotension (in high doses), hypertension, ECG changes, QT prolongation, VT/VF (rare), cardiac arrest, torsades de pointes, and sudden unexplained death

Thioridazine: QT prolongation and torsades de pointes

Trifluoperazine: ECG changes with prolongation of the QT interval and T-wave changes. *Rare*: VF/VT, sudden unexplained death, cardiac arrest, and torsades de pointes have been reported

Zuclopenthixol acetate: as with other antipsychotics avoid drugs that prolong QT

Haloperidol is contraindicated in clinically significant cardiac disorders, QTc interval prolongation, history of ventricular arrhythmias or torsades de pointes, bradycardia or 2nd-3rd-degree heart block, uncorrected hypokalaemia

Table A.16 (Contd.)

Drug name/class/indication	Cardiovascular effects and incidence	Special recommendations for use/notes
Atypical antipsychotic drugs		
(**Amisulpride, aripiprazole, clozapine, olanzapine, paliperidone, quetiapine, sertindole, zotepine**) *Acute and chronic schizophrenia. Many also have antiemetic properties (unlicensed indication)*	Class effect: can cause postural hypotension which can be associated with syncope and reflex tachycardia **Amisulpride**: causes dose-dependent prolongation of the QT interval. Use with *caution* in electrolyte imbalance, conduction disorders, and bradycardia <55bpm. Reduce dose if QTc >500ms **Aripiprazole**: *Uncommon:* tachycardia, orthostatic hypotension. Increased mortality in elderly patients with psychosis associated with Alzheimer's mainly from CV causes (HF, sudden death 3.5% compared to 1.7% with placebo). Reported QT prolongation, bradycardia, ventricular arrhythmias, torsades de pointes, cardiac arrest, and sudden unexplained death **Olanzapine, clozapine, and risperidone**: are associated with a 3-fold increased risk of cerebrovascular events in the >65s with dementia (data from RCTs), whereas **aripiprazole** carries a not statistically significant increase in stroke **Olanzapine**: *Uncommon:* QT prolongation and bradycardia	Recommended that although not all the atypical antipsychotics have been associated with prolongation of the QT interval they should all be used with *caution* when prescribed with drugs that are known to increase the QT interval **Amisulpride**: *Contraindicated* when prescribed with drugs that prolong the QT interval. Use with *caution* if prescribing medication that affects conducting system, e.g. β-blockers **Aripiprazole**: does not prolong QT but *caution* advised when used in patients with a history or family history of prolonged QT. Should be used with *caution* in patients with known CVD (history of MI or ischaemic heart disease, HF, or conduction abnormalities), cerebrovascular disease, conditions which would predispose patients to hypotension (dehydration, hypovolaemia, and treatment with antihypertensive medications), or hypertension **Olanzapine**: advise caution in congenital or acquired prolonged QT, HF, electrolyte abnormalities and hypertrophy

Clozapine: associated with increased risk of myocarditis especially during the first 2 months of treatment. Some cases of myocarditis have been fatal and 14% are associated with eosinophilia. Pericarditis/pericardial effusion and cardiomyopathy have been reported also with fatalities. Rarely circulatory collapse may occur. The minority experience ECG changes similar to those seen with other antipsychotic drugs, including S-T segment depression and flattening or inversion of T waves, which normalize after discontinuation of clozapine. These changes may be associated with myocarditis. Palpitations, bradycardia, hypotension, ventricular arrhythmias, AF

Paliperidone: *Common:* tachycardia, AV block, 1st-degree heart block, bradycardia, bundle branch block, orthostatic hypotension, QT prolongation at high doses. *Uncommon:* palpitations, sinus arrhythmia, AF

Quetiapine: QT prolongation in overdose only. *Common:* syncope, orthostatic hypotension, tachycardia mediated by α₁, α₂ receptor agonism

Risperidone: *Uncommon:* orthostatic hypotension and syncope due to α-blocking activity. Not shown to be associated with prolongation of QTc but caution recommended. *Uncommon:* palpitation, hypertension, hypotension, AV block, MI. *Rare:* VT, angina pectoris, premature atrial beats, T-wave inversion ventricular extrasystoles, ST depression, myocarditis

Sertindole (named patient basis only): known to prolong QT more with higher dose, risk further increased with drugs that also prolong QT or inhibit sertindole metabolism. *Common:* α-blocking activity causes hypotension. QT prolongation, peripheral oedema. *Uncommon:* torsades de pointes, syncope

Ziprasidone: bradycardia, palpitations, hypotension, QT prolongation

Zotepine: *Common:* prolonged QT, tachycardia. Rarely bradycardia

Clozapine: pretreatment ECG recommended. *Caution should be exercised in patients with CVD or a family history of QT prolongation. Myocarditis or cardiomyopathy should be suspected in patients who experience persistent tachycardia at rest, especially in the first 2 months of treatment, and/or palpitations, arrhythmias, chest pain, and other signs and symptoms of HF

Paliperidone: can cause hypotension due to its α-adrenergic-blocking activity. Use with *caution in CVD*

Sertindole and zotepine: *Contraindicated* in significant CVD, congestive HF, cardiac hypertrophy, arrhythmias, bradycardia (<50bpm) or congenital, family history or acquired long QT (QTc >450ms men and 470ms women). ECG monitoring before treatment, at 3 weeks (or 16mg dose), then 3-monthly and before every dose increase. If QTc >500ms stop treatment and evaluate patient

Drugs for mania and depression (Table A.17)

Table A.17 Drugs for mania and depression

Drug name/class/indication	Cardiovascular effects and incidence	Special recommendations for use/notes
Drugs for bipolar disorder/mania (lithium carbonate, lithium citrate)	Rarely reported effects are arrhythmia, oedema, and sinus node dysfunction. QT interval prolongation, ventricular arrhythmias (VF, VT). Sudden unexplained death, cardiac arrest and torsades de pointes have been reported	*Caution with CVD and family history of LQTS. Avoid drugs that prolong QT*
Antidepressants—tricyclics *(only those medications with specific enhanced cardiac effects above the normal are listed)* **(amitriptyline hydrochloride** may have more potent CV effects than other tricyclic antidepressants)	Class effect: hypotension, syncope, postural hypotension, hypertension, tachycardia, palpitations, MI, arrhythmias, heart block, stroke, non-specific ECG changes, and changes in AV conduction. Arrhythmias and severe hypotension with high dosage or overdose **Clomipramine hydrochloride:** *Common:* postural hypotension, sinus tachycardia, and clinically irrelevant ECG changes in patients of normal cardiac status (e.g. T and ST changes), palpitations. *Uncommon:* arrhythmias, increased BP. *Very rare:* conduction disorders (e.g. widening of QRS complex, prolonged QTc interval, PR changes, bundle-branch block), torsades de pointes (particularly in patients with hypokalaemia)	*Contraindicated in recovery phase post MI, arrhythmias particularly any form of heart block. Avoid sympathomimetic agents. Supervise closely in patients with CV disorders. Close monitoring in hyperthyroidism due to increased risk of arrhythmias* Antimuscarinic side effects and cardiotoxicity in overdose. Arrhythmias and heart block occasionally found with use. May be factor in sudden death in patients with CVD

	Nefazodone: *Very common:* hypotension/orthostatic hypotension. *Common:* bradycardia. *Uncommon:* peripheral oedema, tachycardia, hypertension, ventricular extrasystoles, and angina pectoris. *Rare:* AV block, conduction defects, congestive HF **Trazodone hydrochloride:** has fewer antimuscarinic and CV effects. May be arrhythmogenic in patients with pre-existing CVD. Arrhythmias identified include isolated premature ventricular contractions, ventricular couplets, and short episodes (3–4 beats) of VT	In overdose thought to block Na^+ channels and have a quinidine-like effect on the myocardium. The most important ECG feature of toxicity is prolongation of the QRS interval, which indicates a high risk of VT. In very severe poisoning the ECG may be bizarre. *Rarely:* prolongation of the PR interval or heart block may occur as may QT interval prolongation, and torsades de pointes have also been reported **Clomipramine hydrochloride:** liable to prolong QT interval particularly at high doses. Avoid concomitant administration of medications that prolong QT
MAOIs (iproniazide, moclobemide, phenelzine, tranylcypromine)	*Common:* hypotension, arrhythmias, palpitations. May respond to dose reduction. Ventricular extrasystoles and ventricular tachycardia. Hypertensive episodes in patients given tricyclic antidepressants and MAOIs simultaneously	*Caution in CVD, contraindicated in severe CVD*
SSRIs (citalopram, escitalopram, fluoxetine, fluvoxamine maleate, paroxetine, sertraline)	**Citalopram:** minimal CV effects: *Very common:* (>5–20%) palpitations. *Common:* (1–5%) postural hypotension, tachycardia **Escitalopram:** *Uncommon:* tachycardia. *Rare:* bradycardia. Cases of QT prolongation have been reported in patients with pre-existing CVD. No causal relationship established **Fluoxetine:** postural hypotension **Fluvoxamine maleate:** palpitations/tachycardia, bradycardia. *Rarely:* postural hypotension **Paroxetine:** *Uncommon:* sinus tachycardia. *Rare:* bradycardia **Sertraline:** postural hypotension, tachycardia	In overdose: ECG changes including nodal rhythm, prolonged QT intervals, and wide QRS complexes may occur **Sertraline** and **citalopram** are the preferred SSRIs post MI; both have demonstrated safety (SADHART and CREATE trials) and in the case of **sertraline** a possible reduction in MI and death. Those with premorbid or severe depression are more likely to respond to treatment **Fluoxetine:** monitor patients with acute cardiac disease closely, potential for triggering coronary spasm in susceptible patients

Table A.17 (Contd.)

Drug name/class/indication	Cardiovascular effects and incidence	Special recommendations for use/notes
Other antidepressants: **duloxetine, mianserin, mirtazepine, reboxetine, venlafaxine, viloxazine**	**Duloxetine:** palpitations **Mianserin:** orthostatic hypotension **Mirtazepine:** orthostatic hypotension, syncope. *Uncommon:* angina pectoris, MI, bradycardia, ventricular extrasystoles, hypotension **Reboxetine:** *Common:* tachycardia, palpitations, vasodilatation, postural hypotension **Venlafaxine:** increased heart rate (clinical trials suggest 4bpm at high doses). Postural hypotension, clinically significant increases in cholesterol in 5.3% of patients. *Common:* hypertension, palpitation, vasodilatation. *Uncommon:* hypotension/postural hypotension, syncope, arrhythmias (including tachycardia). *Very rare:* torsades de pointes, QT prolongation, VT, VF **Viloxazine:** orthostatic hypotension	**Mirtazepine:** *caution* with CVD, recent MI, angina and conduction disturbance. Overdose: mild hyper/hypotension, tachycardia **Venlafaxine:** *Contraindicated:* in patients with an identified very high risk of a serious cardiac ventricular arrhythmia (e.g. those with a significant LV dysfunction, NYHA class III/IV) or uncontrolled hypertension Overdose: ECG changes (e.g. prolongation of QT interval, bundle branch block, QRS prolongation), sinus and ventricular tachycardia, bradycardia and hypotension

CNS stimulants and drugs for attention-deficit hyperactivity disorder

Atomoxetine: can increase heart rate (mean <10bpm) and BP (mean <5mmHg). *Common:* palpitations and sinus tachycardia. *Rare:* QT prolongation

Dexamfetamine sulphate: cardiomyopathy reported in chronic use. MI, palpitations, and tachycardia. Hypertension and hypotension

Methylphenidate hydrochloride: mildly raised pulse and BP. *Uncommon:* tachycardia, palpitations and hypertension. *Unknown:* angina pectoris, bradycardia, SVT, ventricular extrasystoles

Modafinil: *Common* tachycardia, palpitations, vasodilatation. *Uncommon:* ECG abnormalities, extrasystoles, arrhythmias, bradycardia, hypo/hypertension

Sudden death in adolescents and children with structural heart disease has been reported during the use of CNS stimulants at normal dose. Stimulants in this group are not recommended

Atomoxetine: *Caution* in congenital, positive family history and acquired prolonged QT. Also addition of drugs that can prolong the QT and in hypertension, hypotension, CV, and cerebrovascular disease

Dexamfetamine sulphate: *Contraindicated* in symptomatic heart disease, structural heart disease (linked to sudden death) and moderate to severe hypertensive disease. Use of β-blockers can result in severe hypertension. Overdose can result in arrhythmias and CV collapse

Methylphenidate hydrochloride: *Contraindicated* in patients with arrhythmias, severe angina, and hypertension

Modafinil: not recommended in patients with LVH, cor pulmonale, or mitral valve prolapse who have previously suffered mitral valve prolapse syndrome while taking CNS stimulants

Drugs used in obesity (Table A.18)

Table A.18 Drugs used in obesity

Drug name/class/indication	Cardiovascular effects and incidence	Special recommendations for use/notes
Treatment of obesity (**sibutramine hydrochloride**)	*Common*: most occur in first 4 weeks of treatment. Tachycardia (mean increase 3–7 beats, higher in isolated cases), palpitations, hypertension (mean increase in systolic and diastolic BP 2–3mmHg and higher in isolated cases), vasodilatation (hot flushes). *Uncommon*: AF, paroxysmal SVT, coronary artery spasm	Taken off the market in the UK in January 2010 *Contraindicated*: history of CAD, congestive HF, tachycardia, peripheral arterial occlusive disease, arrhythmia or cerebrovascular disease BP should be monitored and if raised by 10mmHg from baseline on two separate occasions or if previously well controlled hypertension exceeds 145/90mmHg, medication should be stopped Main CV effect through active 1° and 2° metabolites which inhibit noradrenaline, dopamine, and serotonin reuptake

Anti-emetics (Table A.19)

Table A.19 Anti-emetics

Drug name/class/indication	Cardiovascular effects and incidence	Special recommendations for use/notes
Drugs for nausea and vertigo **Cyclizine** *Histamine H₁ receptor antagonist* **Domperidone** and **metoclopramide** *D₂ receptor antagonists*	**Cyclizine**: *Very common*: tachycardia on IV injection, raised BP **Metoclopramide**: *Very rare*: reports of bradycardia, supraventricular arrhythmias and heart block with IV use **Domperidone**: risk of causing torsades de pointes	**Cyclizine**: *Caution* in severe HF May cause a fall in cardiac output associated with an increase in heart rate, mean arterial pressure, and pulmonary wedge pressure
Dolasetron mesilate, granisetron, ondansetron, palonosetron *5-HT₃ receptor antagonists*	**Dolasetron**: cancer patients—*Common*: tachycardia. Surgical patients—*Common*: bradycardia and T-wave changes Reversible ECG changes related to level of active metabolites (PR, QTc, and QRS prolongation). In IV form *very rare* cases of VT, wide complex tachycardia, VF and cardiac arrest	**Dolasetron**: *contraindicated* in patients with markedly prolonged QT, 2nd- and 3rd-degree AV block, concurrent use of class II and III antiarrhythmic agents

Table A.19 (Contd.)

Drug name/class/indication	Cardiovascular effects and incidence	Special recommendations for use/notes
	Granisetron: *Common*: hypertension. *Rare*: hypotension, angina pectoris, AF, and syncope **Ondansetron**: chest pain with or without ST segment depression/elevation cardiac arrhythmias, hypotension and bradycardia have been rarely reported. *Very rare*: with IV administration transient ECG changes including QT prolongation **Palonosetron**: *Uncommon*: tachycardia, bradycardia, arrhythmia, myocardial ischaemia	*Contraindicated* in children and adolescents due to more marked effect on QTc and, very commonly, ECG changes. Sustained SVT, VT, cardiac arrest, and MI reported in this age group *Caution* with underlying cardiac disease, bundle branch block, congestive HF and medications that prolong the QT **Ondansetron/palonosetron**: *Caution* with drugs that prolong the QT, with cardiac rhythm or conduction disturbance and with anti-arrhythmic drugs **Ondansetron**: cause of chest pain thought to be due to coronary artery spasm
Substance P antagonist (aprepitant)	*Uncommon*: bradycardia	
Cannabinoid (nabilone)	Elevated supine and standing heart rates. Causes orthostatic hypotension	*Caution* in elderly, hypertension and heart disease
Hyoscine hydrobromide		*Caution* in patients with CVD Can block vagal inhibitory reflexes

Anticonvulsants (Table A.20)

Table A.20 Anticonvulsants

Drug name/class/ indication	Cardiovascular effects and incidence	Special recommendations for use/notes
Antiepileptics (carbamazepine, oxcarbazepine, gabapentin, pregabalin, phenobarbital, felbamate, fosphenytoin sodium, phenytoin sodium)	**Carbamazepine**: mild anticholinergic activity. *Rare*: cardiac conduction disorders, hypertension, or hypotension. *Very rare*: bradycardia, arrhythmia, AV block with syncope, circulatory collapse, congestive HF, aggravation of CAD, thrombophlebitis, thromboembolism (e.g. pulmonary embolism)	**Carbamazepine**: *Contraindications*: AV block. *Overdose*: tachycardia, hypotension and at times hypertension, conduction disturbance with widening of QRS complex; syncope in association with cardiac arrest. Causes enzyme induction and can increase the rate of metabolism of other drugs (i.e. warfarin and digoxin)
	Oxcarbazepine: *Very rare*: arrhythmias, AV block	**Oxcarbazepine**: serum Na^+ <125mmol/L have been observed in up to 2.7% of treated patients. Warning for patients in HF
	Felbamate: QT prolongation	**Phenobarbital**: prolonged use can cause hypocalcaemia. *Overdose*: CV depression, hypotension and shock
	Gabapentin: *Uncommon*: palpitations, hypertension	**Fosphenytoin sodium/ phenytoin sodium**: parenterally affects ventricular automaticity. *Contraindicated* in bradycardia, SA block 2nd–3rd-degree AV block, Stokes–Adams syndrome. *Caution* in hypotension and myocardial insufficiency. Severe reactions include atrial and ventricular conduction depression and VF/fatality. Hypotension at high infusion doses/rates = recommend reduce dose/rate. Higher risk of hypotension in those with an acute stroke/cerebrovascular event
	Pregabalin: *Uncommon*: tachycardia. *Rare*: 1st-degree AV block, sinus tachycardia, sinus arrhythmia, sinus bradycardia, hypotension, hypertension. *Unknown*: congestive cardiac failure	
	Phenytoin: hypotension, intracardiac conduction delay, arrhythmias	**Phenytoin** causes liver enzyme induction and can increase the rate of metabolism of other drugs (i.e. warfarin and digoxin)

Drugs used in parkinsonism and movement disorders (Table A.21)

Table A.21 Drugs used in parkinsonism and movement disorders

Drug name/class/indication	Cardiovascular effects and incidence	Special recommendations for use/notes
Drugs in parkinsonism (apomorphine hydrochloride (also used in male impotence), bromocriptine, cabergoline, pergolide, pramipexole, ropinirole, rotigotine) *Dopamine receptor agonists*	**Apomorphine hydrochloride:** *Uncommon:* postural hypotension Ergot-derived dopamine receptor agonists **bromocriptine, cabergoline, pergolide, and lisuride** (discontinued) are associated with pericardial as well as pleural and retroperitoneal fibrotic reactions, pericardial effusion, cardiac valvulopathy involving one or more valves (aortic, mitral, and tricuspid). In some cases, symptoms or manifestations of cardiac valvulopathy improved after discontinuation of cabergoline Although no reactions have been reported, it is not known if non-ergot derived agonists can cause these reactions **Pergolide:** atrial premature contractions and sinus tachycardia. *Rare:* Raynaud's phenomenon, chest pain	**Apomorphine hydrochloride:** *Caution in CVD as can cause hypotension. Overdose:* bradycardia and hypotension NB Baseline measurements of echo, CXR, ESR, CRP, renal function tests, and possibly lung function tests should be done. Monitor for chest pain, dyspnoea, and HF. Any suspicion of deterioration in valvular function is an indication to stop cabergoline **Bromocriptine:** *Contraindicated* in uncontrolled hypertension and in non-life threatening conditions if history of CAD or CV condition present. If life-threatening condition present, careful consideration of risk vs. benefit **Cabergoline:** *Contraindicated;* history of fibrotic reactions, cardiac valvulopathy of any kind

Table A.21 (Contd.)

Drug name/class/indication	Cardiovascular effects and incidence	Special recommendations for use/notes
	Bromocriptine: *Rare:* hypertension, MI, stroke, tachycardia, bradycardia, arrhythmia. Fibrosis and serosal inflammatory reactions with ergot derivatives, pleuritis, pleural and pericardial effusion, pleural and pulmonary fibrosis, constrictive pericarditis, and retroperitoneal fibrosis occurred after prolonged use **Pramipexole:** hypotension **Ropinirole:** *Common to very common:* syncope. *Uncommon:* hypotension, postural hypotension (depending on dose and condition treated) **Rotigotine:** *Common:* orthostatic hypotension. *Uncommon:* hypertension, hypotension, AF, palpitations, increased heart rate. *Rare:* SVT	**Pergolide:** *Caution should be exercised when administering pergolide to patients prone to cardiac dysrhythmias or with significant underlying cardiac disease* **Rotigotine** (transdermal patch): *Contraindicated in MRI and cardioversion due to burns from aluminium backing*
Levodopa *Precursor of dopamine*	Occasional reports of cardiac arrhythmias and orthostatic hypotension. Hypotension usually responds to dose reduction	Caution in CVD particularly with history of MI Sudden sleep onset sometimes without warning
Monoamine-oxidase B inhibitors (**rasagiline, selegiline hydrochloride**)	**Rasagiline:** depending on dose, monotherapy vs. adjuvant therapy *Common:* angina pectoris 1.3%. *Uncommon:* cerebrovascular accident 0.7%. MI 0.7% *Common:* postural hypotension 4.7%, *Uncommon:* angina pectoris 0.5%, cerebrovascular accident 0.5%	

	Selegiline hydrochloride: *Rare:* cardiac arrhythmias, palpitations, hypotension	
Catechol-O-methyltransferase inhibitors (amantadine hydrochloride)	*Common:* oedema of ankles. *Occasional:* palpitations, orthostatic hypotension. *Isolated cases:* heart insufficiency/ failure	*Caution* in congestive heart disease as may exacerbate oedema
	QT prolongation and possible risk of ventricular arrhythmias	
Tetrabenazine *Used in movement disorders associated with organic central nervous system conditions e.g. Huntington's chorea*	Mild hypotension	
Botulinum toxin type A *Blocks the release of acetylcholine*	*Rare:* reports of arrhythmias and MI in patients with CV risk and/or disease	
Tizanidine *Centrally acting α₂-adrenergic agonist for the management of spasticity*	*Common:* hypotension. *Rare:* bradycardia, orthostatic hypotension and syncope (at times of peak plasma concentration 2–3h post dosing). QTc prolongation mild	*Contraindicated:* in patients with congenital or acquired prolonged QT syndrome, history of cardiac arrhythmias. Avoid use with drugs known to prolong QT. *Caution:* bradycardia, hypokalaemia, hypomagnesaemia

Drugs used in addiction (Table A.22)

Table A.22 Drugs used in addiction

Drug name/ class/indication	Cardiovascular effects and incidence	Special recommendations for use/notes
Alcohol dependence (disulfiram)		*Contraindicated* in cardiac failure, CAD, previous CVA and hypertension When taken with alcohol acetylaldehyde accumulates in the blood which causes intense flushing, palpitations, tachycardia, hypotension among other non-CV effects
Tobacco smoking cessation (nicotine, varenicline, bupropion)	**Nicotine**: *Uncommon*: palpitations **Varenicline**: *Uncommon*; ECG changes—AF, ST segment depression, and reduction of T-wave amplitude, increased heart rate. palpitations, increased BP **Bupropion**: *Uncommon*: tachycardia, hypertension (can be severe), chest pains. *Rare*: palpitations, vasodilatation, postural hypotension	**Nicotine**: *Avoid* in recent MI, stroke, unstable, Prinzmetal's or worsening angina. If used in these situations do so with close medical supervision as safety data are lacking in these groups *Caution* in severe hypertension, stable angina pectoris, cerebrovascular disease, occlusive peripheral arterial disease, HF *Overdose*: palpitations, tachycardia, arrhythmias and circulatory collapse **Bupropion overdose**: associated with conduction disturbances (QRS and QTc prolongation), arrhythmias, tachycardia
Opioid dependence (lofexidine hydrochloride) *Central alpha 2 adrenergic agonist*	**Lofexidine hydrochloride**: QT prolongation, bradycardia, hypotension **Methadone hydrochloride**: T-wave inversion, QT interval prolongation, torsades de pointes especially in doses >100mg/day reported. Bradycardia, hypotension, palpitations, ventricular arrhythmias	**Lofexidine hydrochloride**: *Caution* in severe coronary insufficiency, bradycardia (<55bpm) monitor pulse rate frequently, recent MI, prolonged QT and drugs that prolong the QT **Methadone hydrochloride**: *Caution* with history of cardiac conduction abnormalities, advanced heart disease, or ischaemic heart disease, family history of sudden death, concomitant use of drugs known to prolong the QT. Risk of cardiac events in electrolyte disturbance and drugs that affect electrolyte balance

Table A.22 (*Contd.*)

Drug name/ class/indication	Cardiovascular effects and incidence	Special recommendations for use/notes
(methadone hydrochloride) **Levacetyl-methadol**	**Levacetylmethadol** hypotension, QT prolongation, and serious arrhythmia (torsades de pointes), ST elevation, angina pectoris, MI	In patients with risk for QT prolongation, routine ECG monitoring advised. Without risk factors but undergoing dose titration at and above 100mg/day monitor ECG before and 7 days after titration **Levacetylmethadol** no longer licensed in USA

Dementia (Table A.23)

Table A.23 Dementia

Drug name/class/ indication	Cardiovascular effects and incidence	Special recommendations for use/notes
Drugs for dementia (donepezil hydrochloride, galantamine, rivastigmine) *Acetylcholinesterase inhibitors (AChE inhibitors)*	**Donepezil hydrochloride:** reports of syncope and seizures—manufacturer recommends considering withdrawing if long sinus pauses or heart block *Common:* hypertension, vasodilatation, hypotension, AF. *Uncommon:* bradycardia. *Rare:* postural hypotension, SA block, bradycardia, AV block, angina **Galantamine:** *Common:* hypertension. *Uncommon:* atrial arrhythmia, myocardial ischaemia/infarction, palpitations, cerebrovascular disease, TIA. *Rare:* severe bradycardia. *Very rare:* AV block, hypotension **Rivastigmine:** *Rare:* angina. *Very rare:* hypertension, cardiac arrhythmias (bradycardia, AV block, AF, tachycardia)	Cholinesterase inhibitors may cause bradycardia due to vagal effects. Intensive CV screening prior to initiating treatment is not deemed necessary as AV block occurs just as frequently in those with a normal pretreatment ECG as those with pre-existing abnormalities. Pulse checks should be carried out after 1 week if heart rate 50–60bpm. Stop treatment if dose increased and avoid if heart rate <50bpm until investigat or definitively treated (i.e. permanent pacemaker). Pulse check should be carried out as part of routine monitoring of those on AChE inhibitors **Donepezil hydrochloride, rivastigmine:** *Caution* in sick sinus syndrome, SA, AV block supraventricular conduction disturbances **Galantamine:** *Caution* in the above and with drugs that slow/impair cardiac conduction, e.g. β-blockers, digoxin, and in electrolyte disturbances. *Caution* in CVD especially post MI, new onset AF, 2nd-degree heart block or greater, UA, congestive HF esp. NYHA III–IV Trials in non Alzheimer's patients showed an increased mortality rate in patients treated with galantamine (1.4% vs. 0.3%). Roughly half the deaths were due to vascular causes (MI, stroke, sudden death)

Miscellaneous drugs

See Table A.24.

Table A.24 Miscellaneous drugs

Drug name/class/indication	Cardiovascular effects and incidence	Special recommendations for use/notes
Adenosine	*Very common:* asystole, bradycardia, sinus pause, AV block, atrial extrasystoles, skipped beats, ventricular excitability (ventricular extrasystoles, non-sustained VT). *Uncommon:* sinus tachycardia, palpitations. *Very rare:* severe bradycardia requiring temporary pacing and not corrected with atropine, AF, ventricular excitability including VT and torsades de pointes. *Unknown:* cardiac arrest	*Contraindicated:* LQTS, sick sinus syndrome. 2nd- or 3rd-degree heart block, severe hypotension or HF *Caution:* in 1st year post heart transplant increased sensitivity to adenosine. CAD with significant stenosis due to potential to cause significant hypotension and hypoperfusion. Hypovolaemia, valvular stenosis, left-to-right shunt, pericardial effusion, carotid artery stenosis with cerebrovascular insufficiency. MI, HF, bundle branch block, AF/flutter accessory bypass tract
Papaverine *Benzylisoquinoline group of alkaloids obtained from opium or synthetically prepared* *Relaxes smooth muscle for relief of cerebral and peripheral ischaemia associated with arterial spasm. Erectile dysfunction*	Vasodilatation, flushing, tachycardia, hypotension, hypertension, cardiac arrhythmias	*Contraindicated:* complete heart block. *Caution:* large doses can depress AV and intraventricular conduction, prolonging refractory period and thereby produce serious arrhythmias through premature systoles
Bepridil hydrochloride *Calcium-channel blocker. Blocks voltage- and receptor-operated calcium channels. Interferes with calcium calmodulin binding, as well as slow calcium and fast inward sodium currents in myocardial and vascular smooth muscle* *Anti-anginal with some type I anti-arrhythmic and antihypertensive properties*	*Common:* sinus tachycardia, bradycardia, hypertension, vasodilatation, peripheral oedema, ventricular premature contractions, VT (torsades de pointes), prolonged QT/QTc interval, HF	*Contraindicated:* recent MI (within 3 months), prolonged QT of any cause, sick sinus syndrome, history of serious ventricular arrhythmias, cardiac insufficiency

(Continued)

Table A.24 (Contd.)

Drug name/class/ indication	Cardiovascular effects and incidence	Special recommendations for use/notes
Protamine *Neutralization of the anticoagulant effect of heparin therapy and the treatment of heparin overdose. Acts by forming a stable protamine–heparin salt*	3 categories of adverse reaction reported: **1** Systemic hypotension via reduction in peripheral vascular resistance **2** Anaphylactoid reactions (oedema of the skin, mucosa, and viscera, decreased systemic vascular resistance, bronchospasm, flushing, severe cardiovascular collapse) **3** Catastrophic pulmonary vasoconstriction; accompanied by right ventricular dilation, pulmonary arterial hypertension, decreased left ventricular filling pressure, and systemic hypotension Also reported reduction in cardiac output when BP drop of >10mmHg occurs, bradycardia Catastrophic pulmonary vasoconstriction and oedema may be associated with protamine use following cardiac surgery	IV injection should not exceed 50mg in 10 min Reactions often related to rate of administration. Hypersensivity reactions can occur in those who have previously received protamine–insulin preparations (isophane insulin) and in those allergic to fish. There are reports of vasectomized and infertile men who have anti-protamine antibodies Some side effects of protamine thought to occur through increased complement activity and thromboxane release. Reduced side effects noted during cardiac surgery when protamine injection bypasses the lungs

Index